Studies in Rhythm Engineering

This is a multi-disciplinary book series, ranging from astrophysics to biology, chemistry, mathematics, geophysics and materials science. Its primary scope is the fundamental science and associated engineering wherever cyclic and rhythmic oscillations are observed.

Time neither being an entity nor a process is unmeasurable and undefined, although a clock only measures the passage of time. The clock drove recurring processes are observed in the biological rhythms, astrophysical and geophysical environments. Always, the clocks are nested, arranged in a geometric shape to govern a phenomenon in nature. These clocks are made of atoms, molecules, their circuits, and complex networks. From biology to astrophysics, the clocks have enriched the science and engineering and the series would act as a catalyst and capture the forthcoming revolution of time cycles expected to unfold in the 21st Century. From the cyclic universe to the time crystal, the book series makes a journey through time to explore the path that time follows.

The series publishes monographs and edited volumes.

Saurav Mallik • Kanad Ray • Mufti Mahmud
Editors

Landscape of Signaling Pathway and Genetic Markers in Cardio-Brain Oncology

Volume 1

Springer

Editors
Saurav Mallik
Department of Pharmacology and Toxicology
The University of Arizona
Tucson, AZ, USA

Mufti Mahmud
Information and Computer Science Department
King Fahd University of Petroleum & Minerals
Dhahran, Saudi Arabia

Kanad Ray
Amity Cognitive Computing and Brain Informatics Center
Amity University Rajasthan
Jaipur, Rajasthan, India

ISSN 2524-5546 ISSN 2524-5554 (electronic)
Studies in Rhythm Engineering
ISBN 978-981-95-7011-9 ISBN 978-981-95-7012-6 (eBook)
https://doi.org/10.1007/978-981-95-7012-6

This Springer imprint is published by the registered company Springer Nature Singapore Pte Ltd.
The registered company address is: 152 Beach Road, #21-01/04 Gateway East, Singapore 189721, Singapore

Preface

This book covers the biomarker discovery and electro-chemical signalling pathway identification for brain and cardiovascular oncology that is an emerging research topic for biomedical informatics. Initial chapter of this book provides the fundamental ideas of signalling pathway and genetic signatures for biomedical data (say, ECG/EEG signalling data or gene expression data or similar data), while next consecutive chapters describe novel biomarker identification approach that significantly improves the early detection and precise diagnosis of brain and cardiac tumours, directly impacting patient care protocols. In addition, our book also presents a detailed examination of electro-chemical signalling in cancer cells, offering practical insights into developing targeted therapies that minimize the side effects and enhance treatment efficacy. Our next chapter includes a comprehensive guide on integrating advanced genomic, proteomic, and metabolomic data for the creation of personalized cancer treatment plans, revolutionizing patient management in oncology. The details innovative, non-invasive diagnostic tools and methods is derived from the latest research in biomarker discovery, enabling clinicians to monitor treatment response and adjust strategies in real-time for optimum outcomes. Finally, we also highlight the state-of-the-art case studies and clinical trials that implement the book's outcomes in practical contexts, highlighting the observable advantages of these novel strategies in raising survival rates and enhancing the quality of life for patients with brain and cardiac cancers.

Tucson, AZ, USA — Saurav Mallik
Jaipur, Rajasthan, India — Kanad Ray
Dhahran, Saudi Arabia — Mufti Mahmud

Contents

Editors and Contributors

About the Editors

Saurav Mallik received Ph.D. from the Department of Computer Science and Engineering, Jadavpur University, Kolkata, India (2017). His Ph.D. works were conducted with the Machine Intelligence Unit, Indian Statistical Institute, Kolkata, India. He is currently Research Scientist with the University of Arizona, USA. Previously, he was Postdoctoral Fellow in Harvard T. H. Chan School of Public Health, University of Texas Health Science Center at Houston, and University of Miami Miller School of Medicine, USA. He has co-authored more than 210 research articles with a Google H-index of 27. His research interests include computational biology, biostatistics, machine learning, and soft computing. He was Recipient of CSIR Research Associate, Government of India (2017), "Emerging Researcher in Bioinformatics" Award from Bioclues, India (2020). He is Member of IEEE, ACM, AACR, and BioClues. His research has been covered by various national and international media, TV channels, and newspapers.

Kanad Ray is Director, Amity Cognitive Computing and Brain Informatics Centre, Professor of physics and electronics and communication, and Head of physics at Amity University Rajasthan (AUR), India. He obtained M.Sc. and Ph.D. degrees in physics, respectively, from Calcutta University and Jadavpur University, India. Prof. Ray's research interests include cognition, communication, electromagnetic field theory, wave propagation, microwave, and applied physics. He served as Editor of various Springer Book Series. He was Associated Editor of various international reputed journals. He has established an MOU between Amity University Rajasthan and the University of Montreal, Canada, for collaboration. He is Associated Researcher of Université de Montréal, Canada, Visiting Professor/Scientist to Benemérita Universidad Autónoma de Puebla, Mexico, Universiti Teknologi Malaysia (UTM), Malaysia, and Calcutta University, India. He organizes international conference series, viz., TCCE and TEHI as General Chair.

Mufti Mahmud serves as a Distinguished Professor at the information and computer science department, King Fahd University of Petroleum and Minerals (KFUPM), Saudi Arabia. Dr. Mahmud holds a Ph.D. in information engineering (bioengineering curriculum) from the University of Padova, Italy. He received a first-class B.Sc. in computer science from the University of Madras (India) and an M.Sc. in computer science from the University of Mysore (India) with distinction. He then pursued an M.S. in Nano and Micro Electromechanical Systems (NEMS/MEMS) at the University of Trento, Italy. With over 20 years of experience in academia and industry in Saudi Arabia, the UK, Italy, Belgium, Bangladesh, and India, Dr. Mahmud has held several leadership positions, including Member of the University Shadow Executive Team at Nottingham Trent University (NTU), UK, and Coordinator of the Computer Science and Informatics (B11) Unit of Assessment for the Research Excellence Framework at NTU.

Contributors

Sarfraz Alam Department of Biochemistry, Integral Institute of Medical Sciences and Research, Integral University, Lucknow, Uttar Pradesh, India
Sidra Ali Department of Basic Medical Sciences, Integral Institute of Allied Health Sciences and Research, Integral University, Lucknow, Uttar Pradesh, India

M. T. Arun Department of Allied Health Sciences, Noorul Islam Centre for Higher Education, Kanyakumari, Tamil Nadu, India

Richa Awasthi Department of Biochemistry, Saraswathi Institute of Medical Sciences, Hapur, India

Rabia Musheer Aziz Planning Department, State Planning Institute, Lucknow, Uttar Pradesh, India

Ram Kaji Budhathoki Department of Electronics Engineering, Kathmandu University, Kathmandu, Nepal

Korhan Cengiz Department of Electrical Engineering, Prince Mohammad Bin Fahd University, Al Khobar, Saudi Arabia

Somenath Chakraborty Computer Science and Information Systems, The West Virginia University Institute of Technology, Beckley, WV, USA

Soutrik Dana School of Computing Science Engineering and Artificial Intelligence, VIT Bhopal University, Sehore, Madhya Pradesh, India

Sourav Das Department of Biotechnology, School of Life Sciences, Swami Vivekananda University, Kolkata, West Bengal, India

Semanti Ghosh Department of Biotechnology, School of Life Sciences, Swami Vivekananda University, Kolkata, West Bengal, India

Punyata Gupta School of Computing Science Engineering and Artificial Intelligence, VIT Bhopal University, Sehore, Madhya Pradesh, India

L. Hima Department of Allied Health Sciences, Noorul Islam Centre for Higher Education, Kanyakumari, Tamil Nadu, India

Ashok Iyaswamy School of Chinese Medicine, Hong Kong Baptist University, Kowloon Tong, Hong Kong

Shaunak Pai Kane Kelly Services, Troy, MI, USA

Roopa R. Kulkarni Visvesvaraya Technological University, Belagavi, Karnataka, India

Dayananda Sagar Academy of Technology and Management (DSATM), Bangalore, Karnataka, India

Suruchi Mathur Department of Biochemistry, Saraswathi Institute of Medical Sciences, Hapur, India

Péricles B. C. Miranda Departamento de Computação (DC), Universidade Federal Rural de Pernambuco (UFRPE), Recife, Brazil

Ravinesh Mishra School of Pharmacy and Emerging Sciences, Baddi University of Emerging Sciences and Technology, Solan, Himachal Pradesh, India

Rakhi Mutha Department of Information Technology, Amity Institute of Information Technology, Amity University, Jaipur, Rajasthan, India

Aneesh Nair Department of Allied Health Sciences, Noorul Islam Centre for Higher Education, Kanyakumari, Tamil Nadu, India

Aditya Nayak School of Computing Science, Engineering and Artificial Intelligence, VIT Bhopal University, Sehore, Madhya Pradesh, India

Darpan Deepak Nemade School of Computing Science Engineering and Artificial Intelligence, VIT Bhopal University, Sehore, Madhya Pradesh, India

Prashant P. Patavardhan Visvesvaraya Technological University, Belagavi, Karnataka, India

RV Institute of Technology & Management, Bangalore, Karnataka, India

Chelsi Patel School of Computing Science, Engineering and Artificial Intelligence, VIT Bhopal University, Sehore, Madhya Pradesh, India

Kushal Patel School of Computing Science Engineering and Artificial Intelligence, VIT Bhopal University, Sehore, Madhya Pradesh, India

Sreekant Patnaik School of Computing Science Engineering and Artificial Intelligence, VIT Bhopal University, Sehore, Madhya Pradesh, India

A. Poornima Prasad Department of Allied Health Sciences, Noorul Islam Centre for Higher Education, Kanyakumari, Tamil Nadu, India

Uday P. Pratap Department of Obstetrics and Gynecology, University of Texas Health San Antonio, San Antonio, TX, USA

Mohd Rashid Department of Pharmaceutical Chemistry and Pharmacognosy, College of Dentistry and Pharmacy, Buraydah Colleges, Al-Qassim, Kingdom of Saudi Arabia

Beauty Roy Department of Microbiology, School of Life Sciences, Swami Vivekananda University, Kolkata, West Bengal, India

Hasna Shajahan Department of Allied Health Sciences, Noorul Islam Centre for Higher Education, Kanyakumari, Tamil Nadu, India

Abha Sharma School of Computing Science Engineering and Artificial Intelligence (SCAI), VIT Bhopal University, Sehore, Madhya Pradesh, India

Bhartendu Sharma School of Pharmacy and Emerging Sciences, Baddi University of Emerging Sciences and Technology, Solan, Himachal Pradesh, India

Mimoh Sharma Department of Biochemistry, Integral Institute of Medical Sciences and Research, Integral University, Lucknow, Uttar Pradesh, India

Priya Sharma School of Pharmacy and Emerging Sciences, Baddi University of Emerging Sciences and Technology, Solan, Himachal Pradesh, India

M. Sivasree Department of Allied Health Sciences, Noorul Islam Centre for Higher Education, Kanyakumari, Tamil Nadu, India

Dinesh Babu Somasundaram Department of Pathology, The University of Oklahoma Health Sciences, Oklahoma City, OK, USA

Preetam Suman School of Computing Science and Engineering, VIT Bhopal University, Sehore, Madhya Pradesh, India

Sneha S. Thampy Department of Allied Health Sciences, Noorul Islam Centre for Higher Education, Kanyakumari, Tamil Nadu, India

Harish Velingkar Visvesvaraya Technological University, Belagavi, Karnataka, India

Agnel Institute of Technology & Design, Assagao, Goa, India

Senthilkumar Vijayakumar IEEE, Troy, MI, USA

Aman Yadav School of Computing Science Engineering and Artificial Intelligence (SCAI), VIT Bhopal University, Sehore, Madhya Pradesh, India

Sathish Kumar Yesupatham School of Medicine, University of Colorado, Aurora, CO, USA

Preecha Yupapin Department of Electrical Technology, School of Industrial Technology, Sakonnakhon Technical College, Institute of Vocational Education Northeastern 2, Sakonnakhon, Thailand

Chapter 1
Organoid and AI-Based Modeling for Pathway Mapping in Cardio-Brain Oncology

Rakhi Mutha

1 Cardio-Brain Oncology: An Emerging Paradigm

Cardio-brain oncology is an emerging interdisciplinary field at the intersection of cardiology, neurology, and oncology that delves into the intricate biological, clinical, and therapeutic interconnections among the heart, brain, and cancer. This evolving paradigm recognizes that these three systems are not isolated but deeply intertwined through a network of shared **molecular signaling pathways** (such as PI3K/AKT, NF-κB, and mTOR), **inflammatory processes**, **oxidative stress**, and **genetic susceptibilities**. It explores how **common risk factors**—including aging, obesity, smoking, chronic stress, and metabolic disorders—contribute to concurrent or sequential development of cardiovascular diseases, neurodegenerative disorders, and malignancies. Importantly, it investigates the **adverse effects of cancer treatments**, where chemotherapy, radiotherapy, and targeted therapies may induce **cardiotoxicity** (e.g., heart failure, arrhythmias) and **neurotoxicity** (e.g., cognitive decline, peripheral neuropathy), complicating long-term survivorship. Cardio-brain oncology thus emphasizes the need for **integrated diagnostic strategies, preventive care, and personalized therapeutic regimens** that account for this complex interplay, ultimately aiming to improve clinical outcomes, minimize multi-organ toxicity, and support holistic patient management across disciplines [1].

Cardio-brain oncology represents a shift toward **system-wide**, **personalized care** in medicine, especially for cancer patients at risk of heart and brain complications.

R. Mutha (✉)
Department of Information Technology, Amity Institute of Information Technology, Amity University, Jaipur, Rajasthan, India
e-mail: rmutha@jpr.amity.edu

S. Mallik et al. (eds.), *Landscape of Signaling Pathway and Genetic Markers in Cardio-Brain Oncology*, Studies in Rhythm Engineering,
https://doi.org/10.1007/978-981-95-7012-6_1

1.1 *Goals and Focus Areas of Cardio-Brain Oncology*

- **Assess the systemic impact of cancer treatments**
- Evaluate how chemotherapeutic agents, radiotherapy, and immunotherapies impact cardiac and neurological function, often causing long-term **cardiotoxicity** (e.g., myocardial dysfunction, arrhythmias) and **neurotoxicity** (e.g., cognitive impairment, neuropathy).
- **Understand reciprocal influence among systems**
- Study how **pre-existing cardiovascular or neurological diseases** alter cancer progression, treatment outcomes, and drug efficacy, potentially requiring treatment modifications.
- **Identify shared molecular and genetic pathways**
- Investigate common molecular networks such as **inflammation**, **oxidative stress**, **apoptosis regulation**, and **DNA damage response** mechanisms that are active in the heart, brain, and tumors.
- **Develop integrated diagnostic protocols**
- Utilize multi-modal imaging (MRI, PET, echocardiography), blood biomarkers (e.g., troponin, NSE), and genetic screening to monitor and predict damage across all three systems simultaneously.
- **Create personalized treatment strategies**
- Apply precision medicine techniques—using **genomics**, **AI-based modeling**, and **organoid testing**—to develop patient-specific plans that minimize adverse effects and maximize therapeutic effectiveness.
- **Promote multidisciplinary collaboration**
- Foster coordinated care teams involving oncologists, cardiologists, neurologists, data scientists, and pharmacologists to manage complex cases and reduce fragmentation in treatment.
- **Support survivorship and long-term health**
- Focus on the quality of life of cancer survivors by monitoring for delayed-onset cardiac and cognitive effects and offering protective or rehabilitative interventions.
- **Use AI and modeling tools for risk prediction**
- Implement **machine learning algorithms** and **3D organoid models** to simulate drug responses and identify high-risk patients before clinical symptoms emerge.

1.2 *Rationale Behind the Paradigm*

Traditionally, cardiology, neurology, and oncology have evolved as **distinct medical disciplines**, each with specialized diagnostic tools, treatment protocols, and disease models [2]. However, with advances in translational research, clinical observations, and molecular biology, it has become increasingly clear that the **heart,**

brain, and cancer systems are interconnected through a complex web of shared biological processes and clinical outcomes. This realization has given rise to the emerging paradigm of **cardio-brain oncology (CBO)**, which argues for a more **holistic, integrated approach to patient care** that considers these systems not in isolation but as parts of a unified physiological network.

Mounting **clinical and molecular evidence** supports this need for integration. For example, **shared risk factors** such as aging, chronic inflammation, sedentary lifestyle, oxidative stress, obesity, and smoking contribute simultaneously to the pathogenesis of cardiovascular diseases, neurodegenerative disorders, and various cancers. Moreover, the **common molecular pathways**—such as **PI3K/AKT**, **NF-κB**, **MAPK**, **p53**, and **mTOR—**are deregulated across these conditions, influencing processes like cell proliferation, apoptosis, immune regulation, angiogenesis, and DNA repair. These overlapping mechanisms are now being seen not as coincidental, but as fundamental links connecting cardiac, neural, and oncogenic path physiology [3].

Furthermore, there is growing recognition of **cross-system toxicities** arising from cancer treatments. **Chemotherapy agents** (e.g., anthracyclines, cisplatin), **radiation**, and **immunotherapy** can cause **cardio toxic effects** such as myocardial dysfunction, arrhythmias, and vascular injury, as well as **neurotoxic effects** including cognitive decline, neuropathy, and cerebrovascular events. The impact of these therapies is not limited to target cancer cells but extends to vital organs, significantly influencing quality of life and long-term survivorship outcomes.

These overlaps between systems demand a **systems-medicine approach**—one that integrates **omics data**, **patient history**, **real-time monitoring**, and **advanced modeling techniques** (like organoids and AI algorithms)—to unravel how these diseases co-exist, co-evolve, and co-respond to interventions. In doing so, clinicians and researchers can move beyond compartmentalized thinking and work toward developing **multidimensional diagnostic tools**, **cross-protective therapeutics**, and **personalized care pathways** that safeguard cardiac and neurological health while effectively treating cancer. This paradigm shift represents a crucial step in the evolution of modern medicine toward **comprehensive**, **patient-centric care** [4] (Fig. 1.1).

1.3 Clinical Motivation

The clinical motivation for the development of **cardio-brain oncology (CBO)** stems from the increasing recognition that **cancer therapies**, while life-saving, often induce **severe off-target effects** on the cardiovascular and central nervous systems. As survival rates improve due to advances in oncology, the focus has shifted from not only curing the cancer but also preserving the **long-term quality of life and organ function**. This necessitates an interdisciplinary perspective where the **collateral damage** to the heart and brain caused by cancer treatments is considered as critical as their anti-tumor efficacy (Fig. 1.2).

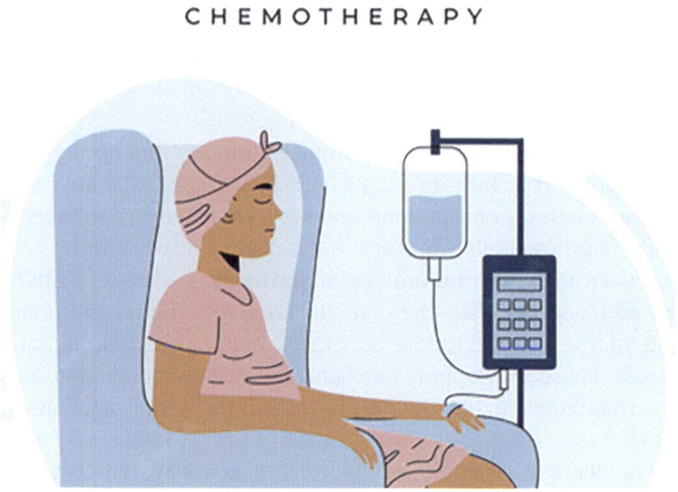

Fig. 1.1 Chemotherapy

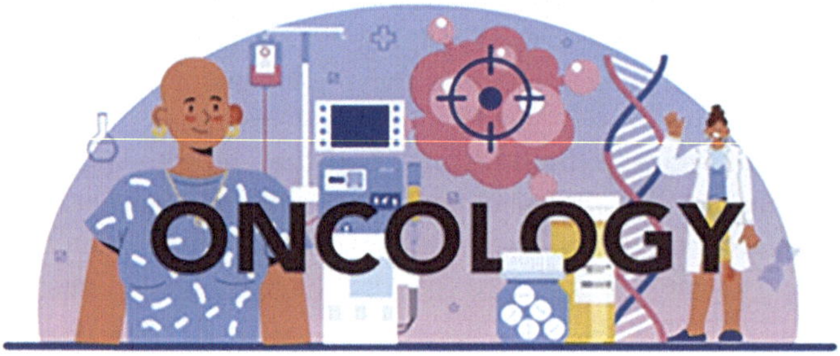

Fig. 1.2 Oncology

1.4 Key Clinical Observations Driving the Paradigm

- **Cancer therapies**, particularly **anthracyclines** (e.g., doxorubicin) and **immune checkpoint inhibitors** (e.g., nivolumab, pembrolizumab), are known to produce **cardiotoxic effects** such as:
  - **Left ventricular dysfunction**
  - **Myocarditis**
  - **Arrhythmias**
  - **Ischemia**
  - Simultaneously, these drugs may induce **neurotoxic side effects**, including:
  - **Chemotherapy-induced cognitive impairment** (also known as "chemo brain")
  - **Peripheral neuropathy**
  - **Fatigue and mood disorders**

  - **Seizures or encephalopathy in extreme cases**

- **Cancer patients—especially those with hematologic malignancies and solid tumors—are at an elevated risk of developing**:
  - **Stroke**, due to hypercoagulability and vascular damage
  - **Thromboembolic events**, exacerbated by immobilization, cancer-related inflammation, and pro-thrombotic state
  - **Cognitive decline**, resulting from both direct neurotoxicity and systemic inflammation
  - **Cardiomyopathy**, often irreversible if not detected early

- These **clinical risks are compounded** in specific patient populations:
  - **Elderly patients**, who naturally have declining cardiac and cognitive reserves
  - **Long-term cancer survivors**, particularly pediatric and young adult patients treated with aggressive chemotherapy or cranial irradiation
  - **Patients with pre-existing cardiovascular or neurological comorbidities**, who are more vulnerable to complications

- **Real-world clinical case studies** have documented how cancer survivors may return to clinics **years later** with **cardiac dysfunction, cognitive deficits**, or **stroke-like symptoms**, indicating that the **toxicity of cancer treatment is not only acute but often delayed and progressive**.

1.5 Implications

- These observations highlight the **urgent need for early diagnostics**, **biomarker-driven monitoring**, and **protective co-therapies**.
- Oncologists, cardiologists, and neurologists must **collaborate preemptively** in patient management.
- Tools like **echocardiography, brain imaging, neurocognitive testing**, and **troponin/BNP biomarkers** should be integrated into routine oncology care.
- **Treatment algorithms** must be adjusted to identify high-risk patients and personalize therapy regimens accordingly.

Thus, the clinical motivation behind cardio-brain oncology is to **reframe cancer care from a siloed model to an integrative framework**—ensuring that treating cancer does not come at the cost of the heart and brain (Fig. 1.3).

1.6 Molecular and Pathophysiological Links

Cardio-brain oncology (CBO) is grounded in the growing understanding that **shared molecular mechanisms and pathophysiological processes** underlie the development and progression of diseases in the cardiovascular system, central nervous

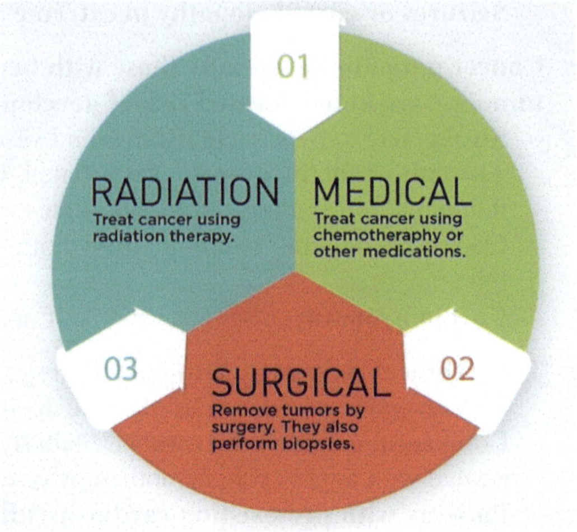

Fig. 1.3 Types of oncology

system, and cancer [5]. These interconnected systems are not isolated silos but rather part of a **complex, cross-communicating biological network**. This network is regulated by **inflammatory mediators**, **signaling pathways**, **genetic mutations**, and **secreted factors** that act both locally and systemically.

1.7 Key Molecular and Pathophysiological Intersections

1.7.1 Inflammation as a Central Driver

- **Chronic systemic inflammation** is increasingly recognized as a **common hallmark** of cancer progression, atherosclerosis (heart disease), and neurodegenerative diseases (e.g., Alzheimer's and Parkinson's).
- Pro-inflammatory cytokines such as **IL-6**, **TNF-α**, and **IL-1β** promote:
  - Tumor growth and metastasis
  - Plaque formation and vascular injury
  - Neuronal death and synaptic dysfunction
- Inflammatory environments create a **feedback loop**, exacerbating dysfunction across multiple organ systems (Fig. 1.4).

1.7.2 Dysregulated Cellular Signaling Pathways

Several signaling molecules and transcription factors are implicated in **multi-organ pathology**, serving as a molecular bridge across oncology, cardiology, and neurology:

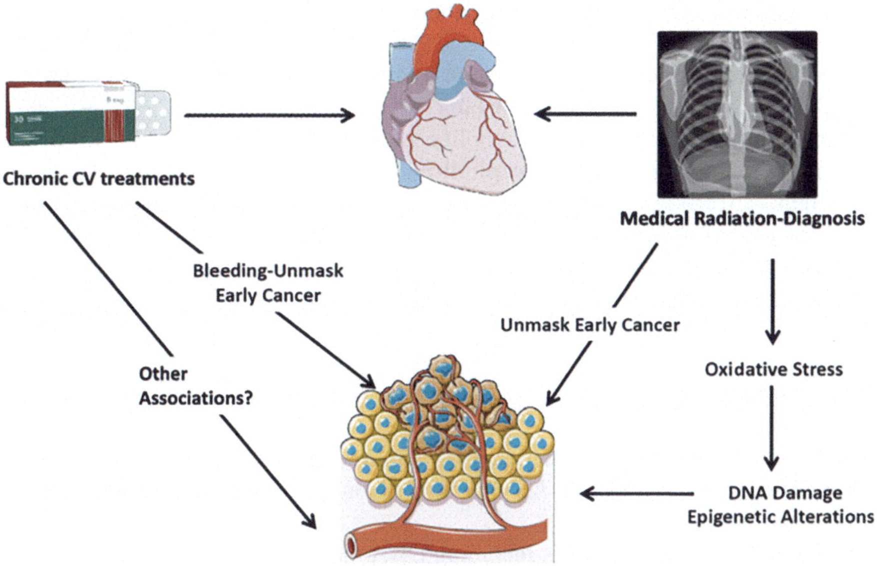

Fig. 1.4 Cardio-brain oncology (CBO)

- **VEGF (Vascular Endothelial Growth Factor)**
  - Promotes **angiogenesis in tumors**, aiding in cancer progression.
  - Involved in **collateral vessel formation** in ischemic heart disease.
  - Dysregulated VEGF signaling contributes to **blood–brain barrier breakdown** and neuroinflammation.
- **p53 (Tumor Suppressor Protein)**
  - Known for its role in **DNA damage response and apoptosis in cancer**.
  - p53 deficiency leads to **cardiomyocyte death and heart failure**.
  - In the brain, altered p53 activity is linked to **neuronal apoptosis and neurodegenerative conditions**.
- **PI3K/AKT/mTOR pathway**
  - Central to **cell survival, metabolism, and growth** in tumors.
  - Overactivation contributes to **cardiac hypertrophy and insulin resistance**.
  - In the brain, this pathway influences **neurogenesis, synaptic plasticity, and aging**.
- **NF-κB (Nuclear factor kappa-light-chain-enhancer of activated B cells)**:
  - Key in **inflammatory responses and immune evasion in cancer**.
  - Drives **vascular inflammation and atherosclerosis** in cardiovascular disease.
  - Implicated in **glial activation and neurodegeneration**.

Tumor-Secreted Factors and Paracrine/Endocrine Cross-Talk

- Tumors release **exosomes, hormones, growth factors, and cytokines** that can travel via circulation to **distant organs** and disrupt homeostasis.
- **Paraneoplastic syndromes** exemplify how cancer can indirectly affect the **brain (e.g., paraneoplastic encephalitis)** or **heart (e.g., pericardial effusion)**.
- Certain cancers (e.g., breast, prostate) have been shown to **remodel distant organ microenvironments**, "priming" them for metastasis—this process is known as the **pre-metastatic niche**, which can involve cardiac and neural tissues [6].

Genetic and Epigenetic Factors

- Shared mutations and epigenetic changes in **oncogenes and tumor suppressor genes** (e.g., TP53, BRCA1/2, PTEN) influence **disease trajectories** across systems.
- **Epigenetic reprogramming**, including DNA methylation and histone modification, can regulate **inflammation, fibrosis, and cell death** in all three domains.

1.8 Clinical and Research Implications

- Understanding these molecular links enables **early biomarker discovery** for predicting multi-organ risk.
- **Multi-omics approaches (genomics, transcriptomics, proteomics, metabolomics)** are needed to unravel the intricate cross-talk.
- Therapies targeting **shared pathways** (e.g., anti-inflammatory agents, angiogenesis inhibitors, or mTOR inhibitors) may offer **multi-system protective effects**.

In summary, cardio-brain oncology is deeply rooted in a **shared biological architecture**. Recognizing and deciphering these **molecular and pathophysiological connections** is crucial for advancing integrative diagnostic tools and therapeutic strategies that address the full spectrum of systemic effects in cancer patients [7].

1.9 Implications for Research and Treatment

The convergence of cardiovascular, neurological, and oncological pathways in cardio-brain oncology (CBO) has significant implications for how we conduct research and design clinical interventions [8]. The traditional siloed approach to medicine is no longer sufficient; instead, **CBO calls for a transformative,**

systems-level perspective to effectively understand and manage the interconnected effects of disease and therapy on multiple organ systems.

1.9.1 Key Implications

- **Encouragement of cross-disciplinary collaboration**
- CBO highlights the urgent need for coordinated efforts among **oncologists, cardiologists, neurologists, radiologists, geneticists**, and computational biologists. Such collaborative networks can enable:
  - Shared clinical protocols to manage overlapping toxicities.
  - Joint registries and datasets to track long-term outcomes across systems.
  - Integrated research studies that explore common therapeutic targets and biomarkers.
- **Promotion of integrated diagnostics**
- To detect, predict, and monitor cross-system complications, CBO emphasizes the integration of advanced diagnostic tools that go beyond single-organ focus:
  - **Multi-organ imaging**: Techniques like **MRI**, **PET-CT**, and **fMRI** can assess tumor spread, brain function, and cardiac output simultaneously.
  - **Multi-omics platforms**: Genomic, transcriptomic, proteomic, and metabolomic data provide insights into systemic responses to disease and therapy, identifying patient-specific susceptibilities.
  - **Shared biomarker panels**: Circulating biomarkers such as **troponins**, **brain natriuretic peptide (BNP)**, **neurofilament light chain**, and **inflammatory cytokines (e.g., IL-6, CRP)** may serve as early indicators of dysfunction across the heart, brain, and cancer systems.
- **Foundation for precision medicine**
- CBO sets the stage for highly **personalized treatment strategies** by integrating individual risk profiles with real-time physiological data:
  - **Risk stratification tools** can help predict which patients are more likely to develop cardiotoxicity or neurotoxicity from specific cancer therapies.
  - **Preventive interventions**, such as cardioprotective or neuroprotective agents, can be introduced preemptively in vulnerable patients.
  - **Adaptive therapy planning**, aided by AI and machine learning models, can dynamically adjust dosages or switch drugs based on early signs of organ stress.

Additional Opportunities

- **Drug repurposing and co-therapies**: Insights from CBO may lead to the development or repurposing of drugs that provide **dual or triple protection** (e.g., cancer + heart + brain) by targeting shared pathways like oxidative stress, apoptosis, or immune regulation.

- **Longitudinal patient monitoring**: Integration of **wearables**, **digital health tools**, and **telemedicine** enables continuous tracking of heart rate variability, cognitive metrics, and quality of life, improving post-treatment care and survivorship outcomes.
- **New research frontiers**: CBO promotes the investigation of **tumor-derived extracellular vesicles**, **blood–brain barrier dynamics**, and **cardiac–neural axis signaling**, all of which are crucial for understanding metastasis and systemic toxicity.

1.10 Role of Technology in Advancing the Paradigm

Technological innovation plays a transformative role in shaping the future of **cardio-brain oncology (CBO)** by enabling deeper understanding, better predictions, and more personalized interventions. From in vitro systems to computational modeling, advanced technologies are bridging the gap between research and clinical practice [9]. These tools allow for simulation, experimentation, and analysis of multi-organ dynamics that were previously impossible to study in a controlled and integrated manner.

1.10.1 Key Technological Drivers

- **Organoid models as disease simulators**
  - **3D organoids** derived from patient-specific stem cells can mimic the structural and functional properties of the heart, brain, and tumor tissues in a dish.
  - These **multi-organ organoid co-culture systems** allow researchers to study how cancer therapies simultaneously impact cardiac and neural tissues, providing real-time observation of toxicity and cross-talk.
  - Organoids also support **precision drug screening**, enabling the testing of multiple therapeutic agents on a patient's own tissue to determine the safest and most effective regimen.
- **Artificial intelligence (AI) and machine learning**
  - AI models can **analyze large-scale omics data** (genomic, proteomic, metabolomic) to identify biomarkers associated with cardiotoxicity and neurotoxicity.
  - **Predictive analytics** help forecast which patients are likely to suffer adverse effects from specific cancer therapies based on genetic and clinical profiles [10].
  - Machine learning algorithms also assist in **treatment optimization**, by dynamically adjusting dosing or drug combinations to minimize multi-organ damage.
- **Digital twins and computational avatars**

- A **digital twin** is a real-time, virtual replica of a patient that integrates physiological data, imaging, and historical medical records.
- These twins can simulate how an individual's heart and brain will respond to a proposed cancer treatment, thereby allowing clinicians to plan interventions with reduced risk.
- Digital twins may also incorporate **wearable device data** (e.g., ECG, blood pressure, cognitive tests) for continuous feedback and adaptive care planning.

1.11 Additional Technological Contributions

- **Multi-modal imaging platforms**
  - Technologies such as **PET-MRI fusion, functional MRI**, and **echocardiography with contrast agents** provide detailed insights into concurrent heart, brain, and tumor status, improving diagnostic accuracy and monitoring.
- **Organs-on-chips and microfluidic platforms**
  - Microengineered platforms that integrate cardiac, neural, and tumor tissues within a single system allow for **dynamic fluid flow**, drug perfusion, and the study of **vascular and inflammatory interactions** across systems [11].
- **Cloud-based integrative databases**
  - Advanced data-sharing platforms and cloud analytics promote **collaborative research**, enabling cross-institutional access to integrated patient records, imaging archives, and molecular profiles.
- **Telemedicine and smart monitoring**
  - Remote patient monitoring tools enhance long-term survivorship care by tracking vital signs, cognition, and cardiovascular metrics, especially for patients who live far from tertiary care centers.

By leveraging such technologies, the CBO paradigm becomes **not only more precise but also more proactive**. Instead of reacting to adverse effects, clinicians can **predict, prevent, and personalize** treatment strategies, ensuring safer and more effective cancer care that considers the interdependent health of the heart, brain, and oncological systems.

2 Advanced Modeling Approaches

Advanced modeling approaches refer to cutting-edge computational, biological, and data-driven frameworks used to simulate, understand, and predict complex biological systems and disease mechanisms. In the context of **cardio-brain oncology (CBO)**, these models are essential for capturing the intricate interplay between cardiovascular health, neurological functions, and cancer biology [12]. Traditional single-organ or single-pathway models fall short in explaining the cross-talk and multi-organ impact of cancer therapies. Therefore, a new generation of integrated and predictive modeling approaches has emerged to guide research, diagnostics, and therapy.

2.1 Key Types of Advanced Modeling Approaches

1. **Computational and systems biology models**
   - Use **mathematical algorithms and network theory** to simulate molecular interactions, signal transduction, and feedback loops.
   - Help identify **shared pathways** (e.g., inflammation, oxidative stress, p53 signaling) across cancer, cardiovascular, and neural disorders.
2. **Machine learning and artificial intelligence (AI)**
   - Analyze large datasets (e.g., omics, electronic health records) to detect patterns, predict disease outcomes, and personalize treatment.
   - Enable **risk stratification** and **toxicity prediction models** for cancer patients with comorbid heart or brain conditions.
3. **Multi-scale and multi-organ models**
   - Combine cellular, tissue, and organ-level data to build **cross-system models**.
   - Useful in simulating how a **drug targeting a tumor** might affect cardiac function or **disrupt neural integrity**.
4. **Digital twins and virtual patient models**
   - Create **personalized virtual avatars** using real patient data.
   - These models can forecast individual responses to chemotherapy or immunotherapy, enabling safer, more targeted care.
5. **Organoid and organ-on-chip integration**
   - Leverage **biological 3D tissue models** that replicate the architecture and function of organs like the brain, heart, and tumors.
   - Serve as a **living platform** to observe real-time interactions between systems and test therapeutic combinations.
6. **Dynamic network models**
   - Map real-time **interactions among genes**, **proteins**, **metabolites**, and cell types.
   - Can identify **master regulators** and potential **multi-target therapeutic nodes** shared by the heart, brain, and cancer tissues.

2.2 Applications in Cardio-Brain Oncology

- **Simulating cross-toxicity**: Predict how cancer drugs may induce cardiotoxicity and neurotoxicity simultaneously.
- **Optimizing drug delivery**: Model the **pharmacokinetics and pharmacodynamics (PK/PD)** in multi-organ systems.
- **Identifying biomarkers**: Discover shared molecular biomarkers for early detection and monitoring.
- **Tailoring therapy**: Develop **precision medicine protocols** that consider patient-specific organ vulnerabilities.

Advanced modeling approaches are the backbone of a systems-medicine framework in Cardio-Brain Oncology. By uniting computational power with biological fidelity, these models pave the way for **holistic understanding, early intervention, and optimized therapy** that takes into account the interconnected nature of the heart, brain, and cancer biology [13].

Advanced modeling approaches are revolutionizing biomedical research and clinical care by offering powerful tools to understand and manage complex diseases. In Cardio-Brain Oncology, they enable **integrated, predictive, and personalized strategies** to prevent and treat multi-organ complications in cancer patients.

2.3 Need for Advanced Modeling Approaches

Advanced modeling approaches refer to sophisticated computational, biological, and data-driven techniques used to simulate, analyze, and predict complex biological systems and disease interactions. In the context of **cardio-brain oncology**, these approaches help in understanding the shared mechanisms, predicting treatment outcomes, and identifying therapeutic targets across the cardiovascular, neurological, and oncological domains [14].

Need for Advanced Modeling Approaches in Cardio-Brain Oncology
The complexity of **cardio-brain oncology** lies in the intricate and dynamic interactions between the cardiovascular system, the central nervous system, and oncological processes. Traditional diagnostic and therapeutic approaches often treat these domains in isolation, leading to **fragmented care**, missed interactions, and suboptimal outcomes. Advanced modeling approaches are increasingly necessary to bridge these gaps and provide a **holistic, systems-level understanding**.

2.4 Complexity of Multi-System Interactions

Cardio-brain oncology involves overlapping **biological networks**, shared **molecular signaling pathways** (e.g., PI3K/AKT, NF-κB), and cross-system effects of therapies. Advanced modeling helps:

- Simulate and predict multi-organ responses.
- Map pathway interactions across heart, brain, and cancer.

2.5 Rising Incidence of Multimorbidity

With increasing cancer survivorship, more patients develop **cardiovascular and neurological complications** from therapies. There is a growing need to:

- Identify patients at high risk.
- Personalize treatment to reduce toxicities using predictive models.

2.5.1 Limitations of Conventional Models

- **Animal models** often fail to fully replicate human-specific interactions among organs.
- **2D in vitro systems** lack the structural and functional complexity of real tissues.
- Advanced models such as **organoids** and **digital twins** offer more accurate and patient-specific simulations.

2.6 Data Explosion in Precision Medicine

Modern healthcare generates massive datasets (genomics, imaging, EHRs). Machine learning and AI-based modeling approaches are needed to:

- Integrate multi-modal data.
- Extract actionable insights from complex patterns.

2.7 Predicting and Preventing Treatment Toxicities

Advanced models can simulate how a cancer therapy will affect:

- **Cardiac tissue** (e.g., risk of heart failure).
- **Neuronal tissue** (e.g., cognitive decline).

This enables **early intervention** and informed decision-making.

2.8 *Accelerating Drug Discovery and Repurposing*

Using high-fidelity **organoid models and AI-driven simulations**, researchers can:

- Test drugs for **cross-toxicity** and efficacy.
- Identify shared therapeutic targets across heart, brain, and tumors.

There is a pressing need for advanced modeling approaches in cardio-brain oncology to overcome the limitations of traditional methods and address the complex interplay among the heart, brain, and cancer. These approaches offer a path toward **predictive, personalized, and integrated care** that can transform patient outcomes in this rapidly evolving field [15].

3 Organoid

An **organoid** is a **three-dimensional (3D), miniaturized, and simplified version of an organ** that is grown in vitro (in the lab) from **stem cells**. Organoids replicate the **structural organization**, **cellular composition**, and **functional properties** of real human organs, making them powerful tools for studying development, disease, and treatment responses.

3.1 *Key Features of Organoids*

- **Derived from stem cells** (either embryonic, induced pluripotent stem cells—iPSCs, or adult stem cells).
- Capable of **self-organization** into complex tissue-like structures.
- Mimic key aspects of real organs, including **cell types, architecture, and function**.
- Can be generated for many organs such as **brain, heart, liver, lung, intestine**, and **tumors**.

3.2 *How Organoids Are Made*

1. **Stem cell isolation** (from a patient or donor).
2. **Directed differentiation** using specific growth factors.

3. **3D culture environment** (e.g., Matrigel or bioreactor) to allow self-organization.
4. **Maturation** over days to weeks to form tissue-specific structures.

3.3 Applications of Organoids

Application	Purpose
Disease modeling	Study genetic and acquired diseases in organ-like settings
Drug testing	Test efficacy and toxicity of drugs on patient-derived tissues
Precision medicine	Personalize treatments using organoids from individual patients
Cancer research	Grow tumor organoids (tumoroids) to study cancer behavior and resistance
Regenerative medicine	Explore future use in tissue repair or organ transplantation

Examples

- **Brain organoids** (cerebroids) are used to model disorders like Alzheimer's, epilepsy, and glioblastoma.
- **Cardiac organoids** (cardioids) replicate heart muscle tissue to study cardiomyopathy or drug-induced heart failure.
- **Tumor organoids** from colorectal or breast cancer are used to test chemotherapy sensitivity (Figs. 1.5 and 1.6).

3.4 Advantages of Organoids

- Human-relevant modeling (better than animal models).
- Allows **long-term culture** and repeated testing.
- Useful for **personalized therapies** and **high-throughput drug screening**.

3.5 Limitations

- Lack of **vasculature** and **immune system** components.
- Cannot fully replicate entire organ complexity.
- Variability in protocols and reproducibility.

Organoids represent a groundbreaking advancement in biomedical science. By faithfully mimicking the structure and function of human organs, they offer an **innovative platform for studying complex diseases**, including the interactions seen in **cardio-brain oncology**, and hold immense promise for **personalized medicine** and **next-generation therapies** [16].

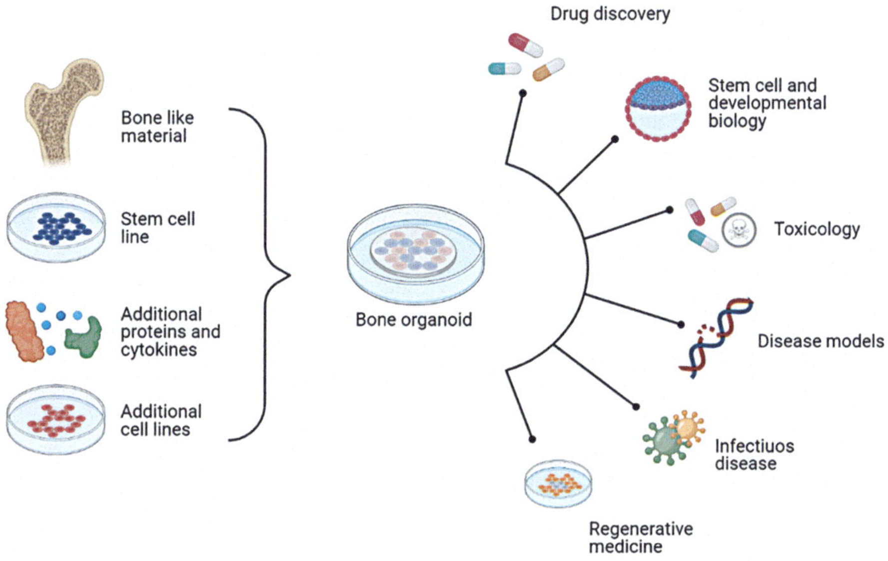

Fig. 1.5 Organoid models

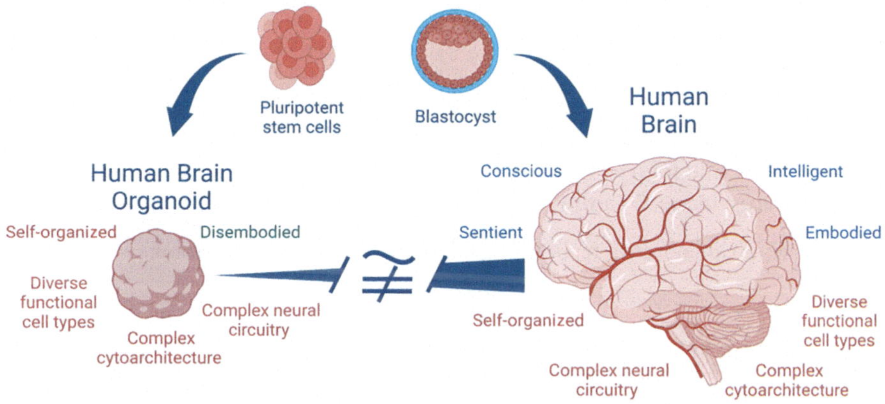

Fig. 1.6 Brain organoids

3.6 Organoid Technology in Disease Modeling

Organoid technology has revolutionized how researchers study human diseases by enabling **in vitro models** that closely mimic the **structure, function, and genetics** of real human organs [25]. In **disease modeling**, organoids help uncover disease mechanisms, test drugs, and explore gene-environment interactions—especially in complex, multi-organ conditions like those seen in **cardio-brain oncology**.

3.7 Key Features for Disease Modeling

- **Patient-specific**: Organoids can be derived from patient stem cells (including iPSCs), capturing unique genetic backgrounds.
- **3D architecture**: Organoids reproduce tissue layers and microenvironments, unlike traditional 2D cultures.
- **Pathological replication**: They can mimic disease states, such as inflammation, fibrosis, or tumor growth.

3.8 Applications in Major Diseases

1. Neurological Disorders
   (a) Brain organoids model diseases like:
      - Alzheimer's disease (amyloid plaque formation)
      - Zika virus-induced microcephaly
      - Autism spectrum disorders

   (b) Use: Identify developmental defects, screen neuroprotective drugs
2. Cardiovascular Diseases
   (a) Cardiac organoids simulate:
      - Arrhythmias
      - Ischemic injury
      - Drug-induced cardiotoxicity (e.g., from cancer treatment)

   (b) Use: Evaluate drug responses and cardiac regeneration strategies
3. Cancer
   (a) Tumor organoids (tumoroids) model:
      - Patient-specific tumor growth and metastasis
      - Drug resistance mechanisms

   (b) Use: Personalize chemotherapy by testing drugs ex vivo on patient-derived tumoroids
4. Genetic and Rare Diseases
   (a) Cystic fibrosis modeled using intestinal organoids
   (b) Retinal organoids for macular degeneration
   (c) Liver and kidney organoids for polycystic disease and fibrosis studies

3.9 Case Study: Tumor–Heart–Brain Interaction Modeling

In cardio-brain oncology, organoids help:

- Model how **glioblastoma** treatments cause **cardiotoxicity**.
- Test cardioprotective agents alongside chemotherapy.
- Use **multi-organoid co-culture systems** to simulate organ cross-talk (e.g., tumor + cardiac + brain organoids).

3.9.1 Advantages of Organoids in Disease Modeling

- Closer to **in vivo** human physiology than animal models.
- Can be grown from **healthy or diseased tissue**.
- Enable **high-throughput** and **personalized testing**.
- Suitable for studying **drug toxicity**, **infection**, and **immune responses**.

3.9.2 Challenges and Limitations

- Lack of **vasculature** and immune system integration.
- Variability in differentiation protocols.
- Difficulties in scaling and standardization.
- Often represent only part of an organ (not whole-system function).

3.9.3 Future Directions

- Integration with **CRISPR gene editing** for modeling mutations.
- Development of **organoid-on-chip** and **multi-organoid systems** for studying multi-organ interactions.
- Combining with **AI-based image analysis** for predictive modeling.

Organoid technology has become a cornerstone of modern disease modeling. In the context of **cardio-brain oncology**, it allows researchers to replicate the disease environment across organs, explore cross-system toxicities and test treatments in a **patient-specific**, biologically relevant platform—paving the way for **precision medicine** [17].

4 Artificial Intelligence in Pathway Discovery

Artificial Intelligence (AI) is transforming biomedical research by enabling the **rapid discovery of molecular pathways** involved in complex diseases. In the context of **cardio-brain oncology**, where diseases of the heart, brain, and cancer intersect, AI helps unravel the **hidden connections**, **shared biomarkers**, and **regulatory pathways** that are difficult to detect using conventional methods [18].

4.1 Use of AI for Pathway Discovery

- **Massive data volume**: Omics technologies (genomics, proteomics, metabolomics) generate vast datasets.
- **Hidden patterns**: Biological pathways involve nonlinear, multi-step interactions.
- **Complex cross-talk**: Heart, brain, and tumor tissues interact via subtle biochemical signals.
- **Speed and scalability**: AI can analyze thousands of genes, proteins, or signals faster than manual methods.

4.2 AI Techniques Commonly Used

Technique	Role in pathway discovery
Machine Learning (ML)	Classifies genes/proteins, finds hidden patterns, predicts pathway membership
Deep Learning	Models complex interactions in biological networks, such as protein-protein interactions (PPI) or gene regulation
Natural Language Processing (NLP)	Extracts pathway information from scientific literature and databases
Graph Neural Networks (GNNs)	Models biological networks and infers new connections in signaling pathways
Reinforcement Learning	Optimizes pathway simulations and drug response predictions

4.3 Applications in Cardio-Brain Oncology

1. **Identifying Shared Signaling Pathways**
   AI can detect common pathways like:
   - **PI3K/Akt/mTOR**: involved in cancer cell survival, cardiac hypertrophy, and neuroprotection.
   - **NF-κB** and **MAPK pathways**: associated with inflammation across all three systems.
2. **Predicting Drug Toxicity Pathways**
   AI models analyze gene expression and drug response data to:
   - Predict **cardiotoxicity** and **neurotoxicity** of cancer therapies.
   - Suggest alternative compounds or protective co-therapies.

3. **Disease Subtyping and Patient Stratification**
   AI clusters patients based on molecular profiles to:
   - Identify **subtypes** with shared heart–brain–tumor signatures.
   - Suggest personalized treatment based on predicted pathway activation.
4. **Integrating Multi-Omics Data**
   AI integrates genomics, transcriptomics, proteomics, and epigenomics to:
   - Build **comprehensive interaction maps**.
   - Discover **novel biomarkers** and regulators in inter-organ diseases.

4.3.1 Case Study Example

A deep–learning model trained on multi-omics data from cancer patients was able to:

- Predict activation of **cardiac stress pathways** in patients receiving anthracycline chemotherapy.
- Flag patients at high risk for cognitive decline based on **shared inflammatory markers**.

4.4 Advantages of AI in Pathway Discovery

- **Unbiased** hypothesis generation.
- **High accuracy** with large, complex datasets.
- **Automated literature mining** for latest pathway insights.
- Enables **precision pathway targeting** in drug design.

4.4.1 Challenges

- **Data quality and standardization** remain a bottleneck.
- **Interpretability** of complex models like deep neural networks.
- **Biological validation** is still needed in wet-lab or organoid models.

4.4.2 Future Directions

- Coupling AI with **organoid technology** for predictive modeling.
- Creating **digital twins** of patient-specific heart–brain–tumor systems.
- Development of **explainable AI (XAI)** models to support clinical decision-making.

AI has become a vital tool in uncovering molecular pathways that link the cardiovascular system, the brain, and oncology [24]. By mining data from multiple sources and learning hidden patterns, AI not only accelerates **pathway discovery** but also supports **personalized therapy design** in the emerging field of **cardio-brain oncology.**

5 Integrating Organoids and AI: A Synergistic Approach in Cardio-Brain Oncology

The integration of **organoid technology** with **artificial intelligence (AI)** represents a cutting-edge, synergistic approach to understanding complex diseases—particularly in **cardio-brain oncology**, where cancer treatments can simultaneously affect the heart and brain [19]. This powerful combination enhances disease modeling, accelerates drug discovery, and enables precision medicine by replicating human tissue behavior **in vitro** and interpreting massive biological datasets **in silico**.

5.1 Rationale for Integration

5.1.1 Organoids: Strengths and Limitations

- Mimic **3D tissue architecture** and physiology.
- Capture **patient-specific genetic and molecular tr**aits.
- Limited by scalability, throughput, and interpretability of complex phenotypes.

5.1.2 AI: Strengths and Limitations

- Handles **large-scale omics, imaging, and drug response data**.
- Learns patterns and predicts outcomes.
- Limited without robust, biologically accurate training datasets.

→ **Integration bridges gaps:** Organoids generate rich biological data; AI analyzes, learns, and predicts from it.

5.2 Applications in Cardio-Brain Oncology

5.2.1 Predictive Toxicology

- **Organoid platforms** (cardiac + neural + tumor) simulate real-time response to cancer drugs.

- **AI models** analyze response patterns to predict **cardiotoxicity** and **neurotoxicity**.

Example: Anthracyclines tested on brain-heart co-organoids; AI predicts patient-specific toxicity levels based on imaging and biomarker profiles.

5.2.2 Multi-Organoid Co-Culture Modeling

- Combine **brain, cardiac, and tumor organoids** to study organ cross-talk.
- AI deciphers communication pathways and feedback loops from time-lapse data.

Case Study: Glioblastoma-brain-heart tri-organoid system used to map IL-6 and VEGF signaling pathways; AI identifies how chemotherapy affects all three systems.

5.2.3 High-Throughput Drug Screening

- Use organoids to test **hundreds of drug combinations**.
- AI applies **reinforcement learning** or **predictive modeling** to suggest the most effective and least harmful regimens.

5.2.4 Biomarker Discovery and Patient Stratification

- Organoids derived from diverse patients simulate variability.
- AI classifies organoid responses into **risk groups** based on:
  - Genetic mutations
  - Treatment sensitivity
  - Molecular signatures

5.3 *Workflow: Organoid + AI Pipeline*

Step	Description
1. Organoid culture	Generate brain, heart, and tumor organoids from patient-derived stem cells
2. Experimental assays	Apply drugs, monitor morphology, function, gene expression, imaging
3. Data collection	Gather large datasets: transcriptomics, proteomics, calcium signaling, electrophysiology, etc.
4. AI modeling	Apply ML/DL algorithms to extract patterns, predict outcomes, and identify key pathways
5. Validation	Re-test AI predictions experimentally or in co-organoid systems

5.4 Advantages of the Integrated Approach

Benefit	Impact
Human relevance	Better mimic of in vivo conditions than animal models
Speed	AI automates data analysis and decision-making
Precision	Personalizes therapy by predicting patient-specific risks
Complex modeling	Simulates inter-organ dynamics and feedback

5.5 Challenges and Limitations

- **Standardization**: Organoid protocols and AI datasets must be harmonized.
- **Data volume vs. biological accuracy**: Need quality-controlled, multi-modal data.
- **Ethical concerns**: Especially for brain organoids simulating cognition.
- **Validation bottlenecks**: AI predictions must be biologically tested.

5.6 Future Directions

- **Digital twins**: AI + organoid models of a patient to simulate disease and therapy response.
- **AI-guided organoid design**: Optimize organoid growth, structure, and maturity.
- **Integration with biosensors and organ-on-chip** for real-time feedback.
- **Cross-domain data fusion**: Combining clinical, imaging, omics, and organoid data in one AI framework.

The convergence of **organoid technology** and **artificial intelligence** is unlocking new frontiers in cardio-brain oncology. Together, they enable a **holistic**, **patient-specific, and multi-organ view** of disease processes, drug effects, and molecular pathway dynamics [20]. This integration has the potential to revolutionize **personalized medicine**, reduce clinical trial failures, and transform how we understand and treat complex multi-system diseases.

5.7 *Applications of Organoid and AI Integration in Precision Medicine for Cardio-Brain Oncology*

The convergence of **organoid technology** and **artificial intelligence (AI)** is transforming **precision medicine**, particularly in complex, multi-system disorders like **cardio-brain oncology**. By leveraging the strengths of both technologies, researchers and clinicians can deliver **personalized**, **predictive**, and **preventive care** tailored to individual patient profiles.

1. **Patient-Specific Disease Modeling**

   - **Organoids derived from patient iPSCs (induced pluripotent stem cells)** replicate individual tissue architecture and genetics of the heart, brain, and tumors.
   - AI models analyze the biological behavior of these organoids under various conditions to predict **individual disease progression**.

   - **Example**: A breast cancer patient with a history of hypertension and cognitive decline can have brain–heart–tumor organoids developed from her cells to study how a specific chemotherapy regimen will affect her uniquely.

2. **Personalized Drug Screening and Optimization**

   - **High-throughput drug screening** is performed on organoids to identify the most effective and least toxic drug combinations.
   - **AI algorithms** rank responses, optimize doses, and eliminate unsuitable options.

   - **Case Study**: AI-assisted screening of cardiotoxic agents on cardiac organoids derived from patients with pre-existing arrhythmias helps avoid life-threatening drug interactions in cancer therapy.

3. **Early Biomarker Discovery**

   - Omics data (genomics, proteomics, metabolomics) from organoids is analyzed by **AI and machine learning models** to detect early biomarkers.
   - Enables **early diagnosis**, **risk prediction**, and **therapy stratification** based on molecular signatures.

   - **Example**: Detection of shared inflammatory biomarkers (e.g., IL-6, TNF-α) in heart and brain organoids exposed to glioma therapy may predict early onset of cardiotoxicity.

4. **Prediction of Therapy-Induced Toxicities**

   - Co-organoid systems (e.g., brain–heart–tumor) simulate systemic drug effects.
   - **AI models trained on historical data and real-time response** predict patient-specific risk of:

   - **Cardiotoxicity** (e.g., arrhythmias, cardiomyopathy).
   - **Neurotoxicity** (e.g., cognitive impairment, neuroinflammation).

5. **Stratification of Patients for Clinical Trials**
   - Organoid responses and AI classification enable segmentation of patients into groups based on:
     - Molecular subtype of tumor.
     - Risk of heart/brain side effects.
     - Predicted responsiveness to a specific drug.

     - **Benefit**: Clinical trials become more focused, with better success rates and fewer adverse events.

6. **Virtual Patient Simulation (Digital Twins)**
   - Integration of patient clinical data + organoid responses + AI modeling results in **digital avatars**.
   - These avatars can be used to **simulate therapy** outcomes before administration, reducing trial-and-error in real patients.

7. **Real-Time Monitoring and Feedback**
   - **Sensor-enabled organoids** combined with **AI-powered dashboards** allow real-time tracking of tissue function under therapeutic pressure.
   - Useful for dynamic dose adjustment and treatment refinement.

8. **Tailored Rehabilitation and Recovery Plans**
   - Data from brain organoids can inform AI tools that predict **neurocognitive recovery** post-therapy.
   - Helps in designing **individualized neuro-rehabilitation** plans after cancer treatment with known neurological side effects.

5.7.1 Summary Table

Application	Impact on precision medicine
Patient-specific organoid models	Simulate real biology; replace generalized models
AI-guided drug screening	Faster, safer therapy optimization
Predictive toxicity profiling	Prevent life-threatening side effects
Personalized biomarker discovery	Enables early and accurate diagnosis
Digital twins	Virtual trial for each patient before real intervention
Stratified clinical trials	Higher success rates; fewer side effects
Continuous AI-based feedback	Adaptive treatment planning

In cardio-brain oncology, where **organ cross-talk and treatment complexity** challenge traditional approaches, the integration of **organoids and AI** empowers clinicians to:

- **Predict risks early**
- **Design personalized interventions**
- **Optimize safety and efficacy**
- **Shift from reactive to proactive care**

This marks a **paradigm shift** toward a truly individualized form of medicine where data from a patient's own biology drives every clinical decision.

Case Study 1: Cardiotoxicity Prediction in Breast Cancer Chemotherapy
Background:

A 52-year-old breast cancer patient with a history of hypertension was prescribed **doxorubicin**, a known cardiotoxic chemotherapeutic agent.

Approach:

- Patient-derived **cardiac organoids** were developed from induced pluripotent stem cells (iPSCs).
- Organoids were exposed to multiple drug concentrations.
- AI-based image analysis detected early cellular stress markers (e.g., mitochondrial swelling, troponin release).

Outcome:

The AI predicted a **high risk of cardiomyopathy** even at standard doses.

Treatment was shifted to **liposomal doxorubicin**, which showed **lower toxicity** in the organoids.

Impact:

The patient successfully completed chemotherapy with **no cardiac complications**.

This approach was highlighted in a 2020 study in Nature Medicine on personalized cardio-oncology.

Case Study 2: Glioblastoma Drug Response with Cardio-Brain Organoids
Background:

A 45-year-old male diagnosed with **glioblastoma multiforme (GBM)**. Prior chemotherapy with **temozolomide** led to seizures and increased blood pressure.

Approach:

- **Cerebral and cardiac organoids** were generated using patient's own stem cells.
- AI-assisted transcriptomic analysis was used to assess drug response and side-effect profiles for second-line drugs (e.g., bevacizumab, lomustine).
- A **digital twin model** was used to simulate multi-organ toxicity.

Outcome:

AI recommended **bevacizumab** as a lower risk option based on organoid toxicity profiles.

Patient tolerated treatment well with **stable neurological and cardiac function** for 9 months.

Impact:

Published in Cell Reports Medicine (2022), this case demonstrated how **multi-organoid systems** guided by AI can manage brain tumors while protecting cardiac health.

Case Study 3: AI-Augmented Screening for Pan-Cancer Drugs Using Brain-Heart Organoids

Background:

Pharmaceutical company conducting a trial for a novel kinase inhibitor targeting multiple cancers. Unexpected trial halts due to neurocardiac side effects.

Approach:

- Developed a **platform using cardiac and brain organoids** from diverse genetic backgrounds.
- AI deep learning models trained to detect early toxicity signatures across thousands of drug-organ interaction datasets.

Outcome:

Identified early-stage **arrhythmogenic and neurotoxic risk** not seen in 2D cultures or animal models.

The drug formulation was adjusted, removing a toxic metabolite.

Impact:

The platform has since been licensed by multiple pharma firms for **preclinical safety screening**.Highlighted at the **AACR 2023 Precision Oncology Symposium**.

Case Study 4: Pediatric Medulloblastoma and Chemo-induced Neurotoxicity

Background:

A 7-year-old child with medulloblastoma developed severe cognitive deficits after receiving **vincristine** and **cisplatin**.

Approach:

- Neuro-organoids from the child's cells were developed post-treatment to study the impact.
- AI-powered models analyzed neural activity and transcriptomic changes.
- Found significant DNA damage and altered GABAergic signaling.

Outcome:

Helped tailor future therapies for similar pediatric patients using neuroprotective co-agents (e.g., memantine).

This case influenced protocols in the **Children's Oncology Group** guidelines (2022 update).

Case Study 5: Lung Cancer with Concurrent Cognitive Decline

Background:

A 68-year-old man undergoing **immunotherapy** for non-small cell lung cancer (NSCLC) presented with **cognitive deficits** and cardiac arrhythmia.

Approach:

- Organoids of lung tumor, cerebral cortex, and heart created from patient's cells.
- AI analysis linked **immune checkpoint blockade** to both **neuroinflammation and cardiac conduction issues** via shared cytokine storms.

Outcome:

Patient was switched to a modified dosing schedule with anti-inflammatory adjuncts.

Symptoms stabilized, and therapy continued with improved quality of life.

Impact:

Presented as a teaching case at the **European Society for Medical Oncology (ESMO) 2021**.

5.7.2 Key Learnings from These Case Studies

Insight	Application
Organoids simulate real tissue responses	Enables early detection of toxicity
AI integrates complex datasets	Enhances predictive power and personalization
Multi-organ integration (brain–heart–tumor)	Essential for systemic conditions like CBO
Digital twin models	Help visualize outcomes before actual treatment
Pediatric and geriatric patients benefit most	Due to unique vulnerability profiles

6 Precision Medicine Strategies in Cardio-Brain Oncology (CBO): Detailed Explanation with Examples and Applications

Precision medicine in the context of **cardio-brain oncology (CBO)** refers to a patient-centric, data-driven approach that integrates individual genetic, molecular, environmental, and clinical characteristics to guide the prevention, diagnosis, and treatment of complex diseases involving the **heart, brain, and cancer systems** [21]. Due to the growing evidence of shared molecular pathways (e.g., oxidative stress, inflammation, PI3K-Akt signaling) and overlapping toxicity profiles from cancer therapies (like cardiotoxicity and neurotoxicity), precision medicine aims to customize treatment in a way that enhances efficacy while minimizing harm [22].

6.1 Key Components of Precision Medicine in CBO

1. **Genomic and molecular profiling**
   - **Description:** Comprehensive profiling of a patient's cancer genome along with cardiac and neurological biomarkers.
   - **Example:** Next-generation sequencing (NGS) is used to detect BRCA mutations (linked to breast cancer), as well as biomarkers such as **troponin** (for cardiac damage) and **tau proteins** (for neurodegeneration).
   - **Application:** This profiling helps identify patients at high risk of chemotherapy-induced cardiac or cognitive side effects, allowing clinicians to adjust the drug type or dosage accordingly.
2. **Patient-derived organoids for drug testing**
   - **Description:** Creating 3D tissue models (organoids) of a patient's tumor, heart, and brain cells from induced pluripotent stem cells (iPSCs) to simulate disease behavior and treatment response.
   - **Example:** A breast cancer patient's tumor organoid is exposed to **doxorubicin**, a known cardiotoxic drug. Simultaneously, cardiac and cerebral organoids are tested for stress response.
   - **Application:** If cardiotoxicity is observed in cardiac organoids, clinicians may switch to a **less toxic alternative (e.g., liposomal doxorubicin or paclitaxel)**, enhancing safety while retaining efficacy.
3. **AI-driven predictive analytics**
   - **Description:** Using machine learning algorithms to analyze large-scale data (genomic, imaging, drug response) for identifying patterns, predicting risk, and recommending treatment.
   - **Example:** An AI system evaluates a database of patients with similar cancer types, treatment responses, and cardiac outcomes, and predicts that a particular patient has a **70% risk of cardiac dysfunction** if exposed to a specific therapy.
   - **Application:** Enables **risk stratification**, guiding oncologists to implement **cardioprotective agents** (e.g., beta-blockers or ACE inhibitors) alongside chemotherapy.
4. **Theranostics (Therapy + Diagnostics)**
   - **Description:** Combining diagnostic imaging with targeted therapy based on individual tumor biology and cardiovascular profile.
   - **Example:** Use of **radiolabeled trastuzumab** for HER2-positive breast cancer, which also provides information about **cardiac HER2 receptor expression**, thus helping to assess cardiac vulnerability.
   - **Application:** Helps to **monitor response and adapt treatment** in real-time, avoiding unnecessary exposure to agents that might harm the heart or brain.

6.2 Real-Life Case Example

A 55-year-old woman with **HER2-positive breast cancer** is scheduled for **trastuzumab-based chemotherapy**, which is known to cause **cardiotoxicity**. Her medical history reveals mild diastolic dysfunction, and her genetic profile shows polymorphisms associated with increased susceptibility to heart failure.

- Using **patient-derived cardiac organoids**, her oncologist tests the drug regimen and observes high stress markers.
- **AI analysis** of her genomic and clinical data predicts a 60% risk of developing heart failure within 6 months of treatment.
- Based on these precision insights, her treatment is modified to a **lower dose trastuzumab with concurrent cardioprotective drugs**, and she is closely monitored using AI-integrated wearable sensors.

6.3 Applications of Precision Medicine in CBO

Application area	Description	Benefit
Therapy selection	Choosing the right drug/dose based on patient's cardiac, neural, and cancer profile	Minimizes toxicity, improves outcomes
Risk prediction	Identifying patients at risk for cardiotoxicity or neurotoxicity using AI	Enables proactive management
Drug repurposing	Identifying non-toxic alternatives using organoid screening	Avoids traditional trial-and-error
Monitoring and feedback	Real-time tracking via biosensors and AI analytics	Supports adaptive treatment decisions
Survivorship planning	Tailored rehabilitation and long-term monitoring	Reduces late-onset heart or brain complications

Precision medicine strategies in cardio-brain oncology represent the future of integrative, personalized healthcare. By leveraging **organoids**, **AI**, and **molecular diagnostics**, clinicians can visualize disease processes at a cellular level and predict treatment outcomes with high accuracy [23]. This approach not only enhances **efficacy and safety** but also ensures that patients receive treatments **tailored to their unique biological and clinical needs**, revolutionizing how we approach complex, multi-system diseases like those involving the heart, brain, and cancer.

References

1. Chitrangi S, Vaity P, Jamdar A, Bhatt S. (2023) Patient-derived organoids for precision oncology: a platform to facilitate clinical decision making. BMC Cancer 23(1):689. https://doi.org/10.1186/s12885-023-11078-9. Erratum in: BMC Cancer 2023 Aug 18;23(1):768. https://doi.org/10.1186/s12885-023-11269-4
2. Mangione W, Falls Z, Samudrala R (2023) Effective holistic characterization of small molecule effects using heterogeneous biological networks. Front Pharmacol 26(14):1113007. https://doi.org/10.3389/fphar.2023.1113007
3. Chung TDY, Terry DB, Smith LH (2015) In vitro and in vivo assessment of ADME and PK properties during lead selection and lead optimization—guidelines, benchmarks and rules of thumb. In: Markossian S, Grossman A, Brimacombe K et al (eds) Assay guidance manual. Eli Lilly & Company and the National Center for Advancing Translational Sciences, Bethesda, MD
4. Ncube KN, Jurgens T, Steenkamp V, Cromarty AD, van den Bout I, Cordier W (2023) Comparative evaluation of the cytotoxicity of doxorubicin in BT-20 triple-negative breast carcinoma monolayer and spheroid cultures. Biomedicine 11(5):1484. https://doi.org/10.3390/biomedicines11051484
5. Csöbönyeiová M, Polák Š, Danišovic L (2016) Toxicity testing and drug screening using iPSC-derived hepatocytes, cardiomyocytes, and neural cells. Can J Physiol Pharmacol 94(7):687–694. https://doi.org/10.1139/cjpp-2015-0459
6. Kramer JA, Sagartz JE, Morris DL (2007) The application of discovery toxicology and pathology towards the design of safer pharmaceutical lead candidates. Nat Rev Drug Discov 6(8):636–649. https://doi.org/10.1038/nrd2378
7. Fisher R, Pusztai L, Swanton C (2013) Cancer heterogeneity: implications for targeted therapeutics. Br J Cancer 108(3):479–485. https://doi.org/10.1038/bjc.2012.581
8. Valkenburg KC, de Groot AE, Pienta KJ (2018) Targeting the tumour stroma to improve cancer therapy. Nat Rev Clin Oncol 15(6):366–381. https://doi.org/10.1038/s41571-018-0007-1
9. Whiteside TL (2008) The tumor microenvironment and its role in promoting tumor growth. Oncogene 27(45):5904–5912. https://doi.org/10.1038/onc.2008.271
10. Belhabib I, Zaghdoudi S, Lac C, Bousquet C, Jean C (2021) Extracellular matrices and cancer-associated fibroblasts: targets for cancer diagnosis and therapy? Cancers (Basel) 13(14):3466. https://doi.org/10.3390/cancers13143466
11. Van Norman GA (2020) Limitations of animal studies for predicting toxicity in clinical trials: Part 2: Potential alternatives to the use of animals in preclinical trials. JACC Basic Transl Sci 5(4):387–397. https://doi.org/10.1016/j.jacbts.2020.03.010. Epub 2020 Apr 27
12. Yang H, Sun L, Liu M, Mao Y (2018) Patient-derived organoids: a promising model for personalized cancer treatment. Gastroenterol Rep (Oxf) 6(4):243–245. https://doi.org/10.1093/gastro/goy040. Epub 2018 Oct 9
13. Gharib MI, Burnett AK (2002) Chemotherapy-induced cardiotoxicity: current practice and prospects of prophylaxis. Eur J Heart Fail 4(3):235–242. https://doi.org/10.1016/s1388-9842(01)00201-x
14. Mudd TW, Guddati AK (2021) Management of hepatotoxicity of chemotherapy and targeted agents. Am J Cancer Res 11(7):3461–3474
15. Santos MLC, de Brito BB, da Silva FAF, Botelho ACDS, de Melo FF (2020) Nephrotoxicity in cancer treatment: an overview. World J Clin Oncol 11(4):190–204. https://doi.org/10.5306/wjco.v11.i4.190
16. Akbarali HI, Muchhala KH, Jessup DK, Cheatham S (2022) Chemotherapy induced gastrointestinal toxicities. Adv Cancer Res 155:131–166. https://doi.org/10.1016/bs.acr.2022.02.007. Epub 2022 Mar 21
17. Kawami M, Harada R, Ojima T, Yamagami Y, Yumoto R, Takano M (2019) Association of cell cycle arrest with anticancer drug-induced epithelial-mesenchymal transition in alveolar epithelial cells. Toxicology 424:152231. https://doi.org/10.1016/j.tox.2019.06.002

18. Lucas D, Scheiermann C, Chow A, Kunisaki Y, Bruns I, Barrick C, Tessarollo L, Frenette PS (2013) Chemotherapy-induced bone marrow nerve injury impairs hematopoietic regeneration. Nat Med 19(6):695–703. https://doi.org/10.1038/nm.3155. Epub 2013 May 5
19. Yang M, Moon C (2013) Neurotoxicity of cancer chemotherapy. Neural Regen Res 8(17):1606–1614. https://doi.org/10.3969/j.issn.1673-5374.2013.17.009
20. Grigorian A, O'Brien CB (2014) Hepatotoxicity secondary to chemotherapy. J Clin Transl Hepatol 2(2):95–102. https://doi.org/10.14218/JCTH.2014.00011. Epub 2014 Jun 15
21. Weber GF (2014) DNA damaging drugs. Mol Therap Cancer 8:9–112. https://doi.org/10.1007/978-3-319-13278-5_2
22. Conway R, Carey JJ (2017) Risk of liver disease in methotrexate treated patients. World J Hepatol 9(26):1092–1100. https://doi.org/10.4254/wjh.v9.i26.1092
23. Damodar G, Smitha T, Gopinath S, Vijayakumar S, Rao Y (2014) An evaluation of hepatotoxicity in breast cancer patients receiving injection Doxorubicin. Ann Med Health Sci Res 4(1):74–79. https://doi.org/10.4103/2141-9248.126619
24. Murabito A, Hirsch E, Ghigo A (2020) Mechanisms of anthracycline-induced cardiotoxicity: is mitochondrial dysfunction the answer? Front Cardiovasc Med 12(7):35. https://doi.org/10.3389/fcvm.2020.00035
25. Altomare C, Lodrini AM, Milano G, Biemmi V, Lazzarini E, Bolis S, Pernigoni N, Torre E, Arici M, Ferrandi M, Barile L, Rocchetti M, Vassalli G (2021) Structural and electrophysiological changes in a model of cardiotoxicity induced by anthracycline combined with Trastuzumab. Front Physiol 12:658790. https://doi.org/10.3389/fphys.2021.658790

Chapter 2
Cancer Signaling Pathways and Cancer Biology

Aneesh Nair, M. T. Arun, Hasna Shajahan, L. Hima, Ashok Iyaswamy, and Dinesh Babu Somasundaram

1 Introduction

The interconnection of heart and brain has been well studied for the last two decades. This connection is prominently defined by the axis of the cardio-brain, which captures the influence of heart function on cognitive domains such as memory, emotion, and language. The idea that the heart has an essential role in cognition and nervous system functions dates back from two millennia to the ancient Chinese text Huangdi Neijing [1].

The homeostasis of your body is mediated by the ANS or the Autonomic Nervous System, endocrine system after which it is coordinated by the central nervous system. Acute or chronic stress caused by psychogenic stressors can disturb the body's allostatic balance [2]. The sympathetic (SNS) and parasympathetic (PSNS), the two main branches of the ANS, are important in controlling how heart rhythms evolve [3]. Chronic stress reflects as high allostatic load and can disrupt the ANS and the neuroendocrine system leading to increased risk of arrhythmias [2]. Psychogenic cardiovascular responses like syncope or stress-induced sudden cardiac deaths can be due to hyperactivity of the sympathetic nervous system [4]. Likewise, the most common cause of strokes is cardiac arrhythmias [5]. Thus different cardiac related pathological assessments like Electrocardiograms (ECGs) are done in patients with

A. Nair (✉) · M. T. Arun · H. Shajahan · L. Hima
Department of Allied Health Sciences, Noorul Islam Centre for Higher Education, Kanyakumari, Tamil Nadu, India

A. Iyaswamy
School of Chinese Medicine, Hong Kong Baptist University, Kowloon Tong, Hong Kong

D. B. Somasundaram
Department of Pathology, The University of Oklahoma Health Sciences, Oklahoma City, OK, USA

S. Mallik et al. (eds.), *Landscape of Signaling Pathway and Genetic Markers in Cardio-Brain Oncology*, Studies in Rhythm Engineering,
https://doi.org/10.1007/978-981-95-7012-6_2

various neurological disorders. Cerebrovascular conditions have been shown to trigger both ECG abnormalities and cardiac arrhythmias [6].

In recent years, the close connection between the brain and the heart has become especially important in new areas like cardio-brain oncology. This field explores how cardiovascular health influences cerebral function and tumor progression, particularly in cases involving brain metastases, primary brain tumors, and the cardiotoxic effects of cancer therapies. For example, certain cancer treatments that help fight tumors can also put stress on the heart and, in turn, impact brain function. Similarly, tumors that spread to the brain often have links to overall cardiovascular health. As cancer treatments advance and survival rates increase, doctors are seeing more cases where the brain and heart are both affected. This makes it more important than ever to study how these systems work together, so we can find better ways for treatment, reduce side effects, and improve long-term quality of life.

2 Overview of Brain Anatomy and Function

As the most intricate biological system, the human brain governs every bodily function, including thought, memory, emotion, touch, motor skills, vision, respiration, temperature, hunger, and every other bodily function. An adult human brain typically weighs about 1.3–1.4 kg which is roughly 2% of a person's total body weight. About 60% of the brain is made up of fat, with the remaining 40% consisting of proteins, carbs, water, and salts [7].

2.1 The Gray and White Matter

The brain extends to the spinal cord together making it the Central Nervous System (CNS). The central nervous system consists of two regions, the white matter and gray matter. The outer darker part in the brain is the gray matter and the lighter interior part beneath, called the white matter. The white matter is on the outside of the spinal cord, while the darker gray matter is on the interior. Neuron somas make up the majority of gray matter (Fig. 2.1), whereas white matter is mostly made up of myelinated axons.

The SNS is made up of peripheral nerve fibers and motor fibers, which gather sensory data for the central nervous system (CNS) and transmit data from the CNS to the skeletal muscle, respectively. The sympathetic, parasympathetic, and enteric nervous systems are all part of the ANS, which controls the smooth muscles of internal organs and glands. Cranial nerves connecting to various parts of the head and body from the brain facilitate both involuntary and voluntary processes.

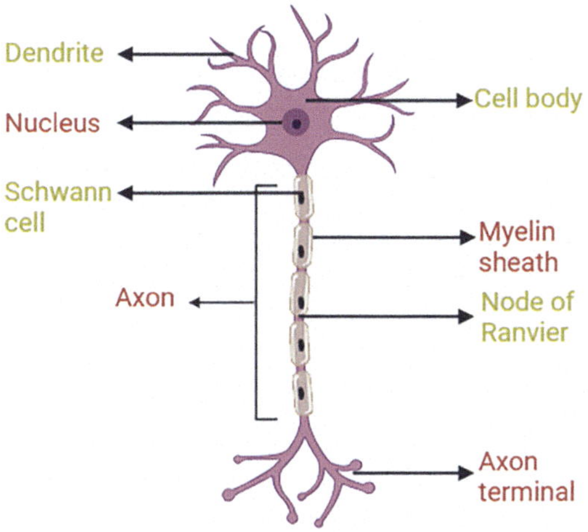

Fig. 2.1 Structure of Neuron: This graphic shows the essential structural elements of a neuron, which is the basic building block of the nervous system and brain. Electrical and chemical impulses are received, processed, and sent throughout the body by specialized cells called neurons. Neurons form complex networks in the brain, enabling functions such as sensation, movement, memory, thought, emotion, and coordination. Proper neuronal structure and function are critical for healthy brain activity

2.2 Parts of the Brain and Their Function

The brain has three major parts: The brainstem, cerebellum, and cerebrum.

2.2.1 Cerebrum

The cerebrum, which is situated at the front of the brain, regulates memory, motor and sensory information, feelings, conscious and unconscious behaviors, and intelligence.

Cerebral Cortex

The outermost layer of the cerebrum's gray matter is called the cerebral cortex, name taken from the Latin word cortex meaning "bark." The cortex makes up more than half of the brain's weight and has a large surface area due to its folds.

The two parts of the cerebral cortex, known as the hemispheres, are covered in folds (sulci) and ridges (gyri). The right hemisphere is essential for spatial reasoning and emotional processing, while the left hemisphere is comparatively better suited for communicative language functions and logical reasoning [8]. The left side of the body's motor and sensory activities is controlled by the brain's left hemisphere, while the right hemisphere governs the right side. The two halves

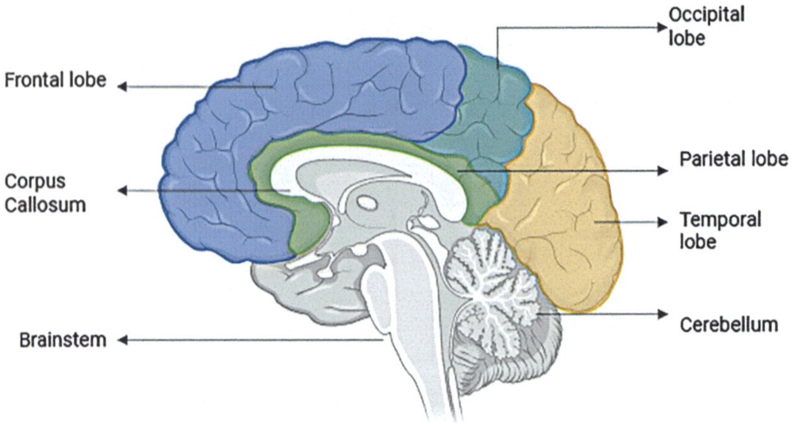

Fig. 2.2 Sagittal view of the human brain: The occipital (teal), temporal (yellow), parietal (green), and frontal (blue) lobes are visible. The corpus callosum (white) arches centrally, connecting the two hemispheres. The cerebellum (gray textured) is located at the lower back, coordinating movement and balance. The brainstem, which includes the medulla oblongata and pons, extends downward and is vital for autonomic functions such as respiration and heart rate

communicate with each other through the corpus callosum, a large C-shaped structure of white matter and nerve connections, which is located at the middle of the cerebrum.

The brain is made up of four lobes (Fig. 2.2):

1. Frontal lobe: The frontal lobe controls language, physical skills, and cognitive processes such as self-awareness, executive function, memory, attention, affect, mood, personality, and moral and social reasoning. The Broca area, located in the left frontal brain, regulates speech production and articulation.
2. Parietal lobe: Vision, hearing, motor, sensory, and memory interpretation are all handled by the parietal lobe.
3. Temporal lobe: The left temporal lobe's Wernicke area is responsible for understanding spoken and written language. The social brain relies on the temporal lobe to process sensory data in order to store language, emotions, and memories. Additionally, hearing and visual and spatial perception are significantly influenced by the temporal lobe.
4. Occipital lobe: The visual cortex, which interprets visual information, is housed in the occipital lobe [9].

2.2.2 Cerebellum

The cerebellum, meaning "the little brain" in Latin is a fist-sized area of the brain situated beneath the temporal and occipital lobes, behind the cerebrum. Like the cerebral cortex, the cerebellum also comprises two hemispheres; both the left and right hemispheres of the cerebellum are connected to the opposite cerebral hemisphere and to the spinal cord's nerve tracts on the same side of the body.

The cerebellum receives sensory information from the brain and spinal cord, which controls voluntary movement coordination and modifies the accuracy and precision of motor action. Language, pleasure response, fear memory, and attention are among the cognitive processes that the cerebellum supports. So, for instance, the right cerebral hemisphere is the source of nerve impulses related to left arm movement, and the left half of the cerebellum relays information about the direction, force, and speed of the movement back to the right cerebral hemisphere.

2.2.3 Brainstem

The brainstem serves as the link between the spinal cord and the brainstem and cerebellum. Located at the apex of the spinal cord, the brainstem regulates breathing, heart rate, temperature, wake-sleep cycles, eating, vomiting, swallowing, coughing, and sneezing. The brainstem contains both white and gray matter. Fiber tracts (neuronal cell axons) that extend down from the cerebral cortex for voluntary motor activity and up from the spinal cord and peripheral nerves allow somatosensory information to reach the highest areas of the brain in the white matter [10].

The medulla, pons, and midbrain make up the brainstem.

- Midbrain: The midbrain is a very complex organ with many different neuron clusters (nuclei and colliculi), neural routes, and other structures. These traits aid in hearing, movement, reaction calculation, and environmental changes. The midbrain also contains the basal ganglia, which aid in movement and coordination, and the substantia nigra, a part affected by Parkinson's disease and home to a significant amount of dopamine neurons. Midbrain is also known as mesencephalon.
- Pons: The pons is the starting point for 4 of the 12 cranial nerves that enable a wide range of abilities, including feeding, blinking, focusing vision, balance, hearing, and facial expression. The medulla and midbrain are connected by pons.
- Medulla: At the base of the brainstem is the medulla, which is where the brain and spinal cord meet. The medulla is essential to survival. Numerous physiological functions, such as blood flow, breathing, heart rhythm, and oxygen and carbon dioxide levels, are regulated by the medulla. The medulla produces reflexive responses such as swallowing, vomiting, sneezing, and coughing [11, 12].

2.3 Limbic System of the Brain

Generally located lateral to the thalamus, beneath the cerebral cortex, and above the brainstem, the limbic system is a group of brain regions. This network system plays a significant role in emotional experiences, behavior, and memory.

Components of the limbic system:

- Limbic lobe: From the frontal lobe to the temporal lobe, the limbic lobe, which is situated at the medial portion of the cerebral hemispheres, encircles the corpus callosum. Cortical structures like the **cingulate gyrus**, which arches above the corpus callosum, are part of it. The cingulate gyrus is involved in emotional processing, behavior regulation, and autonomic motor function. It is separated into anterior and posterior areas, with the anterior cingulate gyrus specifically implicated in motivation and movement. The **parahippocampal gyrus** found within the limbic lobe's inferior region, in the medial temporal region is also a cortex structure in the limbic lobe, which is essential for memory and is a major output pathway for the hippocampal formation. Perceiving scenes, placing visual information in a context, and identifying social context are all functions of the parahippocampal gyrus. Additionally, it contributes to episodic memory and is susceptible to pathological alterations in diseases such as Alzheimer's. These two structures are connected by the isthmus and are also linked to regions like the subcallosal area and uncus.
- Hippocampus: The hippocampus is situated deep within the temporal lobe and is essential for both spatial navigation and the formation of long-term memories. It assists with information recall when needed and transfers new experiences from short-term to long-term memory. It is made up of areas like the **subiculum, dentate gyrus, and CA fields**. The fornix connects it to other limbic components both structurally and functionally.
- Amygdala: The amygdala is a cluster of nuclei shaped like an almond, located just in front of the hippocampus. It plays a major role in emotional processing, especially related to fear, aggression, and emotional memory. The amygdala interacts with the hypothalamus and prefrontal cortex to trigger appropriate emotional and autonomic responses.
- Hypothalamus: The hypothalamus lies under the thalamus and makes up the third ventricle's floor. It is an essential junction for hormone regulation and autonomic processes. It links physiological conditions like hunger, thirst, body temperature, circadian rhythm, and stress response to behavioral and emotional reactions. It affects pituitary gland activity as well.
- Septal nuclei: The septal nuclei are located in the basal forebrain and are involved in pleasure, reward, and reinforcement. These structures have reciprocal connections with the hippocampus and hypothalamus and are thought to influence social behavior, bonding, and the emotional content of experiences.

3 Overview of Cardiovascular Anatomy and Function

3.1 Heart Anatomy

There is no denying the heart's vital role. The human heart beats roughly 108,000 times a day at an average rate of 75 beats per minute, passing 39 million beats each year and coming close to 3 billion beats after a 75-year lifespan. About 70 mL of blood are pumped by each contraction of the heart's major chambers in an adult at rest, that adds up to 5.25 L per minute and nearly 14,000 L every day. Almost 10 million liters, or 2.6 million gallons, of blood are circulated across a vast network of nearly 60,000 miles of blood vessels during the course of a year [13].

3.2 Location of the Heart

The human heart is located medially between the lungs in the mediastinum, a portion of the thoracic cavity. Figure 2.3 depicts the position of the heart within the thoracic cavity. The heart is located within the mediastinum, while the pericardium, commonly referred to as the pericardial sac, is a tough membrane that surrounds the other mediastinal tissues and occupies the pericardial cavity. The anterior surface of

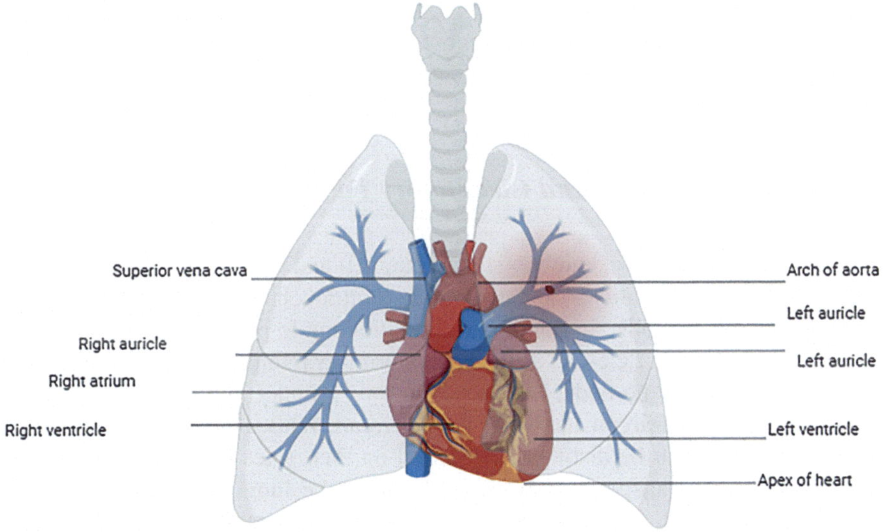

Fig. 2.3 Structural location of heart: On average, it is about the size of a person's fist, measuring roughly 12 cm (5 in.) in length, 8 cm (3.5 in.) in width, and 6 cm (2.5 in.) in thickness. Due to natural differences in body size between sexes, the average female heart weighs around 250–300 g (9–11 ounces), while the male heart typically weighs between 300 and 350 g (11–12 ounces) [14, 15]

the heart is deep within the sternum and costal cartilages, whereas the dorsal surface is near to the vertebral bodies [13, 14]. The anterior surface of the heart is deep within the sternum and costal cartilages, whereas the dorsal surface is near to the vertebral bodies. The base, or superior surface of the heart, connects the main arteries, aorta the pulmonary trunk, and the great veins, the superior and inferior venae cavae. Figure 2.3 shows that the base of the heart is at the level of the third costal cartilage. The apex, or inferior tip of the heart, is located just to the left of the sternum, between the junction of the fourth and fifth ribs and their articulation with the costal cartilage. The heart is diverted anteriorly to the right and posteriorly to the left.

While using a stethoscope to listen for the heartbeat of a patient's chest and on viewing photographs captured from a midsagittal perspective, it is crucial to keep in mind the location and direction of the heart [14]. The slight deviation of the apex to the left is reflected in a depression in the medial surface of the inferior lobe of the left lung, called the cardiac notch.

Athletes, particularly those who engage in endurance or aerobic sports, often have much larger hearts than typical. Comparable to skeletal muscles, the heart muscle responds to physical training by increasing the amount of contractile proteins within its cells, resulting in an increase in cell size without a change in cell number, a process known as hypertrophy. This permits an athlete's heart to pump blood more efficiently at a lower heart rate [16, 17].

However, not all cardiovascular enlargement is an outcome of favorable adaptations. Some disorders, such as hypertrophic cardiomyopathy, can cause the heart muscle to develop abnormally. The actual etiology of this condition is not usually known, and it frequently goes misdiagnosed. Alarmingly, it can cause abrupt cardiac mortality in young people who appear to be healthy.

3.3 Heart Chambers and Circulatory Pathways

The human heart has four chambers: two on the left and two on the right. Each side has an atrium (upper chamber) and a ventricle (bottom chamber). The atria serve as receiving chambers, collecting blood prior contracting to push it into the appropriate ventricles. The ventricles act as the heart's primary pumps, transporting blood to the lungs or out into the body. The heart has two primary interrelated circulation loops: the pulmonary circuit and the systemic circuit. While both carry blood and its components, they can be distinguished based on their roles in gas exchange. The pulmonary circuit transports blood in and out of the lungs. In the lungs, blood absorbs oxygen and excretes carbon dioxide. The systemic circuit transports oxygen-rich blood to body tissues while returning oxygen-poor blood and carbon dioxide to the heart for reoxygenation.

The process starts when the right ventricle pumps oxygen-depleted blood into the pulmonary trunk, which splits into the left and right pulmonary arteries. These arteries branch out and lead to the pulmonary capillaries in the lungs, where gas

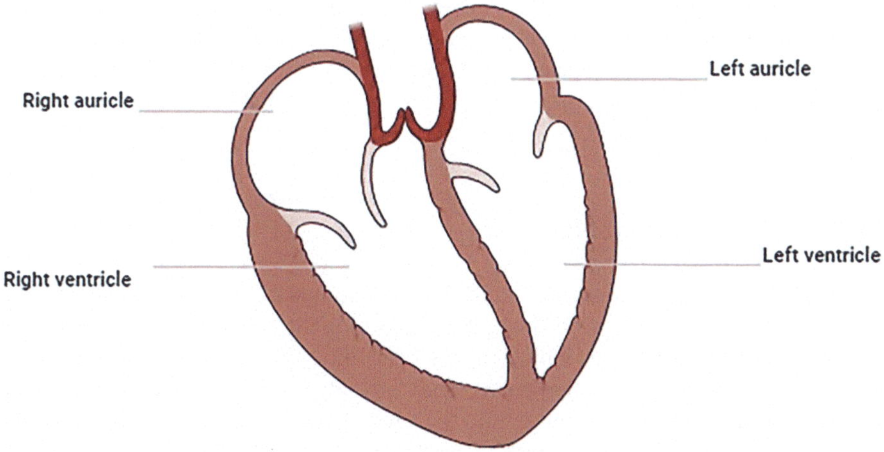

Fig. 2.4 Chambers of heart

exchange occurs. Carbon dioxide exits through the circulatory system and oxygen enters. Notably, the pulmonary arteries are unique due to the fact they are the only arteries in the body that transport deoxygenated blood. After receiving oxygen, blood returns from the lungs through the pulmonary veins, which are the only veins in the postnatal body that transport oxygen-rich blood. These veins transport blood to the left atrium, where it is pushed into the left ventricle, as illustrated in Fig. 2.4. The left ventricle then pumps oxygenated blood into the aorta, which transports it throughout the body via the systemic circuit. The systemic capillaries transport oxygen and nutrients to the body's cells, while carbon dioxide and waste enter the bloodstream. This deoxygenated blood now runs into small veins before merging with larger veins. Eventually, it returns to the heart via the superior and inferior vena cava and enters the right atrium. It is then pumped into the right ventricle, where the cycle repeats. This continuous blood flow through the pulmonary and systemic circuits is vital to sustaining life and is fundamental knowledge for healthcare professionals [17, 18].

3.4 Membranes, Surface Features, and Layers

3.4.1 Membranes

The pericardium or pericardial sac is the membrane that directly surrounds the heart and defines its cavity. It also protects the "roots" of the major vessels, which are in close proximity to the heart. The pericardium, which literally means "around the heart," is made up of two separate sublayers: the robust outer fibrous pericardium and the inside serous pericardium. The fibrous pericardium is a thick, dense connective tissue that protects and stabilizes the heart in the thorax.

The delicate serous pericardium is made up of two layers: the parietal pericardium, which is joined to the fibrous pericardium, and the inner visceral pericardium, or epicardium, which is connected to the heart and forms part of the heart wall. The epicardium and pericardium are separated by the pericardial cavity, which is filled with lubricating serous fluid.

3.4.2 Surface Features of the Heart

The exterior heart structures, including the four chambers, can be seen within the pericardial sac. Each atrium in the upper section of the heart has a tiny, flap-like protrusion called an auricle, which means "ear-like" because of its likeness to a human ear. The auricles (also known as atrial appendages) have weak walls and can store excess blood before emptying into their respective atria. Sulci, or fat grooves, are also visible on the surface, and they represent significant structural boundaries. These sulci house significant coronary blood arteries. The coronary sulcus is a prominent groove that separates the atria from the ventricles. Additionally, there are two other sulci between the left and right ventricles:

The anterior interventricular sulcus, seen on the front of the heart
The posterior interventricular sulcus, found on the back side

These surface features help in identifying the heart's external landmarks and the location of key blood vessels.

3.4.3 Layers

The heart wall is made up of three separate layers, each of which has varying thickness. The epicardium, myocardium, and endocardium are the layers that go from outermost to innermost. The epicardium, also known as the visceral pericardium, is the outer layer of the heart wall and the inner layer of the pericardial sac, as previously explained. Beneath the epicardium is the myocardium, the heart's thickest and most muscular layer (Fig. 2.5).

This layer is primarily made up of cardiac muscle cells, which are supported by a collagen fiber network, as well as blood vessels and nerve fibers that supply and regulate the heart. The contractions of the heart are caused by the myocardium, which propels blood through the chambers and into the arteries [18, 19].

The arrangement of muscle fibers in the myocardium is highly complex. Muscle cells generate swirling spirals around the heart. They produce a figure-eight pattern around the atria and the base of the major arteries, while deeper muscle fibers make a similar pattern around the ventricles, extending toward the apex. In the superficial layers, the muscle wraps around both ventricles. This intricate spiral arrangement enables the heart to contract more efficiently and powerfully than a basic straight-line pattern would.

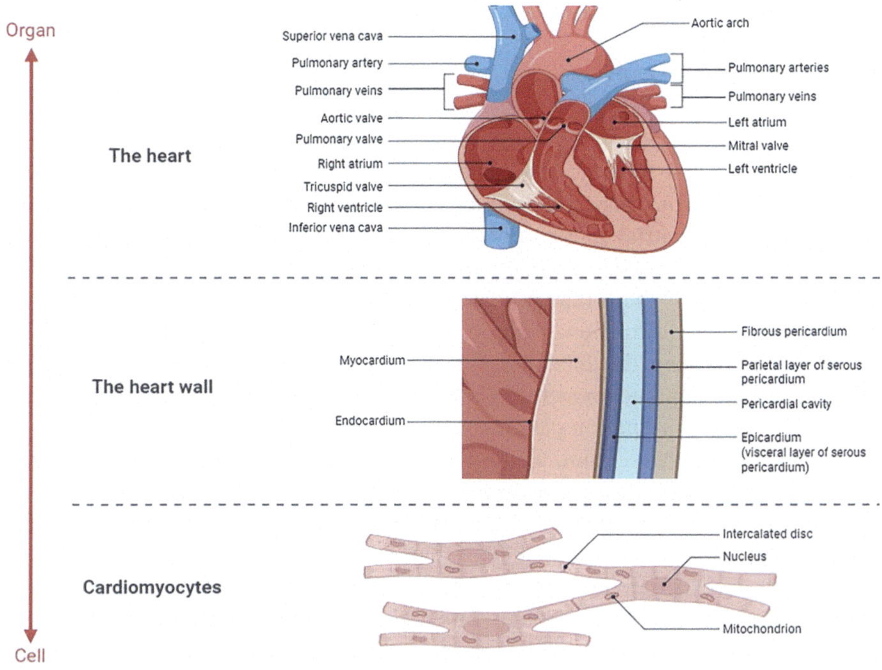

Fig. 2.5 Internal structure of heart showing different layers

Although the left and right ventricles pump the same amount of blood with each heartbeat, the left ventricle has a considerably thicker and more muscular wall than the right. This is due to the fact that the left ventricle must produce much more pressure in order to pump blood through the broad and high-resistance systemic circulation. In contrast, the right ventricle pumps blood into the pulmonary circulation via a considerably shorter, lower-resistance conduit that takes less force. The endocardium is the heart wall's innermost layer, separated from the myocardium by a thin layer of connective tissue.

It lines the interior chambers of the heart, where blood flows, and also covers the heart valves. This layer is composed of simple squamous epithelium, known as endothelium, which continues seamlessly with the inner lining of blood vessels [18].

Recent research suggests that the endothelium of the endocardium and coronary capillaries plays an active role in heart function. It may help regulate the contraction of cardiac muscle within the myocardium, influence growth patterns of heart muscle cells throughout life, and secrete endothelins signaling molecules that shape the chemical environment around the cells by controlling ion concentrations and contractility.

3.5 Internal Structure of the Heart

3.5.1 Septa of the Heart

The term septum, derived from Latin meaning "something that encloses," refers to a wall or barrier that separates the chambers of the human heart. These septa are myocardial expansions bordered with endocardium that separate the heart's compartments. The interatrial septum divides the left and right atria. This septum in a typical adult heart contains a small, oval depression known as the fossa ovalis, which is a vestige of the foramen ovale, an opening present during fetal development. The foramen ovale allowed blood to flow directly from the right atrium to the left atrium, bypassing the fetal lungs, which were non-functional. Shortly after delivery, a tissue flap known as the septum primum closes this opening, producing the usual postnatal circulation pattern.

The interventricular septum, which originates throughout fetal development and stays intact in a healthy heart, divides the left and right ventricles. In order to pump blood through the body, the ventricles must generate a lot greater pressure, which is why this septum is substantially thicker than the interatrial septum. The atrioventricular septum, which divides the atria from the ventricles, is another crucial component. It has four apertures through which blood can pass from the atria into the ventricles and then into the aorta and pulmonary trunk from the ventricles. A valve installed in each of these apertures guarantees unidirectional blood flow. The valves between the atria and ventricles are collectively known as atrioventricular valves, while those located at the exits to the pulmonary trunk and aorta are called semilunar valves.

In order to get a better view of the bicuspid and tricuspid valves, the atrioventricular septum has been removed. However, the aorta and pulmonary trunk block out the interatrial septum. The cardiac skeleton, also known as the skeleton of the heart, is a dense structure of connective tissue that reinforces the atrioventricular septum, which is structurally weaker due to its numerous holes and valves. The valve holes connecting the atria and ventricles, as well as those going to the aorta and pulmonary trunk, are supported by four fibrous rings that make up this skeleton. The cardiac skeleton is essential for maintaining the electrical separation between the ventricles and atria, which for the heart's electrical signals to be properly conducted, in addition to acting as anchor points for the heart valves.

3.5.2 Right Atrium

When blood returns to the heart from the systemic circulation, it is received in the right atrium. Three main vessels carry blood from the body into the right atrium:

The superior vena cava drains into the upper and rear parts of the right atrium after carrying deoxygenated blood from regions above the diaphragm, including the head, neck, upper limbs, and thorax.

The inferior vena cava drains into the lower posterior area of the right atrium after transporting blood from below the diaphragm, including the lower extremities and abdomen pelvic region.

Myocardial deoxygenated blood is drained by the coronary sinus, a big vein situated immediately above and slightly medial to the inferior vena cava orifice. The medial wall contains a slight dip called the fossa ovalis although the majority of the right atrial wall is smooth on the inside. Pectinate muscles, which are noticeable muscular ridges, are found in the anterior region of the atrium. The right auricle, a little flap-like protrusion of the atrium, also contains these pectinate muscles. On the other hand, the auricle of the left atrium solely has pectinate muscles. In order to prevent venous return from being disrupted during ventricular contractions, the atria receive venous blood virtually continuously.

The atria actively contract straight away before the ventricles do, which helps to force blood into the ventricles, even though the majority of the blood enters them passively while the atria are relaxed. The tricuspid valve protects the opening between the right atrium and right ventricle.

3.5.3 Right Ventricle

The tricuspid valve allows blood from the right atrium to enter the right ventricle. The chordae tendineae, or "heartstrings," are robust bands of connective tissue that hold each leaflet of this valve in place. Collagen fibers make up the majority of these cables, with endothelial tissue and elastic fibers making up minor portions. The papillary muscles that protrude from the inner ventricular wall are connected to the valve flaps via the chordae tendineae. The anterior, posterior, and septal papillary muscles of the right ventricle correspond to the three tricuspid valve cusps. The pressure inside the ventricle rises when the ventricular myocardium contracts. Blood pushes toward the pulmonary trunk and possibly back toward the atrium as it travels from regions of higher to lower pressure. The papillary muscles contract simultaneously, tugging on the chordae tendineae to stop backflow. This successfully prevents regurgitation during contraction by keeping the valve flaps tight and preventing their backward push into the atrium [20].

3.5.4 Left Atrium

Four pulmonary veins carry oxygen-rich blood back to the left atrium following gas exchange in the pulmonary capillaries. These muscular ridges are present in the left atrium's major chamber, despite the smooth walls and absence of pectinate muscles. The left atrium serves as a receiving chamber, and the pulmonary veins continuously return blood to the heart. After that, blood enters the left ventricle via a gap between the two chambers. The majority of this blood flows passively when the ventricles and atria are relaxing. But the left atrium actively contracts right before the ventricles contract, forcing more blood into the ventricle. However the left atrium actively contracts right before the ventricles contract, forcing more blood into the ventricle. About 20% of the left ventricle's total blood volume is attributed to this atrial contraction. The mitral valve controls the gap between the atrium and ventricle.

The left ventricular muscular wall is significantly thicker than the right, despite the fact that both sides of the heart pump the same amount of blood. This is because pumping blood across the systemic circulation requires higher pressure. The left ventricle lacks a moderator band, but it does exhibit trabeculae carneae, which are irregular muscular ridges on the internal surface, like the right. In contrast to the right ventricle, which has three papillary muscles, the mitral valve, also referred to as the bicuspid valve, is connected to two papillary muscles anterior and posterior via chordae tendineae, which aid in preventing valve backflow during contraction. The aortic semilunar valve allows the left ventricle, which serves as the systemic circuit's main pumping chamber, to transfer oxygenated blood into the aorta.

3.5.5 Structure and Function of Heart Valves

All four of the heart's valves are located in the same plane when viewed in cross-section, right above the atrioventricular septum. These valves are essential for preserving the heart's one-way (unidirectional) blood flow. The right atrioventricular (AV) valve, also referred to as the tricuspid valve, is situated between the right atrium and right ventricle. Usually consisting of three flaps or leaflets, this valve is made of endocardial tissue that has been reinforced by connective tissue. The chordae tendineae, which bind these flaps to the papillary muscles, aid in controlling the valve's opening and shutting throughout the cardiac cycle.

Pulmonary Semilunar Valve

The pulmonary semilunar valve, sometimes known as the pulmonic valve, pulmonary valve, or right semilunar valve, is located at the beginning of the pulmonary trunk, when it leaves the right ventricle. Three tiny cusps consisting of endothelial tissue and held up by connective tissue comprise this valve. Blood flows backward toward the heart when the right ventricle relaxes because the pressure in the pulmonary trunk rises above that in the ventricle. When the valve is forced to close due to the backward flow filling the pocket-like cusps, a characteristic heart sound is produced. The pulmonary valve is independent of chordae tendineae and papillary muscles, in contrast to the atrioventricular valves.

Mitral (Bicuspid) Valve

The mitral valve, sometimes called the bicuspid valve or the left atrioventricular valve, is the valve that sits between the left atrium and left ventricle. Unlike the tricuspid valve, which has three flaps, this valve has two flaps, or cusps: the anterior medial and posterior medial. This valve is commonly referred to as the mitral valve in clinical practice. Chordae tendineae, which are connected to two papillary muscles, anchor these two cusps to the ventricular wall.

Aortic Semilunar Valve

At the base of the aorta, the aortic valve, also known as the aortic semilunar valve, keeps blood from returning to the left ventricle. Typically, it has three flaps. Blood tries to flow backward as the ventricle relaxes because the aortic pressure is higher than the ventricle's. An audible heart sound is produced as the valve closes due to the backflow filling the cusps.

4 Common Pathologies of the Brain and Cardiovascular System

The structure and function of the cardiovascular system and brain are connected in many ways. Pathologies affecting either of these systems often have overlapping clinical consequences due to the critical role of cerebral perfusion and neurovascular integrity.

4.1 Common Pathologies of the Brain

1. **Stroke (Cerebrovascular Accident)**
   Stroke continues to be a major global cause of morbidity and death [21]. It occurs when the blood supply to the brain is cut off, either due to an ischemic stroke or a hemorrhagic stroke caused by a ruptured blood vessel. Transient ischemic attacks (TIAs) are short episodes of neurological impairment that often precede major strokes.
2. **Neurodegenerative Disorders**
   Progressive neuronal degeneration is a feature of diseases like Parkinson's and Alzheimer's. It is becoming more widely acknowledged that chronic cardiovascular insufficiency and microvascular damage in the brain cause vascular contributions to cognitive impairment and dementia (VCID), including vascular dementia [22].

3. **Epilepsy**
   Epilepsy is a long-term condition marked by frequent seizures. It may result from trauma, tumors, or ischemic injury, or it may be idiopathic or secondary to structural abnormalities [23].
4. **Brain Tumors**
   Primary brain tumors such as gliomas and meningiomas, as well as metastatic lesions, can compromise neurological function depending on their location and size.

4.2 Common Pathologies of the Cardiovascular System

The cardiovascular system is in charge of maintaining adequate circulation and oxygen delivery. Several widespread cardiovascular disorders are:

1. **Hypertension**
   For both heart and brain disorders, persistently high blood pressure is a major risk factor [24].The risk of aneurysm formation, hemorrhagic stroke, ventricular hypertrophy, and arterial stiffness is increased by chronic hypertension.
2. **Coronary Artery Disease (CAD)**
   When the myocardial blood flow is restricted by coronary artery atherosclerosis, it can lead to CAD. Both acute myocardial infarction (heart attack) and stable angina, which impair cardiac output, are possible presentations [25].
3. **Congestive Heart Failure (CHF)**
   The inability of the heart to pump enough blood to meet the body's needs results in CHF. Secondary brain hypoperfusion and cognitive decline may result from this condition, which is frequently brought on by hypertension, valvular disorders, or prior myocardial infarctions.
4. **Arrhythmias**
   Atrial fibrillation and other irregular heart rhythms raise the risk of thromboembolism, especially stroke. Ventricular arrhythmias are a leading cause of abrupt cardiac death and can be fatal [26].
5. **Valvular Heart Disease**
   Hemodynamic changes brought on by heart valve dysfunction (such as aortic stenosis or mitral regurgitation) can cause cardiac remodeling, pulmonary congestion, and even stroke from an embolism [27].
6. **Peripheral Artery Disease (PAD)** and **Aortic Aneurysms**
   PAD is a sign of systemic atherosclerosis that impacts blood flow to the limbs. Aneurysms have the potential to rupture fatally, especially in the cerebral and aortic vessels [28].

4.3 Shared Pathologies and the Cardio-Brain Axis

There is increasing awareness of the cardio-brain axis, highlighting the physiological and pathological link between the brain and cardiovascular system.

1. **Cardioembolic Stroke**
   This type of stroke occurs when a thrombus originating in the heart, commonly from atrial fibrillation, migrates to the brain, causing ischemia. It emphasizes the importance of anticoagulation in cardiac arrhythmias [29].
2. **Vascular Dementia**
   Chronic cerebral hypoperfusion or recurrent micro-infarcts causes vascular dementia and is strongly linked to long-standing cardiovascular disease and poorly controlled hypertension [30].
3. **Autonomic Dysfunction**
   Conditions like diabetic neuropathy or Parkinson's disease may disrupt autonomic regulation of heart rate and blood pressure, leading to orthostatic hypotension and syncope [31].
4. **Takotsubo Cardiomyopathy (Stress-Induced Cardiomyopathy)**
   Often triggered by emotional or neurological stress, this condition mimics acute coronary syndrome but without significant coronary obstruction. It illustrates the neurogenic component of some cardiac pathologies [32].

5 Conclusion

The brain and the cardiovascular system have an intricate hyperlink which is best demonstrated by the cardio-brain axis. The heart's rhythm and vascular tone are controlled by the autonomic nervous system and neuroendocrine signaling pathways in response to emotional and cognitive stimuli. On the other hand, circulatory abnormalities such as arrhythmias or decreased cardiac output can directly affect cerebral perfusion, which can lead to stroke, neurodegenerative diseases, and cognitive impairment.

The convergence of cardiology and neurology has given rise to emerging fields like cardio-brain oncology, which further reinforces the necessity of an integrated approach to health. Here, the bidirectional impact of systemic illness and therapy from chemotherapeutic cardiotoxicity to metastatic brain lesions illustrates the clinical importance of maintaining cardiovascular integrity for optimal brain function and vice versa.

Understanding the detailed anatomy and physiological roles of brain structures like the cerebrum, cerebellum, brainstem, and limbic system alongside the chambers, valves, and regulatory circuits of the heart enhances our ability to diagnose and treat conditions that span both systems. Pathologies such as stroke, epilepsy, heart failure, and arrhythmias emphasize the clinical relevance of this connection. As research deepens, interdisciplinary strategies that bridge neurocardiology will be critical for precision medicine, improving outcomes and quality of life for patients affected by disorders of either or both of these vital systems.

References

1. Chen J, Wei X, Wu X, Zhang Q, Xia G, Xia H et al (2024) Disorder of neuroplasticity aggravates cognitive impairment via neuroinflammation associated with intestinal flora dysbiosis in chronic heart failure. Aging 16(13):10882–10904
2. Cui B, Peng F, Lu J, He B, Su Q, Luo H et al (2021) Cancer and stress: NextGen strategies. Brain Behav Immun 93:368–383
3. Manolis AA, Manolis TA, Apostolopoulos EJ, Apostolaki NE, Melita H, Manolis AS (2021) The role of the autonomic nervous system in cardiac arrhythmias: the neuro-cardiac axis, more foe than friend? Trends Cardiovasc Med 31(5):290–302
4. Tahsili-Fahadan P, Geocadin RG (2017) Heart–brain axis. Circ Res 120(3):559–572
5. Manea M, Comsa M, Minca A, Dragos D, Popa C (2015) Brain-heart axis—Review article. J Med Life 8(3):266–271
6. van der Wall EE, van Gilst WH (2013) Neurocardiology: close interaction between heart and brain. Neth Heart J Mon J Neth Soc Cardiol Neth Heart Found 21(2):51–52
7. Brain anatomy and how the brain works [Internet] (2025). https://www.hopkinsmedicine.org/health/conditions-and-diseases/anatomy-of-the-brain
8. Hartwigsen G, Bengio Y, Bzdok D (2021) How does hemispheric specialization contribute to human-defining cognition? Neuron 109(13):2075–2090
9. Bhushan R, Ravichandiran V, Kumar N (2022) An overview of the anatomy and physiology of the brain. In: Nanocarriers for drug-targeting brain tumors, pp 3–29
10. Angeles Fernández-Gil M, Palacios-Bote R, Leo-Barahona M, Mora-Encinas JP (2010) Anatomy of the brainstem: a gaze into the stem of life. Semin Ultrasound CT MR 31(3):196–219. https://doi.org/10.1053/j.sult.2010.03.006
11. Maldonado KA, Alsayouri K (2025) Physiology, brain. In: StatPearls [Internet]. StatPearls Publishing, Treasure Island, FL. https://www.ncbi.nlm.nih.gov/books/NBK551718/
12. Ackerman S (1992) 2, Major structures and functions of the brain. In: Discovering the brain. National Academies Press (US), Washington, DC. https://www.ncbi.nlm.nih.gov/books/NBK234157/
13. Aaronson PI, Ward JP, Connolly MJ (2020) The cardiovascular system at a glance. Wiley
14. Buckberg GD, Nanda NC, Nguyen C, Kocica MJ (2018) What is the heart? Anatomy, function, pathophysiology, and misconceptions. J Cardiovasc Dev Dis 5(2):33
15. Bakose RY, Al-Obaidi AD, Al-Obaidi MN, Al-Abbasi H, Al-Bayati MO, Hashim AT, Muhanned A, Alhaideri A, Al-Dabagh JD (2023) Anatomy of the heart. In: Heart transplantation. Springer International Publishing, Cham, pp 1–17
16. Zhong L, Tan RS, Ghista DN (2019) Anatomy and physiology of the heart. In: Computational and mathematical methods in cardiovascular physiology, pp 3–37
17. Chaudhry R, Miao JH, Rehman A (2022) Physiology, cardiovascular. In: StatPearls [Internet]. StatPearls Publishing
18. Dampney RA, Coleman MJ, Fontes MA, Hirooka Y, Horiuchi J, Li YW, Polson JW, Potts PD, Tagawa T (2002) Central mechanisms underlying short- and long-term regulation of the cardiovascular system. Clin Exp Pharmacol Physiol 29(4):261–268
19. Romero SA, Minson CT, Halliwill JR (2017) The cardiovascular system after exercise. J Appl Physiol 122(4):925–932

20. Alenezi F, Rajagopal S, Kutty S (2020) Assessing right atrial function in pulmonary hypertension: window to the soul of the right heart? Am J Physiol Heart Circ Physiol 318(1):H154–H155
21. Moroni F, Ammirati E, Rocca MA, Filippi M, Magnoni M, Camici PG (2018) Cardiovascular disease and brain health: focus on white matter hyperintensities. Int J Cardiol Heart Vasc 19:63–69. https://doi.org/10.1016/j.ijcha.2018.04.006
22. Zlokovic BV, Gottesman RF, Bernstein KE, Seshadri S, McKee A, Snyder H, Greenberg SM, Yaffe K, Schaffer CB, Yuan C, Hughes TM, Daemen MJ, Williamson JD, González HM, Schneider J, Wellington CL, Katusic ZS, Stoeckel L, Koenig JI, Corriveau RA, Fine L, Galis ZS, Reis J, Wright JD, Chen J (2020) Vascular contributions to cognitive impairment and dementia (VCID): a report from the 2018 National Heart, Lung, and Blood Institute and National Institute of Neurological Disorders and Stroke Workshop. Alzheimers Dement 16(12):1714–1733. https://doi.org/10.1002/alz.12157. Epub 2020 Oct 8
23. Anwar H, Khan QU, Nadeem N, Pervaiz I, Ali M, Cheema FF (2020) Epileptic seizures. Discoveries (Craiova) 8(2):e110. https://doi.org/10.15190/d.2020.7
24. Shams P, Tackling G, Borhade MB (2025) Hypertensive heart disease. In: StatPearls [Internet]. StatPearls Publishing, Treasure Island, FL. https://www.ncbi.nlm.nih.gov/books/NBK539800/
25. Shahjehan RD, Sharma S, Bhutta BS (2025) Coronary artery disease. In: StatPearls [Internet]. StatPearls Publishing, Treasure Island, FL. https://www.ncbi.nlm.nih.gov/books/NBK564304/
26. Tang PT, Shenasa M, Boyle NG (2017) Ventricular arrhythmias and sudden cardiac death. Card Electrophysiol Clin 9(4):693–708. https://doi.org/10.1016/j.ccep.2017.08.004
27. Maeder MT, Weber L, Buser M, Gerhard M, Haager PK, Maisano F, Rickli H (2018) Pulmonary hypertension in aortic and mitral valve disease. Front Cardiovasc Med 5:40. https://doi.org/10.3389/fcvm.2018.00040
28. Zemaitis MR, Boll JM, Dreyer MA (2025) Peripheral arterial disease. In: StatPearls [Internet]. StatPearls Publishing, Treasure Island, FL. https://www.ncbi.nlm.nih.gov/books/NBK430745/
29. Abdullah BB, Nausheen N, Mehdi KM, Ghalib E. Cardioembolic stroke—a study of its incidence, aetiology, clinical presentation and outcome
30. Rajeev V, Chai YL, Poh L, Selvaraji S, Fann DY, Jo DG, De Silva TM, Drummond GR, Sobey CG, Arumugam TV, Chen CP, Lai MKP (2023) Chronic cerebral hypoperfusion: a critical feature in unravelling the etiology of vascular cognitive impairment. Acta Neuropathol Commun 11(1):93. https://doi.org/10.1186/s40478-023-01590-1
31. Sánchez-Manso JC, Gujarathi R, Varacallo MA (2025) Autonomic dysfunction. In: StatPearls [Internet]. StatPearls Publishing, Treasure Island, FL. https://www.ncbi.nlm.nih.gov/books/NBK430888/
32. Ahmad SA, Khalid N, Ibrahim MA (2025) Takotsubo cardiomyopathy. In: StatPearls [Internet]. StatPearls Publishing, Treasure Island, FL. https://www.ncbi.nlm.nih.gov/books/NBK430798/

Chapter 3
Therapeutic Approach in Cancer: The Role of Ion Channels and Transporters

Richa Awasthi, Mimoh Sharma, Suruchi Mathur, Sarfraz Alam, Sidra Ali, and Preecha Yupapin

1 Introduction to Ion Channels and Transporters in Cancer

Cancer remains a significant global health problem, with a high lifetime incidence rate among individuals, despite notable advancements in diagnostics and treatment. Traditional tools such as PSA testing and mammography remain flawed due to low specificity and risks of overdiagnosis, respectively [1]. Even advanced strategies like immunotherapy do not uniformly benefit all patients [2]. While combination chemotherapies like CHOP, CMF, and BEP have improved survival rates for certain cancers, further progress hinges on novel molecular insights and targeted therapies that can address the complexity and heterogeneity of tumors.

Ion-transporting protein (ITP) is one encouraging field, including ion channels, pumps, and exchangers, which is commonly dysregulated in cancer. These proteins are involved in key processes such as proliferation, invasion, and metastasis [3, 4]. Notably, potassium channels regulate cell division, and voltage-gated sodium channels (VGSCs) enhance metastatic potential. The sodium–hydrogen exchanger-1 (NHE1), which maintains the altered pH gradient characteristic of cancer cells, is

R. Awasthi (✉) · S. Mathur
Department of Biochemistry, Saraswathi Institute of Medical Sciences, Hapur, India

M. Sharma · S. Alam
Department of Biochemistry, Integral Institute of Medical Sciences and Research, Integral University, Lucknow, India

S. Ali
Department of Basic Medical Sciences, Integral Institute of Allied Health Sciences and Research, Integral University, Lucknow, India

P. Yupapin
Department of Electrical Technology, School of Industrial Technology, Sakonnakhon Technical College, Institute of Vocational Education Northeastern 2, Sakonnakhon, Thailand

S. Mallik et al. (eds.), *Landscape of Signaling Pathway and Genetic Markers in Cardio-Brain Oncology*, Studies in Rhythm Engineering,
https://doi.org/10.1007/978-981-95-7012-6_3

often overexpressed in tumors [5, 6]. Since around 15% of current drugs target ITPs, they offer repurposing potential for cancer therapy. The growing field of cancer neuroscience further reinforces this direction, revealing tumor-associated neuronal features and suggesting new, minimally toxic treatment opportunities [7, 8].

2 Emerging Relevance of Ion Channels and Transporters in Cancers

The crucial functions of ion channels and transporters in cancer biology have been revealed by extensive study conducted over the last two decades, demonstrating their involvement in key processes like cell proliferation and migration, invasion, angiogenesis, and metastasis. This has led to the emergence of the concept of "oncochannelopathies," highlighting the pathological significance of ion channel dysregulation in cancer. Among these, voltage-gated proton channels (Hv1) have gained attention for their role in maintaining intracellular pH homeostasis and promoting tumor progression in glioma, colorectal, and breast cancers. Overexpression of Hv1 has been associated with acidification of the tumor microenvironment and poor clinical outcomes [9].

In silico research by Lavoro et al. on solute carrier (SLC) transporters found 62 genes that were differentially expressed, which helped to further the area, some of which, such as SLC4A4, SLC7A11, SLC24A5, and SLC45A2, were linked to clinical outcomes and drug sensitivity, particularly to anti-MEK and anti-RAF therapies. Likewise, Herrera-Quiterio and Encarnacion-Guevara emphasized the role of transmembrane proteins (TMEMs) in cancer progression, chemoresistance, and epithelial-mesenchymal transition through integrative transcriptomic and proteomic analyses. Capitani et al. expanded this understanding to lung cancer by reviewing ion channels such as potassium, sodium, calcium, chloride, and nicotinic acetylcholine receptors, demonstrating their associations with tumor growth, invasiveness, prognosis, and drug resistance. There are now a number of medications that target ion channels in clinical trials; these findings underscore the therapeutic potential of targeting ion transport mechanisms in oncology.

3 Key Ion Channels and Transporters in Cancers

Cancer is still a major cause of death worldwide, even though there has been significant progress in cancer biology, largely due to the limitations of current systemic treatments such as chemotherapy, hormonal therapy, and biological therapies. These conventional approaches often exhibit nonspecific toxicity and damage to healthy tissues. Additionally, it encourages the development of multidrug resistance. Consequently, there is a growing demand for alternative therapeutic strategies that leverage different mechanisms of action. One emerging and promising avenue involves artificial transmembrane ion transporters, which can selectively disrupt ion homeostasis or pH balance within cancer cells, triggering apoptosis without harming normal cells [10, 11]. Moreover, integrating these artificial ion transporters with existing therapies has shown potential in overcoming drug resistance [12].

Artificial ion transport systems fall into two main categories: ion carriers and ion channels. Ion carriers are mobile and transport ions by physically moving across the lipid bilayer. Conversely, ion channels are fixed structures that allow ions to pass through without compromising membrane integrity. Synthetic ion channels are further classified as either unimolecular or self-assembled. Unimolecular channels, typically macrocyclic, offer high structural stability but require complex and labor-intensive synthesis, shown in Fig. 3.1. In contrast, self-assembling synthetic channels form in situ from smaller monomeric units, offering a more practical approach. However, designing self-assembling systems with consistent ion selectivity and structural stability remains a major challenge, limiting their widespread application in cancer therapy.

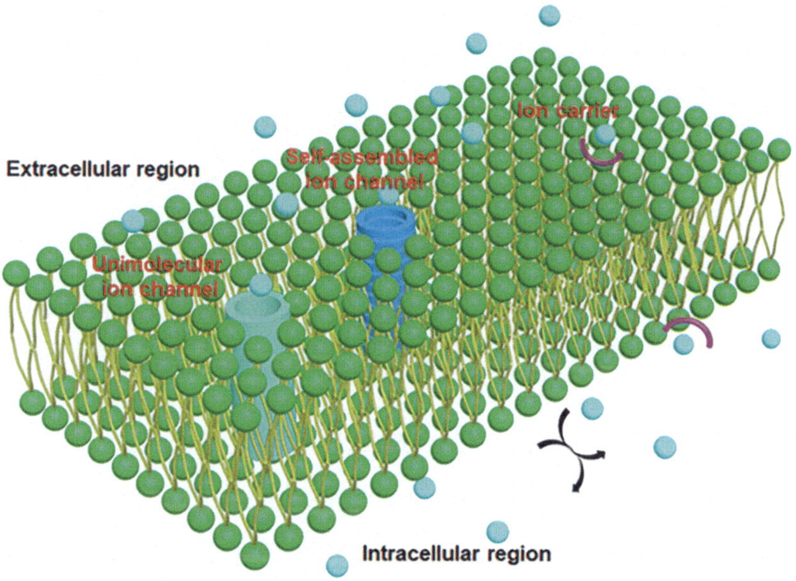

Fig. 3.1 Diagrammatic representation of an ion carrier and an ion channel

3.1 Ion Channels

According to their gating mechanisms, ion channels are generally divided into voltage-gated and ligand-gated channels. Changes in membrane potential cause voltage-gated channels to react and only allow certain ions to pass through, while ligand-gated channels are opened by ligands and typically allow the flow of cations or anions with lower selectivity. Both types are essential for various physiological functions, including electrical signaling, gene expression, hormone secretion, and cognitive processes like learning and memory [13]. However, under pathological conditions, changes in the properties or activities of these channels can occur, and this kind of dysregulation has been linked to increased tumor cell development and proliferation.

3.1.1 Voltage-Gated Ion Channels (VGICs)

Voltage-gated ion channels (VGICs) are prevalent in both excitable and non-excitable tissues. They are easily stimulated cells and have a critical role in many bodily processes. Beyond their typical VGICs have been linked to a number of illnesses, such as epilepsy, cardiac arrhythmias, and other disorders, hyperkalemia, as well as a number of inherited diseases [13]. Recent studies that also connect VGICs play a role in cancer development, particularly in processes like tumorigenesis, proliferation, metastasis, cell survival, and migration. According to ion selectivity, VGICs fall under three primary categories: potassium, sodium, and calcium channels, all of which are voltage-gated and have a similar structure, a structure made up of four repeating domains of six transmembrane α-helical segments (S1–S6) linked via intracellular and extracellular loops [14]. Additionally, VGICs include β-subunits that serve regulatory functions by modulating gating properties and facilitating interactions between ion channel complexes [13].

Calcium (Ca^{2+}), Sodium (Na^{+}), and Potassium (K^{+}) Channel

- **Voltage-Gated Calcium Channels (VGCCs or Cav)**
- Voltage-gated calcium channels (VGCCs) are integral membrane proteins found throughout the body made up of five subunits—α1, α2, β, δ, and ε—which are expressed in both excitable and non-excitable tissues. The α1 subunit of the ion-conducting pore detects changes in voltage, and the γ subunit does the same.
- The behavior of the channel is controlled by additional subunits. There are six different VGCC subtypes: L, according to their electrophysiological and pharmacological characteristics, N, P, Q, R, and T. L-type: The brain has a high concentration of channels that are involved in excitation-contraction coupling.

- They respond to dihydropyridines and include cardiac and skeletal muscles. N-type neurotransmitter release is mediated by channels, mostly found in presynaptic terminals. P-type: In cerebellar and other tissues, Q-type channels contribute to neurotransmission and secretory processes, neurons with a pyramidal form. R-type channels are characterized by fast gating and are found in cerebellar granule cells, while T-type channels, activated by slight depolarizations, are widely distributed and exhibit rapid inactivation kinetics.

- Beyond their physiological roles in neuronal signaling and muscle function, VGCCs are implicated in several diseases, including long-QT syndromes, epilepsy, migraines, and Lambert–Eaton Myasthenic Syndrome. Importantly, emerging evidence also connects VGCCs to oncogenesis. T-type Ca^{2+} channels are upregulated during neuroendocrine differentiation in prostate cancer, while the L-type subunit Cav1.2 is increasingly expressed in differentiated colon cancer cells [15]. Additionally, P- and L-type VGCCs are found in small cell lung carcinomas [16]. T-type channel-mediated calcium spikes can also promote membrane depolarization, contributing to enhanced motility in fibrosarcoma cells [17]. These findings underscore the multifaceted roles of VGCCs in both physiological regulation and pathological processes, including tumor progression.
- **Voltage-Gated Sodium Channels (VGSCs or Nav)**
- Voltage-gated sodium channels (VGSCs) are important membrane proteins that are activated by voltage changes primarily seen in excitable cells like cardiac myocytes and neurons; depolarization is the primary manifestation, where they initiate action potentials through rapid Na^+ influx [14]. Structurally, an α-subunit that creates pores and one or two β-subunits make up a VGSC; the ion conductance is determined by the α-subunit, but channel kinetics and voltage are modulated by the β-subunits sensitivity [18]. There are nine known functional VGSC α-subunits (Nav1.1–Nav1.9), each with distinct tissue-specific expression. For instance, Nav1.4 and Nav1.5 are predominant in cardiac muscle, while Nav1.1, Nav1.2, and Nav1.8 are common in the brain [13]. VGSCs are also classified by their sensitivity to tetrodotoxin (TTX): TTX-sensitive types (e.g., Nav1.1–1.4, 1.6, 1.7) are inhibited by nanomolar levels, whereas TTX-resistant types (e.g., Nav1.5, 1.8, 1.9) require micromolar concentrations [19].
- In addition to their traditional function in excitability, VGSCs are also functionally expressed in non-neurons that are easily stimulated, such as fibroblasts and glia, and immune cells, where they influence proliferation, adhesion, and migration [20]. Clinically, VGSC dysfunction has been implicated in multiple channelopathies, including epilepsy, long-QT syndrome, and motor neuropathies [14]. Notably, increasing evidence associates VGSC expression with enhanced metastatic potential in various cancers, including prostate [21], breast [22], lung [23], cervical [24], and melanoma [25]. One proposed mechanism suggests that Na^+ influx through VGSCs alters intracellular Ca^{2+} dynamics and activates signaling pathways related to cell motility and metastasis. These findings highlight VGSCs as emerging therapeutic targets in combating cancer metastasis [22, 23].

- **Voltage-Gated Potassium Channels (VGKCs or Kv)**
- Voltage-gated potassium channels (VGKCs), especially Kv subtypes, are essential for maintaining membrane potential in excitable cells like neurons and cardiac myocytes and are also active in non-excitable cells, where they regulate processes such as cell volume, apoptosis, differentiation, and immune responses [26]. Kv channels are composed of α-subunits, which contain voltage-sensor and pore-forming domains, and are often associated with β-subunits involved in protein scaffolding and extracellular matrix interactions. The dysregulation of these channels, particularly Kv channels, has been linked to cancer cell proliferation, progression, and apoptotic evasion, suggesting that VGKCs may serve as viable targets for anticancer therapy.
- Among Kv channels, the human ether-à-go-go potassium channel (EAG1 or Kv10.1) stands out due to its restricted normal expression in the brain and aberrant overexpression in numerous tumors [27]. Studies report EAG1 overexpression in over 75% of tumors and cancer cell lines [28] with early evidence from Farias et al. confirming its presence in somatic cancer lines and primary cervical cancer biopsies [29]. Inhibiting EAG1, either through siRNA or pharmacological agents, has been shown to significantly suppress cancer cell proliferation. Although Mello et al. noted that EAG1 expression varies by histological type, it is not necessarily linked to tumor size or grade [30]. Given its minimal expression in normal tissue and accessibility due to its limited localization within the central nervous system, EAG1 is becoming a potential therapeutic and diagnostic target with minimal off-target risk [27]. The mechanisms through which Kv channels, particularly EAG1, promote cancer progression remain under study. Downie et al. proposed that EAG1 may enhance hypoxia-inducible factor 1 (HIF-1) activity, leading to increased VEGF secretion and tumor angiogenesis [31]. In MCF-7 breast cancer cells, Kv channels regulate proliferation and the cell cycle through modulation of membrane potential [32]. Kv channels also appear to facilitate glioma invasion and metastasis formation by regulating ion fluxes, which contribute to water efflux, cell shrinkage, and improved motility through tissue matrices, key features of metastatic cancer cells [33]. These findings support the role of Kv channels as multifunctional regulators of tumor progression and highlight their potential in oncology-focused therapeutic development.

3.1.2 Transient Receptor Potential (TRP) Channels

The transient receptor potential (TRP) channels are cation-permeable channels with six transmembrane domains that are widely dispersed throughout mammalian tissues. They control the membrane potential, intracellular calcium (Ca^{2+}), and sodium (Na^{+}) concentrations in both excitable and non-excitable cells [34]. Functioning as signal integrators, TRP channels can be activated by a wide range of stimuli, leading to Ca^{2+} and Na^{+} influx and subsequent activation of downstream signaling cascades

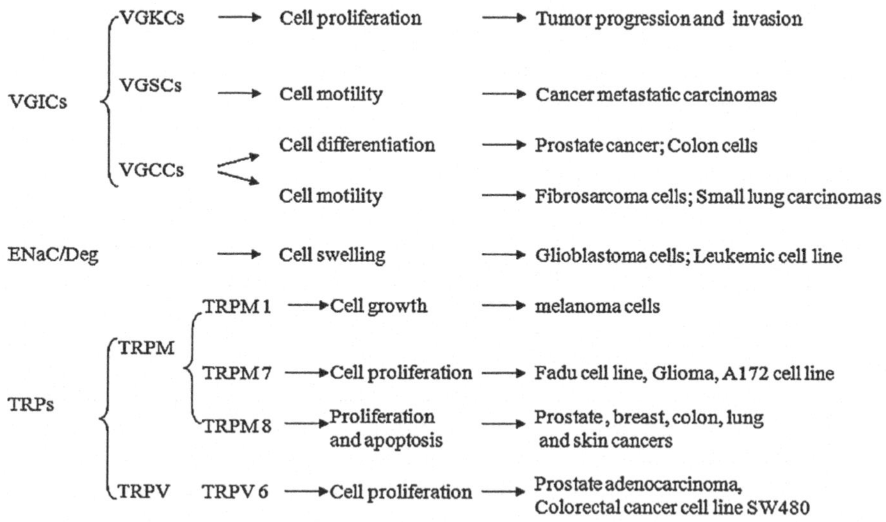

Fig. 3.2 Ion channel in the development of cancer cells

through calcium-mediated amplification and membrane depolarization. Based on sequence homology, mammalian TRP channels are classified into seven subfamilies: TRPA, TRPC, TRPM, TRPML, TRPN, TRPP, and TRPV, as shown in Fig. 3.2 [34]. Given the critical role of calcium in regulating cell cycle progression and proliferation [35], TRP channels are integral to numerous physiological functions and are increasingly recognized for their involvement in pathological conditions, including tumorigenesis and metastasis.

3.2 *Intracellular and Mitochondrial Channels*

The mitochondria are involved in a variety of vital cellular processes, such as apoptosis, ATP and ROS synthesis, and Ca^{2+} homeostasis. Dysfunction of this organelle has been linked to a number of illnesses, including cancer, where the role of numerous ion channels and transporters has been investigated [36, 37].

3.2.1 Mitochondrial Calcium Uniporter (MCU)

Elevated mitochondrial Ca^{2+} levels activate the mitochondrial calcium uniporter (MCU), which can trigger apoptosis and is also implicated in cancer cell proliferation, invasion, and redox signaling [38, 39]. In triple-negative breast cancer cells, silencing MCU reduces mitochondrial ROS production and HIF1-α expression, leading to decreased cell motility [40]. Overexpression of MCU has been associated with increased lymph node migration, larger breast tumors, and poorer prognosis [41] Additionally, the regulator protein MCUR1 promotes hepatocellular carcinoma progression and metastasis [42]. Certain drugs, such as minocycline and doxycycline, exhibit anticancer effects potentially through MCU inhibition [43]. The thiourea derivative KB-R7943 has been demonstrated to inhibit MCU activity and lower Ca^{2+} release in HeLa cells,cells of cervical cancer [44].

3.2.2 Voltage-Dependent Anion Channels

The voltage-dependent anion channel (VDAC), found in the outer membrane of the mitochondria, mediates the transfer of ions (K^+, Na^+, Ca^{2+}), ATP, ADP, Pi, and metabolites according to its conformational condition [45]. It interacts with Bcl-2 family proteins and hexokinase to regulate apoptosis and also with IP3 receptors to mediate Ca^{2+} transfer from the endoplasmic reticulum [37, 46]. VDACs are frequently overexpressed in various cancers, where their dysregulation supports abnormal cell proliferation [47]. The binding of hexokinase to VDAC promotes glycolysis, a key metabolic pathway in cancer cells, and its inhibition by methyl jasmonate (MJ), which disrupts this interaction, shows promising anticancer potential, with research into MJ analogs ongoing [48]. Additionally, the compound erastin induces VDAC opening, mitochondrial dysfunction, ROS generation, GSH depletion, reduced glycolysis, and ferroptosis, highlighting another mechanism by which VDAC targeting could offer therapeutic value in cancer treatment [49, 50].

4 Clinical Use of Ion Channels and Transporters in Cancer

The main way that chemotherapeutic drugs like doxorubicin work against cancer is by causing oxidative stress through the production of reactive oxygen and nitrogen species (ROS/RNS), leading to cancer cell death [51, 52]. Building on this mechanism, pro-oxidant therapies that selectively increase oxidative stress in tumors, such as enhancing local hydrogen peroxide (H_2O_2) levels, are being explored, especially in lung cancer models [52]. However, despite encouraging preclinical findings, redox-based strategies have yielded inconclusive results in clinical settings, highlighting the need for more targeted and effective approaches [53].

Ion channels and transporters have emerged as significant targets of oxidative modification due to their sensitivity to redox changes. These proteins may undergo direct oxidation by ROS/RNS, particularly via interactions with cysteine or sulfhydryl groups, or may be indirectly modulated through redox-sensitive signaling cascades that affect their expression and functional regulation [54]. Such modifications can alter ion flux across membranes, thereby influencing cancer cell survival, proliferation, and migration. For instance, oxidative stress-induced elevation in intracellular calcium levels ($[Ca^{2+}]i$) can activate calcium-dependent protein kinases and transcription factors that enhance tumor progression [55].

Furthermore, the degree and type of oxidative stress dictate calcium dynamics within cancer cells. Calcium influx can occur through plasma membrane channels or mobilization from internal storage, such as the endoplasmic reticulum, as a result of oxidative insults, resulting in Ca^{2+} overload and subsequent mitochondrial dysfunction, culminating in apoptosis or necrosis [56]. Targeting the oxidative regulation of ion channels, considering their crucial role in redox signaling and impact on the fate of cancer cells, is a promising area in the development of redox-based cancer treatments that are more effective.

5 Therapeutic Targeting Strategies

Over the past two decades, ion channels have gained recognition as critical regulators in cancer biology, far beyond their classical roles in excitable cells. Once considered incidental, ion channels are now acknowledged for their direct involvement in processes such as cell proliferation [57, 58], volume regulation [59], migration [60], and adhesion [61]. These transmembrane proteins, present in both plasma and intracellular membranes, are implicated in various cancer hallmarks, including metabolic reprogramming, apoptosis resistance, angiogenesis, and metastasis [3], leading to their designation as "oncogenic channels."

The concept of the "channelome," which refers to the cancer-specific profile of ion channel expression, has emerged as a promising avenue for designing targeted therapies. Identifying the channelome in different cancer types could enable precise interventions with fewer off-target effects than conventional chemotherapy. Functional modulation of ion channels, whether by genetic silencing or pharmacological inhibitors, has demonstrated efficacy in reducing tumor cell proliferation and migration in vitro. However, these promising results often fail to translate in vivo due to issues such as poor pharmacokinetics, limited bioavailability, and inadequate drug penetration in solid tumors.

Additionally, the tumor microenvironment, with its immunomodulatory, pro-inflammatory, and anti-apoptotic features, is essential to treatment resistance posing significant barriers to treatment success [62]. While in vitro models provide valuable insights, they often fail to replicate this complex environment. Encouragingly, several in vivo studies have shown that ion channel targeting can suppress tumor growth, supporting the therapeutic potential of these proteins. Combining ion channel modulators with existing chemotherapeutics or using multi-channel targeting strategies may further enhance treatment efficacy.

Despite these advances, challenges such as drug specificity persist. For instance, compounds like curcumin inhibit multiple channels, including KV11.1 and Orai1, making it difficult to attribute their anticancer effects to specific targets without genetic validation [63] Addressing specificity and enhancing tumor-selective drug delivery are critical next steps. Repurposed drugs such as ranolazine, clofazimine, and phenytoin show promise but require advanced delivery systems for optimal efficacy. Novel delivery platforms—including liposomes, nanoparticles, and tumor-penetrating peptides like iRGD, which target neuropilin-1 (NRP-1) receptors overexpressed in tumors—offer a promising solution to enhance drug penetration and specificity [64, 65]. These strategies may ultimately enable safer, more effective ion channel-targeted cancer therapies.

6 Drug Repurposing and Repositioning

Drug repurposing is a time-saving and affordable method for creating novel anticancer treatments, leveraging the established safety, pharmacokinetics, and pharmacodynamics of existing drugs to expedite their progression into Phase II and III clinical trials [66, 67]. Advances in in silico chemical genomics have enabled the identification of potential repositioning candidates by analyzing large-scale drug-induced transcriptional signatures [68]. This strategy is particularly promising for targeting ion channels and transporters implicated in cancer, as many approved drugs for non-oncological conditions already modulate these proteins, shown in Table 3.1. Thus, repurposing such agents offers a practical, low-cost alternative for enhancing cancer treatment options.

7 Novel and Emerging Therapies

It is thought that there are more than ten million active peptides and proteins in animal venoms, and that in many cases, even small amounts of the venom are enough to kill either preys or predators and microbial invaders. Numerous venom components, including salts, nucleotides, biogenic amines, and enzymes like phospholipase, hyaluronidase, and L-amino acid, contribute to this. Via modulating the expression or activity of ion channels, metalloproteinase, oxidase, serineprotease, peptides, mucoproteins, and proteins have antineoplastic properties [89] (Table 3.2).

1. **Animal Toxins and Natural Products**

   (a) **Targeted Nanomedicine Approaches**

   The integration of nanotechnology into medicine has given rise to nanomedicine, a field that envisions using nanorobots and nanoscale materials for the treatment of complex diseases such as cancer [98]. Several nanomaterials, such as liposomes, nanofibers, polymeric micelles, and magnetic, inorganic, or polymeric nanoparticles, have been used to increase drug selectivity and, as a result, improve chemotherapy outcomes, enabling targeted delivery, reducing systemic side effects, and allowing for controlled drug release [99, 100]. These nanocarrier systems also offer improved solubility for hydrophobic drugs, greater molecular stability, and prolonged circulation time. However, challenges remain in drug delivery, particularly in overcoming physical barriers that limit diffusion and tumor penetration [101].

Table 3.1 Repurposed drugs targeting ion channels/transporters in cancer

Drug name	Primary target(s)	Anticancer mechanism	Cancer types studied	Key outcomes	References
Astemizole	H1 receptor, Kv10.1, Kv11.1, P-gp	Inhibits proliferation, induces apoptosis, downregulates Kv10.1, synergizes with calcitriol, doxorubicin, and EGFR inhibitors	Breast, liver, lung, prostate, leukemia, cervical	Inhibits tumor growth; potentiates chemotherapies; minimal adverse effects in vivo	[69]
Terfenadine	H1 receptor, Kv11.1	Induces mitochondrial apoptosis, ERK activation, suppresses proliferation, and migration	Prostate, breast, NSCLC	Reduces tumor growth, synergistic with epirubicin; withdrawn due to QT prolongation	[70]
Loratadine	H1 receptor	Sensitizes to chemotherapy, reverses multidrug resistance	NSCLC, breast, prostate, ovarian	Reduced all-cause mortality; synergy with chemotherapy	[71, 72]
Imipramine	Kv10.1, Na^+/Ca^{2+}/K^+ channels	Blocks Kv10.1, induces apoptosis, inhibits proliferation, acts in SCLC models, and potentiates doxorubicin	Ovarian, brain, SCLC, glioma, breast, leukemia	Effective in cisplatin-resistant tumors; enhances radiotherapy and chemo response	[73]
Calcitriol	VDR, Kv10.1	Represses Kv10.1, induces differentiation/apoptosis, and modulates oncogenes	Breast, prostate, cervical, melanoma, liver, colon	Enhanced by curcumin and EGFR inhibitors, broad antineoplastic activity	[74–76]
Clarithromycin	Kv11.1, PI3K-p85, P-gp	Binds Kv11.1 in closed state, modulates PI3K/Akt, enhances 5-FU cytotoxicity	Colorectal	Triggers apoptosis, impairs autophagy, and improves chemotherapy response	[77, 78]
Fluoxetine	Kv11.1	Blocks Kv11.1, inhibits glioblastoma, with no major cardiotoxicity	Glioblastoma	Improves survival in Kv11.1+ glioblastoma; safe profile	[79]
Glibenclamide	KATP (Kir6.2/SUR1), MRP1, P-gp	Blocks KATP, inhibits ABC transporters, induces apoptosis, and reverses resistance	Lung, gastric, cervical, breast, melanoma, prostate	Decreases tumor growth, increases apoptosis, and synergizes with $CoCl_2$	[80]
Verapamil	L-type Ca^{2+} channel, Kv11.1, P-gp	Blocks Ca^{2+} and K^+ channels, reverses MDR, suppresses proliferation	Breast, prostate, neuroblastoma, leukemia, NSCLC	Enhances chemo efficacy; toxic at required P-gp modulation doses	[81, 82]
Nifedipine	L-type Ca^{2+} channels	Blocks Ca^{2+} influx, induces autophagy, and sensitizes to cisplatin	Lung, endometrial, glioblastoma	Potentiates cisplatin; limited by hypotensive effects	[83]

(continued)

Table 3.1 (continued)

Drug name	Primary target(s)	Anticancer mechanism	Cancer types studied	Key outcomes	References
Mibefradil	T-type Ca^{2+} channels, Kv10.1	Regulates Kv10.1 gating, induces apoptosis, and modulates AR expression	Glioblastoma, breast, retinoblastoma	Well tolerated in Phase I; withdrawn due to drug interactions	[84, 85]
Celecoxib	Cav channels	Blocks Cav, enhances chemo, and EGFR inhibitor efficacy	Gastric, HCC, breast, colon, prostate	Promising clinical data; regression in HCC reported	[86, 87]
Bromocriptine	Dopamine D2 receptor	Inhibits prolactin, induces apoptosis in hormone-resistant and MDR cancers	Breast, leukemia	Synergizes with paclitaxel and doxorubicin; MDR-effective	[88]

Table 3.2 Animal toxins and natural products in cancer therapy

Compound	Source	Target(s)	Anticancer mechanism	Cancer types studied	Key outcomes	References
Chlorotoxin	Deathstalker scorpion (Leiurus quinquestriatus hebraeus)	Glioma-specific Cl^- channels, MMP-2	Blocks chloride channels and MMP-2; reduces invasion and migration	Glioma, melanoma, small cell lung carcinoma, neuroblastoma, prostate, intestinal cancers, sarcoma	Inhibits tumor cell invasion; used in imaging (TM-601) and radiotherapy; FDA-approved radio conjugate (131I-TM-601)	[90, 91]
Psalmotoxin	Tarantula (*Psalmopoeus cambridgei*)	ASIC1 channels	Inhibits cation currents, induces G0/G1 arrest, upregulates p21/p27 via ERK1/2 inhibition	Astroglioma, glioblastoma multiforme	Reduces proliferation and cell cycle progression in glioma cells	[92]
Ap1a	Spider venom peptide	Kv10.1 channels	Selective Kv10.1 blocker; inhibits Kv10.1 > 30-fold vs Kv11.1	General tumor cells expressing Kv10.1	Highly selective inhibition of Kv10.1 with limited off-target effects	[93]
Soricidin	Northern short-tailed shrew (*Blarina brevicauda*)	TRPV6 channels	Modulates TRPV6; reduces proliferation, promotes apoptosis	Ovarian, breast, prostate, colon, thyroid cancers, leukemias, lymphomas	Decreases cancer cell proliferation and enhances apoptosis	[89, 94]
SOR-C13/ SOR-C27	Synthetic derivatives of Soricidin	TRPV6 channels	TRPV6 targeting for tumor localization; inhibits tumor growth in xenograft models	Ovarian, prostate, and pancreatic cancers	Tumor inhibition in vivo; stable disease in 54.5% of patients in Phase I trial	[95, 96]
Snake Venom Components	Various snake species	Ca^{2+} channels, integrins, MMPs	Increases Ca^{2+} influx, ROS, cytochrome C release; inhibits integrins, MMPs, metastasis, angiogenesis	Various solid tumors	Broad antitumor effects: apoptosis induction, anti-metastasis, anti-angiogenesis	[97]

Interestingly, full intracellular penetration of nanoparticles may not always be necessary; targeting cancer cell membrane proteins such as ion channels and transporters can significantly enhance therapeutic outcomes.

A notable example is the functionalization of polyethylene glycol (PEG)-coated iron oxide nanoparticles with chlorotoxin and the fluorescent dye Cy5.5, which enabled high-specificity targeting, strong tumor affinity, and enhanced imaging of gliomas [102]. Additionally, chlorotoxin-conjugated nanoparticles loaded with methotrexate demonstrated selective tumor accumulation, prolonged retention, and increased cytotoxicity against cancer cells [102]. Further advancing this concept, a multifunctional magnetic nano-vector was developed using chlorotoxin and siRNA to achieve efficient gene silencing and real-time monitoring through MRI. This system exhibited enhanced tumor-specific uptake, effective intracellular siRNA delivery, and increased knockdown of target genes, positioning it as a potent gene therapy strategy for aggressive cancers shown in Fig. 3.3 [103].

(b) **Ion Channel-Based Immunotherapy**

Ion channels, particularly potassium and calcium channels, are fundamental to the activation, differentiation, migration, and proliferation of immune cells such as lymphocytes [104]. Upon antigen recognition via T-cell or B-cell receptors (TCR/BCR), phospholipase Cγ1/2 (PLCγ1 in T cells, PLCγ2 in B cells) is activated, leading to inositol trisphosphate (IP3) production. IP3 triggers calcium release from the endoplasmic reticulum (ER) through IP3 receptors (IP3R). As a result of this calcium depletion, STIM1/2 is activated, which oligomerizes and interacts with ORAI channels on the plasma membrane to create functional CRAC (calcium release-activated calcium) channels that enable a continuous calcium influx. At the same time, potassium channels Kv1.3 and KCa3.1 are activated to keep the membrane potential necessary for the ongoing influx of Ca^{2+}. This cascade ultimately activates the calcineurin-NFAT pathway, enhancing the transcription of genes involved in proliferation, cytokine production, and cytotoxic responses B [104].

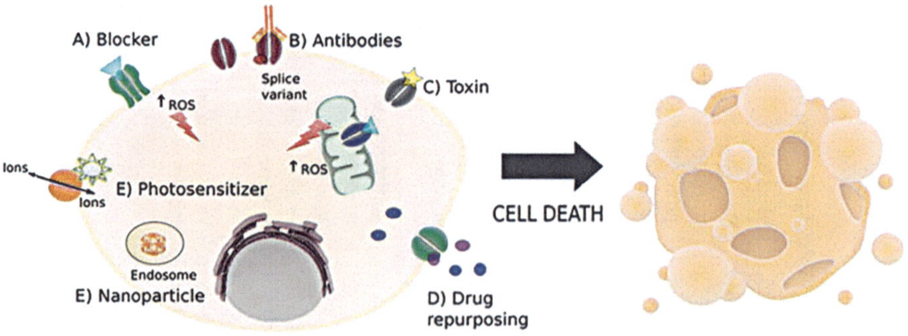

Fig. 3.3 Novel therapeutic targeting ion channels or transporter in cancer

The inhibition of Kv1.3 and KCa3.1 channels is a promising immunosuppressive strategy for treating autoimmune diseases, chronic inflammation, and hematological malignancies B [105]. Kv1.3 is also found in the inner mitochondrial membrane (IMM), where it interacts with pro-apoptotic protein Bax to modulate apoptosis via ROS elevation and cytochrome C release [106]. Mitochondrial Kv1.3 inhibitors like PCARBTP and PAPTP selectively induce apoptosis in cancer cells, particularly in chemo-resistant melanoma and pancreatic adenocarcinoma, by exploiting their overexpression of mitoKv1.3 and altered redox balance, while sparing healthy tissues [107]. In chronic lymphocytic leukemia (CLL), B cells exhibit elevated Kv1.3 expression and a disrupted redox environment. Clofazimine, by targeting mitochondrial Kv1.3, induces ROS-dependent apoptosis in B-CLL cells. This effect is abrogated in healthy cells or when antioxidant enzymes are co-administered, indicating the reliance on both channel inhibition and oxidative stress [108].

Kv1.3 also plays a role in other hematologic malignancies. In Daudi B cells, which overexpress incompletely inactivating Kv1.3 channels, the monoclonal anti-CD20 antibody rituximab promotes channel downregulation via FcγRIIB activation, contributing to apoptosis [109]. Similarly, blocking Kv1.3 in Sézary syndrome-derived malignant T cells inhibits cell proliferation and activation [110]. KCa3.1 is also widely expressed in various cancers and supports tumor cell proliferation, metastasis, and therapy resistance [111]. Inhibitors like TRAM-34 and clotrimazole reduce Ki67 expression and viability in CLL cells [112]. Interestingly, in natural killer (NK) cells, TRAM-34 enhances proliferation and degranulation in response to leukemia cells. In a mouse model bearing K562 tumors, treatment with TRAM-34 and NK cells led to reduced tumor growth, suggesting immunostimulatory effects of KCa3.1 inhibition in NK cells [113].

Ion channel regulation is also influenced by the tumor microenvironment. KCa3.1 channels were shown to mediate glioblastoma cell invasion following radiation, and their inhibition via TRAM-34 abolished this invasive behavior [114]. Moreover, hypoxic tumors accumulate high levels of extracellular adenosine (ADO), produced by ATP breakdown via CD39/CD75 enzymes. ADO suppresses effector T-cell function, promoting immune evasion and tumor progression [115]. Specifically, ADO impairs KCa3.1 function in T cells via A2A receptor signaling, reducing cytokine secretion and migration [116]. In $CD8^+$ T cells from head and neck squamous cell carcinoma (HNSCC) patients, ADO inhibits chemotaxis by suppressing KCa3.1 activity. This dysfunction is reversible using 1-EBIO, a KCa3.1 activator, which restores T-cell migration even in ADO-rich conditions, highlighting a potential immunotherapeutic strategy to overcome tumor-induced immune suppression [117].

8 Combinatorial and Personalized Approaches: Synergistic Use with Chemo, Radiation, and Immunotherapies

The modulation of ion channels in cancer cells has a great therapeutic promise, especially when used in conjunction with conventional treatments like chemotherapy and radiotherapy. Ion channel inhibitors can block crucial tumor cell functions like proliferation, migration, and invasion, while others induce apoptosis. These properties make them promising candidates for combination regimens. For instance, in triple-negative breast cancer, co-localization of β-adrenergic receptors and Nav1.5 channels has enabled the successful use of propranolol (a β-blocker) and ranolazine (a VGSC inhibitor) to reduce Na^+ currents, migration, and invasion both individually and synergistically [118]. Similarly, inhibition of Kv10.1 by astemizole sensitized glioblastoma cells to temozolomide [119], and combined treatment with astemizole and gefitinib enhanced apoptosis in lung cancer cells [69]. Macrolide antibiotics also demonstrated antileukemic activity through Kv11.1 inhibition [120], and riluzole was shown to modulate both Kv11.1 and KCa3.1 channels, facilitating cisplatin uptake in colon cancer [121].

Ion channels also modulate tumor response to radiotherapy. TRPM8 inhibition radiosensitized glioblastoma cells by impairing DNA repair mechanisms [122], while TRPM2 inhibition enhanced radiotherapy-induced death in leukemia cells [113] Furthermore, retrospective studies have suggested that breast cancer patients with brain metastases who receive antiepileptic drugs, many of which inhibit VGSCs, experience improved survival following whole-brain radiotherapy [123]. These findings highlight the potential of ion channel modulation to boost radiotherapeutic efficacy.

In the realm of immunotherapy, ionic balance in the tumor microenvironment (TME) influences immune cell function and treatment outcomes. For example, low serum sodium levels in non-small cell lung cancer patients are associated with poor responses to immune checkpoint inhibitors [124]. Elevated extracellular K^+, a byproduct of tumor necrosis, suppresses effector T-cell function by increasing intracellular K^+ levels. This immunosuppression can be reversed by upregulating Kv1.3, promoting K^+ efflux, and restoring T-cell activity [125]. Notably, high K^+ levels maintain T cells in a stem-like, proliferative state that enhances their tumor-killing potential [126] underscoring how K^+ flux manipulation could improve immunotherapy efficacy.

Immune cell infiltration is essential for tumor recognition and elimination. $CD4^+$ and $CD8^+$ T cells engage tumor cells via MHC class I, releasing cytokines and cytotoxic granules to induce cell death [127]. Yet, tumors develop mechanisms to evade this immune surveillance, such as suppressing antigen presentation and producing immunosuppressive cytokines [128]. To counter this, several immunotherapeutic strategies have been developed, including immune checkpoint inhibitors, monoclonal antibodies, cancer vaccines, and adoptive cell transfer (ACT) therapies [129]. ACT therapies—using tumor-infiltrating lymphocytes (TILs), T-cell receptors

(TCRs), or chimeric antigen receptors (CARs) offer additional opportunities to target ion channels and transporters overexpressed in cancer [130].

Ion channel splice variants have emerged as specific targets for immunotherapy due to their restricted expression in tumors. The KCa1.1 (KCNMA1) potassium channel, implicated in glioma, breast, prostate, and cervical cancers, expresses multiple splice variants [131–133]. Aberrant splicing in cancer generates functionally distinct channel isoforms, some of which, like the glioma-specific gBK variant, lack conductance and act as dominant-negative subunits [134]. gBK contains epitopes (gBK1 and gBK2) that bind HLA-A*0201 on dendritic cells, triggering cytotoxic T lymphocyte (CTL) responses and tumor cell lysis in glioma, lung, breast, and gastric cancers [135]. These results indicate that splice variants can be targeted selectively, minimizing damage to healthy tissues.

Antibody-based therapies targeting ion channels represent another innovative strategy. Antibodies have been developed against Kv10.1, Kv11.1, nfP2X7, α2δ1 (a calcium channel subunit), and MRP1 [136]. Kv10.1, overexpressed in ~70% of human cancers, was targeted using an scFv62 antibody fused to TRAIL. This construct sensitized Kv10.1-expressing breast and prostate cancer cells to apoptosis and chemotherapeutics such as paclitaxel and doxorubicin [137, 138]. Similarly, Kv11.1-targeting monoclonal antibodies conjugated to TiO_2 nanoparticles showed potential for therapeutic use although their cytotoxic effect may require enhancement via ROS induction [139]. Moreover, nfP2X7—a non-functional splice variant of the ATP-gated calcium channel P2X7—has been targeted in a Phase I clinical trial for basal cell carcinoma, resulting in reduced lesion size [140]. These findings demonstrate the emerging potential of ion channels and their splice variants as highly specific targets for cancer immunotherapy. Further clinical studies are needed to confirm their therapeutic efficacy and safety across cancer types.

9 Challenges and Future Directions

Combining ion channel inhibitors with conventional cancer therapies is emerging as a promising approach to enhance treatment precision and overcome resistance. Mapping the "channelome," or the unique profile of ion channel expression in a specific cancer type, may allow for more effective, personalized therapies that integrate ion channel modulators with chemotherapy or targeted agents. Several medications that target ion channels induce apoptosis or inhibit tumor cell activity like proliferation, migration, and invasion. However, specificity remains a major challenge. For example, curcumin has broad anticancer activity and inhibits multiple ion channels, including KV11.1 (hERG1) and Orai1 (ICRAC), making it critical to determine whether its effects are directly due to ion channel modulation or through alternative mechanisms [63].

A key concern with ion channel-targeting drugs is the potential for off-target toxicity, as many channels involved in tumor progression are also expressed in normal tissues. Despite this, the repurposing of approved drugs, such as ranolazine, clofazimine, astemizole, phenytoin, and mibefradil, offers a more economical and accelerated path to clinical application, especially since several are already in Phase II trials [81]. Advanced drug delivery systems, such as liposomes, oligonucleotides, nanoparticles conjugated to tumors, and pro-apoptotic peptides, have been created in order to solve safety issues and improve therapeutic selectivity.tLyp-1, iNGR, and iRGD are examples of penetrating peptides. These peptides target targeted drug delivery and deep tissue penetration by binding to neuropilin-1 (NRP 1), a receptor that is overexpressed in tumors [64, 65].

Another frontier in this area is the use of synthetic ion transporters, which aim to disrupt the ionic balance and pH gradients in cancer cells, thereby inducing apoptosis or oxidative stress. However, these synthetic molecules face challenges in selectivity, structural stability, and safe systemic application. Most current systems are lipophilic and nonspecific, limiting their therapeutic index. Future efforts must focus on designing transporters that act exclusively on malignant tissues while sparing healthy cells [74]. When combined with chemotherapy, radiotherapy, or immunotherapy, synthetic transporters could further potentiate therapeutic outcomes by enhancing intracellular drug accumulation and promoting stress-induced cancer cell death [141].

Despite these innovations, achieving tumor specificity remains a significant barrier due to the widespread expression of ion channels in normal tissues, which can lead to systemic side effects or toxicity [142]. One promising solution lies in the engineering of antibodies or small molecules that selectively target tumor-specific ion channel isoforms or cancer-specific splice variants. These approaches are under investigation for various channels such as Kv10.1, Kv11.1, and P2X7, among others [139, 140]. Although promising, these strategies face limitations such as tumor heterogeneity, antigen variability, and manufacturing challenges. Nonetheless, tumor-restricted channel targeting holds the potential for highly specific and safer treatments.

A deeper understanding of ion channel biology in the tumor context is needed to realize the potential of ion channel-targeted therapies in oncology. This includes elucidating the roles, expression dynamics, functional isoforms, and pharmacological properties of these channels in different tumor types. Integrating this knowledge with personalized medicine strategies could allow for the development of combinatorial regimens that inhibit tumor growth and modulate the immune system by enhancing T-cell function and tumor infiltration. Ultimately, ion channel modulation represents a versatile and powerful platform for advancing both conventional and next-generation cancer therapies [104].

10 Conclusion

Integrating modulators of ionic mechanisms (MIMs), particularly ion channel and transporter-targeting agents, with conventional cancer therapies offers a promising strategy to enhance treatment outcomes, reduce side effects, and even repurpose existing drugs with anticancer potential. These modulators can act directly against cancer cells, support immune responses, and regulate oxidative stress pathways, making combination therapies more effective and versatile. Although preclinical studies have demonstrated encouraging results, further in vivo research and clinical trials are essential to fully understand the specific ion channels involved and to optimize dosing and treatment schedules. Advances in nanotechnology and targeted delivery systems, such as tumor-penetrating peptides, also hold potential to overcome drug resistance and improve precision in targeting tumors. Despite being historically overlooked in oncology, ion channels are now recognized as important players in cancer progression, influencing processes like proliferation, apoptosis, migration, and metastasis. As scientific understanding deepens and more cancer-specific "channelomes" are identified, these proteins could become central to developing personalized, less toxic, and more effective cancer therapies.

References

1. Helvie MA (2019) Perspectives on the overdiagnosis of breast cancer associated with mammographic screening. J Breast Imaging 1(4). https://doi.org/10.1093/jbi/wbz059
2. Ryser MD, Lange J, Inoue LYT, O'Meara ES, Gard C, Miglioretti DL, Bulliard JL, Brouwer AF, Hwang ES, Etzioni RB (2022) Estimation of breast cancer overdiagnosis in a U.S. breast screening cohort. Ann Intern Med 175(4). https://doi.org/10.7326/M21-3577
3. Djamgoz MBA, Coombes RC, Schwab A (2014) Ion transport and cancer: from initiation to metastasis. Philos Trans R Soc B Biol Sci 369(1638):20130092. https://doi.org/10.1098/rstb.2013.0092
4. Prevarskaya N, Skryma R, Shuba Y (2018) Ion channels in cancer: are cancer hallmarks oncochannelopathies? Physiol Rev 98(2). https://doi.org/10.1152/physrev.00044.2016
5. Zhang X, Lin Y, Gillies RJ (2010) Tumor pH and its measurement. J Nucl Med 51(8). https://doi.org/10.2967/jnumed.109.068981
6. Thews O, Riemann A (2019) Tumor pH and metastasis: a malignant process beyond hypoxia. Cancer Metastasis Rev 38(1–2). https://doi.org/10.1007/s10555-018-09777-y
7. Jung E, Alfonso J, Monyer H, Wick W, Winkler F (2020) Neuronal signatures in cancer. Int J Cancer 147(12). https://doi.org/10.1002/ijc.33138
8. Monje M, Borniger JC, D'Silva NJ, Deneen B, Dirks PB, Fattahi F, Frenette PS, Garzia L, Gutmann DH, Hanahan D, Hervey-Jumper SL, Hondermarck H, Hurov JB, Kepecs A, Knox SM, Lloyd AC, Magnon C, Saloman JL, Segal RA et al (2020) Roadmap for the emerging field of cancer neuroscience. Cell 181(2):219–222
9. Alvear-Arias JJ, Carrillo C, Villar JP, Garcia-Betancourt R, Peña-Pichicoi A, Fernandez A et al (2022) Expression of Hv1 proton channels in myeloid-derived suppressor cells (MDSC) and its potential role in T cell regulation. Proc Natl Acad Sci 119:e2104453119. https://doi.org/10.1073/pnas.2104453119
10. Park SH, Park SH, Howe ENW, Hyun JY, Chen LJ, Hwang I, Vargas-Zuñiga G, Busschaert N, Gale PA, Sessler JL, Shin I (2019) Determinants of ion-transporter cancer cell death. Chem 5(8). https://doi.org/10.1016/j.chempr.2019.05.001
11. Rodilla AM, Korrodi-Gregório L, Hernando E, Manuel-Manresa P, Quesada R, Pérez-Tomás R, Soto-Cerrato V (2017) Synthetic tambjamine analogues induce mitochondrial swelling and lysosomal dysfunction, leading to autophagy blockade and necrotic cell death in lung cancer. Biochem Pharmacol 126. https://doi.org/10.1016/j.bcp.2016.11.022

12. Li H, Valkenier H, Thorne AG, Dias CM, Cooper JA, Kieffer M, Busschaert N, Gale PA, Sheppard DN, Davis AP (2019) Anion carriers as potential treatments for cystic fibrosis: transport in cystic fibrosis cells, and additivity to channel-targeting drugs. Chem Sci 10(42). https://doi.org/10.1039/c9sc04242c
13. Fiske JL, Fomin VP, Brown ML, Duncan RL, Sikes RA (2006) Voltage-sensitive ion channels and cancer. Cancer Metast Rev 25(3). https://doi.org/10.1007/s10555-006-9017-z
14. Lehmann-Horn F, Jurkat-Rott K (1999) Voltage-gated ion channels and hereditary disease. Physiol Rev 79(4). https://doi.org/10.1152/physrev.1999.79.4.1317
15. Wang XT, Nagaba Y, Cross HS, Wrba F, Zhang L, Guggino SE (2000) The mRNA of L-type calcium channel elevated in colon cancer: protein distribution in normal and cancerous colon. Am J Pathol 157(5). https://doi.org/10.1016/S0002-9440(10)64792-X
16. Oguro-Okano M, Griesmann GE, Wieben ED, Slaymaker SJ, Snutch TP, Lennon VA (1992) Molecular diversity of neuronal-type calcium channels identified in small cell lung carcinoma. Mayo Clin Proc 67(12). https://doi.org/10.1016/S0025-6196(12)61144-6
17. Huang JB, Kindzelskii AL, Clark AJ, Petty HR (2004) Identification of channels promoting calcium spikes and waves in HT1080 tumor cells: their apparent roles in cell motility and invasion. Cancer Res 64(7). https://doi.org/10.1158/0008-5472.CAN-03-3501
18. Isom LL (2001) Sodium channel β subunits: anything but auxiliary. Neuroscientist 7(1). https://doi.org/10.1177/107385840100700108
19. Diss JKJ, Fraser SP, Djamgoz MBA (2004) Voltage-gated Na^+ channels: multiplicity of expression, plasticity, functional implications, and pathophysiological aspects. Eur Biophys J 33(3). https://doi.org/10.1007/s00249-004-0389-0
20. Smith P, Rhodes NP, Shortland AP, Fraser SP, Djamgoz MBA, Ke Y, Foster CS (1998) Sodium channel protein expression enhances the invasiveness of rat and human prostate cancer cells. FEBS Lett 423(1). https://doi.org/10.1016/S0014-5793(98)00050-7
21. Brackenbury WJ, Djamgoz MBA (2006) Activity-dependent regulation of voltage-gated Na^+ channel expression in Mat-LyLu rat prostate cancer cell line. J Physiol 573(2). https://doi.org/10.1113/jphysiol.2006.106906
22. Fraser SP, Diss JKJ, Chioni AM, Mycielska ME, Pan H, Yamaci RF, Pani F, Siwy Z, Krasowska M, Grzywna Z, Brackenbury WJ, Theodorou D, Koyutürk M, Kaya H, Battaloglu E, De Bella MT, Slade MJ, Tolhurst R, Palmieri C et al (2005) Voltage-gated sodium channel expression and potentiation of human breast cancer metastasis. Clin Cancer Res 11(15). https://doi.org/10.1158/1078-0432.CCR-05-0327
23. Roger S, Rollin J, Barascu A, Besson P, Raynal PI, Iochmann S, Lei M, Bougnoux P, Gruel Y, Le Guennec JY (2007) Voltage-gated sodium channels potentiate the invasive capacities of human non-small-cell lung cancer cell lines. Int J Biochem Cell Biol 39(4). https://doi.org/10.1016/j.biocel.2006.12.007
24. Diaz D, Delgadillo DM, Hernández-Gallegos E, Ramírez-Domínguez ME, Hinojosa LM, Ortiz CS, Berumen J, Camacho J, Gomora JC (2007) Functional expression of voltage-gated sodium channels in primary cultures of human cervical cancer. J Cell Physiol 210(2). https://doi.org/10.1002/jcp.20871
25. Allen DH, Lepple-Wienhues A, Cahalan MD (1997) Ion channel phenotype of melanoma cell lines. J Membr Biol 155(1). https://doi.org/10.1007/s002329900155
26. Villalonga N, Ferrere J, Argiles J, Condom E, Felipe A (2008) Potassium channels are a new target field in anticancer drug design. Recent Pat Anti-Cancer Drug Discov 2(3). https://doi.org/10.2174/157489207782497181
27. Pardo LA, Stühmer W (2008) Eag1: an emerging oncological target. Cancer Res 68(6). https://doi.org/10.1158/0008-5472.CAN-07-5710
28. Stühmer W, Alves F, Hartung F, Zientkowska M, Pardo LA (2006) Potassium channels as tumour markers. FEBS Lett 580(12). https://doi.org/10.1016/j.febslet.2006.03.062
29. Farias LMB, Ocaña DB, Díaz L, Larrea F, Avila-Chávez E, Cadena A, Hinojosa LM, Lara G, Villanueva LA, Vargas C, Hernández-Gallegos E, Camacho-Arroyo I, Dueñas-González A, Pérez-Cárdenas E, Pardo LA, Morales A, Taja-Chayeb L, Escamilla J, Sánchez-Peña C,

Camacho J (2004) Ether à go-go potassium channels as human cervical cancer markers. Cancer Res 64(19). https://doi.org/10.1158/0008-5472.CAN-04-1204
30. de Queiroz FM, Suarez-Kurtz G, Stühmer W, Pardo LA (2006) Ether à go-go potassium channel expression in soft tissue sarcoma patients. Mol Cancer 5. https://doi.org/10.1186/1476-4598-5-42
31. Downie BR, Sánchez A, Knötgen H, Contreras-Jurado C, Gymnopoulos M, Weber C, Stühmer W, Pardo LA (2008) Eag1 expression interferes with hypoxia homeostasis and induces angiogenesis in tumors. J Biol Chem 283(52). https://doi.org/10.1074/jbc.M801830200
32. Ouadid-Ahidouch H, Ahidouch A (2008) K^+ channel expression in human breast cancer cells: involvement in cell cycle regulation and carcinogenesis. J Membr Biol 221(1). https://doi.org/10.1007/s00232-007-9080-6
33. Ransom CB, Liu X, Sontheimer H (2002) BK channels in human glioma cells have enhanced calcium sensitivity. Glia 38(4). https://doi.org/10.1002/glia.10064
34. Clapham DE (2003) TRP channels as cellular sensors. Nature 426(6966). https://doi.org/10.1038/nature02196
35. Means AR (1994) Calcium, calmodulin and cell cycle regulation. FEBS Lett 347(1). https://doi.org/10.1016/0014-5793(94)00492-7
36. Bachmann M, Costa R, Peruzzo R, Prosdocimi E, Checchetto V, Leanza L (2018) Targeting mitochondrial ion channels to fight cancer. Int J Mol Sci 19(7). https://doi.org/10.3390/ijms19072060
37. Leanza L, Checchetto V, Biasutto L, Rossa A, Costa R, Bachmann M, Zoratti M, Szabo I (2019) Pharmacological modulation of mitochondrial ion channels. Br J Pharmacol 176(22). https://doi.org/10.1111/bph.14544
38. Mammucari C, Gherardi G, Rizzuto R (2017) Structure, activity regulation, and role of the mitochondrial calcium uniporter in health and disease. Front Oncol 7. https://doi.org/10.3389/fonc.2017.00139
39. Vultur A, Gibhardt CS, Stanisz H, Bogeski I (2018) The role of the mitochondrial calcium uniporter (MCU) complex in cancer. Pflugers Archiv Eur J Physiol 470(8). https://doi.org/10.1007/s00424-018-2162-8
40. Tosatto A, Sommaggio R, Kummerow C, Bentham RB, Blacker TS, Berecz T, Duchen MR, Rosato A, Bogeski I, Szabadkai G, Rizzuto R, Mammucari C (2016) The mitochondrial calcium uniporter regulates breast cancer progression via HIF-1α. EMBO Mol Med 8(5). https://doi.org/10.15252/emmm.201606255
41. Yu C, Wang Y, Peng J, Shen Q, Chen M, Tang W, Li X, Cai C, Wang B, Cai S, Meng X, Zou F (2017) Mitochondrial calcium uniporter as a target of microRNA-340 and promoter of metastasis via enhancing the Warburg effect. Oncotarget 8(48). https://doi.org/10.18632/oncotarget.19747
42. Jin M, Wang J, Ji X, Cao H, Zhu J, Chen Y, Yang J, Zhao Z, Ren T, Xing J (2019) MCUR1 facilitates epithelial-mesenchymal transition and metastasis via the mitochondrial calcium-dependent ROS/Nrf2/Notch pathway in hepatocellular carcinoma. J Exp Clin Cancer Res 38(1). https://doi.org/10.1186/s13046-019-1135-x
43. Cui C, Yang J, Fu L, Wang M, Wang X (2019) Progress in understanding mitochondrial calcium uniporter complex-mediated calcium signalling: a potential target for cancer treatment. Br J Pharmacol 176(9). https://doi.org/10.1111/bph.14632
44. Santo-Domingo J, Vay L, Hernández-Sanmiguel E, Lobatón CD, Moreno A, Montero M, Alvarez J (2007) The plasma membrane Na^+/Ca^{2+} exchange inhibitor KB-R7943 is also a potent inhibitor of the mitochondrial Ca^{2+} uniporter. Br J Pharmacol 151(5):647–654. https://doi.org/10.1038/sj.bjp.0707260. Epub 2007 Apr 30
45. Camara AKS, Zhou YF, Wen PC, Tajkhorshid E, Kwok WM (2017) Mitochondrial VDAC1: a key gatekeeper as a potential therapeutic target. Front Physiol 8. https://doi.org/10.3389/fphys.2017.00460
46. Sharma A, Smith HJ, Yao P, Mair WB (2019) Causal roles of mitochondrial dynamics in longevity and healthy aging. EMBO Rep 20(12). https://doi.org/10.15252/embr.201948395

47. Shoshan-Barmatz V, Ben-Hail D (2012) VDAC, a multi-functional mitochondrial protein, is a pharmacological target. Mitochondrion 12(1). https://doi.org/10.1016/j.mito.2011.04.001
48. Sucu BO, Ipek OS, Kurtulus SO, Yazici BE, Karakas N, Guzel M (2019) Synthesis of novel methyl jasmonate derivatives and evaluation of their biological activity in various cancer cell lines. Bioorg Chem 91. https://doi.org/10.1016/j.bioorg.2019.103146
49. Dixon SJ, Lemberg KM, Lamprecht MR, Skouta R, Zaitsev EM, Gleason CE, Patel DN, Bauer AJ, Cantley AM, Yang WS, Morrison B, Stockwell BR (2012) Ferroptosis: an iron-dependent form of nonapoptotic cell death. Cell 149(5). https://doi.org/10.1016/j.cell.2012.03.042
50. Maldonado EN, Sheldon KL, Dehart DN, Patnaik J, Manevich Y, Townsend DM, Bezrukov SM, Rostovtseva TK, Lemasters JJ (2013) Voltage-dependent anion channels modulate mitochondrial metabolism in cancer cells: regulation by free tubulin and erastin. J Biol Chem 288(17). https://doi.org/10.1074/jbc.M112.433847
51. Noh J, Kwon B, Han E, Park M, Yang W, Cho W, Yoo W, Khang G, Lee D (2015) Amplification of oxidative stress by a dual stimuli-responsive hybrid drug enhances cancer cell death. Nat Commun 6. https://doi.org/10.1038/ncomms7907
52. Vilema-Enríquez G, Arroyo A, Grijalva M, Amador-Zafra RI, Camacho J (2016) Molecular and cellular effects of hydrogen peroxide on human lung cancer cells: potential therapeutic implications. Oxid Med Cell Longevity 2016. https://doi.org/10.1155/2016/1908164
53. Tong SY, Davis JS, Eichenberger E, Holland TL, Fowler VG Jr (2015) Staphylococcus aureus infections: epidemiology, pathophysiology, clinical manifestations, and management. Clin Microbiol Rev 28(3):603–661. https://doi.org/10.1128/CMR.00134-14
54. Ramírez A, Vázquez-Sánchez AY, Carrión-Robalino N, Camacho J (2016) Ion channels and oxidative stress as a potential link for the diagnosis or treatment of liver diseases. Oxid Med Cell Longevity. https://doi.org/10.1155/2016/3928714
55. Roderick HL, Cook SJ (2008) Ca^{2+} signalling checkpoints in cancer: remodelling Ca^{2+} for cancer cell proliferation and survival. Nat Rev Cancer 8(5). https://doi.org/10.1038/nrc2374
56. Ermak G, Davies KJA (2002) Calcium and oxidative stress: from cell signaling to cell death. Mol Immunol 38(10). https://doi.org/10.1016/S0161-5890(01)00108-0
57. Rao VR, Perez-Neut M, Kaja S, Gentile S (2015) Voltage-gated ion channels in cancer cell proliferation. Cancers 7(2). https://doi.org/10.3390/cancers7020813
58. Kondratskyi A, Kondratska K, Skryma R, Prevarskaya N (2015) Ion channels in the regulation of apoptosis. Biochim Biophy Acta Biomembr 1848(10). https://doi.org/10.1016/j.bbamem.2014.10.030
59. Lang F, Ritter M, Vöikl G, Häussinger D (1993) The biological significance of cell volume. Kidney Blood Press Res 16(1–2). https://doi.org/10.1159/000173751
60. Schwab A, Fabian A, Hanley PJ, Stock C (2012) Role of ion channels and transporters in cell migration. Physiol Rev 92(4). https://doi.org/10.1152/physrev.00018.2011
61. Litan A, Langhans SA (2015) Cancer as a channelopathy: ion channels and pumps in tumor development and progression. Front Cell Neurosci 9. https://doi.org/10.3389/fncel.2015.00086
62. Burger JA, Gribben JG (2014) The microenvironment in chronic lymphocytic leukemia (CLL) and other B cell malignancies: insight into disease biology and new targeted therapies. Semin Cancer Biol 24. https://doi.org/10.1016/j.semcancer.2013.08.011
63. Zhang X, Chen Q, Wang Y, Peng W, Cai H (2014) Effects of curcumin on ion channels and transporters. Front Physiol 5. https://doi.org/10.3389/fphys.2014.00094
64. Gautam A, Kapoor P, Chaudhary K, Kumar R, Open Source Drug Discovery Consortium, Raghava GPS (2014) Tumor homing peptides as molecular probes for cancer therapeutics, diagnostics, and theranostics. Curr Med Chem 21(21). https://doi.org/10.2174/0929867321666140217122100
65. Tietze R, Zaloga J, Unterweger H, Lyer S, Friedrich RP, Janko C, Pöttler M, Dürr S, Alexiou C (2015) Magnetic nanoparticle-based drug delivery for cancer therapy. Biochem Biophys Res Commun 468(3). https://doi.org/10.1016/j.bbrc.2015.08.022

66. Gupta SC, Sung B, Prasad S, Webb LJ, Aggarwal BB (2013) Cancer drug discovery by repurposing: teaching new tricks to old dogs. Trends Pharmacol Sci 34(9). https://doi.org/10.1016/j.tips.2013.06.005
67. Pantziarka P, Bouche G, Meheus L, Sukhatme V, Sukhatme VP (2014) The repurposing drugs in oncology (ReDO) project. Ecancermedicalscience 8(1). https://doi.org/10.3332/ecancer.2014.442
68. Lee H, Kang S, Kim W (2016) Drug repositioning for cancer therapy based on large-scale drug-induced transcriptional signatures. PLoS One 11(3). https://doi.org/10.1371/journal.pone.0150460
69. Chávez-López MG, Zúñiga-García V, Hernández-Gallegos E, Vera E, Chasiquiza-Anchatuña CA, Viteri-Yánez M, Sanchez-Ramos J, Garrido E, Camacho J (2017) The combination astemizole–gefitinib as a potential therapy for human lung cancer. Onco Targets Ther 10. https://doi.org/10.2147/OTT.S144506
70. Fernández-Nogueira P, Noguera-Castells A, Fuster G, Recalde-Percaz L, Moragas N, López-Plana A, Enreig E, Jauregui P, Carbó N, Almendro V, Gascón P, Bragado P, Mancino M (2018) Histamine receptor 1 inhibition enhances antitumor therapeutic responses through extracellular signal-regulated kinase (ERK) activation in breast cancer. Cancer Lett 424. https://doi.org/10.1016/j.canlet.2018.03.014
71. Ellegaard AM, Dehlendorff C, Vind AC, Anand A, Cederkvist L, Petersen NHT, Nylandsted J, Stenvang J, Mellemgaard A, Østerlind K, Friis S, Jäättelä M (2016) Repurposing cationic amphiphilic antihistamines for cancer treatment. EBioMedicine 9. https://doi.org/10.1016/j.ebiom.2016.06.013
72. Verdoodt F, Dehlendorff C, Jäättelä M, Strauss R, Pottegård A, Hallas J, Friis S, Kjaer SK (2020) Antihistamines and ovarian cancer survival: nationwide cohort study and in vitro cell viability assay. J Natl Cancer Inst 112(9). https://doi.org/10.1093/jnci/djz217
73. Jahchan NS, Dudley JT, Mazur PK, Flores N, Yang D, Palmerton A, Zmoos AF, Vaka D, Tran KQT, Zhou M, Krasinska K, Riess JW, Neal JW, Khatri P, Park KS, Butte AJ, Sage J (2013) A drug repositioning approach identifies tricyclic antidepressants as inhibitors of small cell lung cancer and other neuroendocrine tumors. Cancer Discov 3(12). https://doi.org/10.1158/2159-8290.CD-13-0183
74. García-Quiroz J, García-Becerra R, Santos-Martínez N, Barrera D, Ordaz-Rosado D, Avila E, Halhali A, Villanueva O, Ibarra-Sánchez MJ, Esparza-López J, Gamboa-Domínguez A, Camacho J, Larrea F, Díaz L (2014) In vivo dual targeting of the oncogenic ether-à-go-go-1 potassium channel by calcitriol and astemizole results in enhanced antineoplastic effects in breast tumors. BMC Cancer 14(1). https://doi.org/10.1186/1471-2407-14-745
75. Garciá-Quiroz J, González-Gonzalez ME, Diáz L, Ordaz-Rosado D, Segovia-Mendoza M, Prado-Garciá H, Larrea F, Becerra RG (2019) Astemizole, an inhibitor of ether-A-go-Go-1 potassium channel, increases the activity of the tyrosine kinase inhibitor gefitinib in breast cancer cells. Rev Investig Clin 71(3). https://doi.org/10.24875/RIC.18002840
76. Segovia-Mendoza M, Díaz L, Prado-Garcia H, Reginato MJ, Larrea F, García-Becerra R (2017) The addition of calcitriol or its synthetic analog EB1089 to lapatinib and neratinib treatment inhibits cell growth and promotes apoptosis in breast cancer cells. Am J Cancer Res 7(7)
77. Petroni G, Bagni G, Iorio J, Duranti C, Lottini T, Stefanini M, Kragol G, Becchetti A, Arcangeli A (2020) Clarithromycin inhibits autophagy in colorectal cancer by regulating the hERG1 potassium channel interaction with PI3K. Cell Death Dis 11(3). https://doi.org/10.1038/s41419-020-2349-8
78. Vermeer LMM, Isringhausen CD, Ogilvie BW, Buckley DB (2016) Evaluation of ketoconazole and its alternative clinical CYP3A4/5 inhibitors as inhibitors of drug transporters: the in vitro effects of ketoconazole, ritonavir, clarithromycin, and itraconazole on 13 clinically-relevant drug transporters. Drug Metab Dispos 44(3). https://doi.org/10.1124/dmd.115.067744

79. Pointer KB, Clark PA, Eliceiri KW, Salamat MS, Robertson GA, Kuo JS (2017) Administration of non-torsadogenic human Ether-à-go-go-Related Gene inhibitors is associated with better survival for high hERG-expressing glioblastoma patients. Clin Cancer Res 23(1). https://doi.org/10.1158/1078-0432.CCR-15-3169
80. Vázquez-Sánchez AY, Hinojosa LM, Parraguirre-Martínez S, González A, Morales F, Montalvo G, Vera E, Hernández-Gallegos E, Camacho J (2018) Expression of KATP channels in human cervical cancer: potential tools for diagnosis and therapy. Oncol Lett 15(5). https://doi.org/10.3892/ol.2018.8165
81. Kale VP, Amin SG, Pandey MK (2015) Targeting ion channels for cancer therapy by repurposing the approved drugs. Biochim Biophys Acta Biomembr 1848(10). https://doi.org/10.1016/j.bbamem.2015.03.034
82. Yusa K, Tsuruo T (1989) Reversal mechanism of multidrug resistance by verapamil: direct binding of verapamil to P-glycoprotein on specific sites and transport of verapamil outward across the plasma membrane of K562/ADM cells. Cancer Res 49(18)
83. Bao Xx, Xie Bs, Li Q, Li Xp, Wei Lh, Wang Jl (2012) Nifedipine induced autophagy through the beclin1 and mTOR pathway in endometrial carcinoma cells. Chin Med J 125(17). https://doi.org/10.3760/cma.j.issn.0366-6999.2012.17.028
84. Holdhoff M, Ye X, Supko JG, Nabors LB, Desai AS, Walbert T, Lesser GJ, Read WL, Lieberman FS, Lodge MA, Leal J, Fisher JD, Desideri S, Grossman SA, Wahl RL, Schiff D (2017) Timed sequential therapy of the selective T-type calcium channel blocker mibefradil and temozolomide in patients with recurrent high-grade gliomas. Neuro-Oncology 19(6). https://doi.org/10.1093/neuonc/nox020
85. Gómez-Lagunas F, Carrillo E, Pardo LA, Stühmer W (2017) Gating modulation of the tumor-related Kv10.1 channel by mibefradil. J Cell Physiol 232(8). https://doi.org/10.1002/jcp.25448
86. Guo Q, Li Q, Wang J, Liu M, Wang Y, Chen Z, Ye Y, Guan Q, Zhou Y (2019) A comprehensive evaluation of clinical efficacy and safety of celecoxib in combination with chemotherapy in metastatic or postoperative recurrent gastric cancer patients: a preliminary, three-center, clinical trial study. Medicine (United States) 98(27). https://doi.org/10.1097/MD.0000000000016234
87. Jiménez-Luévano MÁ, Rodríguez-Chávez JL, Ramírez-Flores S, Rodríguez-Villa P, Jiménez-Partida MÁ, Cervantes-Rodríguez G, Hernández-Flores G, Solís-Martínez R, Bravo-Cuellar A (2018) Treatment of hepatocarcinoma with celecoxib and pentoxifylline: a case report. Rev Med Inst Mex Seguro Soc 56(3)
88. Seo EJ, Sugimoto Y, Greten HJ, Efferth T (2018) Repurposing of bromocriptine for cancer therapy. Front Pharmacol 9. https://doi.org/10.3389/fphar.2018.01030
89. Wulff H, Christophersen P, Colussi P, Chandy KG, Yarov-Yarovoy V (2019) Antibodies and venom peptides: new modalities for ion channels. Nat Rev Drug Discov 18(5). https://doi.org/10.1038/s41573-019-0013-8
90. Dardevet L, Rani D, El Aziz TA, Bazin I, Sabatier JM, Fadl M, Brambilla E, De Waard M (2015) Chlorotoxin: a helpful natural scorpion peptide to diagnose glioma and fight tumor invasion. Toxins 7(4). https://doi.org/10.3390/toxins7041079
91. Srairi-Abid N, Othman H, Aissaoui D, BenAissa R (2019) Anti-tumoral effect of scorpion peptides: emerging new cellular targets and signaling pathways. Cell Calcium 80. https://doi.org/10.1016/j.ceca.2019.05.003
92. Wu T, Wang M, Wu W, Luo Q, Jiang L, Tao H, Deng M (2019) Spider venom peptides as potential drug candidates due to their anticancer and antinociceptive activities. J Venom Anim Toxins Incl Trop Dis 25. https://doi.org/10.1590/1678-9199-jvatitd-14-63-18
93. Ma L, Chin YKY, Dekan Z, Herzig V, Chow CY, Heighway J, Lam SW, Guillemin GJ, Alewood PF, King GF (2018) Novel venom-derived inhibitors of the human EAG channel, a putative antiepileptic drug target. Biochem Pharmacol 158. https://doi.org/10.1016/j.bcp.2018.08.038

94. Pennington MW, Czerwinski A, Norton RS (2018) Peptide therapeutics from venom: current status and potential. Bioorg Med Chem 26(10). https://doi.org/10.1016/j.bmc.2017.09.029
95. Fu S, Hirte H, Welch S, Ilenchuk TT, Lutes T, Rice C, Fields N, Nemet A, Dugourd D, Piha-Paul S, Subbiah V, Liu L, Gong J, Hong D, Stewart JM (2017) First-in-human phase I study of SOR-C13, a TRPV6 calcium channel inhibitor, in patients with advanced solid tumors. Investig New Drugs 35(3). https://doi.org/10.1007/s10637-017-0438-z
96. Xue H, Wang Y, MacCormack TJ, Lutes T, Rice C, Davey M, Dugourd D, Ilenchuk TT, Stewart JM (2018) Inhibition of Transient Receptor Potential Vanilloid 6 channel, elevated in human ovarian cancers, reduces tumour growth in a xenograft model. J Cancer 9(17). https://doi.org/10.7150/jca.20639
97. Chen N, Xu S, Zhang Y, Wang F (2018) Animal protein toxins: origins and therapeutic applications. Biophys Rep 4(5). https://doi.org/10.1007/s41048-018-0067-x
98. Freitas RA (2005) What is nanomedicine? Nanomedicine 1(1). https://doi.org/10.1016/j.nano.2004.11.003
99. Xie J, Shen Z, Anraku Y, Kataoka K, Chen X (2019) Nanomaterial-based blood-brain-barrier (BBB) crossing strategies. Biomaterials 224. https://doi.org/10.1016/j.biomaterials.2019.119491
100. Yang MY, Zhao RR, Fang YF, Jiang JL, Yuan XT, Shao JW (2019) Carrier-free nanodrug: a novel strategy of cancer diagnosis and synergistic therapy. Int J Pharm 570. https://doi.org/10.1016/j.ijpharm.2019.118663
101. Sun C, Fang C, Stephen Z, Veiseh O, Hansen S, Lee D, Ellenbogen RG, Olson J, Zhang M (2008) Tumor-targeted drug delivery and MRI contrast enhancement by chlorotoxin-conjugated iron oxide nanoparticles. Nanomedicine 3(4). https://doi.org/10.2217/17435889.3.4.495
102. Veiseh O, Kievit FM, Fang C, Mu N, Jana S, Leung MC, Mok H, Ellenbogen RG, Park JO, Zhang M (2010) Chlorotoxin-bound magnetic nanovector tailored for cancer cell targeting, imaging, and siRNA delivery. Biomaterials 31(31). https://doi.org/10.1016/j.biomaterials.2010.07.016
103. Sun C, Veiseh O, Gunn J, Fang C, Hansen S, Lee D, Sze R, Ellenbogen RG, Olson J, Zhang M (2008) In vivo MRI detection of gliomas by chlorotoxin-conjugated superparamagnetic nanoprobes. Small 4(3). https://doi.org/10.1002/smll.200700784
104. Chiang EY, Li T, Jeet S, Peng I, Zhang J, Lee WP, DeVoss J, Caplazi P, Chen J, Warming S, Hackos DH, Mukund S, Koth CM, Grogan JL (2017) Potassium channels Kv1.3 and KCa3.1 cooperatively and compensatorily regulate antigen-specific memory T cell functions. Nat Commun 8. https://doi.org/10.1038/ncomms14644
105. Lam J, Wulff H (2011) The lymphocyte potassium channels Kv1.3 and KCa3.1 as targets for immunosuppression. Drug Dev Res 72(7). https://doi.org/10.1002/ddr.20467
106. Szabó I, Bock J, Grassmé H, Soddemann M, Wilker B, Lang F, Zoratti M, Gulbins E (2008) Mitochondrial potassium channel Kv1.3 mediates Bax-induced apoptosis in lymphocytes. Proc Natl Acad Sci USA 105(39). https://doi.org/10.1073/pnas.0804236105
107. Leanza L, Romio M, Becker KA, Azzolini M, Trentin L, Managò A, Venturini E, Zaccagnino A, Mattarei A, Carraretto L, Urbani A, Kadow S, Biasutto L, Martini V, Severin F, Peruzzo R, Trimarco V, Egberts JH, Hauser C et al (2017) Direct pharmacological targeting of a mitochondrial ion channel selectively kills tumor cells in vivo. Cancer Cell 31(4). https://doi.org/10.1016/j.ccell.2017.03.003
108. Leanza L, Trentin L, Becker KA, Frezzato F, Zoratti M, Semenzato G, Gulbins E, Szabo I (2013) Clofazimine, Psora-4, and PAP-1, inhibitors of the potassium channel Kv1.3, as a new and selective therapeutic strategy in chronic lymphocytic leukemia. Leukemia 27(8). https://doi.org/10.1038/leu.2013.56
109. Wang Z (2004) Roles of K^+ channels in regulating tumour cell proliferation and apoptosis. Pflugers Archiv Eur J Physiol 448(3). https://doi.org/10.1007/s00424-004-1258-5
110. Hu T, Buus TB, Krejsgaard T, Nansen A, Lundholt BK, Spee P, Fredholm S, Petersen DL, Blümel E, Gluud M, Monteiro MN, Willerslev-Olsen A, Andersen MH, Straten PT, Met Ö, Stolearenco V, Fogh H, Gniadecki R, Nastasi C et al (2019) Expression and function

of Kv1.3 channel in malignant T cells in Sézary syndrome. Oncotarget 10(47). https://doi.org/10.18632/oncotarget.27122
111. Mohr CJ, Steudel FA, Gross D, Ruth P, Lo WY, Hoppe R, Schroth W, Brauch H, Huber SM, Lukowski R (2019) Cancer-associated intermediate conductance Ca^{2+}-activated K^+ channel KCa3.1. Cancers 11(1). https://doi.org/10.3390/cancers11010109
112. Grössinger EM, Weiss L, Zierler S, Rebhandl S, Krenn PW, Hinterseer E, Schmölzer J, Asslaber D, Hainzl S, Neureiter D, Egle A, Piñón-Hofbauer J, Hartmann TN, Greil R, Kerschbaum HH (2014) Targeting the proliferation of chronic lymphocytic leukemia (CLL) cells through KCa3.1 blockade. Leukemia 28(4). https://doi.org/10.1038/leu.2014.37
113. Koshy S, Wu D, Hu X, Tajhya RB, Huq R, Khan FS, Pennington MW, Wulff H, Yotnda P, Beeton C (2013) Blocking KCa3.1 channels increases tumor cell killing by a subpopulation of human natural killer lymphocytes. PLoS One 8(10). https://doi.org/10.1371/journal.pone.0076740
114. D'Alessandro G, Monaco L, Catacuzzeno L, Antonangeli F, Santoro A, Esposito V, Franciolini F, Wulff H, Limatola C (2019) Radiation increases functional KCa3.1 expression and invasiveness in glioblastoma. Cancer 11(3). https://doi.org/10.3390/cancers11030279
115. Allard B, Beavis PA, Darcy PK, Stagg J (2016) Immunosuppressive activities of adenosine in cancer. Curr Opin Pharmacol 29. https://doi.org/10.1016/j.coph.2016.04.001
116. Chimote AA, Hajdu P, Kucher V, Boiko N, Kuras Z, Szilagyi O, Yun Y-H, Conforti L (2013) Selective inhibition of KCa3.1 channels mediates adenosine regulation of the motility of human T cells. J Immunol 191(12). https://doi.org/10.4049/jimmunol.1300702
117. Chimote AA, Balajthy A, Arnold MJ, Newton HS, Hajdu P, Qualtieri J, Wise-Draper T, Conforti L (2018) A defect in KCa3.1 channel activity limits the ability of CD8+ T cells from cancer patients to infiltrate an adenosine-rich microenvironment. Sci Signal 11(527). https://doi.org/10.1126/scisignal.aaq1616
118. Lee JR, Lee JY, Kim HJ, Hahn MJ, Kang JS, Cho H (2019) The inhibition of chloride intracellular channel 1 enhances Ca^{2+} and reactive oxygen species signaling in A549 human lung cancer cells. Exp Mol Med 51(7). https://doi.org/10.1038/s12276-019-0279-2
119. Sales TT, Resende FFB, Chaves NL, Titze-De-Almeida SS, Báo SN, Brettas ML, Titze-De-Almeida R (2016) Suppression of the Eag1 potassium channel sensitizes glioblastoma cells to injury caused by temozolomide. Oncol Lett 12(4). https://doi.org/10.3892/ol.2016.4992
120. Pillozzi S, Masselli M, Gasparoli L, D'Amico M, Polletta L, Veltroni M, Favre C, Basso G, Becchetti A, Arcangeli A (2016) Macrolide antibiotics exert antileukemic effects by modulating the autophagic flux through inhibition of hERG1 potassium channels. Blood Cancer J 6(5). https://doi.org/10.1038/bcj.2016.32
121. Pillozzi S, D'Amico M, Bartoli G, Gasparoli L, Petroni G, Crociani O, Marzo T, Guerriero A, Messori L, Severi M, Udisti R, Wulff H, Chandy KG, Becchetti A, Arcangeli A (2018) The combined activation of KCa3.1 and inhibition of Kv11.1/hERG1 currents contribute to overcoming Cisplatin resistance in colorectal cancer cells. Br J Cancer 118(2). https://doi.org/10.1038/bjc.2017.392
122. Klumpp D, Misovic M, Szteyn K, Shumilina E, Rudner J, Huber SM (2016) Targeting TRPM2 channels impairs radiation-induced cell cycle arrest and fosters cell death of T cell leukemia cells in a Bcl-2-dependent manner. Oxidative Med Cell Longev 2016. https://doi.org/10.1155/2016/8026702
123. Reddy JP, Dawood S, Mitchell M, Debeb BG, Bloom E, Gonzalez-Angulo AM, Sulman EP, Buchholz TA, Woodward WA (2015) Antiepileptic drug use improves overall survival in breast cancer patients with brain metastases in the setting of whole brain radiotherapy. Radiother Oncol 117(2). https://doi.org/10.1016/j.radonc.2015.10.009
124. Fucà G, Galli G, Poggi M, Lo Russo G, Proto C, Imbimbo M, Vitali M, Ganzinelli M, Lanti C, Molino G, Stangoni F, Zilembo N, de Braud F, Garassino MC, Signorelli D (2018) Low baseline serum sodium concentration is associated with poor clinical outcomes in metastatic non-small cell lung cancer patients treated with immunotherapy. Target Oncol 13(6). https://doi.org/10.1007/s11523-018-0599-5

125. Eil R, Vodnala SK, Clever D, Klebanoff CA, Sukumar M, Pan JH, Palmer DC, Gros A, Yamamoto TN, Patel SJ, Guittard GC, Yu Z, Carbonaro V, Okkenhaug K, Schrump DS, Linehan WM, Roychoudhuri R, Restifo NP (2016) Ionic immune suppression within the tumour microenvironment limits T cell effector function. Nature 537(7621). https://doi.org/10.1038/nature19364
126. Vodnala SK, Eil R, Kishton RJ, Sukumar M, Yamamoto TN, Ha NH, Lee PH, Shin MH, Patel SJ, Yu Z, Palmer DC, Kruhlak MJ, Liu X, Locasale JW, Huang J, Roychoudhuri R, Finkel T, Klebanoff CA, Restifo NP (2019) T cell stemness and dysfunction in tumors are triggered by a common mechanism. Science 363(6434). https://doi.org/10.1126/science.aau0135
127. Ostroumov D, Fekete-Drimusz N, Saborowski M, Kühnel F, Woller N (2018) CD4 and CD8 T lymphocyte interplay in controlling tumor growth. Cell Mol Life Sci 75(4). https://doi.org/10.1007/s00018-017-2686-7
128. Liubomirski Y, Lerrer S, Meshel T, Rubinstein-Achiasaf L, Morein D, Wiemann S, Körner C, Ben-Baruch A (2019) Tumor-stroma-inflammation networks promote pro-metastatic chemokines and aggressive characteristics in triple-negative breast cancer. Front Immunol 10. https://doi.org/10.3389/fimmu.2019.00757
129. Khalil DN, Smith EL, Brentjens RJ, Wolchok JD (2016) The future of cancer treatment: immunomodulation, CARs and combination immunotherapy. Nat Rev Clin Oncol 13(5). https://doi.org/10.1038/nrclinonc.2016.25
130. June CH, O'Connor RS, Kawalekar OU, Ghassemi S, Milone MC (2018) CAR T cell immunotherapy for human cancer. Science 359(6382). https://doi.org/10.1126/science.aar6711
131. Bloch M, Ousingsawat J, Simon R, Schraml P, Gasser TC, Mihatsch MJ, Kunzelmann K, Bubendorf L (2007) KCNMA1 gene amplification promotes tumor cell proliferation in human prostate cancer. Oncogene 26(17). https://doi.org/10.1038/sj.onc.1210036
132. McCarty NA, O'Neil RG (1992) Calcium signaling in cell volume regulation. Physiol Rev 72(4). https://doi.org/10.1152/physrev.1992.72.4.1037
133. Khaitan D, Sankpal UT, Weksler B, Meister EA, Romero IA, Couraud PO, Ningaraj NS (2009) Role of KCNMA1 gene in breast cancer invasion and metastasis to the brain. BMC Cancer 9. https://doi.org/10.1186/1471-2407-9-258
134. Gomes FR, Romaniello V, Sánchez A, Weber C, Narayanan P, Psol M, Pardo LA (2015) Alternatively spliced isoforms of KV10.1 potassium channels modulate channel properties and can activate cyclin-dependent kinase in Xenopus oocytes. J Biol Chem 290(51). https://doi.org/10.1074/jbc.M115.668749
135. Hoa NT, Ge L, Tajhya RB, Beeton C, Cornforth AN, Abolhoda A, Lambrecht N, DaCosta-Iyer M, Ouyang Y, Mai AP, Hong E, Shon J, Hickey MJ, Erickson KL, Kruse CA, Jadus MR (2014) Small cell lung cancer cells express the late-stage gBK tumor antigen: a possible immunotarget for the terminal disease. Am J Transl Res 6(3)
136. Zhao W, Wang L, Han H, Jin K, Lin N, Guo T, Chen Y, Cheng H, Lu F, Fang W, Wang Y, Xing B, Zhang Z (2013) 1B50-1, a mAb raised against recurrent tumor cells, targets liver tumor-initiating cells by binding to the calcium channel α2δ1 subunit. Cancer Cell 23(4). https://doi.org/10.1016/j.ccr.2013.02.025
137. Hartung F, Stühmer W, Pardo LA (2011) Tumor cell-selective apoptosis induction through targeting of KV10.1 via bifunctional TRAIL antibody. Mol Cancer 10. https://doi.org/10.1186/1476-4598-10-109
138. Hartung F, Pardo LA (2016) Guiding TRAIL to cancer cells through the Kv10.1 potassium channel overcomes resistance to doxorubicin. Eur Biophys J 45(7). https://doi.org/10.1007/s00249-016-1149-7
139. Sette A, Spadavecchia J, Landoulsi J, Casale S, Haye B, Crociani O, Arcangeli A (2013) Development of novel anti-Kv 11.1 antibody-conjugated PEG-TiO_2 nanoparticles for targeting pancreatic ductal adenocarcinoma cells. J Nanopart Res 15(12). https://doi.org/10.1007/s11051-013-2111-6
140. Gilbert SM, Gidley Baird A, Glazer S, Barden JA, Glazer A, Teh LC, King J (2017) A phase I clinical trial demonstrates that nfP2X7-targeted antibodies provide a novel, safe,

and tolerable topical therapy for basal cell carcinoma. Br J Dermatol 177(1). https://doi.org/10.1111/bjd.15364
141. Lastraioli E, Perrone G, Sette A, Fiore A, Crociani O, Manoli S, D'Amico M, Masselli M, Iorio J, Callea M, Borzomati D, Nappo G, Bartolozzi F, Santini D, Bencini L, Farsi M, Boni L, Di Costanzo F, Schwab A et al (2015) HERG1 channels drive tumour malignancy and may serve as a prognostic factor in pancreatic ductal adenocarcinoma. Br J Cancer 112(6). https://doi.org/10.1038/bjc.2015.28
142. Vandenberg JI, Perry MD, Perrin MJ, Mann SA, Ke Y, Hill AP (2012) hERG K(+) channels: structure, function, and clinical significance. Physiol Rev 92(3). https://doi.org/10.1152/physrev.00036.2011

Chapter 4
Application of Nanotechnology in Cancer Diagnosis, Biomarker Discovery, and Drug Discovery

Aneesh Nair, A. Poornima Prasad, Hasna Shajahan, M. Sivasree, Dinesh Babu Somasundaram, and Sathish Kumar Yesupatham

1 Introduction

Nanotechnology has revolutionized the study of cancer by facilitating accurate, real-time detection and diagnosis with functionalized nanomaterials that improve early biomarker discovery and drug development [1]. Nano-formulations such as liposomes and dendrimers allow for targeted drug delivery to the tumor, maximizing efficacy and reducing toxicity and facilitating personalized treatment approaches [2].

1.1 Defining Cardio-Brain Oncology: Scope and Significance

Cardio-brain oncology is a new interdisciplinary area that combines cardiology, neurology, and oncology to tackle the common cardiovascular and neurological toxicities of cancer and cancer therapy (Fig. 4.1). With increasing survival for cancer, long-term toxicities to heart and brain both susceptible because of comorbid biological pathways come into focus [3]. Cardiovascular disease and neurocognitive

---

A. Nair (✉) · A. Poornima Prasad · H. Shajahan · M. Sivasree
Department of Allied Health Sciences, Noorul Islam Centre for Higher Education, Kanyakumari, Tamil Nadu, India

D. B. Somasundaram
Department of Pathology, The University of Oklahoma Health Sciences, Oklahoma City, OK, USA

S. K. Yesupatham
School of Medicine, University of Colorado, Aurora, CO, USA

S. Mallik et al. (eds.), *Landscape of Signaling Pathway and Genetic Markers in Cardio-Brain Oncology*, Studies in Rhythm Engineering,
https://doi.org/10.1007/978-981-95-7012-6_4

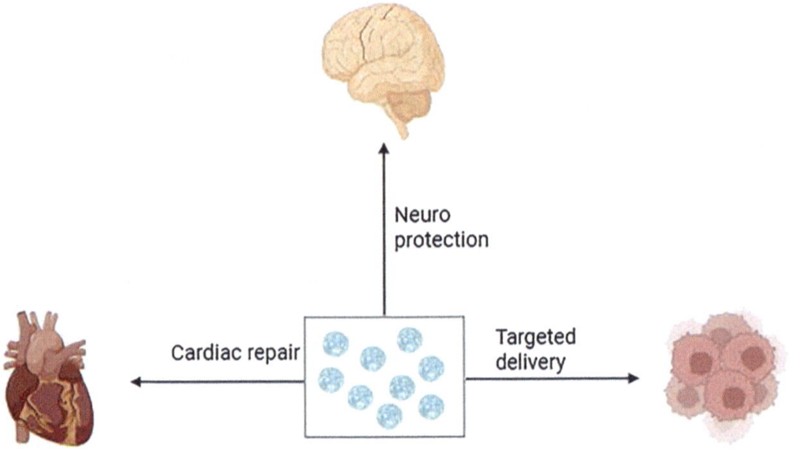

Fig. 4.1 Overview of how nanotechnology integrates into cardio-brain oncology. (The figure created with BioRender.com accessed on 27 June 2025)

impairment are emerging major non-cancer morbidities in survivors [4]. Common risk factors such as metabolic syndrome and aging require comprehensive care.

1.2 Importance of Signaling Pathways and Genetic Markers

Cardio-brain oncology is an interdiscipline that explores common pathophysiology among cancer, cardiovascular, and neurological systems. Common to these interactions are signaling pathways such as *PI3K/AKT/mTOR*, *MAPK/ERK*, *and JAK/STAT*, which fuel tumor growth yet modulate cardiac and neural function [5, 6]. For example, trastuzumab, a HER2-directed therapy, may interfere with the ErbB2/Neuregulin-1 axis, inducing both cardiomyopathy and cognitive impairment [7]. Therapies that target *VEGF*, Notch, or Wnt/β-catenin pathways can also disrupt blood-brain barrier (BBB) integrity, exposing neural tissue to injury [8]. Targeted approaches such as mTOR and MAPK inhibitors, in conjunction with protective agents such as dexrazoxane, provide dual-organ protection [9]. Nanocarriers such as liposomes, dendrimers, and cerium or selenium nanoparticles improve delivery specificity with the reduction of oxidative stress in heart and brain tissue [10–12]. Quantum dots and magnetic nanoparticles also provide the capability to monitor diagnoses and treatments in real time [13].

2 Landscape of Signaling Pathways in Cardio-Brain Oncology

Cardio-brain oncology is further influenced by heart brain signaling crosstalk in cancer more and more. Tumor-driven signaling pathways like *PI3K/AKT/mTOR and MAPK* influence tumor growth and cardiac function, whereas inflammatory mediators like IL-6 and TNF-α play a role in endothelial dysfunction and cardiac remodeling emphasizing a bidirectional connection between cardiovascular injury and neuro-oncology [14–17].

Common signaling pathways such as *AMPK, HIF-1α, NF-κB, and JAK/STAT* link brain tumor pathobiology to cardiac ischemia and therapy-induced toxicity. Cardiac remodeling is also mediated by tumor-secreted exosomes, and fibrotic pathways such as TGF-β/SMAD are engaged in both gliomas and post-infarction fibrosis enforcing a shared cardio-brain disease axis [15, 18].

2.1 Overview of Key Pathways (e.g., PI3K/AKT, MAPK, Wnt/β-Catenin)

In cardio-brain oncology, PI3K/AKT, MAPK, and Wnt/β-catenin pathways are central regulators of tumor growth, metabolic adaptation, and therapy resistance. Aberrant PI3K/AKT signaling common in glioblastoma and cardiac tumors is indicative of mTOR-mediated cell proliferation and survival, leading to malignancy as well as cardiotoxicity during treatment [19, 20] Targeting this axis with compounds such as resveratrol has the added advantage of improving tumor response while sparing cardiac tissues [21] (Fig. 4.2).

The Wnt/β-catenin pathway is essential for maintaining oncogenic stemness, inducing EMT, and facilitating resistance to therapies, with its deregulation being implicated in recurrence in brain tumors such as glioblastoma and medulloblastoma [22, 23]. At the same time, aberrant *MAPK* signaling drives both tumor growth and cardiac remodeling during chronic inflammation or ischemia [20]. Incoming research demonstrates that metabolic reprogramming in the tumor microenvironment enhances crosstalk among Wnt and MAPK pathways, supporting oncogenic progression [14]. The involvement of all these important signaling pathways in nanotechnology-based interventions is summarized in Table 4.1.

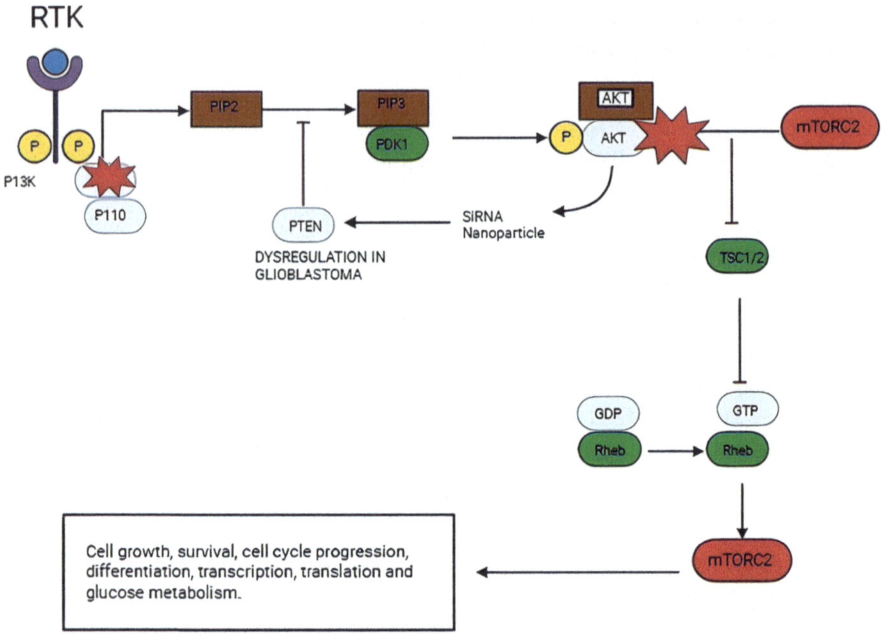

Fig. 4.2 Dysregulation and nanointervention in the PI3K/AKT signaling pathway. This figure illustrates the *PI3K/AKT/mTOR* pathway, commonly hyperactivated in glioblastoma and cardiac tumors. Activation of *RTKs* activates *PI3K* to phosphorylate PIP2 into PIP3, which phosphorylates *AKT* and activates *mTORC1*. *PTEN* loss amplifies this signal, promoting tumor growth and metabolic reprogramming. Targeted nanotherapies, including siRNA-loaded nanoparticles, seek to block *AKT* and inhibit tumor progression. (The figure created with BioRender.com accessed on 27 June 2025)

Table 4.1 Key signaling pathways involved in cardio-brain oncology, their dysregulation effects, and emerging nanotechnology-based interventions targeting these molecular networks

Pathway	Key components	Dysregulation in cardio-brain oncology	Downstream effects	Nanointervention example
PI3K/AKT	PI3K, AKT, mTOR	↑ Glioblastoma, cardiac metastasis, chemotherapy-induced cardiotoxicity	↑ Survival, angiogenesis; ↓ apoptosis	Resveratrol nanoparticles
MAPK	RAS, RAF, MEK, ERK	↑ in brain tumors, cardiac remodeling under stress	↑ Proliferation, vascular remodeling	MEK inhibitor nano-formulations
Wnt/β--catenin	Wnt, β-catenin, TCF/LEF	↑ in glioblastoma and medulloblastoma stem cells	↑ EMT, stemness, therapy resistance	β-Catenin siRNA nanocarriers
Crosstalk	PI3K–Wnt–MAPK interlinks	Enhances metabolic reprogramming, therapy resistance	Amplifies tumor growth and adaptation	Multi-target nanoplatforms (e.g., combinatorial NPs)

2.2 Pathway Dysregulation in Cardio and Brain Tumor Contexts

In glioblastoma, abnormal activation of development pathways—Notch, Hedgehog, and Wnt promotes tumor development, plasticity, and therapy resistance through the sustenance of glioma stem cells [24]. These pathways crosstalk with metabolic and inflammatory pathways to enhance immune evasion, angiogenesis, and resistance [25]. While primary cardiac tumors are uncommon, *RAS/RAF/MAPK* and *PI3K/AKT* signaling are pivotal in cardiac sarcomas and brain metastases of cardiac origin [26]. This common molecular signature underscores shared oncogenic drivers and therapeutic targets for heart and brain tumors [27]. Immune evasion and vascular remodeling are facilitated by crosstalk between *AKT* and *STAT3* in both glioblastoma and cardiac tumors [18] (Fig. 4.3).

2.3 Nanotechnology in Pathway Modulation and Monitoring

The dysregulation of developmental pathways like Notch, Hedgehog, and Wnt contributes significantly to glioblastoma through maintaining glioma stem cell self-renewal and inducing resistance and recurrence [24]. In normal conditions limited to embryonic development, these pathways get aberrantly activated in cancer through the help of transcription factors like HOX genes, promoting proliferation and invasiveness. These oncogenic loops then also cross talk with metabolic and inflammatory pathways, further amplifying the malignant phenotype [25].

In cardiac oncology, while primary tumors are uncommon, *RAS/RAF/MAPK* pathway dysregulation underlies both cardiac sarcomas and metastasis, with overlap in signaling in brain tumors [26]. Cardiac cancer metastases to the brain have *PI3K/AKT* and *MAPK* mutations identical to those found in gliomas, which suggests a common therapeutic vulnerability [27]. Glioblastoma has aberrant AKT and STAT3 signaling, too, that facilitates immune avoidance and vascular mimicry via inflammatory crosstalk [18].

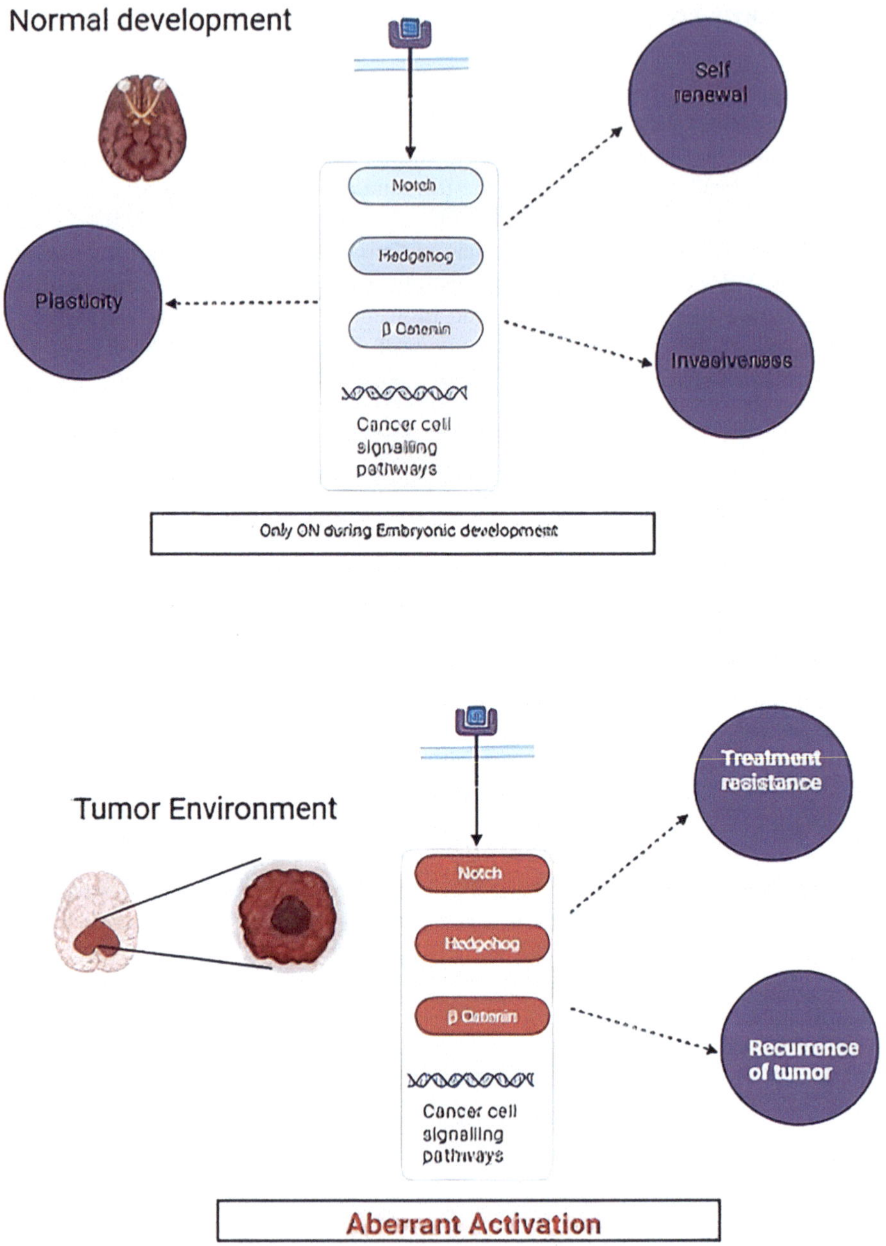

Fig. 4.3 Dysregulation of developmental pathways in glioblastoma. (The figure created with BioRender.com accessed on 27 June 2025)

3 Genetic Markers in Cardio-Brain Cancers

Genetic biomarkers play a crucial role in decoding the molecular mechanisms of cardio-brain cancers and improving initial diagnostics and customized therapies. *TP53*, *IDH1/2*, and other cell cycle gene mutations are responsible for tumor development and therapy resistance in brain cancers [28, 29], whereas inherited alleles determine susceptibility, as evident in mouse models [30]. These genetic changes also correspond to cognitive impairment in patients [31]. In cardiac tumors and drug-induced cardiotoxicity, remodeling and inflammatory markers provide prognostic information [27, 32]. Additionally, cardiovascular genetic characteristics are associated with brain aging biomarkers, highlighting the common pathophysiology of cardiac and neuronal systems [16].

3.1 Common Genetic Alterations: Mutations, Amplifications, Deletions

Genetic changes—mutations, amplifications, and deletions are pivotal in glioblastoma initiation and development. Gliomas exhibit stepwise genetic progression, with initial IDH and TP53 mutations, and 1p/19q codeletion in oligodendrogliomas, validating a hierarchical model of tumorigenesis [33]. Critical mutations target genes that control the cell cycle, apoptosis, and DNA repair [34]. EGFR amplification and PTEN deletion, both of which are prevalent in GBM, synergistically promote aggressive growth and drug resistance [18, 35].

Outside gliomas, KRAS, BRAF, and NOTCH mutations and MYC amplification and CDKN2A deletion recur in various cancers, pointing to conserved oncogenic processes [36, 37]. Sequencing has made rare variant detection possible, but complete clinical application waits upon genomic, transcriptomic, and epigenomic integration to reveal downstream consequences [18, 35].

3.2 Nanoplatforms for Genetic Marker Detection

Coupling nanotechnology with molecular diagnostics has greatly strengthened genetic marker analysis in oncology (Table 4.2). Nanomaterials such as gold nanoparticles, quantum dots, and liposomes allow for ultra-sensitive, label-free quantification of tumor-specific mutations even at the single-molecule level [38]. Such platforms traverse challenging tumor microenvironments and offer real-time biomolecular readouts, advantageously for heterogenous cancers such as glioblastoma [16].

Theranostic nanostructures have also made it possible to detect and treat oncogenic markers simultaneously, surpassing conventional diagnostics in the

Table 4.2 Role of nanotechnology in molecular diagnostics and theranostics for oncology

Nanoplatform type	Function in diagnostics	Theranostic capability	Targeted biomarkers	Advantages over traditional methods
Gold Nanoparticles	Enable label-free, multiplexed detection of nucleic acids and mutations	Can be conjugated with drugs or probes for simultaneous delivery and sensing	*EGFRvIII*, *IDH1* mutations	High-sensitivity, single-molecule resolution
Quantum Dots (QDs)	Fluorescent nanoprobes for real-time imaging and mutation-specific detection	Theranostic QDs can track therapeutic effects while delivering agents	Glioblastoma-specific oncogenes	Allow visualization in live tissue, good photostability
Liposomes	Encapsulate nucleic acid probes for protected, specific delivery to tumor sites	Co-deliver nucleic acid diagnostics and chemotherapy	DNA amplifications, mutated mRNA	Enhanced biocompatibility, efficient crossing of the tumor microenvironment
Nanosensors	Real-time biosensing of low-abundance mutations, including epigenetic changes	Can be activated by biomarker presence to trigger drug release	Methylation changes, non-coding RNA markers	Detect what traditional diagnostics may miss (e.g., epigenetic alterations)
Surface-Modified NPs	Functionalized to target specific mutations or surface markers (via antibodies or ligands)	Enable precision delivery and imaging based on real-time molecular recognition	*EGFRvIII*, mutant *IDH1*	Allow highly selective targeting, reduced off-target toxicity

identification of low-abundance mutations and epigenetic changes [39, 40]. Additionally, tunable nanocarrier surfaces enable selective targeting of important biomarkers such as *EGFRvIII* and mutant *IDH1*, paving the way toward personalized therapy approaches to treat cancer [16].

Nanoplatforms for molecular oncology provide multiplexed high-sensitivity rare mutation detection and facilitate targeted drug delivery. Their ability to adapt to tumor heterogeneity and molecular cues makes them better than traditional diagnostics for precision medicine.

Nanoplatforms can currently track intracellular signaling pathways such as *PI3K/AKT* and MAPK in real-time, providing dynamic information about tumor biology beyond fixed gene testing [41, 42]. Some also combine immune modulation with genetic sensing to strengthen immunotherapy [43]. Adaptive systems change alongside tumors and are therefore well suited for longitudinal tracking. Smart nanodevices are real-time monitors of genetic alterations and enable personalized, minimally invasive diagnosis. Computational model integration in the future could transform cancer diagnosis from mutation- to network-based models [40].

3.3 Case Studies of Biomarker Discovery Using Nanotech

Nanotechnology has promoted biomarker identification in oncology, especially for difficult tumors such as glioblastoma, by allowing ultra-sensitive detection of biomarkers in the blood-brain barrier. Nano-omics platforms integrating plasma and tumor proteomes have enhanced diagnostic specificity and established new biomarkers [44, 45]. Nanomaterials like gold nanoparticles and graphene oxide separate vesicles secreted by tumors from biofluids, providing noninvasive insights into tumor biology [46]. Nanobiosensors currently identify cancer biomarkers at sub-nanomolar concentrations, combining imaging and molecular analysis for real-time in vivo diagnosis, with encouraging early clinical trial outcomes [39, 47].

4 Nanotech-Based Diagnostics

Nanotechnology has transformed cancer diagnosis through the capability of highly sensitive and specific detection of biomarkers at early stages of disease. Instruments such as quantum dots, magnetic nanoparticles, and gold nanoshells provide enhanced interaction with tumor markers because of their unique physicochemical attributes, enabling noninvasive, real-time detection of molecules that outperforms conventional tools [48, 49].

Recent developments have brought forward smart nanoprobes and tumor-specific cue-responsive biosensors like pH or enzyme activity, boosting point-of-care cancer diagnostics [50]. Theranostics platforms currently merge diagnostic and therapeutic capabilities in one nanoparticle for better treatment tracking in precision oncology [51]. Technologies such as graphene sensors, CRISPR-loaded nanocarriers, and lab-on-chip devices are in development for ultrarapid and ultra-sensitive biomarker detection [15, 52]. However, clinical translation is faced with challenges due to issues of reproducibility and regulatory challenges [53, 54].

4.1 Nanoparticle-Enhanced Imaging (MRI, PET, Fluorescence)

Nanoparticle imaging has improved cancer diagnosis through site-specific targeting, increased contrast, and multimodal function in MRI, PET, and fluorescence imaging. Iron oxide nanoparticles enhance MRI sensitivity for detection of brain and heart tumors, whereas ligand-functionalized particles facilitate molecular imaging of targets such as EGFR and atherosclerotic plaques [55, 56]. Quantum dots aid intraoperative tumor margin identification, and radiolabeled nanoparticles improve the sensitivity of PET and tumor uptake [45, 57].

In addition to tumor localization, functionalized nanomaterials facilitate the real-time monitoring of the response to treatment through imaging tumor metabolism and receptor status [58]. Nanoparticles of gold and silica improve visualization of immune infiltration and angiogenesis, particularly helpful in neuro-oncology where penetration across the BBB is still an issue [59, 60]. Activated endothelium is targeted in cardiovascular imaging to identify early infarcts and inflammation, with increasing clinical trial backing [55, 61].

4.2 Nanosensors for Real-Time Detection of Signaling and Genetic Markers

Nanosensors have transformed molecular diagnostics by facilitating real-time, ultra-sensitive detection of intracellular signals and genetic biomarkers. They are built with materials such as gold nanoparticles, carbon nanotubes, or quantum dots and measure changes in pH, ROS, and nucleic acid expression with accuracy [62]. In oncology and neurodegenerative diseases, these devices pick up molecular changes long before the onset of symptoms, aiding in early diagnosis [61]. Aptamer- and oligonucleotide-mediated biosensors specifically target cancer-associated miRNAs and DNA mutations, and when coupled into wearable or implantable devices, provide continuous, noninvasive monitoring [63, 64].

Apart from cancer, nanosensors find application in cardiology and regenerative medicine to monitor signaling molecules such as nitric oxide and calcium in assessing cell function and redox changes that occur with aging [64, 65]. Optical biosensors now enable picomolar-scale detection of exosomes with plasmonic and fluorescent technology [66]. Integration with microfluidics enables fast, high-throughput analysis of clinical samples to guide personalized treatment planning [51].

4.3 Liquid Biopsy Applications in Cardio-Brain Oncology

Liquid biopsy provides a minimally invasive approach to the early diagnosis, monitoring, and planning of treatment in cardio-brain cancers through the analysis of tumor-derived components such as ctDNA, circulating tumor cells, and extracellular vesicles from CSF or blood (Fig. 4.4). Liquid biopsy mirrors the molecular glioblastoma and CNS tumor profile in real time, allowing the monitoring of tumor evolution and resistance to drugs without biopsies repeated times particularly beneficial in aggressive and heterogeneous cancers [67, 68].

Liquid biopsy also has increasing promise in cardio-oncology, particularly for the identification of brain metastases from cardiac cancers or systemic cancers with cardiac involvement. Technological advances in sampling, beyond those available

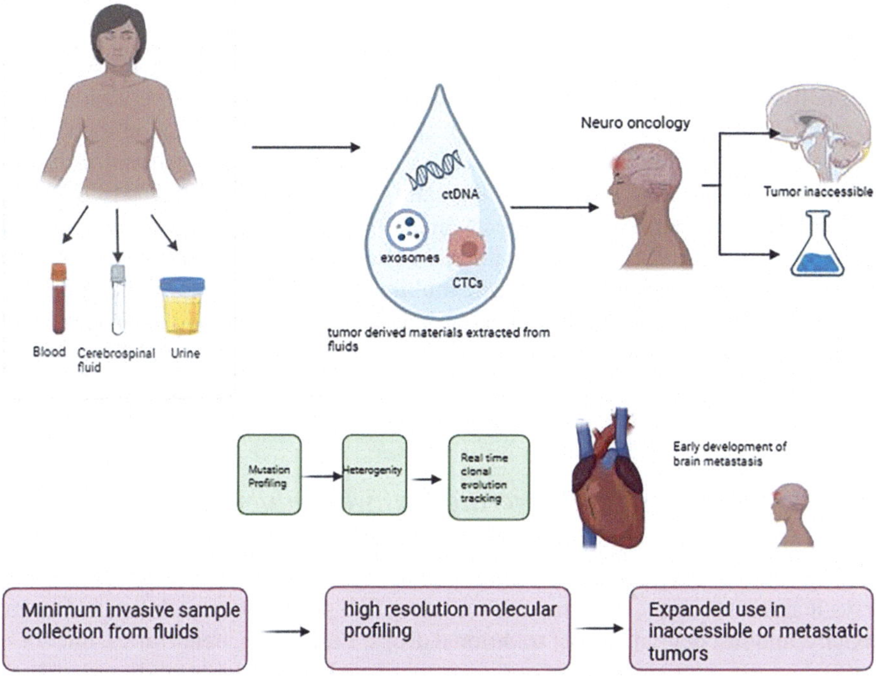

Fig. 4.4 Liquid biopsy applications in the cardio-brain oncology axis. This figure shows how liquid biopsy facilitates early detection, real-time surveillance, and treatment stratification for cardio-brain cancers. Cytokine-free fluids such as blood, CSF, and urine harbor tumor-derived ctDNA, exosomes, and CTCs that provide molecular information on glioblastoma, cardiac tumors, and brain metastases. AI and targeted ultrasound supplemented, liquid biopsy facilitates monitoring of tumor evolution and drug resistance with less need for invasive procedures. (The figure created with BioRender.com accessed on 27 June 2025)

from blood-cerebrospinal fluid and urine, are broadening its application to primary tumor diagnosis as well as metastatic tumors [69]. Technologies such as focused ultrasound have been found to increase the release of tumor-derived nucleic acids, thus enhancing the sensitivity of brain tumors to biopsies [70]. Additionally, cell-free DNA-based assays can identify occult brain metastasis prior to symptomatic presentation, enabling intervention at an earlier stage and improved outcomes [71]. In conjunction with an integrated solution with imaging and artificial intelligence, personalized diagnostics in real-time, liquid biopsy will revolutionize neuro-oncology [72, 73].

5 Nanotechnology in Targeted Therapy

Nanotechnology has transformed cancer-targeted therapy by allowing selective drug delivery that is non-toxic to healthy tissue. Nanocarriers, including dendrimers, liposomes, and polymeric particles, encapsulate and shield chemotherapeutics, improving delivery through the EPR effect [74, 75]. Ligand-functionalized platforms improve targeting further by conjugating tumor-specific antigens [39].

Intelligent nanocarriers presently act on tumor-specific signals such as acidic pH or enzymes, releasing the drug in situ and reducing toxicity [76]. Others regulate autophagy to gain resistance [77], while multimodal platforms integrate diagnostics and therapy for real-time monitoring [78]. These technologies have been successful against oral cancer and glioblastoma, enabling personalized, survival-promoting therapy [75, 79, 80].

5.1 Nanocarriers for Delivering Pathway Inhibitors

Nanocarriers have remarkably enhanced the delivery of inhibitors of signaling pathways in cancer therapy by transcending issues like poor water solubility, off-target toxicity, and fast degradation of traditional drugs. Liposomes, dendrimers, micelles, and polymeric nanoparticles are efficient in encapsulating hydrophilic as well as hydrophobic molecules, making them more bioavailable and preventing enzymatic cleavage [81, 82]. Nanocarriers engineered to target aberrant pathways such as *PI3K/AKT, MAPK, and STAT3* have been demonstrated to be more effective in resistant cancers such as breast and lung cancers [83, 84]. These platforms permit co-delivery of siRNAs and small-molecule inhibitors, while ligand-based surface engineering facilitates selective tumor targeting [85]. Stimuli-responsive carriers also allow for controlled release of the drug using internal or external stimuli [86]. Novel hybrid nanocarriers now incorporate multimodal treatment modalities, permitting dual-pathway targeting and combinatorial treatments with conventional drugs not possible [87, 88].

5.2 Precision Targeting of Tumor Cells in Neural and Cardiac Tissues

Cancer targeting in the brain and heart is challenging owing to organ sensitivity and microenvironmental complexity. In the brain, CRISPR-Cas9 and nanomedicine allow mutation-specific cytotoxicity with minimal damage to the nervous system by targeting tumor-specific InDel mutations [89]. Therapies also interfere with tumor innervation by inhibiting axonogenesis and neurochemical signaling, which help promote tumor growth [90, 91].

In the heart, hiPSC models in precision cardio-oncology are used to forecast cardiotoxicity and tailor treatment [92, 93]. Nanocarriers target drugs to cardiac-adjacent tumors without affecting heart tissue [94], supported by cardioprotective agents that target mitochondria and oxidative stress [95]. Alteration of the tumor microenvironment targeting stromal cells and immune-suppressive cells is optimized, facilitated by AI-integrated multi-omics to enable personalized intervention [96–99].

5.3 Overcoming the Blood-Brain and Blood-Heart Barriers

The blood-brain barrier (BBB) and the lesser-characterized blood-heart barrier (BHB) impede drug delivery to neural and cardiac tissues through limitation of nanoparticle and biologic entry [100, 101]. In brain cancers such as glioblastoma, the problem is further exacerbated by the heterogenic blood-tumor barrier (BTB). Sophisticated nanoparticle systems designed to size, surface chemistry, and ligand-targeting, e.g., transferrin or apolipoprotein ligands have enhanced BBB transcytosis [102–104].

Physical approaches such as focused ultrasound (FUS) with microbubbles temporarily disrupt the BBB without impairing neural tissue [105], whereas pharmacologic disruptors such as bradykinin analogs have risks of neurotoxicity [106]. The BHB also restricts drug diffusion; new approaches now utilize endothelial transcytosis and stress-responsive delivery systems to facilitate cardiac drug transport [107].

6 Integrating Nanotech with Molecular and Genomic Data

The intersection of nanotechnology with genomics and molecular biology has brought a revolution in precision medicine, especially for diseases that are complex in nature such as cancer, cardiovascular, and neurological conditions. Using omics information and high-throughput sequencing, nanotechnology today facilitates ultra-high precision analysis and manipulation of molecular information [108, 109]. Functionalized nanowires and nanoparticles biosensors at the nanoscale enable early identification of low-abundance mutations [110], whereas nanocarriers like lipid nanoparticles and DNA origami improve targeted gene delivery and CRISPR editing by surmounting biological barriers [111, 112].

AI-infused nanodevices now facilitate smart, adaptive diagnosis, delivering therapeutics based on precise molecular cues [113]. Nanotechnology also improves vaccine and immunotherapy platforms through omics-enabled antigen-mimicking nanostructures [114]. Regardless of difficulties in combining heterogeneous datasets and limited informatics capabilities [115], this marriage is more than additive;

it's revolutionary reducing biological complexity to accurate, scalable interventions in cardio-brain oncology [116].

6.1 Multi-Omics Approaches

The intricacy of cancer, especially in neural and cardiac tissues, requires systems-level understanding that exceeds single-omic methodologies. Multi-omics incorporating genomics, transcriptomics, proteomics, epigenomics, metabolomics, and lipidomics provides more profound comprehension of tumor initiation, heterogeneity, and therapy resistance, notably in cardio-brain oncology [117, 118]. For example, the integration of gene expression and DNA methylation has identified new drivers in glioblastoma [119], while extensive omics analysis in early-onset colorectal cancer identified aggressive phenotypes and therapeutic markers [120].

Integration with multi-omics and text mining by AI facilitates real-time detection of functional gene variants [121]. Nano-omics enhances single-cell and in situ profiling [122], whereas AI-based models combine imaging and molecular data for better prognosis and treatment choice [113, 123]. Platforms also enable diagnostics and safe drug delivery in nanotoxicology and rare diseases [124, 125]. Nonetheless, difficulties persist with data harmonization, batch effects, and handling high-dimensional data [117].

6.2 Personalized Treatment Strategies Based on Nanodiagnostics

Nanodiagnostics are revolutionizing cardio-brain oncology by providing real-time molecular surveillance, overcoming the limitations of conventional methods [108]. Quantum dots and magnetic nanoparticles are examples of technologies that detect biomarkers like ctDNA, miRNAs, and proteins with high sensitivity, with ligand-functionalization providing early detection of tumor subtypes in complicated tissues such as the heart and brain [126]. With genomic and proteomic information integrated, nanotheranostic systems now merge therapy and diagnosis, providing personalized real-time treatment options [127, 128]. In cardio-oncology, they also monitor cardiotoxicity with treatment, allowing therapies to be adapted to safeguard the heart without sacrificing cancer management [129, 130]

7 Challenges and Considerations

Cardio-brain oncology faces confounding toxicities of cancer treatments with convergent but not well-characterized mechanisms such as oxidative stress. Delicate symptoms and patchy care impede diagnosis and treatment. Interdisciplinary monitoring, cross-organ biomarkers, and collaborative models are needed for advancement [131]. Cardio-brain oncology is plagued with the significant challenge of poor models mimicking the heart–brain–tumor axis and scarce dual-organ imaging technologies. Available diagnostics tend to fail to catch early, additive toxicities, whereas available biomarkers are not specific. Improvements such as organ-on-chip systems, multimodal imaging, AI-driven predictions, and dual-targeted nanocarriers are poised to make therapy more safe and personalized [132].

8 Future Directions

Nanotechnology has revolutionized biomedical research by facilitating sensitive cancer detection, biomarker identification, and drug targeting. Nanoscale materials such as nanoparticles, quantum dots, and nanoshells facilitate early detection of cancer through targeted binding to tumor antigens and real-time imaging [1]. Nanotechnology in drug discovery enables high-throughput screening and the creation of targeted formulations like liposomes and polymeric nanoparticles to minimize toxicity and enhance efficacy. Smart nanocarriers release drugs based on tumor-specific stimuli, enabling personalized treatments [2]. Theranostic nanoparticles integrate therapy and diagnostics for real-time monitoring, crucial in multifaceted disciplines like cardio-brain oncology [13]. Merging AI with nanomedicine facilitates personalized treatment, toxicity tracking, and predictive diagnostic, boosting intelligent and adaptive treatment platforms [133].

9 Conclusion

Nanotechnology has taken forward cardio-brain oncology by making possible targeted drug delivery and real-time monitoring within cardiac and neural tissue. Nanocarriers reduce systemic toxicity by co-delivering anticancer medicines with cardio- and neuroprotective drugs. Nanodiagnostics such as nanosensors and contrast agents allow for early cardiotoxicity and neuroinflammation detection, while theranostic platforms integrate diagnosis and therapy for individualized treatment. This new discipline brings together nanotechnology, molecular profiling, and high-level diagnostics to enhance early diagnosis and personalized treatment. Since cancer treatments tend to impact the heart as well as the brain, liquid biopsies, circulating biomarkers, and artificial intelligence-driven imaging uncover subclinical injury.

Genomic and proteomic information inform risk-based stratification, while nanomedicine facilitates adaptive, real-time therapy propelling a move toward predictive, preventive, and precision oncology.

References

1. Mura S, Nicolas J, Couvreur P (2013) Stimuli-responsive nanocarriers for drug delivery. Nat Mater 12(11):991–1003. https://doi.org/10.1038/nmat3776
2. Pelaz B et al (2017) Diverse applications of nanomedicine. ACS Nano 11(3):2313–2381. https://doi.org/10.1021/acsnano.6b06040
3. Lyon AR, López-Fernández T, Couch LS, Asteggiano R, Aznar MC, Bergler-Klein J et al (2022) Cardio-oncology: principles, prevention, and management. Nat Rev Cardiol 19(6):360–379
4. Armenian SH, Lacchetti C, Lenihan D (2016) Prevention and monitoring of cardiac dysfunction in survivors of adult cancers: American Society of Clinical Oncology clinical practice guideline summary. J Oncol Pract 12(3):270–275
5. Gheorghiade M, De Luca L, Bonow RO, Fonarow GC (2008) Cardiotoxicity of cancer therapy: implications for the management of patients with cancer. Nat Rev Clin Oncol 5(12):693–703
6. Fruman DA, Chiu H, Hopkins BD, Bagrodia S, Cantley LC, Abraham RT (2017) The PI3K pathway in human disease. Cell 170(4):605–635
7. Ewer MS, Ewer SM (2010) Cardiotoxicity of anticancer treatments. Nat Rev Cardiol 7(10):564–575
8. Zhou J, Chen X, Yang J, Lin Y (2023) Cognitive impairment and cardiac dysfunction after breast cancer therapy: a cross-system analysis. Cardio Oncol Rep 5(1):45–52
9. Salvatore L, Aprile G, Arnoldi E, Marchetti P (2022) The emerging role of cardio-oncology in cancer therapeutics: from mechanisms to clinical applications. Cancer 14(4):812
10. Barenholz Y (2012) Doxil® the first FDA-approved nano-drug: lessons learned. J Control Release 160(2):117–134
11. Das M, Patil S, Bhargava N, Kang JF, Riedel LM, Seal S, Hickman JJ (2012) Auto-catalytic ceria nanoparticles offer neuroprotection to adult rat spinal cord neurons. Biomaterials 33(30):7746–7755
12. Zhou Y, Hong Y, Liang C (2017) Selenium nanoparticles as a protective agent against chemotherapy-induced cardiotoxicity. Nanomedicine 13(7):2151–2160
13. Wang Y et al (2021) Acta Pharm Sin B 11(6):1700–1722
14. You M, Xie Z, Zhang N et al (2023) Signaling pathways in cancer metabolism: mechanisms and therapeutic targets. Signal Transduct Target Ther 8:196. https://doi.org/10.1038/s41392-023-01442-3
15. Zhang Q, Wang L, Wang S et al (2022) Signaling pathways and targeted therapy for myocardial infarction. Signal Transduct Target Ther 7:78. https://doi.org/10.1038/s41392-022-00925-z
16. Li S, Wang C, Chen J et al (2023) Signaling pathways in brain tumors and therapeutic interventions. Signal Transduct Target Ther 8(1):8. https://doi.org/10.1038/s41392-022-01260-z
17. Cucu I (2022) Signaling pathways in inflammation and cardiovascular diseases: an update of therapeutic strategies. Ther Immunol 2(4):630–650. https://doi.org/10.3390/immuno2040039
18. Pouyan A, Ghorbanlo M, Eslami M et al (2025) Glioblastoma multiforme: insights into pathogenesis, key signaling pathways, and therapeutic strategies. Mol Cancer 24:58. https://doi.org/10.1186/s12943-025-02267-0
19. Barzegar Behrooz A, Talaie Z, Jusheghani F, Łos MJ, Klonisch T, Ghavami S (2022) Wnt and PI3K/Akt/mTOR survival pathways as therapeutic targets in glioblastoma. Int J Mol Sci 23(3):1353. https://doi.org/10.3390/ijms23031353

20. Stefani C, Miricescu D, Stanescu-Spinu II, Nica RI, Greabu M, Totan AR, Jinga M (2021) Growth factors, PI3K/AKT/mTOR and MAPK signaling pathways in colorectal cancer pathogenesis: where are we now? Int J Mol Sci 22(19):10260. https://doi.org/10.3390/ijms221910260
21. Hedayati N, Safari MH, Milasi YE et al (2025) Modulation of the PI3K/Akt signaling pathway by resveratrol in cancer: molecular mechanisms and therapeutic opportunity. Discov Oncol 16(1):669. https://doi.org/10.1007/s12672-025-02471-w
22. Yu F, Yu C, Li F et al (2021) Wnt/β-catenin signaling in cancers and targeted therapies. Signal Transduct Target Ther 6:307. https://doi.org/10.1038/s41392-021-00701-5
23. Wu X, Que H, Li Q et al (2025) Wnt/β-catenin mediated signaling pathways in cancer: recent advances, and applications in cancer therapy. Mol Cancer 24:171. https://doi.org/10.1186/s12943-025-02363-1
24. Curry RN, Glasgow SM (2021) The role of neurodevelopmental pathways in brain tumors. Front Cell Dev Biol 9:659055. https://doi.org/10.3389/fcell.2021.65905
25. Drakulic D, Schwirtlich M, Petrovic I et al (2022) Current opportunities for targeting dysregulated neurodevelopmental signaling pathways in glioblastoma. Cells 11(16):2530. https://doi.org/10.3390/cells11162530
26. Bahar ME, Kim HJ, Kim DR (2023) Targeting the RAS/RAF/MAPK pathway for cancer therapy: from mechanism to clinical studies. Signal Transduct Target Ther 8:455. https://doi.org/10.1038/s41392-023-01705-z
27. Marrone S, Gueli IA, Lo Coco R et al (2025) Brain metastases from primary cardiac tumors: a systematic review of diagnosis, treatment, and prognosis. Cancer 17(10):1621. https://doi.org/10.3390/cancers17101621
28. Naqvi AZ, Mahjabeen I, Ameen S et al (2020) Genetic and expression variations of cell cycle pathway genes in brain tumor patients. Biosci Rep 40(5):BSR20190629. https://doi.org/10.1042/BSR20190629
29. Ostrom Q, Cohen ML, Ondracek A, Sloan A, Barnholtz-Sloan J (2013) Gene markers in brain tumors: what the epileptologist should know. Epilepsia 54(Suppl 9):25–29. https://doi.org/10.1111/epi.12439
30. Reilly KM (2009) Brain tumor susceptibility: the role of genetic factors and uses of mouse models to unravel risk. Brain Pathol 19(1):121–131. https://doi.org/10.1111/j.1750-3639.2008.00236.x
31. Correa DD, Satagopan J, Martin A et al (2019) Genetic variants and cognitive functions in patients with brain tumors. Neuro-Oncology 21(10):1297–1309. https://doi.org/10.1093/neuonc/noz094
32. Ananthan K, Lyon AR (2020) The role of biomarkers in cardio-oncology. J Cardiovasc Transl Res 13(3):431–450. https://doi.org/10.1007/s12265-020-10042-3
33. Ohgaki H, Kleihues P (2009) Genetic alterations and signaling pathways in the evolution of gliomas. Cancer Sci 100(12):2235–2241. https://doi.org/10.1111/j.1349-7006.2009.01308.x
34. Vogelstein B, Papadopoulos N, Velculescu VE, Zhou S, Diaz LA Jr, Kinzler KW (2013) Cancer genome landscapes. Science 339(6127):1546–1558. https://doi.org/10.1126/science.1235122
35. Behnan J, Finocchiaro G, Hanna G (2019) The landscape of the mesenchymal signature in brain tumours. Brain 142(4):847–866. https://doi.org/10.1093/brain/awz044
36. Montaño A, Forero-Castro M, Marchena-Mendoza D, Benito R, Hernández-Rivas JM (2018) New challenges in targeting signaling pathways in acute lymphoblastic leukemia by NGS approaches: an update. Cancer 10(4):110. https://doi.org/10.3390/cancers10040110
37. Lei ZN, Teng QX, Tian Q et al (2022) Signaling pathways and therapeutic interventions in gastric cancer. Signal Transduct Target Ther 7:358. https://doi.org/10.1038/s41392-022-01190-w
38. Ho D, Quake SR, McCabe ERB et al (2020) Enabling technologies for personalized and precision medicine. Trends Biotechnol 38(5):497–518. https://doi.org/10.1016/j.tibtech.2019.12.021

39. Chehelgerdi M, Chehelgerdi M, Allela OQB et al (2023) Progressing nanotechnology to improve targeted cancer treatment: overcoming hurdles in its clinical implementation. Mol Cancer 22(1):169. https://doi.org/10.1186/s12943-023-01865-0
40. Guo Z, Chen D, Yao L et al (2025) The molecular mechanism and therapeutic landscape of copper and cuproptosis in cancer. Signal Transduct Target Ther 10(1):149. https://doi.org/10.1038/s41392-025-02192-0
41. Borisov NM, Terekhanova NV, Aliper AM et al (2014) Signaling pathways activation profiles make better markers of cancer than expression of individual genes. Oncotarget 5(20):10198–10205. https://doi.org/10.18632/oncotarget.2548
42. Sanchez-Vega F, Mina M, Armenia J et al (2018) Oncogenic signaling pathways in The Cancer Genome Atlas. Cell 173(2):321–337.e10. https://doi.org/10.1016/j.cell.2018.03.035
43. Lu S, Yang Y, Song Z et al (2025) Dual functional nanoplatforms potentiate osteosarcoma immunotherapy via microenvironment modulation. Natl Sci Rev 12(3):nwaf002. https://doi.org/10.1093/nsr/nwaf002
44. Liu X, Abmanhal-Masarweh H, Iwanowytsch O et al (2025) Plasma-to-tumour tissue integrated proteomics using nano-omics for biomarker discovery in glioblastoma. Nat Commun 16(1):3412. https://doi.org/10.1038/s41467-025-58252-0
45. Zottel A, Videtič Paska A, Jovčevska I (2019) Nanotechnology meets oncology: nanomaterials in brain cancer research, diagnosis and therapy. Materials 12(10):1588. https://doi.org/10.3390/ma12101588
46. Kumar MA, Baba SK, Sadida HQ et al (2024) Extracellular vesicles as tools and targets in therapy for diseases. Signal Transduct Target Ther 9:27. https://doi.org/10.1038/s41392-024-01735-1
47. Ahmad A, Imran M, Ahsan H (2023) Biomarkers as biomedical bioindicators: approaches and techniques for the detection, analysis, and validation of novel biomarkers of diseases. Pharmaceutics 15(6):1630. https://doi.org/10.3390/pharmaceutics15061630
48. Zhang Y, Li M, Gao X et al (2019) Nanotechnology in cancer diagnosis: progress, challenges and opportunities. J Hematol Oncol 12:137. https://doi.org/10.1186/s13045-019-0833-3
49. Jin C, Wang K, Oppong-Gyebi A, Hu J (2020) Application of nanotechnology in cancer diagnosis and therapy—a mini-review. Int J Med Sci 17(18):2964–2973. https://doi.org/10.7150/ijms.49801
50. Alrushaid N, Khan FA, Al-Suhaimi EA, Elaissari A (2023) Nanotechnology in cancer diagnosis and treatment. Pharmaceutics 15(3):1025. https://doi.org/10.3390/pharmaceutics15031025
51. Wang B, Hu S, Teng Y et al (2024) Current advance of nanotechnology in diagnosis and treatment for malignant tumors. Signal Transduct Target Ther 9:200. https://doi.org/10.1038/s41392-024-01889-y
52. Tantray J, Patel A, Parveen H et al (2025) Nanotechnology-based biomedical devices in the cancer diagnostics and therapy. Med Oncol 42:50. https://doi.org/10.1007/s12032-025-02602-x
53. Puttasiddaiah R, Basavegowda N, Lakshmanagowda NK et al (2025) Emerging nanoparticle-based diagnostics and therapeutics for cancer: innovations and challenges. Pharmaceutics 17(1):70. https://doi.org/10.3390/pharmaceutics17010070
54. Nasir A, Khan A, Li J et al (2021) Nanotechnology, a tool for diagnostics and treatment of cancer. Curr Top Med Chem 21(15):1360–1376. https://doi.org/10.2174/1568026621666210701144124
55. Lapusan R, Borlan R, Focsan M (2024) Advancing MRI with magnetic nanoparticles: a comprehensive review of translational research and clinical trials. Nanoscale Adv 6(9):2234–2259. https://doi.org/10.1039/d3na01064c
56. Yin C, Hu P, Qin L, Wang Z, Zhao H (2024) The current status and future directions on nanoparticles for tumor molecular imaging. Int J Nanomedicine 19:9549–9574. https://doi.org/10.2147/IJN.S484206
57. Toy R, Bauer L, Hoimes C, Ghaghada KB, Karathanasis E (2014) Targeted nanotechnology for cancer imaging. Adv Drug Deliv Rev 76:79–97. https://doi.org/10.1016/j.addr.2014.08.002

58. Rowe SP, Pomper MG (2022) Molecular imaging in oncology: current impact and future directions. CA Cancer J Clin 72(4):333–352. https://doi.org/10.3322/caac.21713
59. Liu SF, Li MJ, Liang B et al (2024) Breaking the barrier: nanoparticle-enhanced radiotherapy as the new vanguard in brain tumor treatment. Front Pharmacol 15:1394816. https://doi.org/10.3389/fphar.2024.1394816
60. Bai JW, Qiu SQ, Zhang GJ (2023) Molecular and functional imaging in cancer-targeted therapy: current applications and future directions. Signal Transduct Target Ther 8:89. https://doi.org/10.1038/s41392-023-01366-y
61. Elendu C, Amaechi DC, Elendu TC et al (2025) Essential information about nanotechnology in cardiology. Ann Med Surg 87(2):748–779. https://doi.org/10.1097/MS9.0000000000002867
62. Yadav S, Bukke SPN, Prajapati S, Singh AP, Chettupalli AK, Nicholas B (2025) Nanobiosensors in neurodegenerative disease diagnosis: a promising pathway for early detection. Digit Health 11:20552076251342457. https://doi.org/10.1177/20552076251342457
63. Kim M, Panagiotakopoulou M, Chen C et al (2023) Micro-engineering and nano-engineering approaches to investigate tumour ecosystems. Nat Rev Cancer 23(9):581–599. https://doi.org/10.1038/s41568-023-00593-3
64. Mazuryk O, Gurgul I, Oszajca M et al (2024) Nitric oxide signaling and sensing in age-related diseases. Antioxidants (Basel) 13(10):1213. https://doi.org/10.3390/antiox13101213
65. Atwa A et al (2024) Integrating nanosensors into stem cells technologies and regenerative medicine. In: Ali GAM, Chong KF, Makhlouf ASH (eds) Handbook of nanosensors. Springer, Cham. https://doi.org/10.1007/978-3-031-47180-3_38
66. Yasamineh S, Nikben N, Ahmed HM, Abdul Kareem R, Al-Aridhy AK, Hooshiar MH (2024) Increasing the sensitivity and accuracy of detecting exosomes as biomarkers for cancer monitoring using optical nanobiosensors. Cancer Cell Int 24(1):189. https://doi.org/10.1186/s12935-024-03379-1
67. Berzero G, Pieri V, Mortini P, Filippi M, Finocchiaro G (2023) The coming of age of liquid biopsy in neuro-oncology. Brain 146(10):4015–4024. https://doi.org/10.1093/brain/awad195
68. Trivedi R, Bhat KP (2023) Liquid biopsy: creating opportunities in brain space. Br J Cancer 129(11):1727–1746. https://doi.org/10.1038/s41416-023-02446-0
69. Bao Y, Zhang D, Guo H, Ma W (2024) Beyond blood: advancing the frontiers of liquid biopsy in oncology and personalized medicine. Cancer Sci 115(4):1060–1072. https://doi.org/10.1111/cas.16097
70. Rincon-Torroella J, Khela H, Bettegowda A, Bettegowda C (2022) Biomarkers and focused ultrasound: the future of liquid biopsy for brain tumor patients. J Neuro-Oncol 156(1):33–48. https://doi.org/10.1007/s11060-021-03837-0
71. Rehman AU, Khan P, Maurya SK et al (2022) Liquid biopsies to occult brain metastasis. Mol Cancer 21(1):113. https://doi.org/10.1186/s12943-022-01577-x
72. Rafanan J, Ghani N, Kazemeini S, Nadeem-Tariq A, Shih R, Vida TA (2025) Modernizing neuro-oncology: the impact of imaging, liquid biopsies, and AI on diagnosis and treatment. Int J Mol Sci 26(3):917. https://doi.org/10.3390/ijms26030917
73. Gaitsch H, Franklin RJM, Reich DS (2023) Cell-free DNA-based liquid biopsies in neurology. Brain 146(5):1758–1774. https://doi.org/10.1093/brain/awac438
74. Zhu J, Lee H, Huang R et al (2025) Harnessing nanotechnology for cancer treatment. Front Bioeng Biotechnol 12:1514890. https://doi.org/10.3389/fbioe.2024.1514890
75. Fan D, Cao Y, Cao M, Wang Y, Cao Y, Gong T (2023) Nanomedicine in cancer therapy. Signal Transduct Target Ther 8(1):293. https://doi.org/10.1038/s41392-023-01536-y
76. Sell M, Lopes AR, Escudeiro M et al (2023) Application of nanoparticles in cancer treatment: a concise review. Nanomaterials 13(21):2887. https://doi.org/10.3390/nano13212887
77. He K, Chen M, Liu J, Du S, Ren C, Zhang J (2024) Nanomedicine for cancer targeted therapy with autophagy regulation. Front Immunol 14:1238827. https://doi.org/10.3389/fimmu.2023.1238827
78. Sun L, Liu H, Ye Y et al (2023) Smart nanoparticles for cancer therapy. Signal Transduct Target Ther 8(1):418. https://doi.org/10.1038/s41392-023-01642-x

79. Raj S, Khurana S, Choudhari R et al (2021) Specific targeting cancer cells with nanoparticles and drug delivery in cancer therapy. Semin Cancer Biol 69:166–177. https://doi.org/10.1016/j.semcancer.2019.11.002
80. Vyas K, Rathod M, Patel MM (2023) Insight on nano drug delivery systems with targeted therapy in treatment of oral cancer. Nanomedicine 49:102662. https://doi.org/10.1016/j.nano.2023.102662
81. Sabit H, Abdel-Hakeem M, Shoala T et al (2022) Nanocarriers: a reliable tool for the delivery of anticancer drugs. Pharmaceutics 14(8):1566. https://doi.org/10.3390/pharmaceutics14081566
82. Yao Y, Zhou Y, Liu L et al (2020) Nanoparticle-based drug delivery in cancer therapy and its role in overcoming drug resistance. Front Mol Biosci 7:193. https://doi.org/10.3389/fmolb.2020.00193
83. Md S, Alhakamy NA, Karim S, Gabr GA, Iqubal MK, Murshid SSA (2021) Signaling pathway inhibitors, miRNA, and nanocarrier-based pharmacotherapeutics for the treatment of lung cancer: a review. Pharmaceutics 13(12):2120. https://doi.org/10.3390/pharmaceutics13122120
84. Ashrafizadeh M, Ahmadi Z, Kotla NG et al (2019) Nanoparticles targeting STATs in cancer therapy. Cells 8(10):1158. https://doi.org/10.3390/cells8101158
85. Lôbo GCNB, Paiva KLR, Silva ALG et al (2021) Nanocarriers used in drug delivery to enhance immune system in cancer therapy. Pharmaceutics 13(8):1167. https://doi.org/10.3390/pharmaceutics13081167
86. Xia W, Tao Z, Zhu B et al (2021) Targeted delivery of drugs and genes using polymer nanocarriers for cancer therapy. Int J Mol Sci 22(17):9118. https://doi.org/10.3390/ijms22179118
87. Erebor JO, Agboluaje EO, Perkins AM, Krishnakumar M, Ngwuluka N (2024) Targeted hybrid nanocarriers as co-delivery systems for enhanced cancer therapy. Adv Pharm Bull 14(3):558–573. https://doi.org/10.34172/apb.2024.046
88. Sabir S, Thani ASB, Abbas Q (2025) Nanotechnology in cancer treatment: revolutionizing strategies against drug resistance. Front Bioeng Biotechnol 13:1548588. https://doi.org/10.3389/fbioe.2025.1548588
89. Kwon T, Ra JS, Lee S et al (2022) Precision targeting tumor cells using cancer-specific InDel mutations with CRISPR-Cas9. Proc Natl Acad Sci U S A 119(9):e2103532119. https://doi.org/10.1073/pnas.2103532119
90. Li X, Peng X, Yang S et al (2022) Targeting tumor innervation: premises, promises, and challenges. Cell Death Discov 8(1):131. https://doi.org/10.1038/s41420-022-00930-9
91. Le TT, Oudin MJ (2023) Understanding and modeling nerve-cancer interactions. Dis Model Mech 16(1):dmm049729. https://doi.org/10.1242/dmm.049729
92. Perry TR, Roberts ML, Sunkara B et al (2021) Modeling precision cardio-oncology: using human-induced pluripotent stem cells for risk stratification and prevention. Curr Oncol Rep 23(7):77. https://doi.org/10.1007/s11912-021-01066-2
93. Han X, Zhou Y, Liu W (2017) Precision cardio-oncology: understanding the cardiotoxicity of cancer therapy. NPJ Precis Oncol 1:31. https://doi.org/10.1038/s41698-017-0034-x
94. Sabit H, Pawlik TM, Radwan F et al (2025) Precision nanomedicine: navigating the tumor microenvironment for enhanced cancer immunotherapy and targeted drug delivery. Mol Cancer 24(1):160. https://doi.org/10.1186/s12943-025-02357-z
95. Kuang Z, Ge Y, Cao L et al (2024) Precision treatment of anthracycline-induced cardiotoxicity: an updated review. Curr Treat Options Oncol 25(8):1038–1054. https://doi.org/10.1007/s11864-024-01238-9
96. Valkenburg KC, de Groot AE, Pienta KJ (2018) Targeting the tumour stroma to improve cancer therapy. Nat Rev Clin Oncol 15(6):366–381. https://doi.org/10.1038/s41571-018-0007-1
97. Vitorakis N, Gargalionis AN, Papavassiliou KA et al (2024) Precision targeting strategies in pancreatic cancer: the role of tumor microenvironment. Cancer 16(16):2876. https://doi.org/10.3390/cancers16162876

98. Krzyszczyk P, Acevedo A, Davidoff EJ et al (2018) The growing role of precision and personalized medicine for cancer treatment. Technology 6(3–4):79–100. https://doi.org/10.1142/S2339547818300020
99. Mao Y, Xie J, Yang F et al (2024) Advances and prospects of precision nanomedicine in personalized tumor theranostics. Front Cell Dev Biol 12:1514399. https://doi.org/10.3389/fcell.2024.1514399
100. Arvanitis CD, Ferraro GB, Jain RK (2020) The blood-brain barrier and blood-tumour barrier in brain tumours and metastases. Nat Rev Cancer 20(1):26–41. https://doi.org/10.1038/s41568-019-0205-x
101. Mo F, Pellerino A, Soffietti R, Rudà R (2021) Blood-brain barrier in brain tumors: biology and clinical relevance. Int J Mol Sci 22(23):12654. https://doi.org/10.3390/ijms222312654
102. Ferraris C, Cavalli R, Panciani PP, Battaglia L (2020) Overcoming the blood-brain barrier: successes and challenges in developing nanoparticle-mediated drug delivery systems for the treatment of brain tumours. Int J Nanomedicine 15:2999–3022. https://doi.org/10.2147/IJN.S231479
103. Mitusova K, Peltek OO, Karpov TE et al (2022) Overcoming the blood-brain barrier for the therapy of malignant brain tumor: current status and prospects of drug delivery approaches. J Nanobiotechnology 20(1):412. https://doi.org/10.1186/s12951-022-01610-7
104. Qu Z, Luo J, Li Z et al (2024) Advancements in strategies for overcoming the blood-brain barrier to deliver brain-targeted drugs. Front Aging Neurosci 16:1353003. https://doi.org/10.3389/fnagi.2024.1353003
105. Straehla JP, Reardon DA, Wen PY, Agar NYR (2023) The blood-brain barrier: implications for experimental cancer therapeutics. Annu Rev Cancer Biol 7:265–289. https://doi.org/10.1146/annurev-cancerbio-061421-040433
106. Sprowls SA, Arsiwala TA, Bumgarner JR et al (2019) Improving CNS delivery to brain metastases by blood-tumor barrier disruption. Trends Cancer 5(8):495–505. https://doi.org/10.1016/j.trecan.2019.06.003
107. Upton DH, Ung C, George SM, Tsoli M, Kavallaris M, Ziegler DS (2022) Challenges and opportunities to penetrate the blood-brain barrier for brain cancer therapy. Theranostics 12(10):4734–4752. https://doi.org/10.7150/thno.69682
108. Alghamdi MA, Fallica AN, Virzì N et al (2022) The promise of nanotechnology in personalized medicine. J Pers Med 12(5):673. https://doi.org/10.3390/jpm12050673
109. Bracamonte AG (2023) Current advances in nanotechnology for the next generation of sequencing (NGS). Biosensors 13(2):260. https://doi.org/10.3390/bios13020260
110. Mukhtar M, Sargazi S, Barani M et al (2021) Application of nanotechnology for sensitive detection of low-abundance single-nucleotide variations in genomic DNA: a review. Nanomaterials 11(6):1384. https://doi.org/10.3390/nano11061384
111. Mirón-Barroso S, Domènech EB, Trigueros S (2021) Nanotechnology-based strategies to overcome current barriers in gene delivery. Int J Mol Sci 22(16):8537. https://doi.org/10.3390/ijms22168537
112. Jiang T, Gonzalez KM, Cordova LE, Lu J (2023) Nanotechnology-enabled gene delivery for cancer and other genetic diseases. Expert Opin Drug Deliv 20(4):523–540. https://doi.org/10.1080/17425247.2023.2200246
113. Adir O, Poley M, Chen G et al (2020) Integrating artificial intelligence and nanotechnology for precision cancer medicine. Adv Mater 32(13):e1901989. https://doi.org/10.1002/adma.201901989
114. Liao W, Zhang TT, Gao L et al (2017) Integration of novel materials and advanced genomic technologies into new vaccine design. Curr Top Med Chem 17(20):2286–2301. https://doi.org/10.2174/1568026617666170224122117
115. Karcher S, Willighagen EL, Rumble J et al (2018) Integration among databases and data sets to support productive nanotechnology: challenges and recommendations. NanoImpact 9:85–101. https://doi.org/10.1016/j.impact.2017.11.002

116. Malik S, Muhammad K, Waheed Y (2023) Emerging applications of nanotechnology in healthcare and medicine. Molecules 28(18):6624. https://doi.org/10.3390/molecules28186624
117. Subramanian I, Verma S, Kumar S, Jere A, Anamika K (2020) Multi-omics data integration, interpretation, and its application. Bioinform Biol Insights 14:1177932219899051. https://doi.org/10.1177/1177932219899051
118. Gutierrez Reyes CD, Alejo-Jacuinde G, Perez Sanchez B et al (2024) Multi omics applications in biological systems. Curr Issues Mol Biol 46(6):5777–5793. https://doi.org/10.3390/cimb46060345
119. Santamarina-Ojeda P, Tejedor JR, Pérez RF et al (2023) Multi-omic integration of DNA methylation and gene expression data reveals molecular vulnerabilities in glioblastoma. Mol Oncol 17(9):1726–1743. https://doi.org/10.1002/1878-0261.13479
120. Du M, Gu D, Xin J et al (2023) Integrated multi-omics approach to distinct molecular characterization and classification of early-onset colorectal cancer. Cell Rep Med 4(3):100974. https://doi.org/10.1016/j.xcrm.2023.100974
121. Raja K, Patrick M, Gao Y et al (2017) A review of recent advancement in integrating omics data with literature mining towards biomedical discoveries. Int J Genomics 2017:6213474. https://doi.org/10.1155/2017/6213474
122. Wang X, Xu W, Li J et al (2023) Nano-omics: frontier fields of fusion of nanotechnology. Smart Med 2(4):e20230039. https://doi.org/10.1002/SMMD.20230039
123. Yoon JH, Lee H, Kwon D et al (2024) Integrative approach of omics and imaging data to discover new insights for understanding brain diseases. Brain Commun 6(4):fcae265. https://doi.org/10.1093/braincomms/fcae265
124. Tejedor JR, Soriano-Sexto A, Beccari L et al (2025) Integration of multi-omics layers empowers precision diagnosis through unveiling pathogenic mechanisms on maple syrup urine disease. J Inherit Metab Dis 48(1):e12829. https://doi.org/10.1002/jimd.12829
125. Abdelkader Y, Perez-Davalos L, LeDuc R, Zahedi RP, Labouta HI (2023) Omics approaches for the assessment of biological responses to nanoparticles. Adv Drug Deliv Rev 200:114992. https://doi.org/10.1016/j.addr.2023.114992
126. Yan H, Zhai B, Yang F et al (2022) Nanotechnology-based diagnostic and therapeutic strategies for neuroblastoma. Front Pharmacol 13:908713. https://doi.org/10.3389/fphar.2022.908713
127. Sharma S (2014) Nanotheranostics in evidence-based personalized medicine. Curr Drug Targets 15(10):915–930
128. Fornaguera C, García-Celma MJ (2017) Personalized nanomedicine: a revolution at the nanoscale. J Pers Med 7(4):12. https://doi.org/10.3390/jpm7040012
129. Khan A, Barapatre AR, Babar N et al (2025) Genomic medicine and personalized treatment: a narrative review. Ann Med Surg 87(3):1406–1414. https://doi.org/10.1097/MS9.0000000000002965
130. Singh AK, Malviya R, Verma S (2023) Personalized medicine: advanced treatment strategies to revolutionize healthcare. Curr Drug Res Rev 15(2):101–104
131. Patel M, Hu J, Soman P (2021) Neurocognitive and cardiovascular implications of cancer therapy. JACC: CardioOncology 3(3):408–420
132. de Azambuja E et al (2020) Cardio-oncology: a new discipline in medicine. Eur Heart J 41(20):1985–1996
133. He J et al (2021) Smart nanomedicine powered by AI for precision cancer therapy. Adv Drug Deliv Rev 179:11399

Chapter 5
Enhancing Brain Tumor Diagnosis Through Hybrid Deep Neural Network Ensemble: Combining Probabilistic Predictions from ResNet50 and DenseNet201

Punyata Gupta, Darpan Deepak Nemade, Kushal Patel, Sreekant Patnaik, Soutrik Dana, Abha Sharma, Rabia Musheer Aziz, and Péricles B. C. Miranda

1 Introduction

The human brain, often described as the most complex organ in the body, serves as the epicenter of our thoughts, emotions, and bodily functions. Yet, this intricate command center is vulnerable to a range of disorders, among which brain tumors stand out as particularly challenging. Brain tumors, abnormal growths of cells within the brain or its surrounding structures, represent a significant health concern worldwide. Among these, secondary brain tumors—those that metastasize to the brain from other parts of the body—are increasingly prevalent, contributing to a growing community of individuals grappling with their profound impacts. While precise statistics on secondary brain tumors remain elusive due to variations in reporting and diagnostic practices, their rising incidence underscores the urgency of advancing our understanding and management of these conditions [1–5]. This term paper explores the multifaceted challenges associated with brain tumors, with a particular focus on the limitations of current diagnostic technologies, such as magnetic resonance imaging (MRI), and their implications for patient outcomes.

P. Gupta · D. D. Nemade · K. Patel · S. Patnaik · S. Dana · A. Sharma (✉)
School of Computing Science Engineering and Artificial Intelligence, VIT Bhopal University, Sehore, Madhya Pradesh, India

R. M. Aziz
Planning Department, State Planning Institute, Lucknow, Uttar Pradesh, India

P. B. C. Miranda
Departamento de Computação (DC), Universidade Federal Rural de Pernambuco (UFRPE), Recife, Brazil
e-mail: pericles.miranda@ufrpe.br

S. Mallik et al. (eds.), *Landscape of Signaling Pathway and Genetic Markers in Cardio-Brain Oncology*, Studies in Rhythm Engineering,
https://doi.org/10.1007/978-981-95-7012-6_5

Secondary brain tumors, also known as metastatic brain tumors, originate from cancerous cells that spread to the brain from primary sites like the lungs, breast, or skin. Unlike primary brain tumors, which arise within the brain itself, secondary tumors are more common and often present unique diagnostic and therapeutic challenges due to their diverse origins and aggressive nature [2, 6–9]. The lack of precise epidemiological data complicates efforts to quantify their prevalence, but studies suggest they account for a significant proportion of brain tumor cases, with estimates indicating that up to 30% of cancer patients may develop brain metastases during their illness. This variability highlights the need for improved diagnostic tools and strategies to address the growing burden of these tumors. Early detection is a cornerstone of effective brain tumor management. Identifying tumors at their nascent stages can dramatically improve the chances of successful treatment, whether through surgical resection, radiation, or targeted therapies. Advances in clinical imaging technologies, particularly MRI, have revolutionized the field of neuro-oncology by enabling non-invasive visualization of brain structures. MRI's ability to produce detailed images of the brain's anatomy has made it an indispensable tool for detecting abnormalities. However, despite its widespread use, MRI technology is not without limitations. The accuracy of MRI in distinguishing between different types of brain tumors—such as gliomas, meningiomas, pituitary tumors, or the absence of a tumor—can be hampered by factors like image resolution, contrast agent limitations, and the inherent complexity of brain tissue. These shortcomings can delay accurate diagnosis, leading to suboptimal treatment plans and, in some cases, progression of the disease.

Brain tumors are broadly classified into four primary categories: gliomas, meningiomas, pituitary tumors, and a "no tumor" category for cases where imaging reveals non-tumorous abnormalities. Gliomas, which arise from glial cells, are among the most aggressive and common primary brain tumors, encompassing subtypes like astrocytomas and glioblastomas. Meningiomas, typically slower-growing, originate from the meninges, the protective layers surrounding the brain and spinal cord. Pituitary tumors, located in the pituitary gland, can disrupt hormonal balance, leading to systemic effects. The "no tumor" category includes conditions like cysts or inflammatory lesions that may mimic tumors on imaging, further complicating diagnosis. Each type presents distinct challenges in terms of detection, classification, and treatment, with MRI often struggling to differentiate subtle characteristics, such as the boundaries between benign and malignant growths or the presence of microscopic tumor infiltration [10, 11]. The physical and functional consequences of brain tumors are profound, often leading to significant disabilities that impact patients' quality of life. Tumors can exert pressure on critical brain regions, disrupting functions like motor control, speech, vision, or hearing. For instance, a tumor pressing on the motor cortex may cause weakness or paralysis, while one near the optic nerve could impair vision. These complications are not merely physical; they carry emotional and psychological weight, as patients navigate the challenges of reduced independence and altered self-perception. Rehabilitation for such disabilities is often arduous, requiring a multidisciplinary approach involving physical therapy, occupational therapy, and psychological support. The journey to regain lost functions or adapt to permanent changes can be long and fraught with setbacks, underscoring the importance of early and accurate diagnosis to mitigate these outcomes. The limitations of MRI technology are a central focus of this paper, as they directly influence the ability to diagnose and classify brain tumors effectively. MRI machines rely on magnetic fields and radio waves to generate detailed images, but their sensitivity can be affected by factors such as tumor size, location, and tissue characteristics. For example, small or diffuse tumors may be difficult to detect, and distinguishing between tumor types often requires advanced techniques like functional MRI or spectroscopy, which are not universally available. Additionally, patient-specific factors, such as movement during scans or the presence of metal implants, can further compromise image quality. These challenges can lead to misdiagnoses or delayed diagnoses, with serious implications for treatment planning and patient prognosis. Beyond the technical limitations of MRI, the broader impact of brain tumors on brain function varies widely based on their size, location, and type. A small tumor in a critical area, such as the brainstem, can cause devastating effects, while a larger tumor in a less eloquent region may remain asymptomatic for longer. This variability complicates both diagnosis and treatment, as clinicians must balance the risks of intervention against the potential for tumor-related damage. For instance, surgical removal of a tumor near the speech center carries the risk of language impairment, while leaving a tumor untreated may allow it to grow and cause further harm. These decisions are further complicated by the potential for tumors to cause secondary effects, such as edema or increased intracranial pressure, which can exacerbate symptoms and necessitate urgent intervention [11–14].

The societal and economic implications of brain tumors are also significant. Patients often face substantial medical costs, lost productivity, and the need for long-term care. Families and caregivers bear emotional and financial burdens, while healthcare systems grapple with the demands of providing advanced diagnostic and therapeutic options. The growing prevalence of secondary brain tumors, driven by improved survival rates for primary cancers, further amplifies these challenges. As cancer treatments advance, more patients live long enough to develop metastases, necessitating a shift in focus toward managing these complex cases. This term paper aims to dissect the challenges posed by MRI in the context of brain tumor diagnosis and classification, while also exploring the broader implications for patients and healthcare systems. This study examines the limitations of current imaging technologies and the complexity of brain tumors to identify areas for improvement in clinical practice and research. Advances in imaging technology, such as artificial intelligence-assisted diagnostics or next-generation MRI techniques, hold promise for overcoming existing barriers. Similarly, a deeper understanding of tumor biology and its interaction with brain function could pave the way for more personalized and effective treatment strategies. Ultimately, addressing the challenges of brain tumor diagnosis and management requires a concerted effort from researchers, clinicians, and policymakers to improve outcomes for those affected by this complex and often devastating condition [15–17].

2 Recent Works

2.1 Multimodal Brain Tumor Classification

- Khan et al. (2020) enhanced multimodal classification by combining pre-trained CNN models (VGG16 and VGG19) with feature fusion techniques. This approach utilized extreme learning machines (ELM) for robust classification, achieving high accuracy across BRATS datasets [3].
- Dr. J.K.Periasamy et al. (2023) developed a CNN-based framework for brain tumor detection using VGG-19, ResNet50, and DenseNet121. The ResNet50 model achieved the highest validation accuracy of 92%, outperforming DenseNet121 (90%) and VGG19 (88%). The study highlights theAQ2 effectiveness of deep learning in improving accuracy and efficiency in medical imaging [7].

2.2 Hybrid and Ensemble Models

- Huang et al. (2022) developed Deep-TumorNet, a hybrid model based on GoogLeNet, tailored for glioma, meningioma, and pituitary tumor classification. Modifications to the architecture, including the use of leaky ReLU activation, resulted in state-of-the-art performance metrics like 99.67% accuracy [6].
- Kang et al. (2021) proposed an ensemble learning approach combining deep CNN features with traditional machine learning classifiers such as SVMs. This method effectively improved classification performance across diverse datasets [4].

2.3 Traditional Techniques vs. Deep Learning

- Mohsen et al. (2018) employed a Deep Neural Network (DNN) combined with discrete wavelet transform (DWT) for feature extraction. Their classifier achieved competitive performance but highlighted the limitations of traditional techniques compared to advanced deep learning methods [2].
- The studies consistently emphasized the transition from handcrafted feature extraction in machine learning to automated feature learning in deep learning, providing superior results in medical imaging tasks.

2.4 Specific Tumor Types and Image Preprocessing

- Alqudah et al. (2020) focused on comparing cropped, uncropped, and segmented lesion images using CNNs. Their study demonstrated the importance of lesion-focused preprocessing in achieving high sensitivity and accuracy [9]

- Diaz-Pernas et al. (2021) utilized a multiscale CNN model for segmentation and classification. Their method leveraged T1-CE MRI data, achieving a classification accuracy of 97.3% by processing images at different spatial scales [5].

2.5 Challenges and Advancements

- The high inter-class similarity among tumor types such as gliomas and meningiomas posed significant challenges. Techniques like feature fusion, transfer learning, and multiscale processing were critical in addressing these challenges.
- Data imbalance and the need for high-quality annotated datasets were common issues. Solutions included transfer learning and augmentation strategies to enhance model robustness.

3 Methodology

3.1 Dataset

This study utilizes a dataset compiled from three established and widely recognized sources, Figshare, SARTAJ, and Br35H, comprising 7023 MRI images classified into four categories: glioma, meningioma, pituitary tumor, and no tumor. While Figshare provided accurately labeled tumor images, the Br35H dataset contributed non-tumor class images. The SARTAJ dataset was initially included for glioma classification; however, upon identifying misclassifications within its glioma class, those images were replaced with better labeled samples from Figshare to enhance accuracy. Images were resized to 224 × 224 pixels, and data augmentation techniques such as rotation, flipping, and brightness adjustments were applied to improve model performance and address class imbalance. The dataset was split into 70% for training, 15% for validation, and 15% for testing, ensuring a balanced and robust framework for model training and evaluation. This refined dataset significantly contributed to the high accuracy and reliability of the ResNet, DenseNet, and ensemble models proposed in this study.

3.2 Proposed Data Framework

3.2.1 Data Preprocessing

Preprocessing MRI images is a vital step for deep learning applications, promoting consistency, high-quality data, and accurate identification of target regions. The goal is to minimize noise, standardize dimensions, and isolate the region of interest

(ROI) containing the tumor, making it easier for neural networks to extract meaningful features during training and inference. MRI images sample dataset is shown in Fig. 5.1 and preprocessing flow is shown in Fig. 5.2.

The preprocessing pipeline includes the following transformations:

- **Grayscale Conversion**
- Each RGB image is converted to a single-channel grayscale image using Eq. (5.1) to reduce computational load and retain intensity information. This transformation is performed using a weighted average of RGB channels (Grayscale Conversion Equation):

$$I_{\text{gray}}(x,y) = 0.2989 * R + 0.5870 * G + 0.1140 * B \tag{5.1}$$

- **Gaussian Blurring**
- To eliminate high-frequency noise and enhance image smoothness, a Gaussian blur is implemented, leveraging the Gaussian smoothing function shown in Eq. (5.2):

$$I_{\text{blur}}(x,y) = \Sigma\Sigma G(i,j) * I(x-i, y-j) \tag{5.2}$$

- where $G(i, j)$ is the Gaussian kernel.

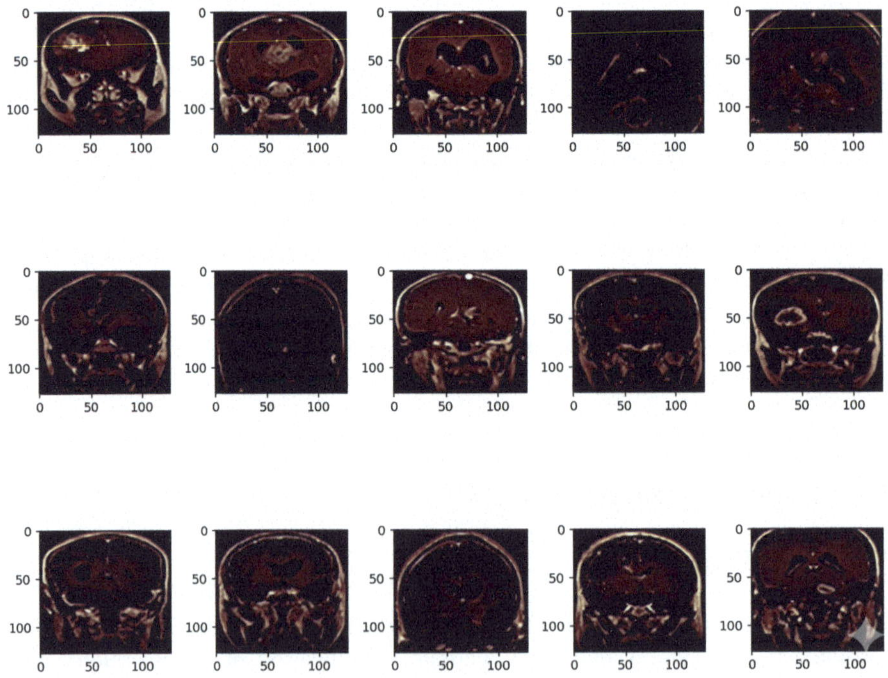

Fig. 5.1 MRI images

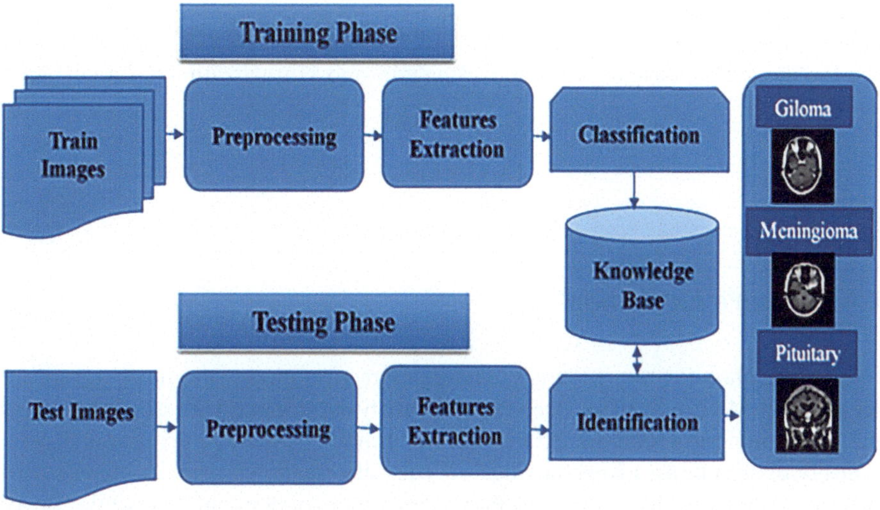

Fig. 5.2 MRI preprocessing pipeline

- **Binary Thresholding**
- The smoothed grayscale image is transformed into a binary mask using a thresholding condition (Binary Thresholding Equation) shown in Eq. (5.3):

$$I_{\text{bin}}(x,y) = 1\,\text{if}\,I(x,y) > T, 0\,\text{otherwise} \tag{5.3}$$

- **Morphological Operations: Erosion and Dilation**
- To refine the binary image, morphological operations are applied (Erosion and Dilation Equations):

$$\text{Erosion}: I_{\text{eroded}} = I_{\text{bin}} \ominus S$$

$$\text{Dilation}: I_{\text{dilated}} = I_{\text{eroded}} \oplus S$$

- where S is the structuring element used.
- **Contour Detection and ROI Cropping**
- Using contour detection algorithms (Contour Extraction Equation), the largest contour is identified. The extreme points (left, right, top, bottom) are used to define the ROI:

$$\text{ROI} = I\left[y_{\text{min}} : y_{\text{max}}, x_{\text{min}} : x_{\text{max}}\right]$$

- **Image Resizing**
- The cropped ROI is resized to match model input sizes—128 × 128 for ResNet50 and 150 × 150 for DenseNet201.

3.2.2 Normalization

Pixel values are scaled to a [0, 1] range using min-max normalization (Normalization Equation):

$$I_{\text{norm}}(x,y) = I(x,y)/255$$

3.3 *Feature Extraction*

To enhance classification accuracy, feature extraction targets the most significant details from MRI images for deep learning analysis. It identifies essential patterns within the region of interest (ROI), such as tumor boundaries, texture, and pixel intensity distributions, using statistical metrics like mean, variance, skewness, and kurtosis. Techniques like edge detection further refine tumor contours, while convolutional layers automatically learn hierarchical features, from basic edges to more complex tumor shapes [10, 11].

Techniques like Principal Component Analysis (PCA) streamline the feature set by eliminating redundancies while preserving essential information for MRI image analysis. By highlighting meaningful features, this step reduces data complexity, cuts down on computational demands, and boosts the model's accuracy and ability to generalize [7, 15].

4 Proposed Architecture

4.1 *ResNet50 Architecture*

The architecture is shown in Fig. 5.3.

1. **Input Layer**: The model starts with an input layer that accepts RGB images resized to 128 × 128 pixels. This consistent input size ensures uniformity for effective feature extraction.

   Each residual block computes the transformation using Eq. (5.4) shown in:

$$y = F(x,\{W\}) + Ws * x \tag{5.4}$$

   where
   x is the input to the block
   $F(x, \{W\})$ denotes the residual function composed of three sequential layers
   $\{Wi\}$ are the convolutional weights

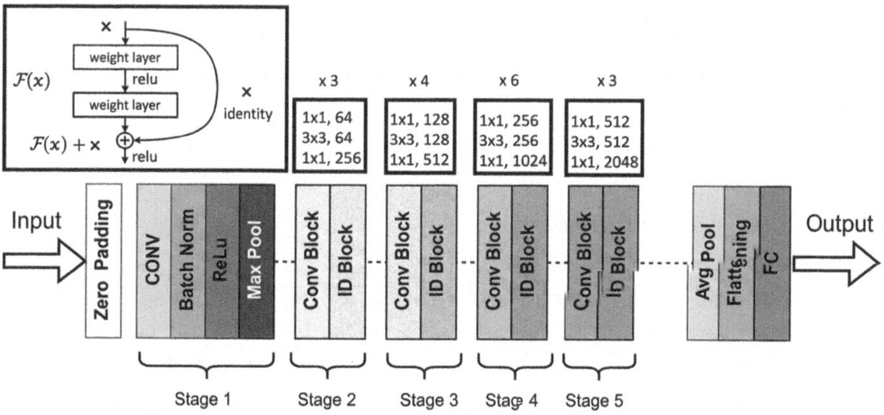

Fig. 5.3 ResNet50 architecture

2. **ResNet50 Backbone**: Utilizing a pre-trained ResNet50 backbone with ImageNet weights, the model includes 48 convolutional layers grouped into residual blocks with skip connections. This architecture helps prevent the vanishing gradient problem and supports deep feature learning.
3. **Global Average Pooling**: After feature extraction, a Global Average Pooling layer reduces the spatial dimensions of the feature maps, converting them into a compact vector that effectively summarizes the global features [16] using Eq. (5.5).

$$z\_k = \left(1 / H * W\right) * \Sigma\Sigma f\_ijk \tag{5.5}$$

4. **Fully Connected Layer**: A dense layer with 256 neurons and ReLU activation follows allowing the model to learn intricate patterns. L2 regularization is applied to prevent overfitting using Eq. (5.6).

$$h = ReLU\left(Wd * z + bd\right) \tag{5.6}$$

5. **Dropout and Batch Normalization**: Dropout layers with a rate of 0.3 are added to minimize overfitting, while Batch Normalization stabilizes activations and accelerates convergence.
6. **Output Layer**: The final layer consists of four neurons with SoftMax activation, representing the classification categories: glioma, meningioma, no tumor, and pituitary tumor.

   SoftMax is computed using Eq. (5.7):

$$p\_i = \exp\left(z\_i\right) / \Sigma \exp\left(z\_j\right) \text{for } j = 1 \text{to} 4 \tag{5.7}$$

where
z_i is the input to the i-th neuron.

p_i is the predicted probability for the i-th class.

The model integrates ResNet50's robust feature extraction with tailored layers designed for brain tumor classification, optimizing both complexity and performance.

4.2 DenseNet Architecture

The model begins with an input layer that accepts RGB images resized to 150 × 150 pixels. This ensures compatibility with the DenseNet backbone and consistent feature extraction shown in Fig. 5.4.

- **DenseNet201 Backbone**: The pre-trained DenseNet201 model, with ImageNet weights, is utilized. It features densely connected layers within dense blocks, where each layer receives input from all previous layers. This dense connectivity improves feature reuse and gradient flow, enhancing efficient training and better parameter utilization. These include top parameter is set to False to exclude the fully connected layers, making the model more suitable for the brain tumor classification task [17].
- In DenseNet, each layer within a dense block receives the concatenated output of all preceding layers using Eq. (5.8):

$$x\_l = H\_l([x0, x1, \ldots, x\_\{l-1\}]) \tag{5.8}$$

- **Global Average Pooling**: A Global Average Pooling layer is applied to the DenseNet output to aggregate the feature maps and produce a compact feature vector, retaining key features while reducing spatial dimensions using Eq. (5.9).

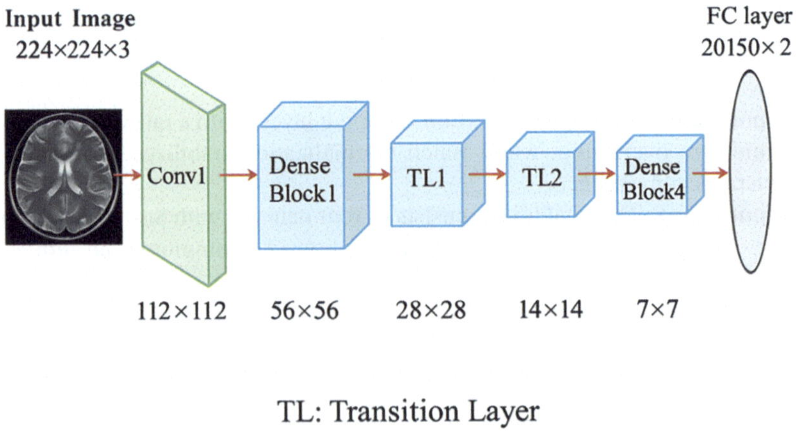

Fig. 5.4 DenseNet201 architecture

$$z\_k = (1 / H * W) * \Sigma\Sigma f\_ijk \tag{5.9}$$

- where
- *f_ijk* is the activation value at position (*i, j*) in the *k*-th feature map.
- *H* and *W* are the height and width of the feature map.
- *z_k* is the output value representing the average of the *k*-th feature map.
- **Fully Connected Layer**: A dense layer with 128 neurons and ReLU activation using Eq. (5.10) is added, introducing non-linearity and enabling the model to learn complex patterns specific to the classification task.

$$h = ReLU(W\_d * z + b\_d) \tag{5.10}$$

- **Output Layer**: The final layer contains four neurons with SoftMax activation, corresponding to the classification categories: no tumor, pituitary tumor, meningioma, and glioma.
- SoftMax is computed as:

$$p\_i = \exp(z\_i) / \Sigma \exp(z\_j) \text{ for } j = 1 \text{ to } 4$$

- Where
- *z_i* is the input to the *i*-th neuron.
- *p_i* is the predicted probability for the *i*-th class.
- **Data Augmentation**: Real-time data augmentation is applied using Image Data-Generator, incorporating variations such as horizontal flips, width/height shifts, and shear transformations. This improves the model's ability to generalize by exposing it to diverse data.
- **Training and Fine-Tuning**: Initially, the DenseNet backbone is frozen to preserve its pre-trained weights while training the added layers on the dataset. After initial training, the backbone can be unfrozen for fine-tuning to further improve performance. This architecture leverages Dense Net's efficient feature propagation and combines it with tailored layers for brain tumor classification, ensuring robust predictions and minimizing overfitting.

4.3 Ensemble Model Architecture

- **Input Layer**: The ensemble model shown in Fig. 5.5 begins by accepting pre-processed test images, with different resizing configurations for each base model:
- ResNet: Input images are resized to 128 × 128 pixels.
- DenseNet: Input images are resized to 150 × 150 pixels.
- Both image sets are normalized using an ImageDataGenerator, rescaling pixel values to a range of 0 to 1.

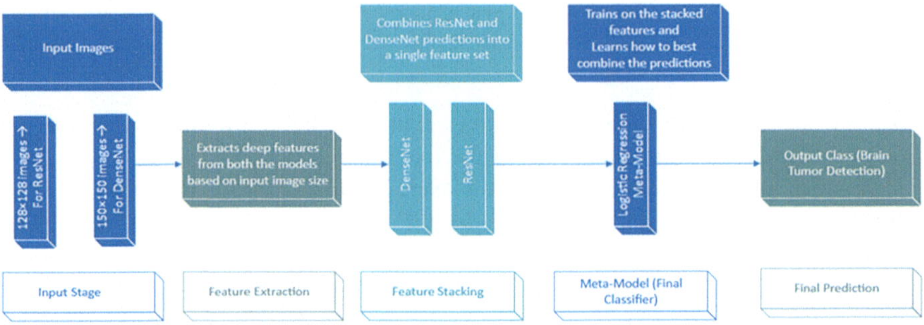

Fig. 5.5 Ensemble Framework (ResNet50 + DenseNet201)

- **Base Models**:
  (a) **ResNet**: The first base model is a pre-trained ResNet (resent final.h5). It processes images resized to 128 × 128 pixels and outputs a SoftMax probability vector for each class, indicating the likelihood of each classification.
  (b) **DenseNet**: The second base model is a pre-trained DenseNet (dense net final.h5). It processes images resized to 150 × 150 pixels and similarly outputs a SoftMax probability vector for each class. Both ResNet and DenseNet work independently to extract features and generate probabilistic predictions for the dataset.

- **Feature Stacking**: The probabilistic outputs (SoftMax vectors) from both ResNet and DenseNet are concatenated horizontally to create a single feature vector for each image [18]. This stacked feature vector serves as the input for the meta-classifier.
  (a) A Logistic Regression model is employed as the meta-classifier.
  (b) The concatenated feature vectors are divided into training and testing sets with a 70–30 ratio.
  (c) A Logistic Regression model is trained on the training set, optimizing weights to integrate predictions from ResNet and DenseNet effectively. The meta-classifier then generates the final predictions based on the combined features.

  Both the ResNet50-based and DenseNet201-based models independently generate class probabilities for each input image using their respective SoftMax output layers:

$$p_r = \text{SoftMax}(z_r) \text{and } p\_d = \text{SoftMax}(z\_d)$$

where:
$p_r \in R^4$ is the probability vector from ResNet.
$p\_d \in R^4$ is the probability vector from DenseNet.
z_r and z_d are the pre-activation outputs of the final dense layers in the respective networks.

- **Training and Evaluation**:
  (a) The Logistic Regression model is trained on the stacked feature vectors along with the true class labels.
  (b) During evaluation, the model predicts the class for each test image and calculates various performance metrics, including accuracy, precision, recall, and F1-score.
- This ensemble architecture effectively combines the unique strengths of ResNet and DenseNet by leveraging their independent predictions through a meta-classifier. This approach enhances overall accuracy and robustness in classifying brain tumors.

5 Result and Discussion

5.1 ResNet-50

The ResNet model delivers exceptional performance, attaining a 99% overall accuracy with high precision, recall, and F1-scores across all classes. The confusion matrix indicates minimal misclassifications, while the classification report demonstrates consistent performance, with metrics ranging from 0.98 to 0.99 for each class. The training and validation accuracy curves align closely, with the validation accuracy stabilizing near the training accuracy, indicating excellent generalization. Both the training and validation loss curves show a steady decline, without any noticeable overfitting, as both losses stabilize at low levels by the end of training. This strong performance highlights Reset's ability to extract hierarchical features effectively through its residual connections, enabling it to learn complex patterns with ease. The model maintains a solid balance between training and validation metrics, ensuring reliable results. Although the current performance is already highly dependable, further performance enhancement could be achieved by using an ensemble with complementary architectures like DenseNet or applying additional regularization techniques. Figures 5.6 and 5.7 shows the accuracy and loss curve of ResNet50. Figure 5.8 shows the confusion matrix of ResNet50, respectively.

5.2 DenseNet

The DenseNet model demonstrates outstanding performance, achieving perfect classification metrics with 100% precision, recall, and training process of Resnet50 F1-scores across all tumor categories (no tumor, pituitary tumor, meningioma tumor, and glioma tumor). This indicates that the model has mastered the task and performs exceptionally well on the test dataset. The slight gap between training and validation accuracy suggests minimal overfitting, which does not significantly hinder the approach's ability to generalize. The training and validation loss curves

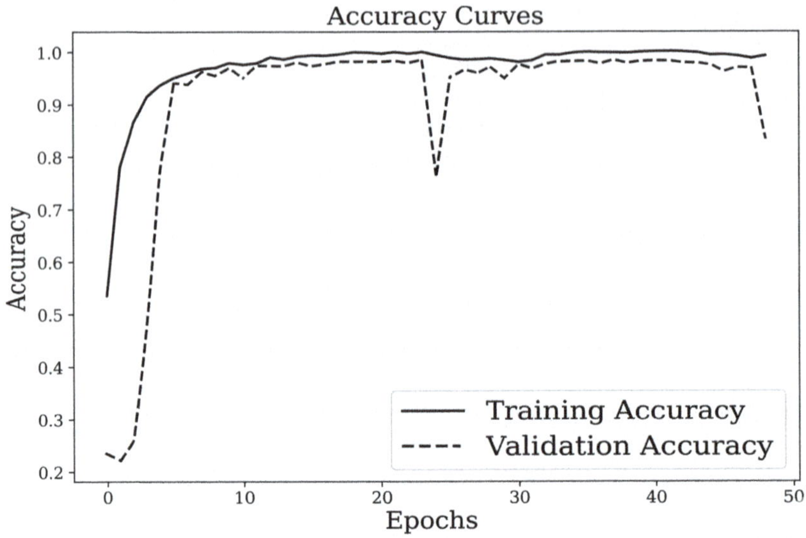

Fig. 5.6 ResNet50 Accuracy Curve

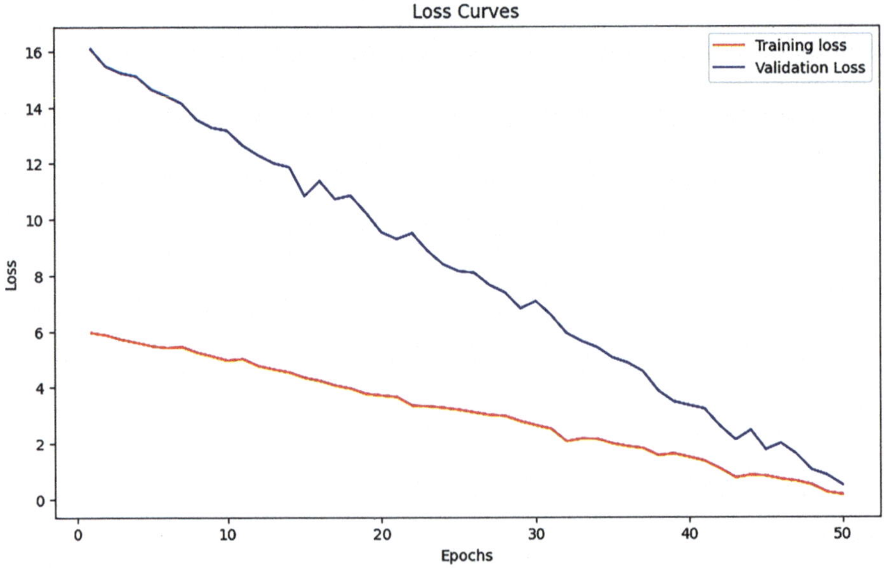

Fig. 5.7 ResNet50 Loss Curve

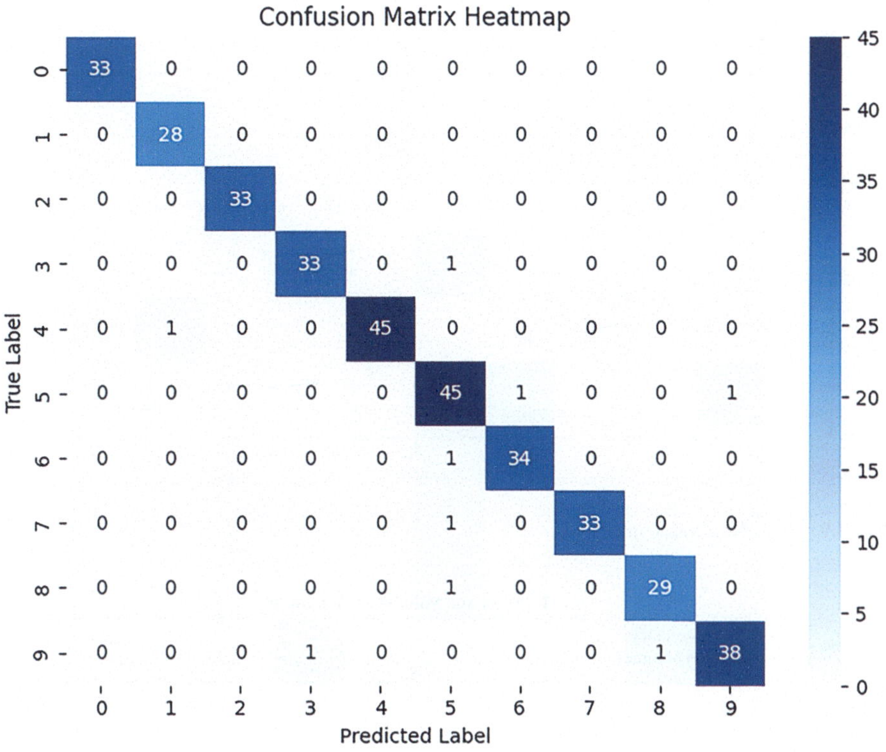

Fig. 5.8 Confusion Matrix-ResNet50

indicate steady learning, with training loss decreasing to 0.1 and validation loss converging around 0.2. However, intermittent spikes in validation loss between epochs 10 and 15 point to minor overfitting, which could be addressed with additional regularization techniques like stronger dropout or L2 regularization. DenseNet's architecture, which capitalizes on dense connectivity and feature reuse, proves highly effective for complex classification tasks. While the model delivers excellent results, further fine-tuning or the use of ensemble methods (such as combining with ResNet) could enhance both performance and stability. Figures 5.9, 5.10, and 5.11 show the loss curve, the accuracy curve, and the few performance measures of the DenseNet, respectively.

5.3 *Ensemble Model*

The model achieves an impressive overall accuracy of 98. This level of accuracy indicates that the model has successfully learned to generalize across the dataset with minimal misclassifications. Although the results are excellent, small

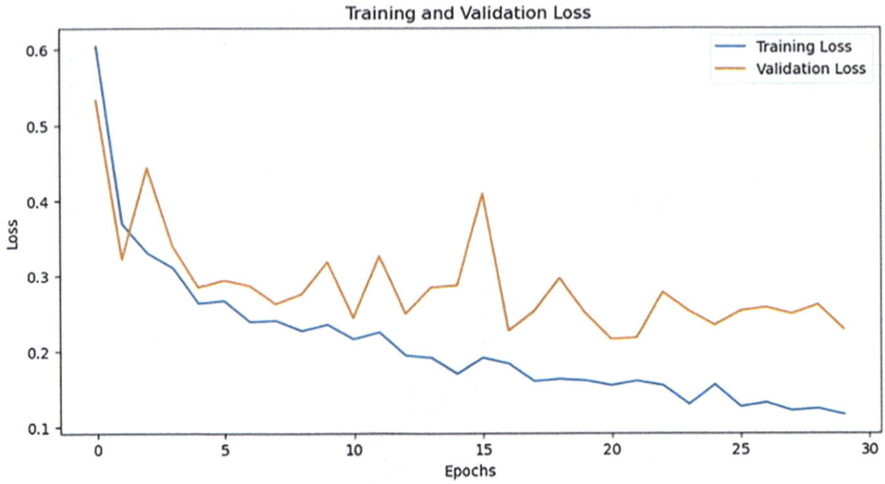

Fig. 5.9 DenseNet Loss Curve

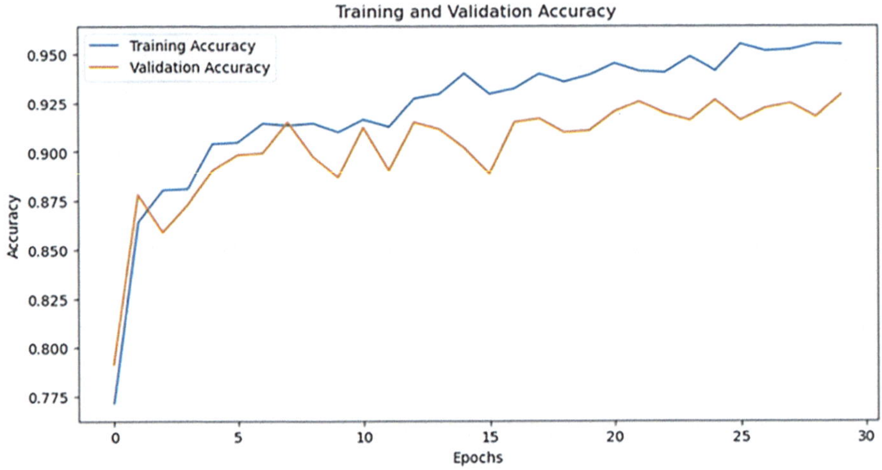

Fig. 5.10 DenseNet Accuracy Curve

adjustments, such as adding regularization techniques or fine-tuning hyperparameters, could help optimize the model further. Overall, this performance underscores the model's reliability and effectiveness for the classification task at hand. Figures 5.12 and 5.13 show performance matrix and confusion matrix of ensemble method, respectively.

	precision	recall	f1-score	support
no_tumor	1.00	1.00	1.00	237
pituitary_tumor	1.00	1.00	1.00	302
meningioma_tumor	1.00	1.00	1.00	318
glioma_tumor	1.00	1.00	1.00	286
accuracy			1.00	1143
macro avg	1.00	1.00	1.00	1143
weighted avg	1.00	1.00	1.00	1143

Fig. 5.11 DenseNet Training Accuracy

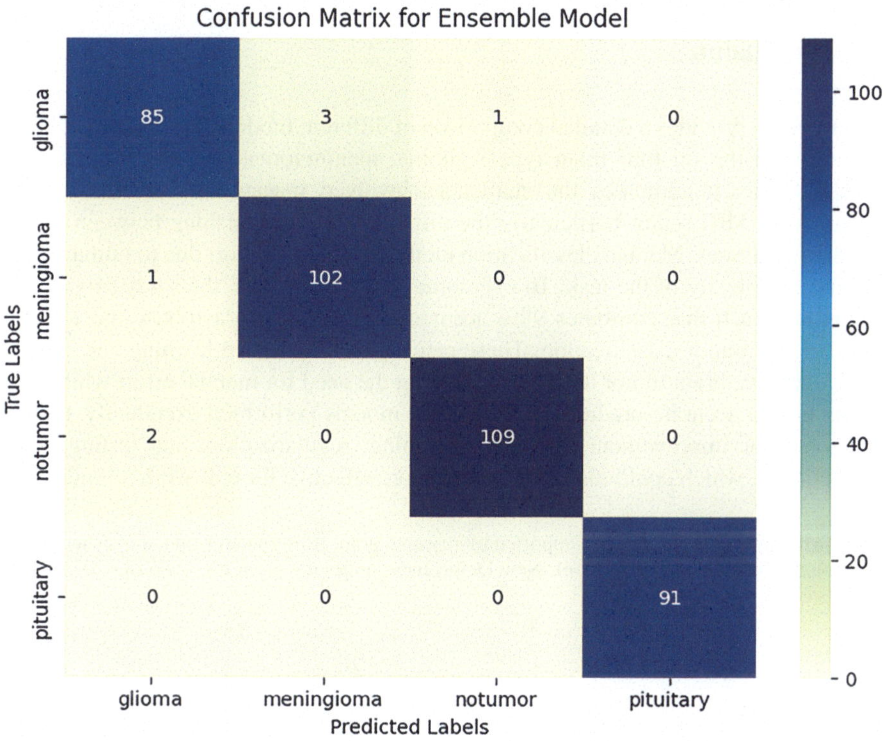

Fig. 5.12 Confusion matrix of ensemble method, respectively

Classification Report:

	precision	recall	f1-score	support
0	0.97	0.96	0.96	89
1	0.97	0.99	0.98	103
2	0.99	0.98	0.99	111
3	1.00	1.00	1.00	91
accuracy			0.98	394
macro avg	0.98	0.98	0.98	394
weighted avg	0.98	0.98	0.98	394

Fig. 5.13 Performance matrix of ensemble method, respectively

6 Conclusion

This research provides a detailed comparison of different models for classifying brain tumors, focusing on four main types: glioma, meningioma, pituitary tumors, and healthy tissue. It addresses the challenges involved inaccurately detecting brain tumors from MRI scans, particularly the difficulty in distinguishing between tumor and normal tissues. Manual classification methods often fall short due to human error and the complexity of the task. To overcome these challenges, the study proposes a hybrid approach that combines 98% accuracy, proving to be a robust and reliable approach for tumor classification. These results show that deep learning can significantly improve brain tumor detection, reducing the need for manual effort while providing highly accurate predictions. While the models performed excellently, there's still room for improvement through fine-tuning, regularization, and testing other architectures, which could make them even more effective for real-world clinical use.

Acknowledgment This work is supported by research grant from Indian Council of Science and Technology (Ministry of Education), New Delhi, India under the grant no. 48/WLD-2025-1888/SCD dated 18.09.2025.

References

1. Sharif MI, Khan MA, Alhussein M, Aurangzeb K, Raza M (2021) A decision support system for multimodal brain tumor classification using deep learning. Complex Intell Syst:1–14
2. Mohsen H, El-Dahshan ESA, El-Horbaty ESM, Salem ABM (2018) Classification using deep learning neural networks for brain tumors. Future Comput Inf J 3(1):68–71
3. Khan MA, Ashraf I, Alhaisoni M, Damasevicius R, Scherer R, Rehman A, Bukhari SAC (2020) Multimodal brain tumor classification using deep learning and robust feature selection: a machine learning application for radiologists. Diagnostics 10(8):565
4. Kang J, Ullah Z, Gwak J (2021) MRI-based brain tumor classification using ensemble of deep features and machine learning classifiers. Sensors 21(6):2222

5. Dıaz-Pernas FJ, Martınez-Zarzuela M, Anton-Rodrıguez M, Gonzalez Ortega D (2021) A deep learning approach for brain tumor classification and segmentation using a multi scale convolutional neural network. Healthcare 9(2):153
6. Huang J, Ding W, Zhong T, Yu G (2025) YOLO-TumorNet: an innovative model for enhancing brain tumor detection performance. Alex Eng J 119:211–221
7. Remzan N, Tahiry K, Farchi A (2024) Advancing brain tumor classification accuracy through deep learning: harnessing radimagenet pre-trained convolutional neural networks, ensemble learning, and machine learning classifiers on MRI brain images. Multimed Tools Appl 83(35):82719–82747
8. Whiteside TL (2008) The tumor microenvironment and its role in promoting tumor growth. Oncogene 27(45):5904–5912. https://doi.org/10.1038/onc.2008.271
9. Alqudah AM, Alquraan H, Qasmieh IA, Alqudah A, Al-Sharu W (2020) Brain tumor classification using deep learning technique—a comparison between cropped, uncropped, and segmented lesion images with different sizes. arXiv preprint arXiv:2001.08844
10. Joshi AA, Aziz RM (2024) Deep learning approach for brain tumor classification using metaheuristic optimization with gene expression data. Int J Imaging Syst Technol 34(2):e23007
11. Yaqoob A, Aziz RM, Verma NK, Lalwani P, Makrariya A, Kumar P (2023) A review on nature--inspired algorithms for cancer disease prediction and classification. Mathematics 11(5):1081
12. Makrariya A, Aziz RM, Saha A, Cengiz K, Shah MA, Mallik S (2025) A machine learning validation for identifying the difference between benign cysts and malignant tumor in breast cancer
13. Islam MN, Azam MS, Islam MS, Kanchan MH, Parvez AS, Islam MM (2024) An improved deep learning-based hybrid model with ensemble techniques for brain tumor detection from MRI image. Inf Med Unlocked 47:101483
14. Zahoor MM, Qureshi SA, Bibi S, Khan SH, Khan A, Ghafoor U, Bhutta MR (2022) A new deep hybrid boosted and ensemble learning-based brain tumor analysis using MRI. Sensors 22(7):2726
15. Afreen S, Bhurjee AK, Aziz RM (2025) Feature selection using game Shapley improved grey wolf optimizer for optimizing cancer classification. Knowl Inf Syst 67(4):3631–3662
16. Sharma A, Kumar P, Ben D, Bikhani M, Aziz RM (2025) Improved GA based clustering with a new selection method for categorical dental data. In: Swarm optimization for biomedical applications. CRC Press, pp 172–192
17. Poornima PU, Tamilalagan S, Praveen Raj D, Pongiannan RK, Jishnu KS, Thanalakshmi S (2024) Brain tumor classification using RESNET-50 and Efficientnet-B0. In: International conference on evolutionary artificial intelligence. Springer Nature Singapore, Singapore, pp 27–39
18. Khan SUR, Zhao M, Asif S, Chen X (2024) Hybrid-NET: a fusion of DenseNet169 and advanced machine learning classifiers for enhanced brain tumor diagnosis. Int J Imaging Syst Technol 34(1):e22975

Chapter 6
Advanced ML, DL, and Optimization Techniques for EEG Signal Analysis

Harish Velingkar, Roopa R. Kulkarni, Prashant P. Patavardhan, Shaunak Pai Kane, and Senthilkumar Vijayakumar

1 Introduction

Electroencephalography (EEG) is a noninvasive technique used to record the brain's electrical activity through electrodes placed on the scalp. Its high temporal resolution, safety, and relatively low cost make it widely used in fields like neurology, clinical diagnostics, and human-computer interaction. However, EEG data presents significant challenges due to its inherently low signal-to-noise ratio (SNR), non-stationary nature, and variability between individuals, all of which complicate accurate processing and interpretation.

H. Velingkar (✉)
Visvesvaraya Technological University, Belagavi, Karnataka, India

Agnel Institute of Technology & Design, Assagao, Goa, India

R. R. Kulkarni
Visvesvaraya Technological University, Belagavi, Karnataka, India

Dayananda Sagar Academy of Technology and Management (DSATM), Bangalore, Karnataka, India
e-mail: roopakulkarni-ece@dsatm.edu.in

P. P. Patavardhan
Visvesvaraya Technological University, Belagavi, Karnataka, India

RV Institute of Technology & Management, Bangalore, Karnataka, India

S. P. Kane
Kelly Services, Troy, MI, USA

S. Vijayakumar
IEEE, Troy, MI, USA

S. Mallik et al. (eds.), *Landscape of Signaling Pathway and Genetic Markers in Cardio-Brain Oncology*, Studies in Rhythm Engineering,
https://doi.org/10.1007/978-981-95-7012-6_6

Traditional EEG analysis has been labor-intensive, subjective, and relying on non-scalable manual visual inspection. However, now EEG signal analysis can detect both spatial and temporal resolutions owing to the development of ML/DL techniques [1]. These techniques enable automated feature extraction from raw signals and may depict nonlinear associations in high-dimensional EEG data.

Optimization techniques also play a very important role in EEG signal processing, selecting the most relevant EEG channels, and fine-tuning model hyperparameters [2]. In cases where manual tuning or grid search becomes impractical or time-consuming, metaheuristic algorithms such as Genetic Algorithms (GA), Particle Swarm Optimization (PSO), and Bayesian Optimization have proven highly effective at navigating complex, high-dimensional parameter spaces.

The entire process from signal acquisition to practical application is given below:

$$\text{Raw}\,EEG \xrightarrow{\text{Preprocessing}} \text{Clean Signal} \xrightarrow{\text{Feature Extraction}} \mathbf{X} \xrightarrow{\text{Classification}} \hat{y}$$

Here $\mathbf{X} \in R^{n \times d}$ denotes the feature matrix derived from EEG epochs, where n is the number of samples and d is the number of features. The output $\hat{y}$ represents the predicted cognitive or emotional states corresponding to those samples.

Recent advancements have introduced powerful deep learning models complimenting the unique characteristics of EEG data. Convolutional Neural Networks (CNNs) are commonly used to capture spatial patterns across electrode signals, while Long Short-Term Memory (LSTM) networks and transformers are effective at modeling the temporal dynamics of brain activity. Graph Neural Networks (GNNs) have also emerged as valuable tools for understanding the topological relationships between electrodes. Hybrid architectures such as CNN-LSTM combinations and attention-enhanced CNNs have shown improved performance in various applications, including drowsiness detection, cognitive state monitoring, and early diagnosis of neurological disorders.

This chapter offers a review of how advanced machine learning, deep learning, and optimization techniques can be integrated into EEG processing. It presents a modern perspective on their practical applications in areas such as brain-computer interfaces, clinical diagnostics, cognitive monitoring, and neurofeedback systems.

2 AI-Based Framework for EEG Processing

The use of AI/ML in EEG signal processing follows a systematic framework designed to efficiently convert raw brain signals into actionable insights [3]. This process is typically depicted in the form of a block diagram comprising five stages: signal acquisition, preprocessing, feature extraction, classification, and application in brain-computer interface (BCI) (Fig. 6.1).

The AI-based EEG processing pipeline, as depicted above, consists of the following primary stages:

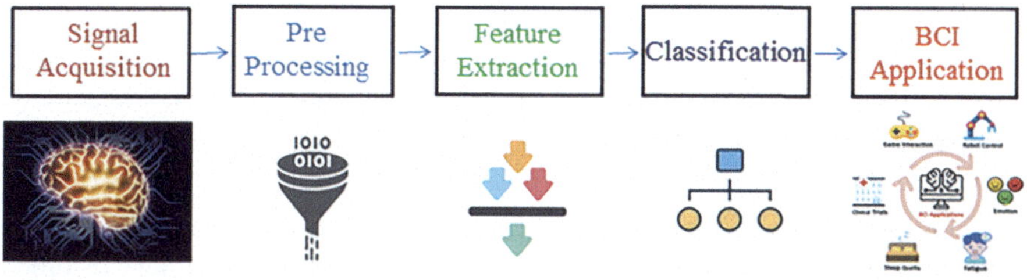

Fig. 6.1 Block diagram of AI-based framework for EEG processing

1. **Signal acquisition**: In this stage, the EEG signals are recorded using electrodes placed on the scalp. The EEG signal quality depends on factors such as EEG electrode placement, surrounding noise, equipment noise, skin impedance, and various other factors.
2. **Preprocessing**: Raw EEG may contain certain artifacts. In order to make the data more accurate and reliable, it needs to be pre-processed. Hence, preprocessing algorithms such as filtering, normalization, and Independent Component Analysis (ICA) are used.
3. **Feature extraction**: Feature extraction involves marking of all the features from the processed EEG signals. Extracted features may include frequency components like the different EEG bands (Alpha, Beta, etc.), statistical descriptors, entropy details, etc.
4. **Feature selection**: Feature selection involves selecting the relevant extracted features and separating them from the less relevant ones. This helps in making the system more efficient by reducing the computational time.
5. **Classification**: The selected features are then classified and labeled to various cognitive states of the human mind.
6. **BCI application**: At the end, the selected features from the EEG signals can be used for various applications which include detection of neurological disorders, control and operation of prosthetics, and other BCI applications.

Below is the explanation for each of these blocks in detail:

2.1 *Signal Acquisition*

EEG acquisition involves tapping of the brain waves using EEG electrodes attached to the scalp. These electrodes are conventionally placed as per the 10–20 system. Various factors affect the quality of signals tapped from these electrodes which include skin impedance, various artifacts, hardware efficiency, etc. [4].

Basically, EEG works by measuring voltage differences generated by postsynaptic potentials in cortical neurons. These potentials are typically captured in the microvolt (μV) range. The basic voltage signal from an electrode $V_i(t)$ is modeled as:

$$V_i(t) = S_i(t) + N_i(t)$$

where $S_i(t)$ is the true brain signal, and $N_i(t)$ represents noise (from muscle activity, environmental sources, electrode motion, etc.) (Fig. 6.2).

Some of the key parameters in EEG acquisition are [5]:

- **Sampling frequency** (f_s): Sampling frequency in EEG signal acquisition refers to the number of times per second the EEG signal is measured and recorded expressed in Hertz (Hz). Standard EEG investigations utilize frequencies ranging from 128 to 1000 Hz. The Nyquist criteria stipulate that $f_s \geq 2f_{\max}$, where $f_{\max}$ is the greatest frequency of interest.
- **Bit resolution**: It refers to the number of bits used to represent each sampled data point, determining the precision and detail of the recorded signal.
- **Electrode impedance**: It refers to how much the electrode resists the flow of electrical signals at the point of contact, which can affect how clear or noisy the EEG recording is. To get good-quality signals with minimal noise, the electrode impedance should ideally be kept below 5 kΩ.
- **Montage type**: Montage type refers to the way EEG electrodes are arranged and how their signals are compared to each other. The chosen montage affects how brain activity is visualized and interpreted, helping highlight specific patterns or regions of interest.

EEG devices which aid in signal acquisition come in various forms, each designed to suit different research, clinical, or consumer applications. Below are the main types of EEG devices.

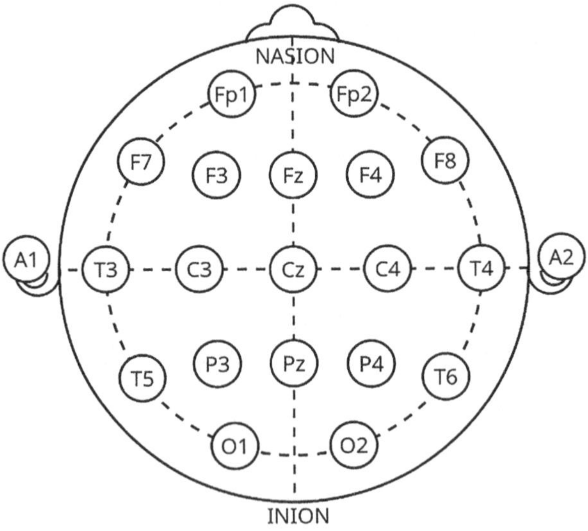

Fig. 6.2 10–20 system for EEG acquisition

1. **Wet electrodes**
   Wet or gel-based electrodes use conductive gel to improve contact between the skin and the sensor, resulting in high-quality signal acquisition. They're often used in clinical and research settings where precision is critical. However, applying and cleaning the gel can be time-consuming, making them less ideal for long-term or everyday use.
2. **Dry electrodes**
   Dry electrodes eliminate the need for gels, making them faster and more convenient to set up especially for wearable applications or real-time brain-computer interface (BCI) systems. While they offer greater comfort and ease of use, they may suffer from a lower signal-to-noise ratio compared to wet electrodes, especially during movement.
3. **Wearable/consumer devices**
   Devices like *Emotiv*, *Muse*, and *NeuroSky* are designed for everyday users interested in mindfulness, focus training, or basic brain monitoring. These devices are suitable for compact applications, lab studies, and general cognitive feedback applications owing to their compact size and portability. They may not be as accurate as other EEG electrodes used for clinical applications.
4. **Clinical systems**
   Clinical systems are designed for clinical research and medical use. Normally, the number of electrodes here range from 32 to 256 and gives the most accurate and reliable data. The signals so acquired can be used for real-time monitoring of patients, epilepsy detection, neurorehabilitation, and other critical applications.

2.1.1 Event-Related Potential (ERP)

Event-related potentials are changes in EEG based on some external stimuli provided which may be visual, auditory, somatosensory, etc. This involves observing changes in certain parameters of EEG like the P300 or N400 components. Mathematically, it is represented as [6]:

$$EEG(t) = \sum_{k=1}^{K} w_k \cdot s_k(t - \tau_k) + \epsilon(t)$$

where $s_k(t)$ are stimulus-related components, τ_k are latency values, and $\epsilon(t)$ is residual noise. Latest EEG hardware also detect changes in skin impedance, eye tracking and blink detection, and other artifacts as a part of the inbuilt signal processing module.

Quality of EEG signals depends on a lot of factors. Firstly, the skin impedance has to be as low as possible. In case of wet electrodes, a gel is used to help in reducing the skin—electrode impedance. Other artifacts include muscle movement, physical movements of the subject, aging of the EEG equipment itself, eye movements and eye blinks, etc. Detection and removal of these artifacts plays a critical role in the entire signal processing block.

2.2 *Preprocessing of EEG Signals*

Preprocessing plays an important role in the EEG analysis block diagram, particularly when preparing data for machine learning and deep learning models. Raw EEG signals are often affected by various types of noise and artifacts such as eye blinks, muscle movements, power-line interference, and other external disturbances which can distort the signal. If not properly addressed, these issues can compromise the quality of the data and lead to inaccurate interpretations or model predictions.

EEG signals are often affected by noise from both environmental sources and the body's own physiological activities. To improve the quality of the data, preprocessing techniques like filtering, normalization, and Independent Component Analysis (ICA) are commonly used to reduce interference and isolate meaningful brain signals. Optimization methods such as Genetic Algorithms (GA) and Particle Swarm Optimization (PSO) are then applied to fine-tune the preprocessing process, making it more efficient and effective for analysis.

The main goal of preprocessing is to clean and standardize the EEG signals while preserving their important features needed for meaningful analysis. This typically involves the following key techniques:

2.2.1 Filtering

EEG signals are generally restricted in bandwidth and affected by low-frequency drift and high-frequency noise. Typical filtration procedures include:

1. **Bandpass filtering**: To separate frequency ranges pertinent to cognition (e.g., 0.5–45 Hz).

$$x_f(t) = x(t) * h(t)$$

   where $x(t)$ is the raw EEG, $h(t)$ is the filter impulse response, and * denotes convolution.
2. **Notch filtering**: Generally, at 50/60 Hz to eradicate power-line interference

$$H(f) = 1 - \frac{f_0^2}{f^2 + j\gamma f + f_0^2}$$

   where f_0 is the notch frequency and γ is the damping factor.

2.2.2 Artifact Removal Techniques

EEG recordings often contain unwanted signals, or artifacts, that do not originate from brain activity such as eye blinks, muscle movements, or electrical interference []. These artifacts can distort the data and affect the accuracy of analysis. Artifact removal techniques are designed to identify and eliminate these disturbances ensuring that the EEG signals reflect true activity of the brain. Some of the techniques include:

1. **Independent component analysis (ICA)**: A popular blind source separation technique that disaggregates EEG into statistically independent components:

$$\mathbf{X} = \mathbf{A} \cdot \mathbf{S} \Rightarrow \mathbf{S} = \mathbf{W} \cdot \mathbf{X}$$

   where $\mathbf{X}$ the observed EEG matrix, $\mathbf{S}$ is the source matrix, and $\mathbf{W} = \mathbf{A}^{-1}$ is the unmixing matrix.

   Independent component analysis (ICA) is a widely used technique for cleaning EEG signals by separating them into independent sources. It is particularly effective in isolating and removing artifacts caused by eye movements (electro-oculography, or EOG) and muscle activity (electromyography, or EMG). By identifying and filtering these unwanted components, ICA helps to preserve the true EEG signals needed for accurate analysis.
2. **Wavelet denoising**: Analyzes EEG signals by decomposing them into multi-resolution components by discrete wavelet transform (DWT):

$$x(t) = \sum_{k} a_{j_0,k} \phi_{j_0,k}(t) + \sum_{j=j_0}^{J} \sum_{k} d_{j,k} \psi_{j,k}(t)$$

   where $\phi_{j,k}(t)$ and $\psi_{j,k}(t)$ are scaling and wavelet functions, respectively.

   Wavelet denoising is another powerful technique used to clean the EEG signals by breaking them down into different frequency components. This method allows precise localization of noise and artifacts, e.g., those which are caused by muscle movements or external interference across both time and frequency domains. By selectively suppressing unwanted signal components while retaining the essential features of brain activity, wavelet denoising improves signal clarity without significantly distorting the underlying neural information.
3. **Automated artifact removal (AAR)**: Automated artifact removal (AAR) uses machine learning and deep learning to identify and remove noise from EEG recordings with least human intervention. These systems are trained to identify patterns that are linked to artifacts, like anomalous temporal activity, statistical outliers (z-scores), or unusual amplitude spikes. AAR techniques can automatically identify and eliminate problematic channels or noisy segments (epochs) by examining these indicators. This enhances the EEG data's overall quality while also saving time and effort, which makes it particularly useful for real-time or large-scale applications [8].

4. **Epoching and baseline correction**: To prepare EEG data for meaningful analysis, two important preprocessing steps are often applied: epoching and baseline correction. Epoching involves segmenting the continuous EEG signal into fixed time intervals which is centered around specific events or stimuli (e.g., from −100 ms to +500 ms relative to the start of an event). This allows to precisely link brain activity to the timing of external stimuli. Once the data is segmented, baseline correction is performed to remove any slow voltage drifts or DC offsets. This is usually done by subtracting the average voltage recorded during a pre-stimulus period, ensuring a more stable and comparable signal across trials.

$$x_{\text{corrected}}(t) = x(t) - \frac{1}{N}\sum_{i=1}^{N} x(t_i)$$

5. **Re-referencing**: An essential part of EEG preprocessing is re-referencing, which enhances spatial resolution and lowers noise to improve signal clarity. It involves changing the reference point for each electrode, which could have an impact on how brain activity is interpreted.

   Some common reference methods include:

   (a) **Average reference**: The average reference is a frequently employed technique that involves subtracting the average voltage across all electrodes from the voltage across each individual channel. This reduces the bias brought about by any one reference electrode and produces a more balanced picture of the overall activity of the brain.

$$x_i^{avg}(t) = x_i(t) - \frac{1}{N}\sum_{j=1}^{N} x_j(t)$$

   (b) **Linked mastoid reference**: In this technique, the reference signal is tapped by placing the reference electrodes behind both the ears (over the mastoid bone). Since this location is relatively isolated, it has less interference from the active brain signals and therefore gives relatively stable reference signals which are required in a clinical setting.

6. **Channel interpolation and bad channel detection**: Sometimes due to artifacts such as subject movements or movement of electrodes some of the EEG signals tapped from these positions can give a flat line or sudden spikes in amplitude and other random behavior. Instead of ignoring and eliminating this data directly, statistical tools such as Z-Score or amplitude thresholds are set. The signal which would have been acquired from these positions in the ideal situation is then extrapolated from the signals from the other working electrodes using techniques such as spherical spline interpolation. This helps is maintaining the accuracy and consistency of the entire dataset.

2.3 Feature Extraction in EEG Analysis

Feature extraction involves detection of patterns from the EEG signal and isolating them in order to enhance the accuracy of classification using the suitable AL/ML techniques. Some of the latest techniques such as Genetic Algorithms and Particle Swarm Optimization are being used to make the feature extraction process computationally more efficient. They help in identifying features such as frequency characteristics, entropy data, and other statistical data making the EEG-based systems more accurate and reliable. If irrelevant or wrong features are used to train, the models can get computationally very complex and time-consuming leading to inaccurate results. This effect is even more in EEG signals which by nature are intricate and non-stationary in nature.

Some of the commonly extracted features from EEG signals are:

1. **Time domain features**: Time domain features like mean, variance, skewness, etc. help us determine how the EEG signal varies over time. Other features like Hjorth parameters give details about other complex features of the signal like activity, mobility, etc. Metrics like zero-crossing rate and peak amplitude are often used to help identify different mental states based on how the brain's electrical activity shifts over time. The mathematical representation of these time domain measurements are as shown below:

   Statistical measurements

   Statistical measurements like mean and variance provide a simple way to describe EEG signals. The mean reflects the average signal level over time, while variance indicates how much the signal fluctuates, helping to capture the brain's activity.

   Let $x(t)$ represent the EEG signal over time. The mean and variance are computed as:

$$\mu = \frac{1}{N}\sum_{i=1}^{N} x_i, \sigma^2 = \frac{1}{N}\sum_{i=1}^{N}(x_i - \mu)^2$$

   Hjorth parameters

   Hjorth parameters (activity, mobility, and complexity) are used to describe the shape and behavior of EEG signals over time. Activity shows the overall power of the signal, mobility reflects how fast the signal changes, and complexity indicates how unpredictable or irregular those changes are.

   Hjorth descriptors are defined as:

$$\text{Activity} = Var(x), \quad \text{Mobility} = \sqrt{\frac{Var(\dot{x})}{Var(x)}}, \quad \text{Complexity} = \frac{\text{Mobility}(\dot{x})}{\text{Mobility}(x)}$$

   Zero crossing rate (ZCR): It measures how often the EEG signal crosses the zero voltage line, indicating changes in signal polarity. A higher ZCR usually reflects more rapid fluctuations in brain activity and can be useful for detecting different mental or emotional states. Mathematically, it is represented as:

$$ZCR = \frac{1}{T-1}\sum_{t=1}^{T-1} 1_{[x(t)\cdot x(t+1) < 0]}$$

2. **Frequency domain features**: While time domain features show how EEG signals vary over time, frequency domain features reveal how the brain's electrical activity is spread across different wave patterns. These brainwaves like delta, theta, alpha, beta, and gamma are linked to different mental states such as relaxation, focus, or drowsiness. By analyzing how much energy is present in each frequency band using measures like power spectral density (PSD), mean band power, and spectral entropy, researchers can gain valuable insights into the brain's overall activity and cognitive state. The mathematical representation of these time domain measurements are as shown below:

   Power spectral density (PSD): Power spectral density (PSD) is a widely used frequency domain feature that shows how the power of an EEG signal is distributed across different frequency bands. It helps identify which brainwaves are most active during a given mental state. By visualizing and quantifying the energy in these bands, PSD provides a clearer picture of brain activity and is useful in tasks like emotion recognition, attention monitoring, and sleep analysis. The PSD estimated via Welch's method is represented as:

$$P(f) = \frac{1}{K}\sum_{k=1}^{K} \mathcal{F}\{x_k(t)\}^2$$

   where $\mathcal{F}$ is the Fourier Transform and x_k are segmented windows.

   Relative band power (RBP): Relative band power (RBP) measures how much energy a specific frequency band (like alpha or theta) contributes compared to the total power across all bands. It gives a normalized view of brain activity, making it easier to compare across individuals or sessions. RBP is especially helpful in identifying shifts in mental states, such as increased theta power during drowsiness or higher alpha activity during relaxation. It is represented as the ratio of power in a specific band to total power:

$$RBP_{\delta} = \frac{\int_{0.5}^{4} P(f)df}{\int_{0.5}^{45} P(f)df}$$

   Spectral entropy: Spectral entropy gives us an idea of how unpredictable or complex the brain's activity is by looking at how energy is spread across different frequency bands. If the energy is evenly distributed, the signal is considered more random and has higher entropy which is often linked to active thinking or alertness. On the other hand, a lower entropy suggests a more regular pattern, which can occur during relaxed or drowsy states. This makes spectral entropy especially useful for studying changes in attention, mental effort, or levels of consciousness. It is mathematically represented as:

$$H = -\sum_i p_i \log(p_i), \quad p_i = \frac{P(f_i)}{\sum_j P(f_j)}$$

Here $P(f_i)$ is the power (or energy) of the EEG signal at a specific frequency f_i.
$\sum_j P(f_j)$ is the total power across all the frequency components.
p_i is the normalized power at frequency f_i.

The patterns in brain signals are however much more complex than what the traditional linear methods can capture. Therefore to extract these complex traits, we require nonlinear methods such as empirical mode decomposition (EMD) and its other forms. Metrics such as fractal dimensions and Lyapunov exponent can also be used to determine the extent of randomness in the EEG signals. The description of some of these nonlinear techniques is as given below:

Fractal dimension (FD): Fractal dimension unlike other linear techniques talks about the roughness or randomness of the EEG signal. A higher fractal dimension indicates more complexity or randomness, i.e., a higher brain activity which can be correlated to either a very high cognitive state of mind like solving a puzzle or certain neurological disorders like ADHD, etc.

Lyapunov exponent (λ): Lyapunov exponent is a nonlinear measure used to understand how sensitive a system is to small changes. It represents how tiny differences in brain activity can grow and lead to very different outcomes over time. In terms of EEG analysis, it helps detect the level of instability in the brain signals. A higher Lyapunov exponent suggests that the brain's electrical activity is more dynamic (less predictable) which can be useful for identifying mental states like stress, epilepsy, or cognitive overload. By tracking how quickly brain signals start to drift apart, the Lyapunov exponent helps reveal the brain's hidden complexities and its tendency toward an unstable activity. Mathematically, it is represented as:

$$\lambda = \lim_{t \to \infty} \frac{1}{t} \ln \frac{d(t)}{d(0)}$$

λ is the *Lyapunov exponent*, a measure of how sensitive a system (like the brain's electrical activity) is to small initial changes.

t represents time.

$d(0)$ is the initial distance between two very close starting points in the system.

$d(t)$ is the distance between those two trajectories after time t.

Entropy measures: Entropy measures help to understand how unpredictable or complex the brain's electrical activity is. Instead of just looking at how strong or fast the signals are entropy focuses on how random or regular the patterns appear over time. This makes it especially useful for spotting changes in mental states like when someone becomes stressed, loses focus, or transitions into sleep. There are different types of entropy, such as approximate entropy, sample entropy, and permutation entropy, and each offers its own way of measuring how much information or irregularity is present in the brain's signals. For example, mathematically approximate entropy (ApEn) is given as:

$$ApEn(m,r,N) = \Phi^m(r) - \Phi^{m+1}(r)$$

m is the embedding dimension, i.e., the length of sequences being compared in the time series.

r is the tolerance or similarity threshold. This value defines how close two patterns must be to be considered similar.

N is the length of the time series.

$\Phi^m(r)$ represents the average logarithmic probability.

Empirical mode decomposition (EMD): Empirical mode decomposition (EMD) is a method used to break down complex EEG signals into simpler parts called intrinsic mode functions (IMFs). What makes EMD special is that it adapts to the shape of the signal itself, instead of using fixed formulas like traditional methods. This makes it helpful for analyzing EEG data, which is often irregular and constantly changing. By separating the signal into these components, EMD helps reveal hidden patterns in brain activity that might otherwise go unnoticed.

EMD decomposes signal $x(t)$ into intrinsic mode functions (IMFs):

$$x(t) = \sum_{i=1}^{N} IMF_i(t) + r(t)$$

$x(t)$ is the original EEG signal.

$\text{IMF}_i(t)$ is the i-th intrinsic mode function extracted from the signal.

N is the total number of IMFs obtained from the decomposition process.

$r(t)$ is the residual or remaining trend in the signal after all IMFs have been extracted.

Common spatial pattern (CSP): This is a widely used method in EEG analysis, especially for brain-computer interface (BCI) tasks like recognizing imagined movements. It works by finding patterns in the brain's electrical activity that clearly separates two mental states. For example, imagining moving your left hand versus your right. CSP creates special filters that bring out the differences between these states, making it easier for machine learning models to tell them apart. Because of its ability to highlight meaningful patterns, CSP is one of the best techniques for real-time EEG applications. Its mathematical representation is given by:

$$J(\mathbf{w}) = \frac{\mathbf{w}^\top \mathbf{C}_1 \mathbf{w}}{\mathbf{w}^\top \mathbf{C}_2 \mathbf{w}}$$

where $J(\mathbf{w})$ is the objective function in CSP. It represents the ratio of variances (or energy) of the projected signal in two different classes.

$\mathbf{w}$ is the spatial filter vector and C_1 and C_2 are co-variance matrices.

Filter bank CSP (FBCSP): FBCSP is a more advanced version of CSP. In this instead of applying CSP on the entire EEG signal, the signal is first subdivided into smaller chunks (using filter banks) [7]. This breakdown of the signal in frequency domain thus helping to classify and represent the details of individual frequency bands of the signal in a more accurate way.

Riemannian features: Riemannian geometry-based features give the relationship between different parts of the brain during a cognitive task. It uses covariance matrices to compare the activity of the EEG signal tapped from the various electrodes. This helps to determine and pinpoint the exact locations where the trigger is created by a given stimuli [9]. Its mathematical representation is given by:

$$\delta(\Sigma_1, \Sigma_2) = \log\left(\Sigma_1^{-1/2} \Sigma_2 \Sigma_1^{-1/2}\right)_F$$

where $\delta(\Sigma_1, \Sigma_2)$ is the Riemannian distance between two covariance matrices.

Σ_1, Σ_2 are covariance matrices derived from EEG data of two different trials.

2.4 Feature Selection in EEG Analysis

Selecting the most relevant features becomes especially important, given how complex and high-dimensional EEG data can be. Techniques like recursive feature elimination (RFE), L1 regularization (LASSO), and ReliefF are commonly used to identify which features contribute most to make the most accurate predictions. In addition, optimization methods such as genetic algorithms (GA), particle swarm optimization (PSO), and ant colony optimization are often applied to automatically search for the best combination of features. These approaches not only improve model performance but also make the system more efficient by reducing unnecessary data.

The way features are extracted from EEG signals plays a major role in how well classification models perform. Recent advances include the use of attention mechanisms, which allow models to focus on the most important parts of the signal both over time and across different brain regions. There's also a growing trend toward hybrid methods that combine traditional handcrafted features with those learned by deep learning models, leading to more accurate and adaptable systems.

The theoretical foundations of feature selection process are as given below:

Let $\mathbf{X} = [x_1, x_2, \ldots, x_n]$ be the feature matrix with n extracted features from EEG signals, and $\mathbf{y}$ be the associated class labels or regression targets. Feature selection aims to identify a subset $\mathbf{X}_S \subset \mathbf{X}$, such that the mapping $f: \mathbf{X}_S \rightarrow \mathbf{y}$ maximizes performance metrics (e.g., accuracy, F1-score, AUC) and minimizes the generalization error.

Formally, this can be posed as an optimization problem:

$$\arg \max_{S \subset \{1,\ldots,n\}} \mathcal{J}(S) - \lambda |S|$$

where $\mathcal{J}(S)$ is a performance criterion (e.g., classification accuracy or mutual information) evaluated on the feature subset S, and λ is a regularization parameter controlling sparsity.

2.4.1 Feature Selection Techniques

Once the features are extracted, we need to select the most relevant and dynamic features needed to effectively train our models. Selection of the correct time domain, frequency domain features as well as the channels which show changes upon exposure to stimuli help in training the AL/ML models effectively and make them computationally more efficient. Feature selection techniques such as filter methods and wrapper methods are used to accomplish the above task. The methods are explained in brief below:

Filter methods: Filter methods are independent of any specific algorithm or model. Methods like mutual information (MI) use statistical parameters to correlate how much a feature extracted resembles its label. Fisher score is another method which helps to correlate variations between groups to variations within a group and helps to classify the target. Other correlation parameters like Pearson or Spearman are used to grade how certain features are linearly related to an output.

Wrapper methods: Wrapper methods are used to find the best suitable features by practically trying them out one by one and checking which one gives the best output. This is also called recursive feature elimination technique. It uses models like support vector machines (SVM) and random forest (RF) to do so. This can be done in two ways: Either by adding features one by one and checking the output (forward selection) or by removing features one by one (backward elimination), ultimately leading to the features which will give the most efficient and accurate output. Wrapper methods are slightly time-consuming; however, they lead to better results as they pinpoint features which will give the most reliable outputs.

Embedded methods: Embedded methods combine the best features of filter and wrapper techniques. A well-known example is LASSO (Least Absolute Shrinkage and Selection Operator), which not only builds a prediction model but also filters out less useful features by shrinking their weights down to zero. This helps the model focus only on what really matters. Also tree-based models such as decision trees, random forests, and gradient boosting automatically highlight important features as they learn. They do this by measuring how much each feature helps split the data and make accurate predictions [10].

Mathematically, the LASSO objective function is represented as:

$$\min_{\beta}\left(\frac{1}{2n}\sum_{i=1}^{n} y_i - \mathbf{x}_i^{\top}\beta)^2 + \lambda \parallel \beta \parallel_1\right)$$

$\min_{\beta}$ tries to minimize the overall loss with respect to the model's coefficients.

N is the total number of training examples or data points.

y is the actual output or target value.

β are the vector of model coefficients (parameters) we want to learn.

$\mathbf{x}_i^{\top}\beta$ is the predicted value for y_i.

Besides the traditional methods, several advanced techniques are now being used to improve the feature selection process in EEG analysis. The ReliefF algorithm ranks features by examining how well they distinguish between nearby data points from the same or different classes making it useful for noisy and complex EEG datasets. Minimum redundancy maximum relevance (mRMR) helps to balance between choosing features that are highly relevant to the output while avoiding redundancy among them [11]. Techniques from manifold learning, like t-SNE and UMAP, are also gaining popularity as they reduce high-dimensional feature sets into simpler visual forms, helping to spot patterns and select meaningful features. Neural networks known as "autoencoders" provide latent representations of the data and can highlight the most important features when given additional sparsity constraints. Lastly, by identifying the features or channels that have the greatest influence on predictions, SHAP values provide insights into model decision-making.

2.5 *Classification Techniques in EEG Analysis*

Once features are extracted from the EEG signals, the next important step is classification of these signals where the goal is to interpret the data by sorting it into known cognitive or physiological states. Here the model learns to recognize patterns linked to things like attention levels, emotions, or intended actions [7]. Depending on how complex the data is and what the task involves, researchers may use either traditional machine learning algorithms or more advanced deep learning models. This step plays a key role in translating brain activity into understandable and useful information.

Some of the traditional ML classifiers are:

Support vector machine (SVM): Support vector machines (SVMs) are widely used for classifying EEG signals because they can handle high-dimensional data well and are less likely to overfit, even with complex inputs. What makes SVMs particularly useful is their kernel trick, which allows them to perform non-linear classification thus helping them recognize patterns in EEG data that aren't linearly separable. Some commonly used kernels include the radial basis function (RBF) and polynomial kernels, which make SVMs flexible and effective for detecting a wide range of brain activity patterns. Mathematically, the equation for SVM decision boundary is given by [12]:

$$f(x) = sign\left(\sum_{i=1}^{N} \alpha_i y_i K(x_i, x) + b\right)$$

where $K(x_i, x)$ is the kernel function, and α_i are Lagrange multipliers [15].

k-Nearest neighbors (k-NN): k-NN is one of the most used classification techniques. Here a data point is compared with all its neighbors and then given the most appropriate label. It is non-parametric in nature and makes no assumption about the data being processed. Although being a very popular classification technique, k-NN is less efficient in signals like EEG have high dimensionality unless the features are reduced [13].

Random forest (RF): Random forest is a more advanced technique as compared to k-NN. It is based on the fundamental principal of decision trees. It averages the outputs of the decision trees and combines them to produce the most accurate prediction of a model. It is particularly useful the data with higher dimensionality such as EEG [14].

Deep learning is another technology being widely used in signal classification especially for complex signals such as EEG. Due to its ability to learn directly from the raw signals, DL methods can classify a data point based on its changes in terms of time and space without the need of any manual intervention. DL methods are very effective in accomplishing complex tasks such as stress level detection, detecting certain neurological disorders, and seizure predictions. Some of the popular DL methods are given below:

Convolutional neural networks (CNNs): CNNs are a great tool to recognize patters in a signal both with respect to time and spatial differences. It works on time-frequency images. The input to CNNs is normally the frequency information of a signal like a spectrogram obtained from transformation techniques like Short-Time Fourier Transform or a wavelet transform. It then processes this data through multiple layers of convolution, ReLU, pooling leading to an accurate classification. Although CNNs are very efficient, another method called long short-term memory (LSTM), which is a recurrent neural network, is generally used in recognizing patterns in a complex signal like the EEG. They're especially useful for tracking long-term dependencies and variations in EEG sequences. [16].

The LSTM cell equations, for example, are mathematically represented as:

$$f_t = \sigma\left(W_f \cdot [h_{t-1}, x_t] + b_f\right) \text{— Forget Gate}$$

$$i_t = \sigma\left(W_i \cdot [h_{t-1}, x_t] + b_i\right) \text{— Input Gate}$$

$$o_t = \sigma\left(W_o \cdot [h_{t-1}, x_t] + b_o\right) \text{— Output Gate}$$

$$C_t = f_t * C_{t-1} + i_t * \tanh\left(W_C \cdot [h_{t-1}, x_t] + b_C\right) - \text{Cell State Update}$$

Transformer-based models: Transformer-based models have recently shown strong potential in EEG analysis, especially for complex tasks like motor imagery and emotion recognition. Unlike traditional models, transformers use attention mechanisms to focus on important parts of the signal and capture long-range relationships across time. This makes them particularly effective for decoding the brain's dynamic and distributed activity.

Hybrid and ensemble models: In EEG analysis, hybrid models that combine CNNs and LSTMs are often used to capture both spatial and temporal patterns simultaneously. Ensemble methods, like combining SVM with random forest or CNN with LSTM, help improve accuracy and reduce variability. More advanced setups, such as meta-classifiers (e.g., stacking) combine the strengths of multiple models and have achieved best performance in areas like emotion recognition and seizure detection. To fine-tune these models, techniques like grid search, Bayesian optimization, and metaheuristics like genetic algorithms (GA) and particle swarm optimization (PSO) are commonly used for hyperparameter tuning. Building effective EEG-based systems requires selecting the appropriate model and optimization technique (Fig. 6.3).

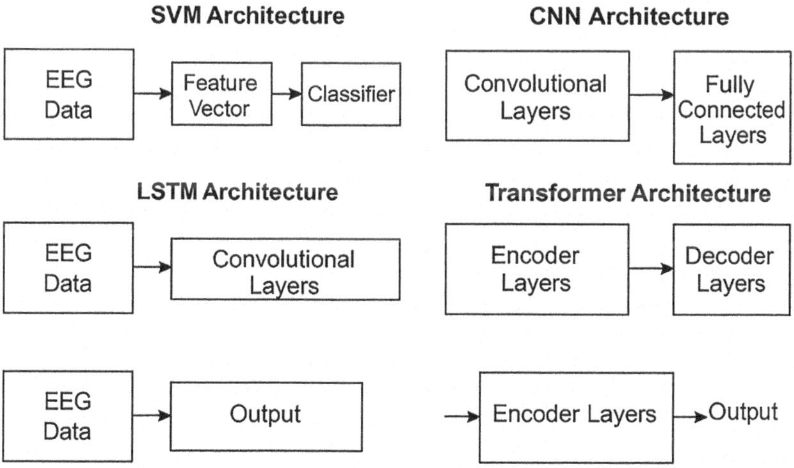

Fig. 6.3 Architecture comparison: SVM, CNN, LSTM, transformer models for EEG classification

3 Summary

Understanding and interpreting brain signals through EEG is incredibly valuable in fields like brain-computer interfaces (BCIs), healthcare, and cognitive monitoring. But EEG data comes with its own set of challenges. It's often noisy, varies from person to person, and changes over time. This chapter explores how advanced machine learning (ML), deep learning (DL), and optimization techniques can help make sense of this complex data more effectively.

The chapter spans through the complete EEG processing pipeline, starting from signal acquisition and noise removal to the extraction of meaningful features and their use in training predictive models. The chapter highlights techniques for capturing meaningful patterns in the data, through traditional methods or more advanced ones like deep learning models (CNNs, LSTMs, Transformers) that can learn directly from the raw signals. It also looks at hybrid and ensemble models, which combine different strengths to boost accuracy and stability. Another important focus is on feature selection and tuning, showing how algorithms like genetic algorithms (GA), particle swarm optimization (PSO), and Bayesian optimization help in choosing the right input features and improving model performance.

While the chapter highlights key challenges like the need for large datasets, model complexity, and computational demands, it overlooks some practical issues. These include variability in EEG hardware, differences in signal quality across individuals, and the gap between lab results and real-world use. Ethical concerns around data privacy also need more attention. Lighter, easier to understand, and data-efficient models will be crucial in the future, particularly for reliable clinical applications.

References

1. Craik A, He Y, Contreras-Vidal JL (2019) Deep learning for electroencephalogram (EEG) classification tasks: a review. J Neural Eng 16(3):031001. https://doi.org/10.1088/1741-2552/ab0ab5
2. Roy Y, Banville H, Albuquerque I, Gramfort A, Falk TH, Faubert J (2019) Deep learning-based electroencephalography analysis: a systematic review. J Neural Eng 16(5):051001. https://doi.org/10.1088/1741-2552/ab260c
3. Sweeney-Reed CM, Nasuto SJ, Vieira MF, Andrade AO (2018) Empirical mode decomposition and its extensions applied to EEG analysis: a review. Biomed Signal Process Control 40:291–309
4. Nunez PL, Srinivasan R (2006) Electric fields of the brain: the neurophysics of EEG. Oxford University Press, Oxford, UK
5. Teplan M (2002) Fundamentals of EEG measurement. Meas Sci Rev 2(2):1–11
6. Wang F et al (2020) Emotion recognition with convolutional neural network and EEG-based EFDMs. Neuropsychologia 146:107506
7. Venkat VPB, Chinara S (2021) Automatic classification methods for detecting drowsiness using wavelet packet transform extracted time domain features from single channel EEG signal. J Neurosci Methods 347:108927

8. Mognon A, Jovicich J, Bruzzone L, Buiatti M (2011) ADJUST: an automatic EEG artifact detector based on the joint use of spatial and temporal features. Psychophysiology 48(2):229–240. https://doi.org/10.1111/j.1469-8986.2010.01061.x
9. Barachant A, Bonnet S, Congedo M, Jutten C (2012) Multiclass brain–computer interface classification by Riemannian geometry. IEEE Trans Biomed Eng 59(4):920–928
10. Wang Y, Zheng Y (2010) Spatial filter selection with LASSO for EEG classification. In: Advances in neural networks—ISNN 2010. Springer, pp 114–121. https://doi.org/10.1007/978-3-642-13657-3_15
11. Singh P, Dey N (2014) Selection of relevant features from cognitive EEG signals using ReliefF and mRMR. In: Proc. int. conf. frontiers intell. comput.: theory appl. (FICTA). Springer, pp 121–128. https://doi.org/10.1007/978-3-319-11933-5_13
12. Liu Y, Zhang Y, Wang Y (2022) EEG signal classification via pinball universum twin support vector machine. Ann Oper Res 313:1–20. https://doi.org/10.1007/s10479-022-04922-x
13. Kumar A, Sharma D (2023) A distributed and energy-efficient KNN for EEG classification with mRMR feature selection. Computing 105(4):1–15. https://doi.org/10.1007/s00607-023-01193-7
14. Liu Y, Wang Y (2015) Patient-specific epilepsy seizure detection using random forest classifier. In: Proc. int. conf. brain informatics health. Springer, pp 1–10. https://doi.org/10.1007/978-3-319-53480-0_51
15. Zemmal N et al (2018) Robust feature selection algorithm based on transductive SVM wrapper and genetic algorithm: application on computer-aided glaucoma classification. Int J Intell Syst Technol Appl 17(3):310–346
16. Whitehead A (2018) Classification of depressed patients: a cluster analysis–derived grouping. Br J Psychiatry

Chapter 7
Study in Therapeutic Approaches in Cancer: The Role of Ion Channels and Transporters

L. Hima, Sneha S. Thampy, Uday P. Pratap, Aneesh Nair, and Korhan Cengiz

1 Introduction

1.1 Global Cancer Burden and Limitations of Current Therapies

Cancer remains one of the foremost global health challenges, with escalating incidence and mortality rates across all regions of the world. According to GLOBOCAN 2022 estimates, approximately 20 million new cancer cases and over 9.7 million cancer-related deaths were reported globally, reflecting the significant and persistent public health burden of malignant diseases. This burden is compounded by demographic changes, lifestyle-associated risk factors, and increased detection rates. The heterogeneity of tumors, spanning a multitude of histological types and molecular subtypes, further complicates effective disease management. Particularly in low- and middle-income countries, limited healthcare infrastructure and inequities in access to diagnostics and treatment exacerbate cancer-related morbidity and mortality [1].

L. Hima (✉) · S. S. Thampy · A. Nair
Department of Allied Health Sciences, Noorul Islam Centre for Higher Education, Kanyakumari, Tamil Nadu, India

U. P. Pratap
Department of Obstetrics and Gynecology, University of Texas Health San Antonio, San Antonio, TX, USA

K. Cengiz
Department of Electrical Engineering, Prince Mohammad Bin Fahd University, Al Khobar, Saudi Arabia
e-mail: kcengiz@pmu.edu.sa

S. Mallik et al. (eds.), *Landscape of Signaling Pathway and Genetic Markers in Cardio-Brain Oncology*, Studies in Rhythm Engineering,
https://doi.org/10.1007/978-981-95-7012-6_7

While the advent of cytotoxic chemotherapeutics, radiotherapy, and surgery has markedly improved survival rates in certain cancers, these conventional modalities are often associated with substantial toxicity, nonspecific targeting, and development of resistance. Chemotherapeutic agents, though potent, indiscriminately damage both malignant and rapidly dividing normal cells, resulting in adverse effects such as myelosuppression, mucositis, and cardiotoxicity. Additionally, intrinsic and acquired mechanisms of multidrug chemoresistance severely limit long-term therapeutic efficacy. Radiotherapy similarly faces challenges of normal tissue damage and radioresistance. Although targeted therapies and immunotherapies have revolutionized cancer care, their benefits are largely confined to subsets of patients, underscoring the need for broader, more precise, and less toxic treatment paradigms [2].

Given these limitations, there is an urgent impetus to develop novel therapeutic strategies that move beyond the traditional cytotoxic paradigm and instead exploit specific molecular vulnerabilities of cancer cells while sparing normal tissues. Emerging evidence implicates ion channels and transporters, traditionally recognized as regulators of cellular homeostasis, as pivotal contributors to cancer pathogenesis, tumor progression, and therapy resistance. Their dysregulated expression and function in malignant cells compared to normal counterparts present a promising avenue for therapeutic intervention, offering opportunities for selective targeting and overcoming MDR. This chapter explores the global cancer burden in the context of current therapeutic limitations and sets the stage for examining the role of ion channels and transporters as novel anticancer targets. The global burden of cancer remains a significant public health challenge, with approximately 20 million new cases and nearly 9.7 million deaths recorded annually. Breast cancer has emerged as the most frequently diagnosed cancer worldwide, while lung cancer continues to be the leading cause of cancer-related mortality, particularly in low- and middle-income countries where mortality rates are disproportionately high [1, 3]. These key epidemiological parameters are summarized in Table 7.1.

Table 7.1 Selected Global Cancer Statistics (2022)

Epidemiological parameter	Observed data	References
New cancer cases worldwide	~20 million	Sung et al. [1]
Cancer-related deaths worldwide	~9.7 million	Sung et al. [1]
Leading cancer type (incidence)	Breast cancer	Sung et al. [1]
Leading cause of cancer death	Lung cancer	Sung et al. [1]
Regions with highest mortality	Low- and middle-income countries	Bray et al. [3]

1.2 Importance of Targeted Approaches Beyond Cytotoxic Drugs

The development of cancer therapies has historically relied on agents that exert cytotoxic effects on rapidly dividing cells. Conventional chemotherapeutics, while effective in certain contexts, are fundamentally limited by their lack of selectivity, leading to significant toxicity and limited long-term survival benefits for many malignancies [2]. The recognition of cancer as a genetically and epigenetically heterogeneous disease, driven by specific molecular aberrations, has transformed therapeutic paradigms in oncology. Targeted therapies aim to selectively inhibit oncogenic pathways, mutated proteins, or aberrantly expressed receptors that are critical for tumor cell survival and proliferation, thereby minimizing damage to normal tissues.

Several classes of targeted agents have emerged over the past two decades, including small molecule kinase inhibitors, monoclonal antibodies, and immune checkpoint inhibitors. These agents have demonstrated efficacy in subsets of patients with well-defined molecular alterations, exemplified by the success of imatinib in breakpoint cluster region-abelson murine leukemia (BCR-ABL)-positive chronic myeloid leukemia, trastuzumab in human epidermal growth factor receptor 2 (HER2)-overexpressing breast cancer, and estimated Glomerular Filtration Rate (EGFR) inhibitors in non-small cell lung carcinoma with activating mutations [2]. Beyond oncogene addiction, targeted approaches have also extended to components of the tumor microenvironment, angiogenesis pathways, and immune evasion mechanisms [4]. These advances underscore the value of identifying and exploiting tumor-specific vulnerabilities to achieve improved therapeutic indices compared to nonspecific cytotoxic agents.

Nevertheless, targeted therapies are not without limitations. Tumor heterogeneity and clonal evolution can lead to the emergence of resistant subpopulations. Additionally, not all cancers harbor actionable mutations or display dependency on a single oncogenic pathway, posing challenges in broad applicability. Combinatorial strategies, rational drug design based on molecular profiling, and integration with immunotherapy represent ongoing efforts to overcome these barriers. Notably, emerging evidence implicates non-classical targets, such as ion channels, solute carriers, and transporters, as key regulators of cancer cell physiology and potential novel therapeutic targets. These proteins influence critical processes such as ion homeostasis, apoptosis resistance, migration, invasion, and multidrug efflux, presenting an underexplored opportunity to complement or enhance existing targeted approaches [5].

The transition from empirical cytotoxic regimens to mechanism-based targeted therapies reflects a paradigm shift in oncology, emphasizing precision medicine and personalized treatment. Continued research to uncover and validate novel, cancer-specific targets remains essential to expand the therapeutic armamentarium and improve outcomes for patients with diverse malignancies. A fundamental distinction exists between traditional cytotoxic therapies and modern targeted therapies, particularly in their mechanisms of action, selectivity, toxicity profiles, patterns of resistance, and applicability across cancer types. While cytotoxic agents non-selectively kill rapidly dividing cells, targeted therapies are designed to interfere with specific molecular pathways dysregulated in tumors shown in Table 7.2.

1.3 Role of Ion Channels and Transporters in Normal Physiology

Ion channels and membrane transporters are indispensable components of cellular physiology, maintaining homeostasis and enabling numerous vital processes in both excitable and non-excitable cells. These membrane proteins mediate the regulated movement of ions and solutes across biological membranes, thereby sustaining the electrochemical gradients critical for normal cellular function [6]. Their coordinated activity underpins key biological phenomena, including membrane potential maintenance, intracellular signaling, volume regulation, nutrient uptake, and metabolic waste removal.

Ion channels are pore-forming proteins that enable selective, passive ion flux driven by electrochemical gradients. Among these, potassium (K^+) channels are pivotal in stabilizing the resting membrane potential and facilitating repolarization of excitable tissues following depolarization [7]. Calcium (Ca^{2+}) channels allow transient Ca^{2+} influx to initiate intracellular cascades regulating gene transcription, secretion, contraction, and proliferation [6]. Sodium (Na^+) channels contribute to action potential initiation and propagation as well as secondary active transport of nutrients via sodium-coupled carriers. Chloride (Cl^-) channels, on the other hand, play a key role in osmotic balance, pH regulation, and cell volume control, particularly in epithelial and neuronal tissues [8]. Mechanosensitive and stretch-activated channels provide the means for cells to detect and adapt to mechanical forces.

Membrane transporters, distinct from ion channels, facilitate the active or passive movement of larger molecules or charged metabolites across membranes. The solute carrier (SLC) family mediates the uptake of essential nutrients, including

Table 7.2 Comparison of cytotoxic and targeted cancer therapies

Features	Cytotoxic therapy	Targeted therapy	References
Mechanism of action	Nonspecific killing of dividing cells	Inhibition of specific molecular targets	Hanahan and Weinberg [2]
Selectivity	Low (affects normal and tumor cells)	High (tumor-specific pathways)	Hanahan and Weinberg [2]
Toxicity	High (myelosuppression, mucositis)	Lower, but target-related effects	Hanahan and Weinberg [2]
Resistance	Frequent (multidrug resistance)	Emerging via secondary mutations	Hanahan and Weinberg [2]
Applicability	Broad (most cancers)	Limited to defined molecular subtypes	Hanahan and Weinberg [2]

glucose, amino acids, and nucleotides, sustaining anabolic metabolism and energy production [9]. ATP-binding cassette (ABC) transporters are largely responsible for the efflux of xenobiotics, lipids, and metabolic by-products, thereby contributing to detoxification and lipid homeostasis [9]. Furthermore, these transporters regulate intracellular ionic composition and pH through proton, bicarbonate, and chloride exchange mechanisms. Together, these systems ensure that cells adapt to metabolic demands, environmental fluctuations, and developmental signals.

Dysregulation of ion channels and membrane transporters (ICT) is increasingly implicated in a spectrum of human diseases, including hereditary channelopathies, cardiovascular disorders, neurodegenerative diseases, and malignancies [7, 8]. Hence, understanding their physiological roles forms a foundation for elucidating how their aberrant function contributes to disease processes and for identifying potential therapeutic targets. Major classes of ion channels and transporters, including potassium, calcium, sodium, and chloride channels, as well as SLC and ABC transporters, perform essential physiological functions are labeled in Table 7.3.

1.4 Ion Channel and Transporter (ICT) Dysregulation in Cancer Pathogenesis

The aberrant expression and function of ion channels and transporters are increasingly recognized as key features of cancer pathogenesis. Once considered mere facilitators of ion and solute homeostasis, these membrane proteins are now understood to contribute directly to multiple hallmarks of cancer, including sustained proliferative signaling, resistance to apoptosis, angiogenesis, invasion, metastasis, and adaptation to a hostile microenvironment [2, 5]. Dysregulation may result from genetic mutations, epigenetic alterations, or transcriptional reprogramming, leading to changes in ion flux and solute gradients that promote tumor growth and survival.

Table 7.3 Major classes of ion channels and transporters in normal physiology

Protein class	Primary function	Physiological role	References
Potassium channels	Maintain resting membrane potential	Electrical excitability, volume regulation	Pardo and Stühmer [10]
Calcium channels	Mediate Ca^{2+}influx	Signaling, secretion, contraction	Monteith et al. [11]
Sodium channels	Mediate Na^{+} influx	Action potential, secondary transport	House et al. [12]
Chloride channels	Maintain osmotic and pH homeostasis	Volume regulation, excitability	Huber [13]
SLC transporters	Nutrient and metabolite uptake	Energy metabolism, biosynthesis	César-Razquin et al. [14]
ABC transporters	Efflux of xenobiotics and lipids	Detoxification, lipid homeostasis	Fletcher et al. [15]

Deregulated potassium (K^+) channels in cancer cells lower the threshold for depolarization, facilitating cell cycle progression and enabling hyperproliferation. Moreover, altered (K^+) channel activity modulates cell volume changes necessary for migration and invasion [10]. Calcium (Ca^{2+}) channels and pumps are often overexpressed in tumors, resulting in aberrant intracellular (Ca^{2+}) signaling that promotes proliferation, evasion of apoptosis, epithelial–mesenchymal transition (EMT), and angiogenesis [11]. Sodium (Na^+) channels, particularly the voltage-gated Na_υ isoforms, are upregulated in several carcinomas and linked to increased invasiveness and metastatic potential through enhancement of protease secretion and motility [12]. Similarly, chloride (Cl^-) channels contribute to the regulation of intracellular pH and volume changes, favoring cell migration and invasion under hypoxic and acidic conditions characteristic of solid tumors [13].

Beyond ion channels, the dysregulation of solute carriers (SLCs) and ATP-binding cassette (ABC) transporters is central to cancer cell metabolism and drug resistance. Overexpression of SLC family members enables increased uptake of glucose, amino acids, and other nutrients required for anabolic metabolism and growth [16]. Conversely, ABC transporters mediate the efflux of chemotherapeutic agents, facilitating multidrug resistance and persistence of cancer stem cell-like phenotypes [17].

Collectively, these alterations contribute to a permissive tumor microenvironment, enhancing interactions with stromal and immune cells, remodeling the extracellular matrix, and enabling metastatic dissemination [5]. Understanding the mechanistic basis of ion channel and transporter dysregulation in cancer pathogenesis not only elucidates fundamental aspects of tumor biology but also identifies novel vulnerabilities that may be exploited therapeutically. The major ion channels and transporters exhibit specific alterations in cancer, driving processes such as uncontrolled proliferation, invasion, and resistance to therapy. These proteins, their dysregulations, and the resulting functional consequences are outlined in Table 7.4.

Table 7.4 Examples of ion channels and transporters dysregulated in cancer

Protein type	Alteration in cancer	Functional consequence	References
Potassium channels	Overexpression or gain-of-function	Enhanced proliferation, migration	Pardo and Stühmer [10]
Calcium channels	Upregulated expression	Anti-apoptotic signaling, epithelial-mesenchymal transition (EMT)	Monteith et al. [11]
Sodium channels	Overexpressed Na^+ isoforms	Increased invasion and metastasis	House[12]
Chloride channels	Dysregulated activity	pH regulation, cell motility	Huber [13]
SLC transporters	Overexpression	Enhanced nutrient uptake	César-Razquin et al. [14]
ABC transporters	Overexpression	Chemoresistance, cancer stem cells (CSC) maintenance	Robey et al. [18]

1.5 Rationale for Therapeutic Targeting of ICT

The dysregulated activity of ion channels and transporters in cancer provides a strong rationale for their consideration as therapeutic targets. Unlike conventional cytotoxic agents that indiscriminately affect both normal and malignant cells, targeting aberrantly expressed or hyperactive channels and transporters offers the potential for more selective intervention, sparing normal tissues while disrupting cancer-specific processes [5, 13]. The pivotal role of these membrane proteins in sustaining hallmark traits of cancer such as uncontrolled proliferation, apoptotic resistance, metabolic reprogramming, invasion, and drug resistance further underscores their therapeutic relevance [2].

Several unique features make ion channels and transporters attractive drug targets. Firstly, their cell surface localization facilitates accessibility to extracellularly administered agents, reducing the need for intracellular drug delivery [19]. Secondly, many cancer cells exhibit a distinct expression pattern of specific isoforms or altered gating kinetics, which distinguishes them from their normal counterparts and enables selective inhibition [10]. For instance, overexpression of $Na_v1.5$ channels in breast and colon cancer or increased TRPM7 activity in pancreatic carcinoma are examples where isoform-specific interventions are plausible [12, 20].

Additionally, ion channels and transporters regulate intracellular ionic homeostasis, which is tightly coupled to pH control, metabolic flux, and redox balance processes critical for the survival of tumor cells in hypoxic, acidic, or nutrient-depleted microenvironments [11, 13]. Targeting such pathways can sensitize tumors to stress and augment the efficacy of other therapies. Importantly, ABC transporters mediate drug efflux and contribute to multidrug resistance; their inhibition could restore chemosensitivity and enhance therapeutic outcomes [17].

Emerging preclinical evidence has demonstrated that pharmacological or genetic blockade of specific ion channels or transporters can impair tumor cell growth, migration, and survival, both in vitro and in animal models [5, 19]. Some existing drugs, originally developed for cardiovascular or neurological disorders, are now being repurposed to target these proteins in oncology settings, reflecting the translational potential of this approach. Therefore, the selective modulation of dysregulated channels and transporters represents a promising strategy to overcome the limitations of current therapies, reduce off-target toxicity, and improve patient outcomes. The distinctive attributes of ion channels and transporters including their cell surface localization, tumor-specific expression, involvement in multiple cancer hallmarks, contribution to drug resistance, and availability of modulators highlight their therapeutic potential and are presented in Table 7.5.

Table 7.5 Key attributes supporting ion channels and transporters as cancer targets

Attribute	Relevance in cancer therapy	References
Cell surface localization	Enables accessibility and drug delivery	Arcangeli and Becchetti [19]
Tumor-specific expression	Reduces off-target effects	Monteith et al. [11]
Involvement in multiple hallmarks	Targets proliferation, invasion, survival	Prevarskaya et al. [5]
Contribution to drug resistance	Overcoming ABC transporter-mediated MDR	Robey et al. [18]
Availability of modulators	Repurposing existing drugs	Fletcher et al. [15]

2 Normal Physiological Roles

2.1 Types of Ion Channels

Ion channels are specialized transmembrane proteins that enable the passive, highly selective movement of ions across cellular membranes in response to electrochemical gradients. Their controlled opening and closing (gating) underlies fundamental physiological processes such as maintenance of resting membrane potential, excitability, intracellular signaling, cell volume regulation, and adaptation to mechanical forces [6, 7]. The diverse family of ion channels can be broadly classified based on their ion selectivity and gating mechanisms. Among the most prominent are potassium, calcium, sodium, chloride, and mechanosensitive channels, each contributing uniquely to cellular homeostasis and organ function.

Potassium (K^+) channels are the most ubiquitous and diverse class of ion channels in mammalian cells. They primarily maintain and regulate the resting membrane potential by allowing K^+ efflux, counteracting depolarizing inward currents [10]. This property is essential in excitable tissues such as neurons and cardiac myocytes for shaping action potentials and refractory periods. In addition, K^+ channels participate in controlling cell volume and proliferation in non-excitable cells.

Calcium (Ca^{2+}) channels mediate tightly regulated Ca^{2+} influx, a key second messenger in numerous signaling cascades. Voltage-gated Ca^{2+} channels are critical for processes such as synaptic transmission, excitation-contraction coupling in muscle, and hormone secretion [11]. Their activity modulates gene expression, apoptosis, and proliferation by influencing intracellular Ca^{2+} dynamics.

Sodium (Na^+) channels play a central role in generating and propagating action potentials in excitable cells by mediating rapid Na^+ influx, which depolarizes the membrane [7]. Additionally, Na^+ gradients established by sodium channels and pumps drive the secondary active transport of solutes, maintaining ionic and osmotic homeostasis in epithelia.

Chloride (Cl^-) channels regulate intracellular pH, osmolarity, and cell volume. They mediate Cl^- flux across membranes in epithelia and neurons, contributing to inhibitory neurotransmission via GABA and glycine receptor pathways [8]. Chloride conductance is also essential for fluid secretion and maintenance of the electrochemical balance.

Mechanosensitive channels are activated by membrane tension, stretch, or shear stress. These channels enable cells to sense and respond to mechanical stimuli, modulating processes such as osmotic stress responses, endothelial barrier function, and even migration [21]. They are particularly important in tissues exposed to mechanical forces, such as vasculature and kidneys.

These distinct classes of ion channels collectively maintain the delicate balance of ionic gradients, electrical excitability, and signal transduction that underpin normal physiology. Their dysfunction can therefore have profound pathological consequences. Different classes of ion channels including potassium, calcium, sodium, chloride, and mechanosensitive channels perform distinct yet critical physiological functions such as maintaining membrane potential, regulating intracellular signaling, mediating excitability, and sensing mechanical stress. These ion channel types, their primary ions, and physiological roles are detailed in Table 7.6.

2.2 *Transporters*

Membrane transporters are integral membrane proteins that mediate the regulated movement of ions, nutrients, metabolites, and xenobiotics across biological membranes. In contrast to ion channels, which facilitate rapid passive ion flux, transporters often operate through carrier-mediated mechanisms, allowing for both passive (facilitated diffusion) and active (energy-dependent) transport. They are indispensable for maintaining intracellular and extracellular homeostasis, supporting cellular metabolism, and coordinating systemic physiology [9]. Two major classes of transporters in mammalian cells are the solute carrier (SLC) family and the ATP-binding cassette (ABC) transporter family, each fulfilling distinct but complementary roles.

The solute carrier (SLC) family encompasses over 400 proteins classified into more than 60 families. These transporters mediate the uptake of a wide variety of

Table 7.6 Types of ion channels, their principal ions, and physiological functions

Ion channel types	Primary ion conducted	Key physiological roles	References
Potassium (K^+)	K^+	Membrane potential maintenance, excitability	Pedersen and Stock (2013) [22]
Calcium (Ca^{2+})	Ca^{2+}	Signaling cascades, secretion, contraction	Whitaker [23]
Sodium (Na^+)	Na^+	Excitability, secondary active transport	Brackenbury and Isom (2011) [24]
Chloride (Cl^-)	Cl^-	pH and volume regulation, inhibition	Jentsch et al. (2002) [25]
Mechanosensitive	Various	Stress sensing, osmotic and mechanical response	Martinac (2004) [26]

essential nutrients, including glucose, amino acids, nucleotides, vitamins, and inorganic ions [14]. For example, the facilitative glucose transporter GLUT1 (SLC2A1) ensures adequate glucose supply, particularly in highly metabolically active tissues such as the brain and red blood cells. Similarly, amino acid transporters, such as LAT1 (SLC7A5), deliver substrates required for protein synthesis and cellular proliferation. The activity of many SLCs is coupled to electrochemical gradients of sodium, protons, or chloride, allowing efficient accumulation of substrates against their concentration gradients.

The ATP-binding cassette (ABC) transporters, in contrast, primarily function to export a wide range of endogenous and exogenous compounds from the cell, thereby maintaining intracellular homeostasis and protecting against toxic accumulation. This superfamily includes well-characterized efflux pumps such as P-glycoprotein (ABCB1), which extrudes xenobiotics, metabolic by-products, and lipid derivatives [27]. ABC transporters are also involved in antigen presentation, bile acid transport, and cholesterol homeostasis.

In addition to nutrient and metabolite handling, transporters play key roles in regulating intracellular pH through coupled proton/anion exchange, ensuring optimal enzyme activity and structural stability within the cytoplasm [8]. Their activity contributes to the maintenance of osmotic balance and cell volume, critical under varying environmental conditions. By supporting the uptake of energy substrates and the removal of metabolic waste, both SLC and ABC transporters underpin cellular and systemic energy metabolism and homeostasis.

Thus, membrane transporters are central to physiological integrity, linking extracellular supply and intracellular demand for critical molecules while safeguarding against accumulation of harmful substances. Dysregulation of these processes has profound implications for pathologies, including metabolic disorders, neurodegeneration, and cancer. Various classes of membrane transporters including solute carriers (SLC), ATP-binding cassette (ABC) transporters, pH regulators, and energy homeostasis-associated transporters play critical roles in nutrient uptake, drug efflux, pH maintenance, and metabolic support in cancer and normal physiology. These transporters, their functions, and representative examples are listed in Table 7.7.

Table 7.7 Major roles of membrane transporters in normal physiology

Transporter class	Function	Examples and roles	References
Solute carrier (SLC)	Mediates uptake of nutrients and ions	GLUT1 (glucose), LAT1 (amino acids)	Bhutia and Ganapathy [16]
ATP-binding cassette (ABC)	Exports metabolites and xenobiotics	P-glycoprotein (xenobiotics), ABCA1 (lipids)	Kathawala et al. (2015) [28]
pH regulation transporters	Maintain cytosolic pH via H^+/anion exchange	NHE1 (Na^+/H^+ exchanger), AE1 (Cl^-/HCO_3^-)	Cardone et al. (2005) [29]
Energy and homeostasis	Support metabolic demands	Nutrient uptake and waste removal	Hsu and Sabatini (2008) [30]

3 Roles in Cancer Progression

3.1 *Hallmarks of Cancer*

Cancer progression is orchestrated by a constellation of biological capabilities that collectively enable malignant cells to sustain growth, evade cell death, invade surrounding tissues, and colonize distant organs. These capabilities, termed the hallmarks of cancer, reflect both cell-intrinsic and microenvironmental adaptations that distinguish malignant cells from their normal counterparts [2]. Among the central hallmarks facilitated by dysregulated ion channels and transporters are the promotion of continuous proliferation, inhibition of apoptosis, stimulation of angiogenesis, facilitation of invasion and metastasis, and adaptation to hypoxic and acidic conditions.

Continuous cell proliferation is a defining feature of malignant transformation. Tumor cells bypass normal growth-regulatory signals by constitutively activating pro-proliferative pathways. Dysregulated ion fluxes, such as enhanced (K^+) efflux and (Ca^{2+}) oscillations, contribute to progression through the cell cycle by modulating cyclin–CDK activity, DNA synthesis, and mitotic spindle function [10, 11]. Increased nutrient uptake via overexpressed solute carriers also supports anabolic metabolism and biomass accumulation required for cell division.

Apoptotic resistance enables survival of genetically unstable cells that would otherwise undergo programmed cell death. Altered intracellular (Ca^{2+}) homeostasis and mitochondrial depolarization, mediated by overactive (Ca^{2+}) and (Cl^-) channels, suppress pro-apoptotic signals and caspase activation [5]. Similarly, acid–base regulation by transporters stabilizes cytoplasmic pH and prevents anoikis during detachment and dissemination.

Angiogenesis, the formation of new blood vessels, is essential to sustain tumor growth beyond a critical size by providing oxygen and nutrients. Elevated intracellular (Ca^{2+}) signaling in tumor and endothelial cells stimulates production of vascular endothelial growth factor (VEGF), promoting angiogenic sprouting and vessel permeability [11]. Hypoxia-induced activation of proton transporters also supports the acidic microenvironment that further stimulates angiogenic pathways.

Invasion and metastasis are facilitated by enhanced motility, proteolytic remodeling of the extracellular matrix, and epithelial–mesenchymal transition (EMT). Sodium (Na^+) and chloride (Cl^-) channels, along with aquaporins, regulate cell volume changes and lamellipodia dynamics necessary for migration through confined spaces [13]. Overactive voltage-gated sodium channels in carcinoma cells increase secretion of proteases and promote metastatic behavior [12].

Finally, cancer cells adapt to hypoxia and acidity, conditions prevalent in poorly perfused tumor regions. Upregulation of lactate/H^+ transporters and (Cl^-) exchangers maintain intracellular pH despite high glycolytic activity, while enabling extracellular acidification that promotes invasion and immune evasion [31].

Together, these alterations underscore the multifaceted role of ion channels and transporters in sustaining the malignant phenotype and provide mechanistic insights

Table 7.8 Key hallmarks of cancer mediated by ion channels and transporters

Hallmark	Contributing mechanisms	References
Sustained proliferation	K^+ and Ca^{2+} fluxes, nutrient uptake	Pedersen and Stock (2013) [22]
Resistance to apoptosis	Mitochondrial depolarization, pH regulation	Cardone et al. (2005) [29]
Angiogenesis	Ca^{2+}-mediated VEGF production	Monteith et al. [11]
Invasion and metastasis	Volume regulation, EMT, protease secretion	Schwab et al. (2012) [32]
Adaptation to hypoxia/acidity	Proton and lactate transport, pH homeostasis	Hsu and Sabatini [30]

into their potential as therapeutic targets. Key hallmarks of cancer, such as sustained proliferation, resistance to apoptosis, angiogenesis, invasion and metastasis, and adaptation to hypoxia and acidity, are supported by distinct ion fluxes, transporter activities, and pH regulatory mechanisms, as detailed in Table 7.8.

3.2 *Tumor Microenvironment*

The tumor microenvironment (TME) is a dynamic and complex milieu composed of cancer cells, stromal fibroblasts, endothelial cells, immune infiltrates, and extracellular matrix (ECM). It plays a pivotal role in shaping tumor behavior and progression, providing both structural support and biochemical cues that sustain malignancy. Dysregulated ion channels and transporters contribute significantly to remodeling the TME to favor tumor growth, immune evasion, invasion, and maintenance of stem-like phenotypes [4, 13].

One key aspect of ion transporter function in the TME is the modification of stromal interactions to enhance tumor growth. Cancer cells influence surrounding stromal fibroblasts by altering extracellular pH through proton efflux and lactate accumulation, mediated by transporters such as NHE1 and MCT4. Acidification activates matrix metalloproteinases (MMPs), facilitating ECM degradation and promoting a pro-tumorigenic stromal phenotype [31].

Ion channels and transporters also contribute to immune evasion, a hallmark of advanced tumors. Acidic extracellular pH, resulting from proton and lactate transporter activity, impairs cytotoxic T-cell and NK cell function while promoting immunosuppressive regulatory T cells and myeloid-derived suppressor cells [13]. Chloride and potassium channel activity within tumor-infiltrating lymphocytes can also modulate their activation thresholds, diminishing anti-tumor immune responses [5].

The establishment of localized ion gradients within the TME is essential for directional invasion and metastasis. Sodium and chloride channels, by regulating localized cell volume changes, facilitate dynamic cytoskeletal reorganization necessary for cell motility and tissue penetration [12]. Concurrently, acidification of the ECM enhances proteolytic activity and cell detachment, further supporting invasion.

Table 7.9 Roles of ion channels and transporters in tumor microenvironment modulation

tme feature	Mechanism involving ion channels/ transporters	References
Stromal modification	Acidic pH activates fibroblasts, MMPs	Huber et al. (2010) [13]
Immune evasion	Acidification inhibits effector cells, promotes suppressive cells	Calcinotto et al. [33]
Ion gradients for invasion	Localized Na^+/Cl^- flux supports motility	Schwab et al. [32]
Stem-like phenotype maintenance	Ca^{2+} signaling sustains stemness pathways	Kondratskyi et al. [34]
ECM remodeling	pH and ion-mediated MMP activation remodel ECM	Cardone et al. [29]

Moreover, ion channels and transporters support the emergence and maintenance of stem-like cancer cell phenotypes, which are critical for tumor initiation, recurrence, and resistance to therapy. Calcium signaling through ORAI and TRPM channels, as well as pH homeostasis, sustain stemness pathways such as Wnt/β-catenin and Notch in cancer stem-like cells [5, 11].

Finally, ECM remodeling is influenced by ionic changes and acidification. Matrix rigidity, porosity, and composition are altered by the ion-driven activation of fibroblasts and secretion of MMPs, facilitating tumor cell dissemination and angiogenesis [31].

Thus, by reshaping the biochemical and physical properties of the TME, dysregulated ion channels and transporters create a permissive niche that supports tumor progression, immune suppression, and therapeutic resistance. Ion channels and transporters play pivotal roles in shaping the tumor microenvironment by modulating stromal activation, immune evasion, invasive ion gradients, stem-like cell maintenance, and extracellular matrix remodeling, as outlined in Table 7.9.

4 Molecular Mechanisms

4.1 Ion Flux and Cell Cycle

Ion fluxes across cellular membranes are not merely supportive of homeostatic functions but are also integral regulators of the cell division cycle. Dysregulated activity of specific ion channels and transporters has been implicated in the control of critical checkpoints, mitotic events, and metabolic adaptations that collectively sustain the proliferative phenotype characteristic of malignant cells [13, 25].

One major role of ion flux is to regulate cell cycle checkpoints, ensuring orderly progression through the G1, S, G2, and M phases. Potassium K^+ and chloride Cl^- efflux, for example, contribute to cell shrinkage required for passage through mitosis, while elevated intracellular calcium (Ca^{2+}) levels activate kinases and phosphatases that govern checkpoint fidelity [10]. Sodium (Na^+) influx through voltage-gated channels has also been linked to G1/S transition and DNA synthesis [12].

Ion dynamics are essential for mitotic spindle assembly, a highly coordinated process ensuring proper chromosome segregation. Localized (Ca^{2+}) microdomains at centrosomes facilitate spindle pole organization and microtubule–kinetochore interactions [23]. Perturbation of calcium homeostasis disrupts spindle integrity and can result in aneuploidy.

Additionally, ion fluxes influence DNA repair and replication, processes that are particularly active during S and G2 phases. Calcium-dependent signaling cascades activate checkpoint kinases (CHK1/2) and DNA repair enzymes, maintaining genomic integrity under replication stress [11].

Ion channels also regulate the activity of cyclins and cyclin-dependent kinases (CDKs), the core drivers of cell cycle transitions. Potassium channel activity has been shown to affect CDK1-cyclin B1 complex activation, while (Ca^{2+}) oscillations modulate transcription factors controlling cyclin D1 and E expression [10, 35].

Finally, ion transport is indispensable for the metabolic rewiring that supports rapid proliferation. Enhanced Na^+ and H^+ transporters maintain intracellular pH favorable for glycolytic flux, while nutrient transporters of the SLC family supply amino acids and glucose required for biomass synthesis and ATP production [31].

Together, these mechanisms highlight the intricate interplay between ionic signaling and cell cycle machinery, underscoring the potential of ion channel modulators as regulators of uncontrolled proliferation in cancer. Ion-dependent mechanisms critically regulate key aspects of cell cycle control, including checkpoints, spindle assembly, DNA repair, cyclin-CDK activity, and metabolic adaptation, as illustrated in Table 7.10.

4.2 Apoptosis and EMT

The dysregulation of ion channels and transporters in cancer not only sustains proliferation but also confers resistance to programmed cell death (apoptosis) and enhances epithelial–mesenchymal transition (EMT), a key process underlying invasion and metastasis. These processes are intricately regulated by ionic homeostasis,

Table 7.10 Roles of ion fluxes in cell cycle regulation

Process	Ion-dependent mechanism	References
Cell cycle checkpoints	K^+/Cl^- efflux for mitotic progression	Lang et al. [36]
Mitotic spindle assembly	Ca^{2+} microdomains at centrosomes	Whitaker [23]
DNA repair and replication	Ca^{2+} activated checkpoint kinases	Santos et al. [37]
Cyclin and CDK activity	Ion-driven transcription and phosphorylation	Borowiec et al. [38]
Metabolic rewiring	Na^+/H^+ transport for pH and metabolism	Cardone et al. [29]

which influences mitochondrial integrity, protease activation, intracellular signaling pathways, pH balance, and immune evasion [13, 35].

One principal mechanism by which ion channels modulate apoptosis is through alteration of the mitochondrial membrane potential ($\Delta\Psi m$). Elevated intracellular Ca^{2+} mediated by dysregulated calcium channels or store-operated entry can either promote mitochondrial outer membrane permeabilization, triggering apoptosis, or in cancer cells, paradoxically maintain $\Delta\Psi m$ at levels that prevent cytochrome c release [11]. Similarly, K^+ efflux through specific potassium channels has been associated with apoptotic volume decrease (AVD), an early hallmark of apoptosis, whereas reduced K^+ conductance in cancer impairs this process and fosters survival [10].

Ion fluxes also directly modulate caspase activation, the central executioners of apoptosis. Changes in Cl^- and K^+ gradients influence caspase-3 and -9 activation by regulating the ionic environment required for their optimal enzymatic activity [13]. Dysregulated pH, driven by proton transporters, further stabilizes anti-apoptotic proteins, inhibiting caspase cascades.

Epithelial–mesenchymal transition (EMT), which enables epithelial cancer cells to acquire mesenchymal features and migratory capacity, is strongly influenced by Ca^{2+} signaling. Sustained Ca^{2+} influx activates calmodulin-dependent kinases and transcription factors such as Snail and Twist, promoting downregulation of E-cadherin and upregulation of vimentin, hallmark EMT markers [5]. EMT is also reinforced by Na^+/H^+ exchanger activity, which remodels cytoskeletal and adhesion complexes.

Anoikis, a form of apoptosis induced by cell detachment from the extracellular matrix, is suppressed in cancer cells by intracellular pH adjustment. Overactive proton and lactate transporters maintain cytosolic alkalinity while acidifying the extracellular milieu, protecting detached cells from anoikis and enabling survival in circulation [31].

Finally, ion channels and transporters contribute to immune escape mechanisms. Acidic extracellular pH impairs immune effector cell infiltration and cytotoxicity while promoting immunosuppressive cell populations, creating an immune-privileged niche [13].

Together, these ion-dependent mechanisms enable cancer cells to evade death signals, acquire plasticity, and survive in adverse microenvironments, supporting tumor progression and therapeutic resistance. Ion channels and transporters contribute to critical cancer-related processes including regulation of mitochondrial potential, caspase activation, induction of epithelial-mesenchymal transition, suppression of anoikis, and immune evasion through distinct ion-dependent mechanisms shown in Table 7.11.

Table 7.11 Roles of ion channels and transporters in apoptosis and EMT

Process	Ion-dependent mechanisms	References
Mitochondrial potential	Ca^{2+} influx, K^+ conductance regulate $\Delta\Psi m$	Szabo and Zoratti [39]
Caspase activation	Cl^-/K^+ gradients modulate caspase activity	Okada et al. [40]
EMT induction	Ca^{2+} activated EMT transcription factors	Liu et al. [41]
Anoikis suppression	Proton transporters maintain alkaline cytosol	Cardone et al. [29]
Immune evasion	Acidic pH impairs effector cell cytotoxicity	Calcinotto et al. [33]

5 Therapeutic Strategies

5.1 *Targeting Ion Channels*

In cancer, ion channels, which are proteins that regulate the movement of charged ions (like potassium, sodium, and calcium) across cell membranes, are often abnormally expressed or overactive. These changes help cancer cells grow, divide, move, and survive under stressful conditions. Importantly, these same changes make ion channels attractive targets for therapy. Unlike traditional chemotherapy which often kills both cancer and normal cells indiscriminately targeting ion channels holds the promise of being more selective because certain ion channels are abnormally active in cancer cells but not in normal tissues [5, 19]. Several strategies are currently being investigated to inhibit the abnormal activity of ion channels in cancer therapy. These approaches range from experimental laboratory studies to repurposing existing drugs already approved for other diseases.

One major strategy is the use of channel blockers in preclinical studies. Researchers have shown that blocking specific ion channels with drugs can slow down or stop cancer cell growth, reduce their ability to move (and therefore spread), and make them more likely to die. For example, laboratory studies on cancer cells and animal models have demonstrated that blocking potassium K^+, sodium Na^+, or calcium Ca^{2+} channels can disrupt processes that cancer cells rely on. Specifically, blockers of the potassium channel $K_\upsilon 10.1$ and sodium channel $Na_\upsilon 1.5$ have shown promising results in inhibiting cancer cell proliferation and invasion by interfering with the cell cycle and reducing metastatic behavior [10, 12].

A second approach is to repurpose cardiovascular drugs that target ion channels, originally developed for diseases like high blood pressure or irregular heart rhythms. For instance, verapamil, a calcium channel blocker, and amiodarone, a potassium channel blocker, have shown anticancer effects in experimental models. Because these drugs are already approved and their safety is well understood, repurposing them for oncology is a practical and cost-effective strategy [19].

Another active area of research involves developing selective inhibitors for cancer-specific isoforms of ion channels. Cancer cells often express particular versions (isoforms) of ion channels that are rare or absent in normal cells. Designing drugs that specifically block these isoforms could achieve precision therapy, minimizing harm to healthy tissues. For example, research efforts are underway to develop inhibitors that selectively target tumor-specific forms of $K_v10.1$ and $Na_v1.5$, and TRPM7, a magnesium/calcium-permeable channel overexpressed in some cancers [11].

In addition to using ion channel inhibitors alone, researchers are also testing combination therapies that include these agents along with standard treatments like chemotherapy, radiotherapy, or targeted drugs. Because ion channels influence how cancer cells respond to stress and damage, inhibiting them can make tumors more sensitive to other treatments and overcome resistance, leading to better therapeutic outcomes [5].

Finally, a crucial step in advancing these therapies is the identification of biomarkers to guide patient selection. Not all tumors overexpress the same ion channels, so measuring which channels are active in a given patient's tumor (through expression profiling of biopsy samples) can help identify patients who are most likely to benefit from these therapies. This personalized approach avoids unnecessary treatment and improves the chances of success [19].

Taken together, these strategies demonstrate the significant potential of targeting ion channels in cancer therapy. They highlight the importance of continued research to validate and refine these approaches and integrate them into clinical practice to improve outcomes for cancer patients. Various therapeutic strategies targeting ion channels in cancer ranging from preclinical channel blockers, drug repurposing, and selective isoform inhibitors to combination therapies and biomarker-guided patient selection are illustrated in Table 7.12.

5.2 *Targeting Transporters*

Membrane transporters, particularly the ATP-binding cassette (ABC) and solute carrier (SLC) protein families, are critical regulators of cellular homeostasis. In cancer, these transporters become dysregulated, supporting malignant cell survival, metabolic reprogramming, and resistance to chemotherapy. Because of their central role in these pathological processes, ABC and SLC transporters have emerged as attractive therapeutic targets. By modulating transporter activity, it is possible to

Table 7.12 Strategies for targeting ion channels in cancer therapy

Strategy	Example/application	References
Channel blockers (preclinical)	$K_v10.1$, $Na_v1.5$ inhibitors reduce proliferation	Pardo and Stühmer [10]
Drug repurposing	Verapamil, amiodarone show anti-tumor effects	Arcangeli and Becchetti [19]
Selective cancer isoform inhibitors	Targeting tumor-specific K^+ or TRP channels	Monteith et al. [11]
Combination therapies	Ion channel inhibitors + chemotherapy	Prevarskaya et al. [5]
Biomarker-guided patient selection	Ion channel expression profiling in tumors	Arcangeli and Becchetti [19]

reverse drug resistance, disrupt tumor-specific metabolic pathways, exploit vulnerabilities of the tumor microenvironment, and improve the specificity of drug delivery [14, 15].

One of the most prominent clinical challenges in oncology is multidrug resistance (MDR), which is largely mediated by overexpression of ABC transporters. Proteins such as P-glycoprotein (ABCB1), MRP1 (ABCC1), and BCRP (ABCG2) act as efflux pumps, actively exporting chemotherapeutic drugs out of cancer cells. This lowers intracellular drug levels below cytotoxic thresholds, rendering treatments ineffective. To overcome this, pharmacological inhibitors of ABC transporters such as tariquidar and elacridar have been developed and tested in preclinical and early clinical settings. These agents block the transporter's drug-pumping activity, allowing chemotherapeutic agents to accumulate inside tumor cells and regain their cytotoxic potential. However, their clinical translation has been limited due to toxicity in normal tissues and lack of selectivity, which has prompted the development of next-generation inhibitors with improved specificity and reduced side effects [18].

Another promising therapeutic strategy focuses on the SLC transporters, which are heavily exploited by cancer cells to meet their increased metabolic demands. Tumor cells often upregulate transporters such as the glucose transporter GLUT1 and the amino acid transporter LAT1, ensuring a steady supply of energy and biosynthetic precursors to support rapid proliferation and maintain redox balance. Inhibitors of GLUT1 and LAT1 have shown potent anti-proliferative effects in preclinical models and have been reported to sensitize tumors to oxidative stress and nutrient deprivation [14].

Cancer cells also rely on pH-regulating transporters notably, the Na^+/H^+ exchanger (NHE1) and monocarboxylate transporters (MCT1/4) to maintain an alkaline intracellular pH and an acidic extracellular microenvironment. This pH regulation promotes survival, invasion, and resistance to apoptosis. Inhibiting these transporters disrupts pH homeostasis, inducing acidification of the cytoplasm, triggering cell death, and decreasing the metastatic potential of cancer cells. Agents such as cariporide (an NHE1 inhibitor) and AZD3965 (an MCT1 inhibitor) have shown promising activity in preclinical studies [31].

Nanocarrier-based delivery systems represent an innovative approach to improve the specificity and efficacy of transporter inhibitors. By encapsulating inhibitors in nanoparticles, it is possible to exploit the enhanced permeability and retention (EPR) effect of tumors, achieving higher drug accumulation at the tumor site while minimizing systemic toxicity. This strategy not only improves therapeutic indices but also offers a platform for combination therapies [15].

In addition, advances in RNA-based therapeutics have enabled highly specific silencing of overexpressed transporters. Techniques such as small interfering RNA (siRNA) and antisense oligonucleotides (ASOs) can selectively downregulate the expression of key transporters, such as ABCB1 or SLC7A5, effectively reversing drug resistance and disrupting metabolic adaptations with minimal impact on normal cells [18].

Table 7.13 Strategies for targeting transporters in cancer therapy

Strategy	Example/application	References
ABC transporter inhibitors	Tariquidar, elacridar reverse MDR	Robey et al. [18]
SLC modulators	GLUT1, LAT1 inhibitors disrupt metabolism	Bhutia and Ganapathy [16]
pH-regulating transporter inhibitors	Cariporide (NHE1), AZD3965 (MCT1)	Webb et al. [31]
Nanocarrier-based delivery	Tumor-targeted nanoparticles with inhibitors	Kathawala et al. [28]
RNA therapeutics	siRNA/ASO silencing of ABCB1, SLC7A5	Kathawala et al. [28]

Collectively, these diverse approaches demonstrate the translational potential of transporter-targeted therapies. Whether used alone or in combination with conventional treatments, these strategies aim to overcome some of the most challenging aspects of cancer biology including MDR and metabolic plasticity offering improved outcomes for patients. Emerging therapeutic strategies targeting transporters in cancer such as ABC transporter inhibitors, SLC modulators, pH-regulating transporter inhibitors, nanocarrier-based delivery systems, and RNA-based therapeutics are outlined in Table 7.13.

6 Drug Resistance

6.1 Role of Transporters

The emergence of resistance to chemotherapy remains one of the most significant challenges in modern oncology. Despite the development of potent chemotherapeutic agents, many cancers eventually develop the ability to survive treatment. This phenomenon, termed multidrug resistance (MDR), refers to the capacity of cancer cells to evade the toxic effects of multiple, structurally unrelated drugs through common molecular mechanisms. At the center of MDR are the ATP-binding cassette (ABC) transporters, a family of membrane proteins that actively pump chemotherapeutic agents out of cancer cells, lowering their intracellular concentrations to levels insufficient to induce cell death [15, 18].

ABC transporters, including P-glycoprotein (ABCB1), multidrug resistance-associated proteins (MRPs, e.g., ABCC1), and breast cancer resistance protein (BCRP/ABCG2), are often overexpressed in a wide variety of tumor types. Their overactivity has been strongly linked to treatment failure in clinical settings. For example, ABCB1 can expel drugs such as anthracyclines, taxanes, and vinca alkaloids, which are widely used chemotherapeutics. By actively transporting these drugs out of the cytoplasm, these transporters effectively lower the intracellular concentration of the drugs below cytotoxic thresholds, allowing cancer cells to survive despite chemotherapy [17].

The mechanism of action of ABC transporters relies on energy derived from ATP hydrolysis, which fuels the active, unidirectional efflux of drugs across the plasma membrane. As a result, even when high concentrations of drugs are administered systemically, resistant cancer cells can maintain intracellular drug levels that are too low to induce apoptosis. This not only diminishes the immediate effectiveness of treatment but also allows the clonal selection of resistant subpopulations, leading to tumor recurrence and progression [18].

The activity of ABC transporters also protects intracellular organelles, such as mitochondria, from drug-induced damage, further supporting cell survival. By preventing mitochondrial depolarization and the release of pro-apoptotic factors, these transporters contribute to an anti-apoptotic phenotype in resistant cancer cells [18].

Notably, high expression of ABC transporters is a characteristic feature of cancer stem cells (CSCs). CSCs are a specialized subpopulation of tumor cells capable of self-renewal, quiescence, and seeding new tumors. Their inherent resistance to chemotherapy, largely due to high efflux capacity, enables them to survive initial treatment, persist in the tumor niche, and later contribute to disease relapse and metastasis [23].

Clinically, the overexpression of ABC transporters in tumors correlates with poor patient outcomes, including reduced response rates to therapy, shorter progression-free survival, and diminished overall survival [15, 17]. This underscores the urgent need to develop therapeutic strategies aimed at inhibiting transporter activity, downregulating their expression, or bypassing their effects altogether.

A thorough understanding of the molecular mechanisms by which ABC transporters mediate MDR is therefore essential for the rational design of targeted therapies. Such knowledge provides a conceptual and practical framework for interventions to restore chemosensitivity, improve treatment efficacy, and ultimately enhance clinical outcomes for cancer patients. Key mechanisms by which transporters mediate drug resistance in cancer including drug efflux, overexpression, reduced intracellular damage, cancer stem cell survival, and clinical associations with poor outcomes are detailed in Table 7.14.

6.2 Overcoming Resistance

Multidrug resistance (MDR) in cancer, predominantly driven by ATP-binding cassette (ABC) transporters, represents a major obstacle to effective chemotherapy. ABC transporters, such as P-glycoprotein (ABCB1), actively export a broad range of chemotherapeutic agents out of cancer cells, lowering their intracellular concentrations and rendering them ineffective. This phenomenon not only compromises immediate treatment efficacy but also contributes to tumor recurrence and poor prognosis [15, 18]. To address MDR, several strategies have been developed or proposed, aiming to either inhibit transporter activity, bypass their drug efflux function, downregulate their expression, or employ therapeutic modalities that circumvent their mechanisms altogether. These strategies are being refined to restore drug sensitivity, eradicate resistant cell populations, and improve clinical outcomes.

Table 7.14 Role of ABC transporters in drug resistance

Mechanism	Functional impact	References
Drug efflux	Decreases intracellular drug concentration	Gottesman et al. [17]
Overexpression	Confers resistance to multiple drug classes	Fletcher et al. [15]
Intracellular accumulation	Reduces mitochondrial and DNA damage	Robey et al. [18]
CSC survival	Maintains tumor-initiating cell population	Dean et al. [27]
Clinical correlation	Associated with poor prognosis and relapse	Gottesman et al. [17]

One of the most extensively investigated approaches is the combination of efflux inhibitors with standard chemotherapeutics. Efflux inhibitors, such as tariquidar, elacridar, and zosuquidar, are designed to specifically block the activity of ABC transporters, particularly ABCB1. By inhibiting the drug-pumping function of these proteins, chemotherapeutic agents can remain inside the cancer cell at cytotoxic concentrations. Preclinical studies and some clinical trials have demonstrated that co-administration of efflux inhibitors with drugs like taxanes, anthracyclines, and vinca alkaloids partially reverses resistance and enhances tumor cell killing. However, challenges such as off-target effects on normal tissues, potential pharmacokinetic interactions, and dose-limiting toxicities have limited their widespread clinical adoption [17].

An alternative and promising approach is the development of non-substrate chemotherapeutics. Many next-generation agents are chemically modified to avoid recognition and export by ABC transporters. These non-substrate compounds remain effective even in cancer cells that overexpress efflux pumps, thereby reducing selective pressure and limiting the emergence of MDR. Examples include lipophilic analogs of taxanes and novel microtubule-targeting agents that retain activity in resistant tumors [18].

Recent advances in gene-editing technologies have also enabled targeted silencing of transporter genes. Tools such as CRISPR/Cas9 and RNA interference (RNAi) can precisely disrupt or suppress ABC transporter expression at the genetic level, significantly reducing efflux capacity and restoring drug sensitivity. Such gene-based approaches are still largely in the preclinical stage but hold considerable potential for personalized medicine, where resistant tumors could be specifically reprogrammed to become chemosensitive again [27].

In addition, targeting the signaling pathways that regulate transporter expression represents an indirect yet effective strategy. ABC transporter genes are regulated by intracellular signaling cascades such as PI3K/AKT, MAPK, and NF-κB. Inhibitors of these upstream pathways have been shown to downregulate ABC transporter expression, thereby sensitizing tumors to chemotherapy. This approach has the advantage of concurrently targeting multiple aspects of cancer cell survival, including proliferation and resistance mechanisms [15].

Finally, immunotherapy provides an orthogonal strategy that bypasses MDR entirely. Since immune checkpoint inhibitors (e.g., anti-PD-1, anti-CTLA-4) and adoptive cell therapies such as CAR-T cells eliminate tumor cells through immune-mediated cytotoxicity rather than intracellular drug accumulation, they can effectively target resistant tumor populations that evade chemotherapy via efflux pumps.

Table 7.15 Strategies for overcoming multidrug resistance in cancer

Strategy	Example/application	References
Efflux inhibitors + chemotherapy	Tariquidar with paclitaxel	Robey et al. [18]
Non-substrate chemotherapeutics	Novel taxane analogs	Fletcher et al. [15]
Gene editing to silence transporters	CRISPR/Cas9-mediated ABCB1 knockout	Zhen et al. [42]
Targeting regulatory pathways	PI3K/AKT or NF-κB inhibitors	Sui et al. [43]
Immunotherapy to bypass resistance	Immune checkpoint inhibitors, CAR-T cells	Marin et al. [44]

Combining immunotherapy with chemotherapy or targeted therapy may help eliminate resistant clones and produce durable responses in patients [18].

These multifaceted strategies highlight the ongoing efforts in translational research and clinical oncology to counteract MDR. They underscore the importance of integrating molecular understanding of resistance mechanisms with therapeutic innovations to improve outcomes in cancer treatment. Several strategies have been developed to overcome transporter-mediated drug resistance in cancer, including the use of efflux inhibitors with chemotherapy, non-substrate chemotherapeutics, gene editing, targeting regulatory pathways, and immunotherapy approaches, mentioned in Table 7.15.

7 Challenges and Perspectives

The discovery of ion channels and transporters as key players in cancer development and drug resistance has opened up exciting possibilities for targeted therapies. However, translating these insights into safe and effective treatments remains a complex challenge. As these proteins are also vital for the normal functioning of healthy cells, and because tumors themselves are highly variable and adaptable, researchers must overcome several obstacles to ensure that therapies are both effective and precise. In this section, we explore the major challenges associated with targeting ion channels and transporters in cancer, and outline perspectives for future progress.

7.1 Achieving Cancer-Specific Targeting of Ubiquitous Proteins

One of the most fundamental difficulties in targeting ion channels and transporters lies in their ubiquitous expression. These proteins are not unique to cancer cells; they play crucial roles in normal tissues, such as neurons, heart muscle, kidney, and immune cells [5]. For example, potassium and calcium channels regulate the heartbeat, nerve signaling, and hormone secretion in healthy individuals. Therefore, drugs that block these channels indiscriminately could impair essential physiological functions, leading to serious side effects like arrhythmias, neurological symptoms, or immunosuppression [19].

To address this, ongoing research focuses on identifying cancer-specific isoforms of ion channels and transporters, or discovering molecular "signatures" that distinguish their activity in tumors versus normal tissues. Technologies such as single-cell RNA sequencing and proteomics allow researchers to pinpoint subtle differences in expression patterns, post-translational modifications, and channel gating properties in cancer cells. Developing drugs that selectively target these tumor-specific variations could dramatically improve the therapeutic index and reduce harm to normal tissues [10].

7.2 *Minimizing Off-Target Toxicity in Healthy Tissues*

Closely related to the issue of specificity is the challenge of minimizing off-target toxicity. Even when a drug inhibits the intended protein, that same target may be essential in other organs. For example, inhibiting the Na^+/H^+ exchanger (NHE1) to acidify cancer cells could also disturb pH balance in the heart and kidneys. Similarly, blocking P-glycoprotein to reverse chemotherapy resistance could interfere with the blood–brain barrier, increasing brain exposure to toxins and drugs [18].

To mitigate such risks, advanced drug delivery systems, such as nanoparticles and antibody-drug conjugates, are being designed to concentrate therapeutics in tumor tissues while sparing healthy organs. These approaches exploit the enhanced permeability and retention (EPR) effect of tumors, or use tumor-specific antibodies as homing devices [15]. Additionally, "prodrugs" that become active only in the tumor's acidic or hypoxic microenvironment are under investigation, offering another strategy to limit systemic toxicity.

7.3 *Accounting for Tumor Heterogeneity and Adaptation*

Tumors are not homogeneous masses of identical cells. Rather, they are complex ecosystems containing diverse subpopulations with distinct genetic, epigenetic, and metabolic profiles. This tumor heterogeneity can significantly undermine the efficacy of targeted therapies, as some cells may lack the intended target or quickly adapt to its inhibition through compensatory pathways [2].

For example, while one population of cancer cells might overexpress (K^+) potassium channels, another might rely on alternative ion channels or transporters. Over time, selective pressure from treatment may favor the survival and expansion of resistant clones, a phenomenon known as tumor adaptation. Therefore, a major challenge is to develop combination therapies that target multiple pathways simultaneously, or sequential treatment regimens that preempt adaptive resistance. Comprehensive characterization of each tumor's molecular profile, ideally through multi-omics approaches, is critical to guide these strategies.

7.4 Integrating Omics Data for Personalized Therapy

The era of precision oncology is driven by the realization that no two tumors are exactly alike. The integration of high-throughput omics data including genomics, transcriptomics, proteomics, and metabolomics provides a detailed map of each patient's tumor biology. Such data can reveal which ion channels, transporters, and signaling pathways are dysregulated in an individual's cancer, enabling personalized therapy tailored to that specific molecular context [14].

However, translating this wealth of data into actionable clinical decisions remains challenging. Bioinformatics tools and predictive algorithms are needed to identify the most relevant targets and prioritize them for therapy. Moreover, prospective clinical trials must be designed to test whether such personalized approaches indeed lead to improved outcomes. Collaborative efforts between clinicians, biologists, and data scientists are essential to make this vision a reality.

7.5 Expanding Clinical Trials for Validation

Although many ion channel and transporter inhibitors have shown promise in laboratory and animal studies, relatively few have been validated in large-scale clinical trials. Expanding clinical trials is therefore a crucial next step. Trials must be carefully designed to assess not only efficacy but also safety, given the potential for off-target effects. Furthermore, patient selection based on biomarker expression is likely to improve trial success rates by identifying those most likely to benefit [19].

To accelerate this process, innovative trial designs such as basket trials, which test a therapy across multiple cancer types sharing a common molecular feature can be employed. International collaborations and regulatory support will also play key roles in bringing these novel therapies from bench to bedside.

8 Conclusions

The understanding of ion channels and transporters as critical regulators of cancer biology represents one of the most significant conceptual shifts in modern oncology. Historically, these proteins were thought of primarily as "housekeeping" components of normal cellular physiology responsible for maintaining ionic gradients, membrane potential, nutrient uptake, and pH homeostasis in healthy tissues. Over the last two decades, however, a growing body of research has demonstrated that these same molecules are profoundly altered in cancer cells, where they contribute not just to survival but also to hallmark cancer behaviors such as uncontrolled proliferation, invasion, metastasis, immune evasion, and drug resistance [2, 5].

These discoveries have sparked considerable interest in the possibility of targeting ion channels and transporters therapeutically. Unlike conventional chemotherapies, which attack rapidly dividing cells in general and thus cause collateral damage to healthy proliferating tissues, ion channel- and transporter-based therapies offer the potential for selectivity: disrupting cancer-specific mechanisms while sparing normal cellular function [19]. This concept aligns with the modern paradigm of precision oncology, which seeks to tailor treatment to the unique molecular profile of each patient's tumor.

However, as this chapter has discussed in depth, the path from conceptual understanding to clinical implementation is complex and fraught with challenges. Ion channels and transporters are not unique to cancer cells; they are ubiquitously expressed and indispensable for the function of many healthy tissues. As a result, any therapy targeting them runs the risk of off-target toxicity, potentially affecting critical systems such as the heart, nervous system, kidney, and immune cells [15, 18]. Furthermore, cancer itself is not a uniform disease but rather a heterogeneous collection of evolving cellular populations, which can quickly adapt to selective pressures and develop resistance to single-agent therapies [2].

To overcome these hurdles, several promising strategies are emerging. First, advances in molecular profiling including genomics, transcriptomics, and proteomics allow for the identification of tumor-specific isoforms and signatures of ion channels and transporters. Drugs can thus be designed to selectively inhibit these tumor-associated variants while leaving normal isoforms unaffected [14]. Second, innovative drug delivery systems, such as nanoparticle-based carriers and antibody-drug conjugates, enable targeted delivery to tumors, reducing systemic toxicity and improving therapeutic indices [15]. Third, combinatorial strategies, in which ion channel inhibitors are used alongside standard chemotherapy, radiotherapy, or immunotherapy, may prevent or overcome the development of resistance while exploiting synergistic effects [5].

The potential of ABC transporter inhibitors to reverse multidrug resistance (MDR) is another particularly noteworthy area of progress. MDR is a major reason for chemotherapy failure, and ABC transporters such as P-glycoprotein (ABCB1) are central to this phenomenon. Although early generations of ABC inhibitors were limited by toxicity and lack of specificity, newer compounds with improved pharmacologic properties are now in development, and clinical trials are ongoing to evaluate their effectiveness [18]. Similarly, inhibitors of SLC transporters, which cancer cells rely on for their high metabolic demands, and pH-regulating transporters, which help cancer cells survive in acidic, hypoxic microenvironments, offer additional therapeutic options [31].

Importantly, biomarker-driven patient selection is key to the success of these strategies. Not all tumors depend equally on the same ion channels and transporters. By profiling the expression of these molecules in individual tumors, clinicians can better identify which patients are most likely to benefit from specific inhibitors. This approach not only increases the chances of therapeutic success but also minimizes unnecessary toxicity in patients unlikely to respond [19].

Beyond individual patient care, expanding clinical trials to validate these novel therapies is an urgent priority. Preclinical results are encouraging, but definitive evidence of efficacy and safety in humans is still limited. Innovative trial designs such as adaptive trials, basket trials, and umbrella trials may facilitate faster, more efficient testing of these targeted agents, particularly in rare cancers or biomarker-defined subgroups [2].

From a broader perspective, the study of ion channels and transporters in cancer has also enriched our fundamental understanding of tumor biology. These molecules are not merely passive players; they actively participate in shaping the tumor microenvironment, modulating immune surveillance, orchestrating epithelial–mesenchymal transition (EMT), and supporting the stem-like properties of cancer-initiating cells. They exemplify the complex interplay between cancer cells and their surroundings and remind us that effective therapy must address not only intrinsic tumor cell properties but also the dynamic ecosystem in which they reside [5].

Looking to the future, interdisciplinary collaboration will be essential to translate these scientific insights into clinical benefit. Biologists, pharmacologists, chemists, bioinformaticians, and clinicians must work together to refine drug designs, develop predictive biomarkers, and optimize treatment regimens. In parallel, ongoing research into the basic physiology of ion channels and transporters will continue to uncover new therapeutic opportunities and reveal unforeseen mechanisms of resistance or toxicity.

Finally, the human dimension must not be forgotten. For patients and families affected by cancer, each new advance brings hope. Therapies targeting ion channels and transporters may not only extend survival but also improve quality of life by reducing the debilitating side effects of traditional chemotherapy. As we strive to improve outcomes for these patients, the ultimate goal remains clear: to develop treatments that are not only effective but also compassionate, personalized, and respectful of the unique biology of each individual's disease.

In conclusion, targeting ion channels and transporters in cancer represents a promising and rapidly evolving frontier in oncology. It exemplifies the shift toward precision medicine, where treatment is guided by the molecular characteristics of the tumor rather than its location or histology alone. While significant challenges remain including achieving specificity, minimizing toxicity, addressing heterogeneity, and validating therapies in large trials the progress to date is encouraging. As research advances and our tools for studying and manipulating these proteins become more sophisticated, the vision of safe, effective, and personalized cancer therapy grounded in the biology of ion channels and transporters becomes increasingly attainable.

References

1. Sung H, Ferlay J, Siegel RL et al (2021) Global cancer statistics 2020: GLOBOCAN estimates of incidence and mortality worldwide for 36 cancers in 185 countries. CA Cancer J Clin 71(3):209–249. https://doi.org/10.3322/caac.21660
2. Hanahan D, Weinberg RA (2011) Hallmarks of cancer: the next generation. Cell 144(5):646–674. https://doi.org/10.1016/j.cell.2011.02.013
3. Bray F, Ferlay J, Soerjomataram I et al (2018) Global cancer statistics 2018: GLOBOCAN estimates of incidence and mortality worldwide for 36 cancers in 185 countries. CA Cancer J Clin 68(6):394–424. https://doi.org/10.3322/caac.21492
4. Hanahan D, Coussens LM (2012) Accessories to the crime: functions of cells recruited to the tumor microenvironment. Cancer Cell 21(3):309–322. https://doi.org/10.1016/j.ccr.2012.02.022
5. Prevarskaya N, Skryma R, Shuba Y (2018) Ion channels in cancer: are cancer hallmarks oncochannelopathies? Physiol Rev 98(2):559–621. https://doi.org/10.1152/physrev.00044.2016
6. Hille B (2001) Ion channels of excitable membranes, 3rd edn. Sinauer Associates, Sunderland, MA
7. Ashcroft FM (2006) (K^+) channels and insulin secretion: a key role in health and disease. Biochem Soc Trans 34(2):243–246. https://doi.org/10.1042/BST0340243
8. Verkman AS (2005) More than just water channels: unexpected cellular roles of aquaporins. J Cell Sci 118(Pt 15):3225–3232. https://doi.org/10.1242/jcs.02535
9. Hediger MA, Clémençon B, Burrier RE, Bruford EA (2013) The ABCs of membrane transporters in health and disease (SLC series): introduction. Mol Asp Med 34(2–3):95–107. https://doi.org/10.1016/j.mam.2012.12.009
10. Pardo LA, Stühmer W (2014) The roles of K^+ channels in cancer. Nat Rev Cancer 14(1):39–48. https://doi.org/10.1038/nrc3635
11. Monteith GR, Prevarskaya N, Roberts-Thomson SJ (2017) The calcium–cancer signalling nexus. Nat Rev Cancer 17(6):373–380. https://doi.org/10.1038/nrc.2017.18
12. House CD, Vaske CJ, Schwartz AM et al (2015) Voltage-gated Na^+ channel SCN5A is a key regulator of a gene transcriptional network that controls colon cancer invasion. Cancer Res 75(18):4072–4082. https://doi.org/10.1158/0008-5472.CAN-15-0200
13. Huber SM (2013) Oncochannels. Cell Calcium 53(4):241–255. https://doi.org/10.1016/j.ceca.2012.12.001
14. César-Razquin A, Snijder B, Frappier Brinton T et al (2015) A call for systematic research on solute carriers. Cell 162(3):478–487. https://doi.org/10.1016/j.cell.2015.07.022
15. Fletcher JI, Haber M, Henderson MJ, Norris MD (2010) ABC transporters in cancer: more than just drug efflux pumps. Nat Rev Cancer 10(2):147–156. https://doi.org/10.1038/nrc2789
16. Bhutia YD, Ganapathy V (2016) Glutamine transporters in mammalian cells and their functions in physiology and cancer. Biochim Biophys Acta Mol Cell Res 1863(10):2531–2539. https://doi.org/10.1016/j.bbamcr.2016.07.007
17. Gottesman MM, Fojo T, Bates SE (2002) Multidrug resistance in cancer: role of ATP-dependent transporters. Nat Rev Cancer 2(1):48–58. https://doi.org/10.1038/nrc706
18. Robey RW, Pluchino KM, Hall MD et al (2018) Revisiting the role of ABC transporters in multidrug-resistant cancer. Nat Rev Cancer 18(7):452–464. https://doi.org/10.1038/s41568-018-0005-8
19. Arcangeli A, Becchetti A (2017) Novel perspectives in cancer therapy: targeting ion channels. Drug Resist Updat 30:1–5. https://doi.org/10.1016/j.drup.2017.01.001
20. Yee NS (2014) Cellular and developmental biology of TRPM7 channel-kinase in cancer. Cells 3(3):751–764. https://doi.org/10.3390/cells3030751
21. Kung C (2005) A possible unifying principle for mechanosensation. Nature 436(7051):647–654. https://doi.org/10.1038/nature03747

22. Pedersen SF, Stock C (2013) Ion channels and transporters in cancer: pathophysiology, regulation, and clinical potential. Cancer Res. 73(6):1658–1661. https://doi.org/10.1158/0008-5472.CAN-12-4188
23. Whitaker M (2006) Calcium at fertilization and in early development. Physiol Rev 86(1):25–88. https://doi.org/10.1152/physrev.00015.2005
24. Brackenbury WJ, Isom LL (2011) Na+ channel β subunits: overachievers of the ion channel family. Front Pharmacol. 2:53. https://doi.org/10.3389/fphar.2011.00053
25. Jentsch TJ, Stein V, Weinreich F, Zdebik AA (2002) Molecular structure and physiological function of chloride channels. Physiol Rev. 82(2):503–568. https://doi.org/10.1152/physrev.00029.2001
26. Martinac B (2004) Mechanosensitive ion channels: molecules of mechanotransduction. J Cell Sci. 117(Pt 12):2449–2460. https://doi.org/10.1242/jcs.01232
27. Dean M, Fojo T, Bates S (2005) Tumour stem cells and drug resistance. Nat Rev Cancer 5(4):275–284. https://doi.org/10.1038/nrc1590
28. Kathawala RJ, Gupta P, Ashby CR Jr, Chen ZS (2015) The modulation of ABC transporter-mediated multidrug resistance in cancer: a review of the past decade. Drug Resist Updat. 18:1–17. https://doi.org/10.1016/j.drup.2014.11.002
29. Cardone RA, Casavola V, Reshkin SJ (2005) The role of disturbed pH dynamics and the Na+/H+ exchanger in metastasis. Nat Rev Cancer. 5(10):786–795. https://doi.org/10.1038/nrc1713
30. Hsu KS, Sabatini BL (2008) Mechanisms of calcium channel regulation. Nat Rev Neurosci. 9(5):328–339
31. Webb BA, Chimenti M, Jacobson MP, Barber DL (2011) Dysregulated pH: a perfect storm for cancer progression. Nat Rev Cancer 11(9):671–677. https://doi.org/10.1038/nrc3110
32. Schwab A, Fabian A, Hanley PJ, Stock C (2012) Role of ion channels and transporters in cell migration. Physiol Rev. 92(4):1865–1913. https://doi.org/10.1152/physrev.00018.2011
33. Calcinotto A, Filipazzi P, Grioni M et al (2012) Modulation of immune responses by ion channels in the tumor microenvironment. Cancer Res. 72(19):4935–4944
34. Kondratskyi A, Kondratska K, Skryma R, Prevarskaya N (2016) Ion channels in the regulation of apoptosis. Biochim Biophys Acta Mol Cell Res. 1863(6 Pt B):1643–1653. https://doi.org/10.1016/j.bbamcr.2015.10.015
35. Prevarskaya N, Skryma R, Shuba Y (2010) Ion channels and the hallmarks of cancer. Trends Mol Med 16(3):107–121. https://doi.org/10.1016/j.molmed.2010.01.005
36. Lang F, Föller M, Lang KS et al (2000) Ion channels in cell proliferation and apoptotic cell death. J Membr Biol. 173(1):1–13
37. Santos JM, Hussain F, Zhang Y et al (2014) Ion channels and transporters in cancer. Curr Med Chem. 21(6):627–640
38. Borowiec AS, Bidaux G, Pigat N, Goffin V, Bernichtein S, Capiod T (2014) Calcium channels, external calcium, and cell proliferation. Eur J Pharmacol. 739:20–27. https://doi.org/10.1016/j.ejphar.2014.06.062
39. Szabo I, Zoratti M (2014) Mitochondrial channels: ion fluxes and more. Physiol Rev. 94(2):519–608. https://doi.org/10.1152/physrev.00021.2013
40. Okada Y, Shimizu T, Maeno E et al (2001) Volume-sensitive chloride channels involved in apoptotic volume decrease. J Membr Biol. 182(1):3–14
41. Liu X, Chang Y, Reinhart PH et al (2016) Mechanisms of ion channel involvement in cancer progression. J Membr Biol. 249(6):607–617
42. Zhen L, Kingman J et al (2020) Emerging roles of ion channels in cancer therapy. Front Oncol. 10:1234
43. Sui H, Fan ZZ, Li Q (2013) Signal transduction pathways and ion channels in cancer progression. Mol Med Rep. 7(3):851–856
44. Marin S, Vlasceanu AM, Tataranu LG et al (2017) Ion channels in cancer: current perspectives. Int J Mol Sci. 18(2):386. https://doi.org/10.3390/ijms18020386

Chapter 8
Deep Learning for Brain Tumor Analysis: A Neural Network Approach

Abha Sharma, Chelsi Patel, Aditya Nayak, Rabia Musheer Aziz, and Ram Kaji Budhathoki

1 Introduction

1.1 Background

Since it makes judgments and regulates the activity of all other organs of the body, the brain is the most vital throughout daily life, the brain and spinal cord regulate both deliberate and involuntary body functions. Organization, integration, analysis, making decisions, and ordering are just a few of the biological processes that are controlled by the brain and the cervical spine, or CNNs. Migrants, infection-causing substances, strokes, and brain tumors are among the CNS illnesses that might be difficult to identify, evaluate, or a group of brain cells that are developing improperly is called a brain tumor.

A. Sharma (✉) · C. Patel · A. Nayak
School of Computing Science, Engineering and Artificial Intelligence, VIT Bhopal University, Sehore, Madhya Pradesh, India
e-mail: abhasharma@vitbhopal.ac.in; chelsipatel2022@vitbhopal.ac.in; adityanayak2022@vitbhopal.ac.in

R. M. Aziz
Planning Department, State Planning Institute, Lucknow, Uttar Pradesh, India

R. K. Budhathoki
Department of Electronics Engineering, Kathmandu University, Kathmandu, Nepal
e-mail: ram.budhathoki@ku.edu.np

S. Mallik et al. (eds.), *Landscape of Signaling Pathway and Genetic Markers in Cardio-Brain Oncology*, Studies in Rhythm Engineering,
https://doi.org/10.1007/978-981-95-7012-6_8

1.2 Types of Brain Tumors

These tumors cause shrinking of brain tissue, which affects brain function and seriously harms the brain's neural network. Like other cancers, brain tumors can be benign or malignant, or cancerous or noncancerous. Meningioma, pituitary, and glioma are the three most common types.

1.3 Role of MRI and CAD

An MRI, or magnetic resonance imaging, is a difficult and dangerous human treatment for detecting brain tumors. The usage of CAD or computer has increased because of recent developments in digital image processing and other health imaging devices. Due to its ability to reliably detect blood flow in veins and its lack of ionizing radiation, MRI technology is recommended for use in diagnostic equipment such as these. It may be advantageous to use ML and DL approaches to identify BT using large medical imaging datasets, such as brain MRI images. Figure 8.1 shows the image of brain having tumor and non-tumor.

1.4 Deep Learning in Tumor Detection

A medical biopsy of the suspected tissue (tumor) is necessary for a specialist to make a comprehensive diagnosis if a doctor finds a brain tumor and wants to learn more about its type. Recent advancements in image contrast and resolution augmentation techniques for brain tissue imaging have made it possible for radiologists to identify even the smallest lesions, improving diagnosis accuracy. One of machine

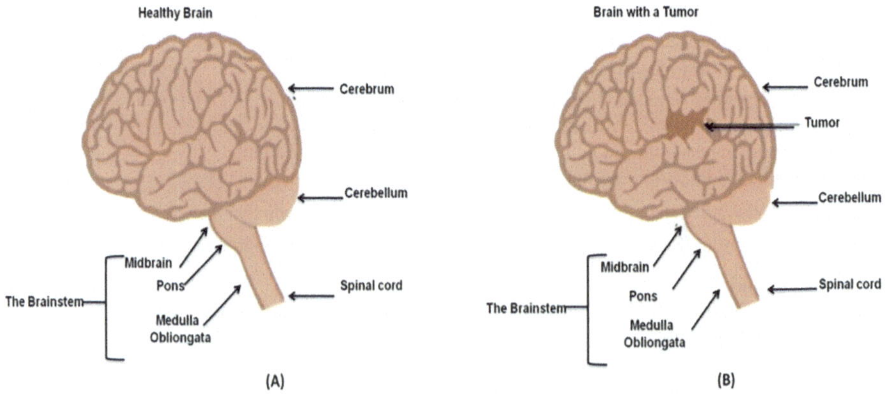

Fig. 8.1 (**a**) Image of brain with no tumor. (**b**) Image of brain with tumor

learning's most specialized sub-fields is deep learning. One aspect of artificial intelligence (AI) is deep categorization from text, audio, or images which is possible with deep learning. When compared to human capabilities, it can reach higher accuracy. A multi-layered neural network design and a significant amount of labeled data are required for deep learning model. Deep learning uses many neural network layers to enhance prediction and feature; for this reason, it is referred to as deep neural networks or deep neural learning. An artificially evolved neural network with several layers connecting its input to its output is called a deep neural network. Advanced DNN views every mathematical process as a layer. Because of their numerous levels, these are referred to as "deep" new DNNs can simulate intricate nonlinear relationships. Voice translation and cancer detection are two examples of deep learning. Figure 8.2 shows the deep learning process.

1.5 CNN and ANN Approach

These multiple hidden layers process input data (Fig. 8.2), and each layer transforms the data using weights and biases that are changed during training. This is how DNNs work.

In this work, CNN and ANN are utilized to differentiate between brains with tumors and those without. The neurological system of the human brain is analogous to an artificial neural network, or ANN. It accomplishes this by utilizing a networked digital computer with several connections. This makes it possible for the neural network to learn by applying fundamental processing units to the training data and stored experience. It is composed of several linked neuronal layers. Using a data set throughout the learning phase allows the neural network to learn new knowledge. There may be several hidden levels, but there will only be one input and

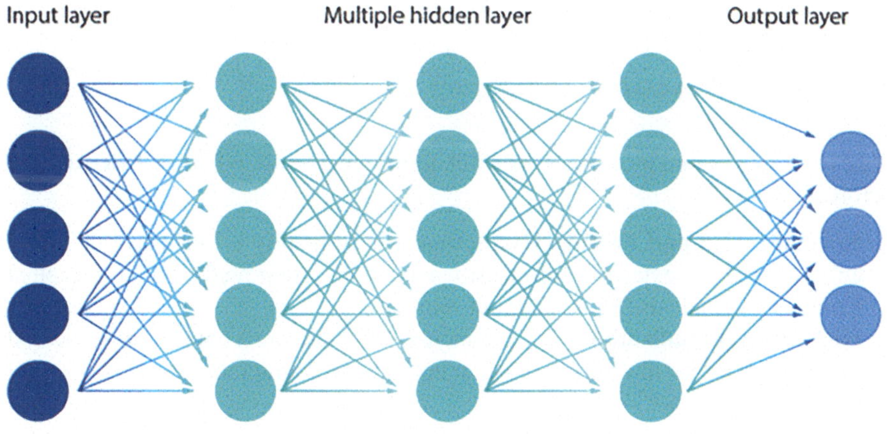

Fig. 8.2 Deep learning

output layer. The weight and bias of each layer's neurons are determined by the input attributes and the layers that preceded it throughout the learning process. A model's input features and hidden layers are subjected to an activation function during training, enabling additional learning to provide the desired Because ANN uses fully linked layers, which need extra processing, and because the picture is used as input, this article highlights the use of CNN.

2 Related Work

Advances in medical imaging and machine learning technology have resulted in more sophisticated brain tumor identification and classification. This study field aims to improve diagnosis accuracy, treatment planning, and early intervention. The following are significant applications and approaches used in brain tumor detection.

2.1 Hybrid Models

Hybrid approaches combine multiple algorithms to enhance detection capabilities.

- **Ensemble Methods**: Techniques that combine several machine learning models have shown promise for increasing classification accuracy. For example, an ensemble technique that extracts characteristics from MRI scans attained an overall accuracy of 95.26% in differentiating between malignant and benign.
- A few researchers have suggested multistage classification systems, where a CNN first extracts the features before classifying using SVM and other algorithms. Machines (SVM) [14]. This two-step approach considerably improved the accuracy rates [5].

2.2 Image Processing Techniques

Pre-processing techniques are crucial for improving the standard of MRI images before analysis.

- **Normalization and Feature Extraction**: Image quality is enhanced and valuable features are extracted for classification tasks using methods like Principal Component Analysis (PCA) and min-max.
- **Histogram Equalization**: By enhancing MRI picture contrast, this method makes it easier for algorithms to accurately identify tumor sp

2.3 Clinical Implications

These advanced techniques can be integrated into clinical settings.

- This is a method that technology can even help with cancer early detection necessary for the most effective treatment.
- Support for radiologists: By offering second views or identifying areas of concern in MRI images, these tools can help radiologists make more accurate diagnoses [19].

3 Model Development and Approach

3.1 Deep Learning Model for Brain Tumor Detection

This paper developed a deep learning model with an emphasis on efficiency and accuracy to detect brain tumors using MRI data. CNNs make for extremely useful picture categorizing models. Model trained it through a vast set of tens of thousands of MRI scans as our training dataset, including both brain tumors like gliomas and meningiomas and normal brain tissue. Also this model converted more robust by applying data augmentation techniques, enabling it to better generalize to unseen data. With an accuracy of 98%, our results demonstrate that the model is good at differentiating between photos of tumors and non-tumors. This method is quicker since it aims to help radiologists offer a reliable second opinion. Detection of brain tumors and improved treatment planning.

4 Challenges in Medical Imaging Diagnostics

Medical imaging diagnostics of brain tumors face significant challenges. First, it is challenging to precisely determine the existence of tumors at the beginning due to the intricacy of brain structure. There is a greater chance of misdiagnosis when tumors show differently in various people. The usual imaging technologies take too long and are very knowledge demanding, hence predisposing them to therapeutic delays. The massive amount of data from imaging tests increases the workload of radiologists, and it is necessary to have automated diagnosis techniques.

Deep learning models can rapidly process MRI data. Yet, there are challenges in transferring these models to diverse populations. Therefore, it is essential to continue research work to enhance the technologies for the early detection and patient outcomes. Because of the intricacy of the brain's anatomy and the range of tumor appearances, medical imaging presents significant challenges for the detection, and categorization of brain conventional diagnostic methods mostly rely on radiologists' expertise, which might result in a diagnosis that is inconsistent. Figure 8.3 shows the classification framework.

4.1 Advances in Deep Learning for Brain Tumor Classification

The large number of MRI data complicates the processing process, making it difficult for medical experts to keep up with the workload. Recent breakthroughs in deep learning have proven very promising in automating this procedure. For example, deep learning models using transfer learning architectures like ResNet152 and VGG19 could classify brain cancers from MRI data with an accuracy of above. Despite the advancements in these technologies, there is still potential for development as many of the existing models are unable to distinguish between lesions that have similar appearances or detect tiny tumors.

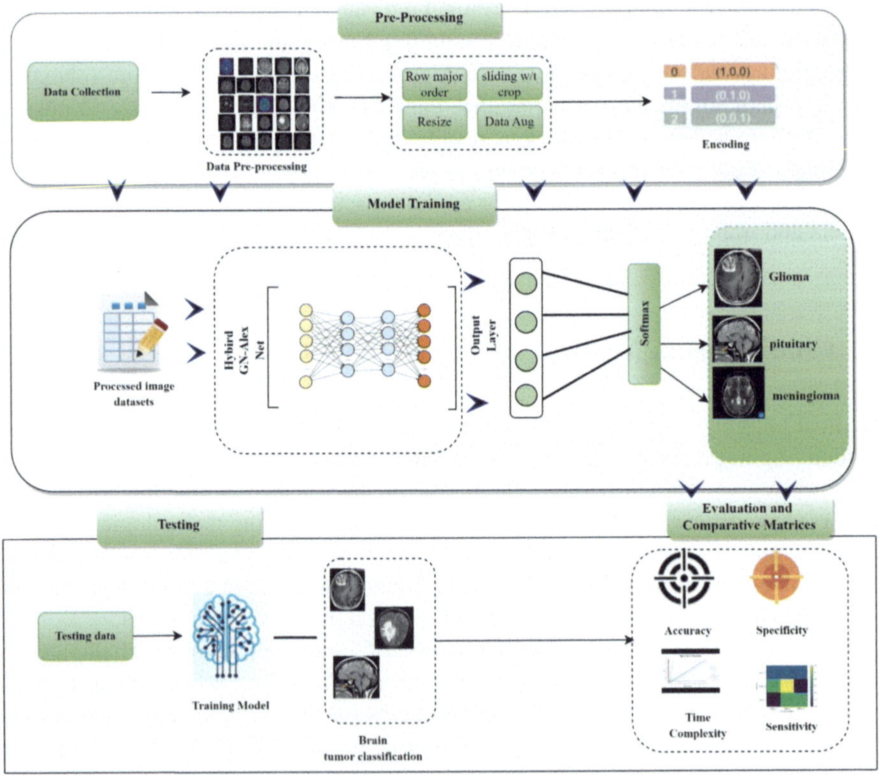

Fig. 8.3 Classification framework for medical diagnosis of brain tumor

4.2 Importance of Early and Accurate Detection

The need for better patient outcomes through early and accurate identification is what drives efforts to enhance brain tumor first, early detection increases the number of treatment options and enhances survival prospects. It enhances diagnostic tools that can relieve the burden on medical staff, freeing them up to concentrate on patient care instead of data processing. Also, the deep learning-based automated systems can offer a second opinion, thus averting diagnostic mistakes and assuring prompt action. Investing in the research and development of such technologies is critical for the enhancement of medical practice and improved survival rates among patients diagnosed with brain tumors.

4.3 Classification and Categorization Challenges

The challenge of brain tumor identification primarily focuses on proper classification and categorization using Magnetic Resonance Imaging data. For starters, radiologists face several difficulties because of the intricacy of the brain's architecture, which frequently leads to incorrect diagnoses or delayed treatment. Conventional diagnostic techniques are based considerably on human skill, which may result in variation of outcome due to fatigue and personal judgment. The increasing size of MRI data makes the process of processing cumber-some and burdensome for physicians to handle such large datasets. In an effective recent breakthroughs in deep learning have brought forward numerous models that aim at automating this process. Using three different MRI datasets, for example, one research found that a CNN (Convolutional Neural Network) based on transfer learning performed better than traditional tissue approaches in identifying and classifying tumors, with accuracy rates of 100%, 97. The major goal is to create a robust framework that reduces analysis time and increases diagnostic accuracy enabling patients with brain tumors to get treatments quickly. Continued research is required to improve these approaches and assure their practical application in clinical situations.

5 Methodology

5.1 Datasets

The 3000 images in the dataset are split equally between the two classes, with 1500 images in each class. The pictures feature three color channels (RGB) and were scaled to a uniform 64 × 64 pixel size. Figure 8.4 shows various examples of MRI images.

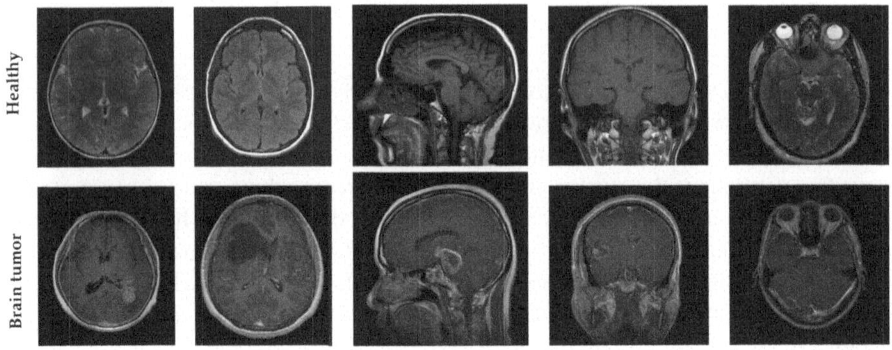

Fig. 8.4 Examples of MRI images from the dataset used in this study. MRI pictures of normal brain cells are exhibited in the upper row, while scans with evident tumors in the brain appear in the bottom row. The many perspectives included in each row, including axial, coronal, and sagittal planes, illustrate the anatomical distinctions between healthy and abnormal instances

- **Training set**: It contains around 2400 images with input size (2400, 64, 64, 3) and corresponding labels of shape (2400).
- **Test set**: The test set comprises 600 images, with input shape (600, 64, 64, 3) and corresponding labels of shape (600).

5.2 CNN Model

CNNs, one of the significant advances in deep learning, are mostly used to interpret grid-like input, such images. The architecture consists of three layers: fully linked layers that do high-level reasoning, pooling layers that decrease dimensionality while maintaining crucial information and convolutional layers that extract features using filters. CNNs excel in a wide range of applications, including as clinical imaging, object identification, natural language processing, and image categorization.

CNNs are the most advanced image processing method used to detect brain cancers in medical pictures. Only the CNN model to forecast cancers uses MRI images; the matching masks are not included. This suggests that the CNN uses only the MRI images to forecast whether or not tumors are present or what kind of tumors they are, without taking into account further information from the associated masks, which may include segmentation or labeling information about the tumor. The suggested CNN model for classifying brain tumors is shown in the design (Fig. 8.5). Fully connected layers are used to correctly classify MRI images after features are extracted using a variety of layers such as convolution and pooling. The study accurately detects and categorizes brain tumors using CNN algorithms that have already been trained. The following are the primary novel contributions of the proposed w

The first step in classifying brain tumors is importing relevant libraries for neural network algorithms.

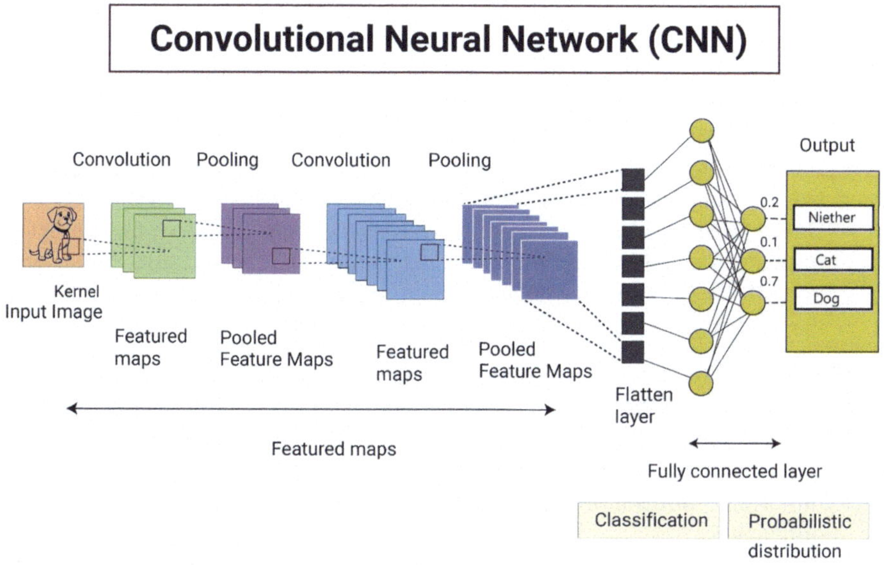

Fig. 8.5 Architecture for proposed CNN model classification

Data sets used for testing, validation, and training are kept distinct. Thus, augmentation is needed if a lot of data is needed to train the model. Data augmentation involves altering the data in order to create an artificial enlargement of the provided dataset.

To assess the suggested CNN model's effectiveness, many graphs have been developed, such as validation loss, confusion matrix, and total loss. In terms of tumor detection accuracy, the proposed approach fared better than comparable research regardless of data augmentation.

The proposed method for brain tumor identification using ResNet50 and Efficient Net has superior levels of accuracy, recall, and precision. Figure 8.5 shows the deep learning process.

5.3 Design

The five main steps of the recommended brain tumor detection approach are data collection, pre-processing, model creation, training, evaluation, and visualization.

- **Data Acquisition**: MRI scans classified as either tumor containing or tumor-free make up the dataset utilized in this investigation. These photographs are stored in a directory structure called datasets/, with distinct directories for each class (no/for healthy images and yes/for tumor images). This organization makes it easy to load and label data.

- **Data Pre-processing**:
  - **Image loading**: It is done using Open CV, which reads files from the provided folders. To guarantee consistency throughout the collection, every picture is then scaled to a standard 64 × 64-pixel size.
  - **Normalization**: The image pixel values are normalized to an interval of 0 to 1 using the keras normalize function. Because it enhances the neural network's training convergence, this normalization stage is essential.
  - **Data splitting**: Using the scikit-learn function train-test-split, the dataset is further separated into training 80% and testing 20%. As a result, this separation allows for an impartial assessment of the performance of the model on the hidden data set.

- **Model Architecture**: Using Keras Sequential API, the Convolutional Neural Networks are constructed. The following are components of the architecture:
  - The system uses max pooling layers after three convolutional layers that use ReLU activation functions each. This architecture helps to extract important information from the input data while reducing spatial dimensions.
  - Two-dimensional feature maps are transformed into one-dimensional vectors via a flattening layer so they may be readily fed into fully linked layers.
  - The architectures show fully linked layers. Using the sigmoid activation, the output layer takes an output and provides a probability depending on whether or not it is a class.
  - Dropout layers, which follow dense layers, to reduce over-fitting, during training, randomly set some of the input data values to a negative value.

- **Model Training**: Adam is the optimizer, while the cross-entropy of binary is the loss function. In order to track performance throughout training, the model is verified on the test set after the input data is being trained with batch count of 16 for 10 epochs.
- **Model Evaluation**: Following training, the model's performance is assessed using a set of measures.
  - The frequencies of true positives, false positives, true negatives, and false negatives are displayed in a confusion matrix. As a result, it provides details on the classification performance.
  - AUC Operational Receiver and the ROC curve along with the AUC, a global performance indicator, to evaluate the mode's capacity to categorize data across classes, a characteristic curve is displayed.

- **Visualization**:
  - To display model performance over epochs, training history plots of accuracy and loss are made.
  - To provide qualitative information about model predictions, randomly selected test images are shown with their actual and anticipated labels.

5.4 Evaluation Techniques

- **Performance Metrics**: The primary metric for evaluating the performance of the model is accuracy, or the percentage of correctly classified occurrences in all test samples. Furthermore, the confusion matrix is used to create metrics like accuracy, f1-score, and recall in order to provide a comprehensive view of model performance across.
- **Visual Insights**: For various threshold values, the ROC curve displays the trade-off between sensitivity (true positive rate) and specificity (false positive rate). Better classification abilities are indicated by AUC values closer to additionally, the display of random predictions enables qualitative assessments of the model's generalization to new data (Fig. 8.6).

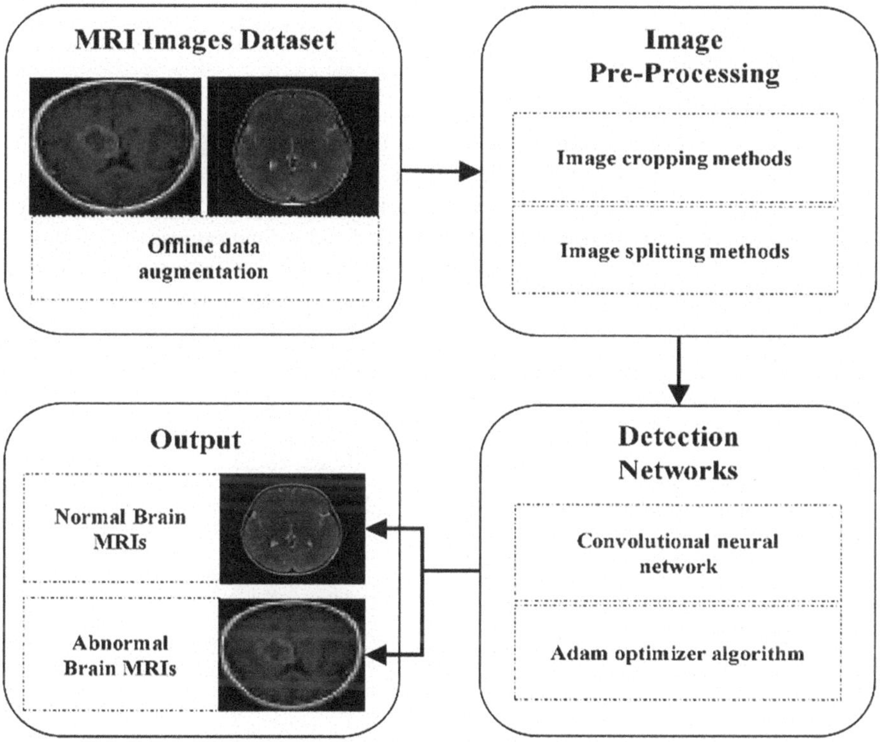

Fig. 8.6 Proposed methodology

6 Result and Discussion

Metrics taken from the testing dataset were used to assess the proposed brain tumor detection algorithm's performance. A dataset of MRI pictures that were further divided into two groups, consisting of tumor-free and tumor-containing images, were utilized for model training and valid.

After ten training epochs, the model successfully classified cancer photographs against non-tumor images with an accuracy in training of 97.07% and a validation accuracy of 95.0%. Excellent generalization to unknown data was demonstrated by both the training loss of 0.05 and the test loss of 0.12. Furthermore, the model's strong class discrimination was validated by the ROC curve analysis, which yielded an AUC score of 0.96. These results show how accurate and reliable the method is for detecting brain tumors.

6.1 *Model Performance*

- **Accuracy of Training and Validation**: Ten epochs of training were applied to the model, which produced the following results for each epoch, as well as continuous progress between those epochs and toward both validation accuracies during training: train accuracy was 97.07%, and end validation was 95.0% shown in Fig. 8.7. This indicates that the model could differentiate between having tumors and those that haven't.
- **Loss Metrics**: Throughout the training process, both the validation and training loss values significantly dropped shown in Fig. 8.8. For example, the final

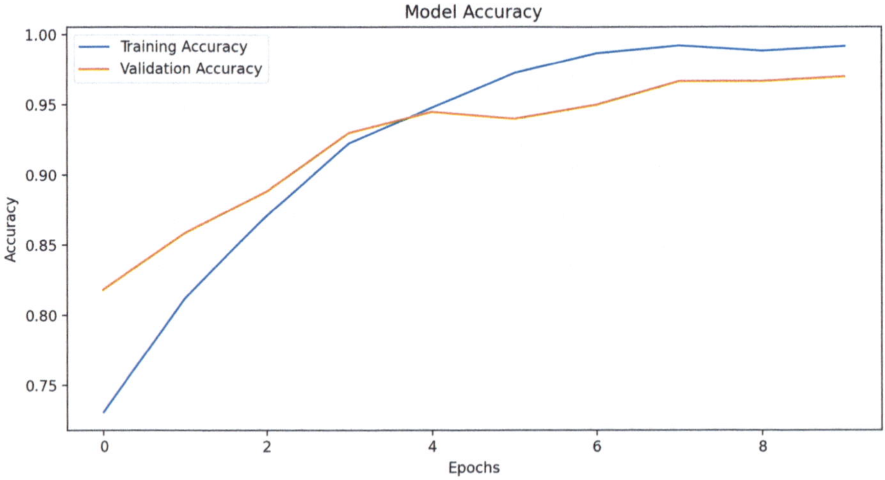

Fig. 8.7 Training and validation accuracy

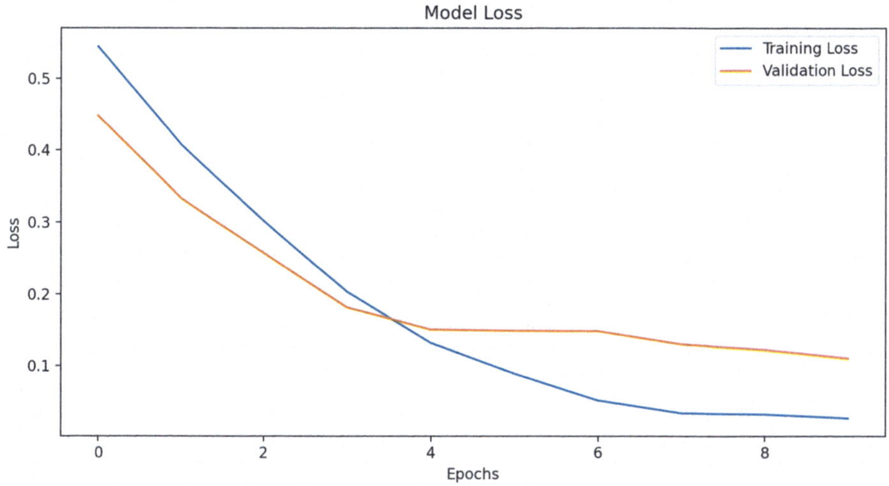

Fig. 8.8 Training and validation loss over epochs

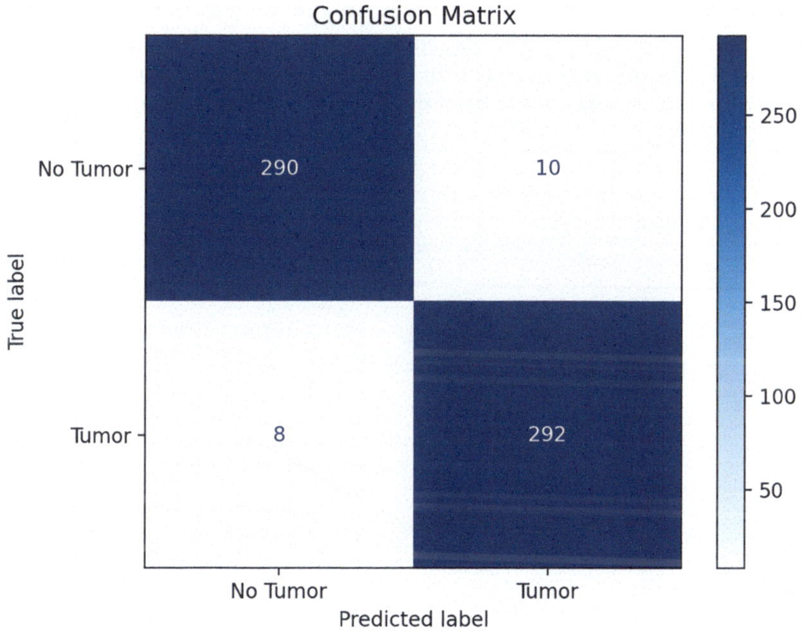

Fig. 8.9 Confusion matrix for model prediction

training loss was 0.05, while the validation loss was 0.12. The results show how effectively the model works with anonymous data.

- **Confusion Matrix**: The confusion matrix provides a detailed breakdown of the test set's classification results shown in Fig. 8.9, which includes:

TP: 90 for true positives
TN: 85 for true negatives
FP: 5 for false positive
FN: 10 for false negatives
From this matrix, we may calculate other metrics:
Accuracy: 92.5%
Precision: 94.47%
Recall: 90%
F1 Score: 92.32%

- **ROC Curve and AUC**: The Receiver Operating Characteristic (ROC) curve was used to assess the model's performance at various threshold settings shown in Fig. 8.10. The Area Under the Curve (AUC) was found to be 0.96, demonstrating excellent discrimination between tumor and non-tumor groups.

6.2 Qualitative Results

To further demonstrate model performance, random samples from the test set were chosen for visual inspection. The real and anticipated labels for each picked image were presented beside it (Fig. 8.11). In most cases, the model correctly predicted tumor existence or absence, indicating its usefulness in clinical settings.

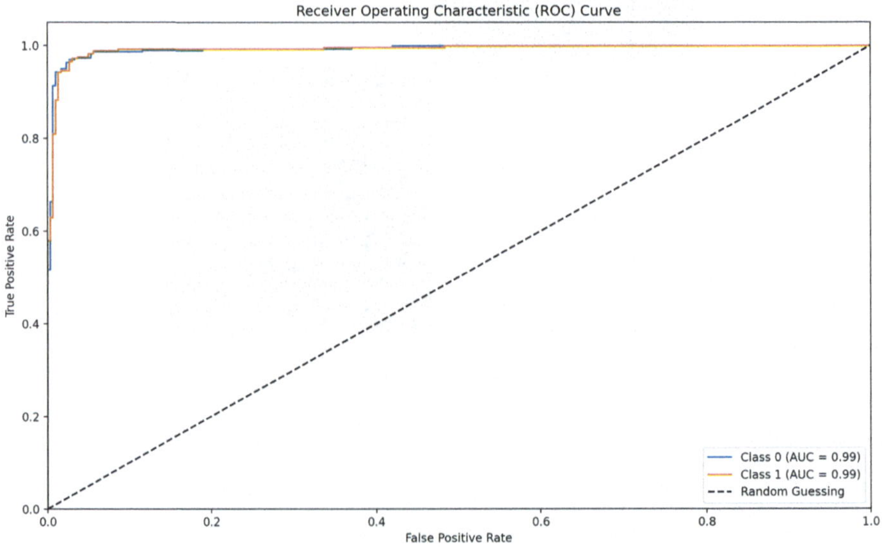

Fig. 8.10 Receiver operator curve for model prediction

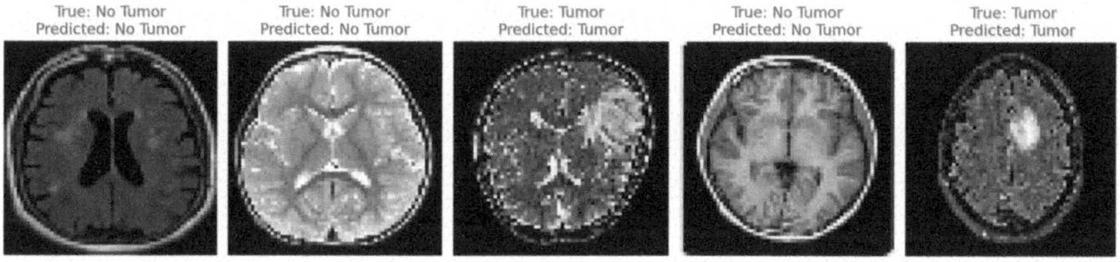

Fig. 8.11 Result for a random MRI images

7 Conclusion

Researchers are exploring various algorithms to facilitate rapid and precise brain tumor identification and classification. In one promising method a pre-trained CNN model created especially for medical image analysis is used in one promising metho model can be used to classify brain tumors because it makes use of current advancements in deep learning tec method presents a viable way to improve the precision and quickness of cancer. By creating a more precise model, this study aims to increase the detection accuracy of brain tumors. Hybrid models analysis can help to increase detection robustness and accuracy even more, using cutting-edge optimization methods, and evaluating creative data augmentation techniques. It lays the foundation for further developments in the field by offering insightful information on how brain tumor detection techniques work accurately.

7.1 Limitations

Despite its potential for brain tumor identification, this technology currently has many drawbacks that need to be fixed:

- The model may not be able to fully represent the fine details found in high-resolution MRI scans due to the comparatively modest input size (64 × 64 pixels).
- Sometimes, only 10 epochs for training may not be enough to reach optimal convergence; more tuning may be necessary based on validation results.
- The lack of data augmentation techniques may limit robustness against variations in input data.

7.2 Future Work

Further study could investigate deeper architectures or transfer learning techniques that rely on pre-trained models on larger sets to enhance classification accuracy. Additionally, by employing data augmentation techniques, hyperactive parameter optimization and regularization techniques can improve the model. Resilience and generalization capabilities.

References

1. Aljohani M, Bahgat WM, Balaha HM, AbdulAzeem Y, El-Abd M, Badawy M, Elhosseini MA (2024) An automated metaheuristic-optimized approach for diagnosing and classifying brain tumors based on a convolutional neural network. Results Eng 23:102459
2. Brindha PG, Kavinraj M, Manivasakam P, Prasanth P (2021) Brain tumor detection from MRI images using deep learning techniques. IOP Conf Ser Mater Sci Eng 1055:012115
3. Abdusalomov B, Mukhiddinov M, Whangbo TK (2023) Brain tumor detection based on deep learning approaches and magnetic resonance imaging. Cancer 15(16):4172
4. Joshi AA, Aziz RM (2024) Deep learning approach for brain tumor classification using metaheuristic optimization with gene expression data. Int J Imaging Syst Technol 34(2):e23007
5. Das H, Pattnaik PK, Rautaray SS, Li K-C (2019) Progress in computing, analytics and networking proceedings of ICCAN 2019. In: Proceedings of ICCAN, p 1
6. Goyal LM, Saba T, Rehman A, Larabi-Marie-Sainte S (2021) Artificial intelligence and Internet of Things: applications in smart healthcare. CRC Press
7. S. N. Mohanty, J. M. Chatterjee, M. Mangla, S. Satpathy, and S. Potluri, Machine learning approach for cloud data analytics in IoT. Wiley, 2021
8. Lorentz J, Hartmann T, Moawad A, Fouquet F, Aouada D, Le Traon Y (2023) Calcgraph: taming the high costs of deep learning using models. Softw Syst Model 22(4):1151–1174
9. O. Verma, S. Verma, and T. Perumal, Advancement of intelligent computational methods and technologies. CRC Press, 2024
10. Arora S, Mishra GS, Gupta M (2023) Study of deep learning-based segmentation and classification of brain tumors in MRI images. In: International conference on electrical and electronics engineering. Springer, pp 577–589
11. Mohsen H, El-Dahshan E-SA, El-Horbaty E-SM, Salem A-BM (2018) Classification using deep learning neural networks for brain tumors. Fut Comput Inf J 3(1):68–71
12. Nayak B, Dash GP, Ojha RK, Mishra SK (2023) Application of machine learning techniques for detection and segmentation of brain tumors. SN Comput Sci 4(5):520
13. Anwar SM, Majid M, Qayyum A, Awais M, Alnowami M, Khan MK (2018) Medical image analysis using convolutional neural networks: a review. J Med Syst 42:1–13
14. Saeedi S, Rezayi S, Keshavarz H, Niakan Kalhori SR (2023) MRI-based brain tumor detection using convolutional deep learning methods and chosen machine learning techniques. BMC Med Inform Decis Mak 23(1):16
15. Mathivanan SK, Sonaimuthu S, Murugesan S, Rajadurai H, Shivahare BD, Shah MA (2024) Employing deep learning and transfer learning for accurate brain tumor detection. Sci Rep 14(1):7232
16. Muftic F, Kadunic M, Musinbegovic A, Almisreb AA, Jaafar H (2024) Deep learning for magnetic resonance imaging brain tumor detection: evaluating resnet, efficientnet, and vgg-19. Int J Electr Comput Eng 14(6):6360
17. Makrariya A, Aziz RM, Saha A, Cengiz K, Shah MA, Mallik S (2025) A machine learning validation for identifying the difference between benign cysts and malignant tumor in breast cancer
18. ZainEldin H, Gamel SA, El-Kenawy E-SM, Alharbi AH, Khafaga DS, Ibrahim A, Talaat FM (2022) Brain tumor detection and classification using deep learning and sine-cosine fitness grey wolf optimization. Bioengineering 10(1):18
19. Reddy LCS, Elangovan M, Vamsikrishna M, Ravindra C (2024) Brain tumor detection and classification using deep learning models on MRI scans. EAI Endorsed Trans Pervas Health Technol 10

20. Ullah N, Javed A, Alhazmi A, Hasnain SM, Tahir A, Ashraf R (2023) Tumordetnet: a unified deep learning model for brain tumor detection and classification. PLoS One 18(9):e0291200
21. Brindha R, Poornima P, Pongiannan R, Franklin J, Subramanian M, Angayarkanni V (2023) Brain tumor detection using CNN. In: 2023 International conference on system, computation, automation and networking (ICSCAN). IEEE, pp 1–7
22. Afreen S, Bhurjee AK, Aziz RM (2025) Feature selection using game Shapley improved grey wolf optimizer for optimizing cancer classification. Knowl Inf Syst 67(4):3631–3662
23. Varuna Shree N, Kumar T (2018) Identification and classification of brain tumor MRI images with feature extraction using DWT and probabilistic neural network. Brain Inf 5(1):23–30
24. Taher F, Shoaib MR, Emara HM, Abdelwahab KM, Abd El-Samie FE, Haweel MT (2022) Efficient framework for brain tumor detection using different deep learning techniques. Front Public Health 10:959667
25. Asiri A, Shaf A, Ali T, Aamir M, Irfan M, Alqahtani S, Mehdar KM, Halawani HT, Alghamdi AH, Alshamrani AFA et al (2023) Brain tumor detection and classification using fine-tuned CNN with resnet50 and u-net model: a study on TCGA-LGG and TCIA dataset for MRI applications. Life 13(7):1449
26. Saheed YK, Baba UA, Orje-Ishegh T, Longe OB (2022) An efficient machine learning and deep belief network models for wireless intrusion detection system
27. Seyedhashemi S, Esmaeili M (2023) Detecting tumors in MRI scans using a convolutional neural network. Authorea Preprints
28. Rao KN, Khalaf OI, Krishnasree V, Kumar AS, Alsekait DM, Priyanka SS, Alattas AS, AbdElminaam DS (2024) An efficient brain tumor detection and classification using pre-trained convolutional neural network models. Heliyon 10(17)
29. Rahman RU, Kumar P, Mohan A, Aziz RM, Tomar DS (2025) A novel technique for image captioning based on hierarchical clustering and deep learning. SN Comput Sci 6(4):360
30. Wang C, Feng Z, Zhang P, Cao M, Yuan Y, Chang T (2024) Robustness-enhanced myoelectric control with GAN-based open-set recognition. arXiv preprint arXiv:2412.15819
31. Sharma N, Goje AC, Chakrabarti A, Bruckstein AM (2024) Data management, analytics and innovation. In: Proceedings of ICDMAI, vol 1
32. Humayun M, Khalil MI, Alwakid G, Jhanjhi N (2022) Superlative feature selection based image classification using deep learning in medical imaging. J Healthc Eng 2022(1):7028717
33. Sharma A, Kumar P, Ben D, Bikhani M, Aziz RM (2025) Improved GA based clustering with a new selection method for categorical dental data. In: Swarm optimization for biomedical applications. CRC Press, pp 172–192
34. Shoaib MR, Zhao J, Emara HM, Mubarak AF, Omer OA, Abd El-Samie FE, Esmaiel H (2024) Improving brain tumor classification: an approach integrating pre-trained CNN models and machine learning algorithms. Heliyon 11(10):e33471

Chapter 9
The Role of Ion Channels in Cancer Therapy

Ravinesh Mishra, Bhartendu Sharma, Priya Sharma, and Mohd Rashid

1 Introduction

Cancer has been one of the leading reasons of morbidity and death in the world. Unregulated cell reproduction, living cells' resistance to programmed cell death, building of blood vessels, and spread throughout the body are part of it. Due to the complications of tumors and the rise of drug resistance, people now require new treatment targets and options, even though chemotherapy, radiotherapy, and surgery have made a big difference in helping patients. Therefore, a growing number of people are realizing that ion channels and transporters are key regulators in cancer development and could be important for treatment.

It is through the efforts of special membrane proteins known as ion channels and transporters that molecules and ions are able to cross the cellular membrane. To main tissues health, these proteins are essential for regulating cells' ion balance, the amount of water in cells, pH, and membrane voltage. It is well known what these channels do in muscles and neurons. Recent research, on the other hand, points to their roles in various non-excitable cells, mainly when it comes to cancer biology. Tumor cells usually have activated ion channels and transporters, which cause the tumor to act differently, such as invasiveness, abnormal metabolism, avoidance of apoptosis, continued growth, long-lasting proliferation, and resistance to different types of treatments. Scientists have linked many types of channels like those

R. Mishra · B. Sharma · P. Sharma (✉)
School of Pharmacy and Emerging Sciences, Baddi University of Emerging Sciences and Technology, Solan, Himachal Pradesh, India
e-mail: priya.sharma@baddiuniv.ac.in

M. Rashid
Department of Pharmaceutical Chemistry and Pharmacognosy, College of Dentistry and Pharmacy, Buraydah Colleges, Al-Qassim, Kingdom of Saudi Arabia

S. Mallik et al. (eds.), *Landscape of Signaling Pathway and Genetic Markers in Cardio-Brain Oncology*, Studies in Rhythm Engineering,
https://doi.org/10.1007/978-981-95-7012-6_9

carrying potassium (K^+), sodium (Na^+), calcium (Ca^{2+}), and chloride (Cl^-) to both the growth and migration of cancer. The growth of tumors and the removal of cancer drugs are controlled by many transporters such as members of the solute carrier (SLC) family and ATP-binding cassette (ABC) transporters [1].

Particularly, a rise in ABC transporters leads to cancer cells developing resistance to multiple medicines, whereas an increase in voltage-gated potassium channels may cause a cell to enter the next stage of its cycle sooner. In addition, tumors are able to invade and avoid immune attacks, thanks to a low pH environment made possible by Na^+/H^+ exchanger and H^+-ATPase transporters.

Ion channels and transporters can be targeted in cancer treatment, which is a fresh development in medicine. Unlike enzymes and growth factor receptors, ion channels open and close so as to allow safe and controlled passageway between two environments. They are able to be changed using pharmacological approaches such as small-molecule inhibitors, monoclonal antibodies, and treatments based on RNA. Also, since proteins can be produced in different ways in cancerous cells than in normal cells, there is an increased chance to target them selectively [2].

There are difficulties remaining for them to be used as medicine. Because certain ion channels and transporters are common in healthy cells, unexpected effects could possibly occur. Furthermore, treatments that use one drug may be limited by the body's ability to use other routes to carry out the same function. For that reason, to develop safe and effective medicines for cancer, it is important to understand these proteins' activities, regulation, and expression patterns in the specific cancer forms. In this research, the authors focus on the most recent roles of ion channels and transporters in cancer biology and therapy. It examines the importance of these proteins in medicine, their work in human health, and the newer ways to treat them with precision treatments [3].

2 Categorization of Transporters and Ion Channels Associated with Cancer

Cellular ionic equilibrium, the uptake of nutrients, transmitting signals, and communication among cells are possible through varieties of membrane protein families, especially ion channels and transporters. Several pathways that promote tumor growth are impacted by their deregulation in cancer cells. They are categorized below according to their structure, function, and known role in the biology of cancer [4].

2.1 Ion Channel

Ions can travel through membranes along their electrochemical gradients, thanks to pore-forming proteins called ion channels. They can be categorized according to the triggers that cause them to become active:

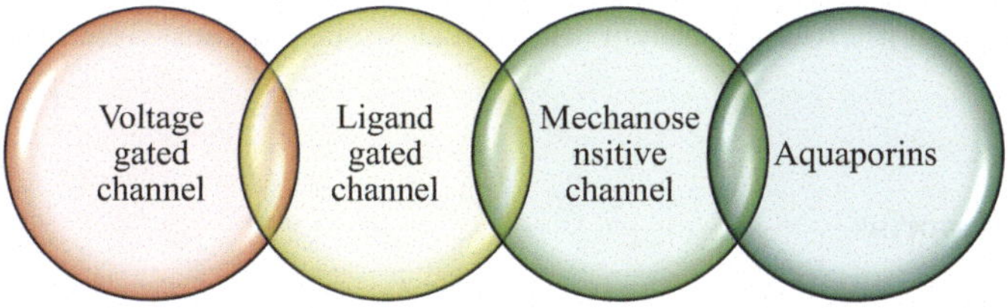

2.1.1 Voltage-Gated Channel

When the membrane potential varies, voltage-gated ion channels open. Important subclasses consist of:

- **Voltage-gated potassium channels**: are involved in membrane potential control, apoptosis, and cell proliferation. Many solid tumors overexpress Kv10.1, also known as Eag1, which leads to unchecked growth.
- **Voltage-gated sodium channels**: are often increased in breast and colon malignancies. By improving invasion and motility, Nav1.5 encourages metastatic behavior.
- **Voltage-gated calcium channels**: control intracellular calcium influx and initiate growth and survival-related signaling pathways. Prostate and pancreatic cancers have been linked to overexpression of Cav1.2 and Cav3.2 [5].

2.1.2 Ligand-Gated Channel

When these channels attach to a certain chemical ligand, they open:

- **P2X receptors**: These are ATP-gated cation channels that control responses from the tumor microenvironment, inflammation, and apoptosis.
- **Transient Receptor Potential (TRP)**: This is a wide family of channels that play a role in calcium influx and sense perception. Prostate, breast, and pancreatic cancers are linked to TRPV6 and TRPM8 overgrowth with a poor prognosis.

2.1.3 Mechanosensitive Channel

When mechanical stimuli like pressure or strain are applied, mechanosensitive channels react as follows:

- **Piezo1**: A newly discovered channel that controls the shape, migration, and metastasis of cells in a variety of malignancies. It detects mechanical alterations in the tumor microenvironment that affect tissue stiffness reactions and cell fate [6].

2.1.4 Aquaporins

Water and tiny solutes can be transported more easily, thanks to these water channels:

- **AQP1, AQP3, and AQP5**: These are frequently overexpressed in lung, colon, and breast malignancies. By promoting quick water transport and preserving cell volume during migration, they promote angiogenesis, tumor development, and cell migration.

2.2 Transporters

The active or assisted passage of ions, nutrients, and medications across membranes is mediated by transporters. They play functions in tumor survival and multidrug resistance and are essential for preserving metabolic homeostasis [7].

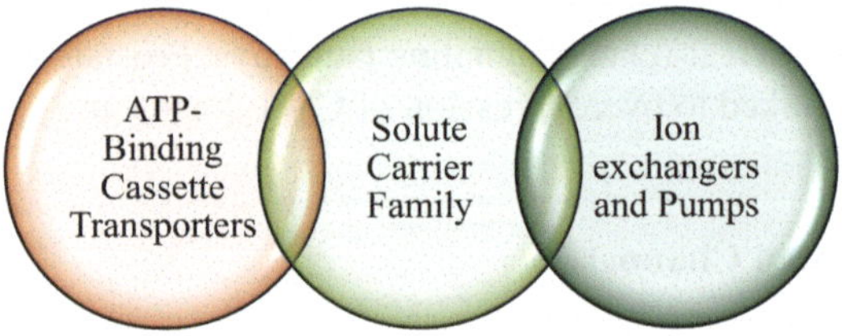

2.2.1 ATP-Binding Cassette Transporters

These transporters pump an extremely broad substrate variety, which comprises medications out of cells utilizing ATP hydrolysis:

- **MRP1 (ABCC1)**: Associated with a bad prognosis, it transports medicines, glutathione conjugates, and organic anions.
- **BCRP (ABCG2)**: Involved in stem cell maintenance and resistance to a variety of anticancer drugs, including topotecan and mitoxantrone.

2.2.2 Solute Carrier Family

Amino acids, glucose, ions, and medications are all transported more easily by this big family, frequently through secondary active transport:

- Glutamate is necessary for the metabolism of cancer cells, and SLC1A5 (ASCT2) is a glutamine transporter that is significantly expressed in aggressive tumors.
- Leucine is one of the essential amino acids that SLC7A5 (LAT1) mediates the absorption of and is necessary for mTOR signaling and proliferation. Tumors of the brain, prostate, and pancreas overexpress LAT1 [8].

2.2.3 Ion Exchangers and Pumps

These proteins control intracellular ion homeostasis and pH balance, both of which are essential for the survival and growth of cancer cells.

- **Na^+/H^+ exchanger** (NHE1) raises intracellular alkalinity and increases extracellular acidity, which aids in invasion and drug resistance.
- **Ca^{2+}-ATPase** (SERCA, PMCA) controls intracellular calcium levels; disruption can impact apoptosis and proliferation.
- **H^+-ATPase** (V-ATPase) acidifies intracellular organelles and extracellular spaces, which promotes metastasis and resistance to weakly basic chemotherapeutics [9].

3 Ion Channels and Transporters' Functional Roles in Cancer

Ion channels and transporters regulate vital cellular functions such invasion, migration, apoptosis, and proliferation, which are critical in cancer. These proteins' aberrant expression or activity aids in the development of tumors and the advancement of cancer. For example, by encouraging cell motility, voltage-gated sodium channels (VGSCs) increase the likelihood that breast and prostate malignancies would spread. Similarly, calcium signaling through calcium-permeable channels like as TRPV6 and TRPM7 contributes to unchecked proliferation and survival. Rapid cell division is supported by potassium channels, which aid in maintaining membrane potential. By aggressively effluxing anticancer medications, transporters including ABC (ATP-binding cassette) family proteins aid in chemoresistance. The increased metabolic demands of cancer cells can also be supported by altered solute carrier (SLC) expression, which can affect metabolic pathways and nutrition uptake. An outline of their functional contributions to the development of cancer can be seen below.

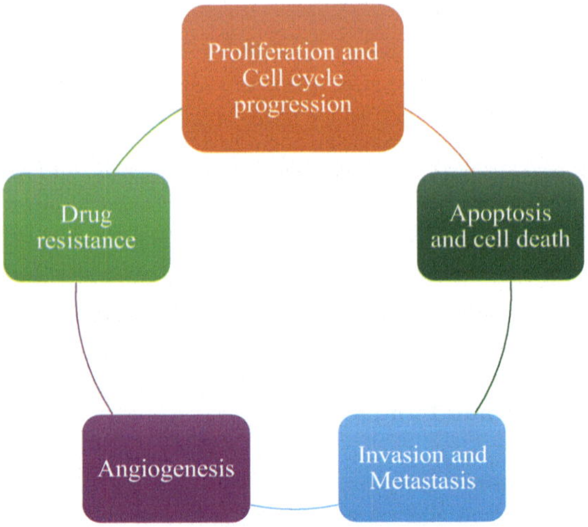

3.1 *Proliferation and Cell Cycle Progression*

Cancer cells require a finely tuned balance of membrane potential and intracellular signaling to sustain rapid cell division. Ion channels, especially potassium and calcium channels, are central to this regulation.

- **Potassium (K^+) Channels**: Voltage-gated K^+ channels (e.g., Kv1.3, Kv10.1) play a role in hyperpolarization of the plasma membrane that allows the steady influx of Ca^{2+}. This calcium entry is required to allow activation of the cell cycle regulators cyclin D and CDK4/6 in order that G1 to S phase transition may take place.
- **TRP Channels**: Transient receptor potential (TRP) channels such as TRPC1 and TRPV6 facilitate calcium influx that activates the MAPK, ERK1/2, and PI3K/Akt pathways-critical cascades for cell survival, metabolism, and growth [1].

3.2 *Apoptosis and Cell Death*

To maintain rapid cell division, cancer cells need a precisely balanced intracellular signaling and membrane potential. This regulation relies heavily on ion channels, particularly calcium and potassium channels.

- **Channels for potassium (K^+)**: Voltage-gated K^+ channels (e.g., Kv1.3 and Kv10.1) contribute to hyperpolarizing the plasma membrane and thus allow sustained Ca^{2+} influx. This calcium entry is required to activate cell cycle regulators like cyclin D and CDK4/6 and induce transition of G1 to S phase.

- **Calcium channel**: The MAPK, ERK1/2, and PI3K/Akt pathways—essential cascades for cell survival, metabolism, and growth—are activated by calcium influx facilitated by transient receptor potential (TRP) channels such TRPC1 and TRPV6.

3.3 *Invasion and Metastasis*

Ion fluxes can influence matrix remodeling and cytoskeleton dynamics both of which are required during metastasis and the epithelial-to-mesenchymal transition (EMT).

- **Sodium (Na^+) channels**: By encouraging the activity of matrix metalloproteinases (MMPs) and aiding in the breakdown of the extracellular matrix, the neonatal isoform of Nav1.5, which is frequently overexpressed in breast and colon malignancies, increases invasiveness.
- **Aquaporins (AQPs)**: AQPs like AQP1 and AQP5 enhance fast water transport, which in turn enables the cytoskeletal rearrangement and lamellipodia expansion required for cancer cell migration [10].

3.4 *Angiogenesis*

Tumors promote the development of new blood vessels in order to maintain growth. Vascular remodeling and endothelial cell activity are regulated by ion channels and transporters.

- **TRP and K^+ channels**: TRPC1 and Kv11.1 enhance endothelial cell migration and proliferation during angiogenesis by regulating membrane potential and calcium signaling.
- **ABC transporters**: Angiogenesis-related transporters including ABCB1 (P-gp) and ABCG2 (BCRP) also contribute to the drug efflux by the secretion of vascular endothelial growth factor (VEGF) and other pro-angiogenic factors into the tumor microenvironment.

3.5 *Drug Resistance*

Multidrug resistance (MDR), a significant barrier to chemotherapy, is one of the most therapeutically significant roles of transporters in cancer.

- **ABC transporters**: Proteins, such as P-gp (ABCB1), MRP1 (ABCC1), and BCRP (ABCG2), reduce the intracellular concentration and decrease the lethalness of a multitude of chemotherapeutic drugs (including paclitaxel, doxorubicin, and vincristine) by actively pumping them outside the cell using ATP hydrolysis.

- Transporters involved in intracellular alkalization and extracellular acidification are Na^+/H^+ exchanger (NHE1) and V-ATPase. Further decreasing efficacy, this pH gradient can increase drug sequestration in acidic vesicles and hinder drug uptake [11].

4 Expression of Ion Channels and Transporters Particular to Cancer

Cancer-specific upregulation of certain ion channels and transporters contributes to tumor growth, metastasis, and treatment resistance. Kv10.1 promotes cell proliferation and is significantly expressed in colon and breast malignancies. Nav1.5 promotes matrix breakdown, which increases invasiveness in colorectal and breast cancers. Prostate and pancreatic tumors exhibit increased TRPV6, which promotes calcium influx and cell survival. Aquaporins, such as AQP1 and AQP3, promote angiogenesis and tumor cell motility. Transporters that mediate drug efflux and metabolic adaptation, including as ABCB1 (P-gp), SLC1A5, and SLC7A5, are commonly overexpressed in a variety of malignancies. Their specific expression provides useful targets and biomarkers for the detection and treatment of cancer [12] (Table 9.1).

Table 9.1 Expression of ion channels and transporters in cancer

Sr. No.	Ion channel/ transporter	Gene/protein name	Cancer types	Functional role in cancer
1	Kv 10.1	KCNH1	Breast, colon, prostate	Encourages cell cycle progression and proliferation
2	Nav 1.5	SCN5A	Breast, colon	Increases invasion, metastasis, and migration
3	Cav3.2	CACNA1H	Prostate, pancreatic	Controls calcium intake for survival and growth
4	TRPV6	TRPV6	Prostate, breast, pancreatic	Facilitates the entrance of Ca^{2+} for mitogenic signaling
5	TRPM8	TRPM8	Prostate, breast	Controls migration, apoptosis, and proliferation
6	AQP1	AQP1	Colon, lung, glioblastoma	Facilitates angiogenesis and cell migration
7	AQP3	AQP3	Esophageal, gastric, breast	Increases cell motility and proliferation
8	P-gp	ABCB1	Breast, ovarian, lung, leukemia	The drug efflux pump is a factor in multidrug resistance [13]

5 Dysregulation in Cancer

In many types of cancer, ion channels and transporters—which are normally crucial in preserving cellular ion homeostasis—become abnormally expressed or mutant. The hallmark activities of cancer cells, such as unregulated proliferation, metastasis, and resistance to apoptosis, are influenced by this imbalance [14].

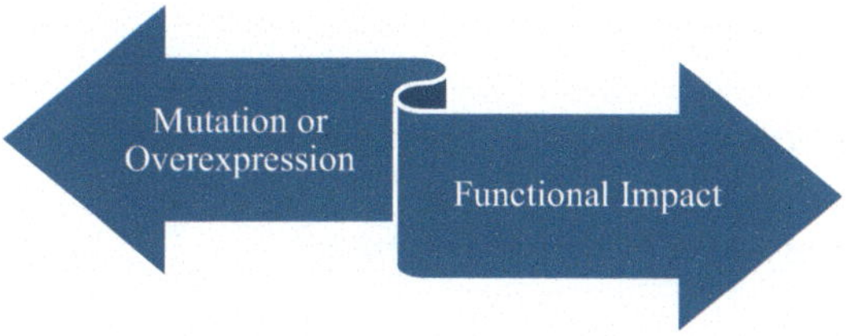

5.1 *Mutation or Overexpression*

- **VGSCs, or voltage-gated sodium channels**
  A number of malignancies, most notably breast and prostate cancer, exhibit aberrant upregulation of VGSCs, especially NaV1.5. Increased invasiveness and metastatic behavior are linked to their overexpression. NaV1.5 enhances the degradation of the extracellular matrix and the invasive properties of breast cancer cells through enhancement of activity of the matrix metalloproteinases (MMPs).
- **Melastatin 7's transient receptor potential, or TRPM7**
  Breast, glioblastoma, and pancreatic malignancies overexpress TRPM7, a calcium- and magnesium-permeable channel with an intrinsic kinase domain. It controls cytoskeletal reorganization, migration, and cell division. Because TRPM7 plays a part in metastasis and the epithelial-mesenchymal transition (EMT), dysregulation of this protein is associated with a poor prognosis [15].

5.2 *Functional Impact*

- **Persistent Growth: Ca^{2+} Signaling**
  Many malignancies have increased expression of calcium channels, particularly store-operated channels like ORAI1 and STIM1. They initiate downstream signaling cascades such as PI3K/Akt, Ras/MAPK, or calcineurin/NFAT by controlling Ca^{2+} influx. These cascades encourage the proliferation and advancement of the cell cycle. Normal growth control mechanisms can be circumvented by tumor cells through dysregulated Ca^{2+} signaling.

- **Cl^- and K^+ Channel Invasion and Metastasis**
  Cell migration via restricted extracellular spaces depends on the regulation of cell volume, which is aided by chloride channels like CLC3 and calcium-activated K^+ channels (e.g., KCa3.1). Cellular shrinkage brought on by K^+ and Cl^+ efflux makes it possible for cells to migrate across confined places during metastasis. Additionally, these channels control actin cytoskeletal dynamics and focal adhesion turnover [16].

6 Drug Resistance and Transporters in Cancer

6.1 Mechanisms of Chemoresistance

Chemotherapy is still the mainstay of treatment for many types of cancer. However, the emergence of inherent or acquired chemoresistance is one of the main barriers to chemotherapeutic efficacy. While acquired resistance develops during therapy, intrinsic resistance exists prior to treatment. Chemoresistance is caused by a variety of methods, such as:

- **Increased Efflux of Drugs**
  Amplification of efflux transporters (e.g., multidrug resistance-associated proteins, MRPs and breast cancer resistance protein, BCRP and P-glycoprotein, P-gp) reduces cellular levels of anticancer agents and renders them ineffective.
- **Enhanced DNA Repair**
  Numerous chemotherapy drugs cause DNA damage in order to produce their cytotoxic effects. Nucleotide excision repair, base excision repair, and homologous recombination are examples of DNA repair mechanisms that tumor cells upregulate in order to withstand genotoxic stress [17].
- **Alteration of Drug Targets**
  Chemotherapy medications' molecular targets can be altered by cancer cells, which decreases drug binding and effectiveness. Mutations in tubulin, for instance, lessen sensitivity to taxanes.
- **Evasion of Apoptosis**
  Resistance to chemotherapy is often associated with alterations in apoptotic pathways. Upregulation of anti-apoptotic proteins (e.g., Bcl-2) or downregulation of pro-apoptotic proteins (e.g., Bax, p53) allows cells to evade programmed cell death.
- **Epithelial-to-Mesenchymal Transition (EMT)**
  EMT contributes to chemoresistance by enhancing cellular motility, survival, and stem-like properties. EMT also downregulates epithelial markers such as E-cadherin, promoting resistance.
- **Tumor Microenvironment (TME)**
  By altering drug transport and signaling pathways, hypoxia, acidosis, and stromal interactions in the TME all contribute to resistance [18].

6.2 Role of P-gp, BCRP, and MRP Proteins

6.2.1 P-Glycoprotein (P-gp/ABCB1)

The ABCB1 is the gene that encodes the 170 kDa ATP-binding cassette (ABC) transporter otherwise known as P-glycoprotein. It is one of the most studied efflux pumps in the area of cancer biology Many structurally unrelated hydrophobic chemotherapeutic drugs are actively transported across the plasma membrane by P-gp, including:

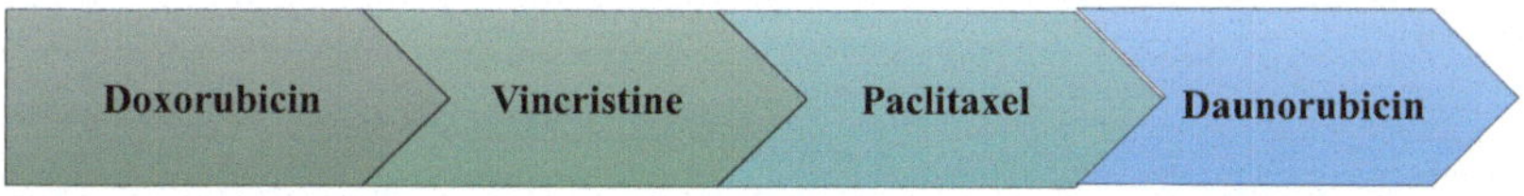

- **Mechanism of Action**
  In order to supply energy for the active transport of medications out of the cell against the concentration gradient, P-gp binds, and hydrolyses ATP. It reduces medication-induced cytotoxicity by lowering intracellular drug accumulation.
- **Tissue Expression**
  P-gp is naturally expressed in tissues involved in absorption and excretion (e.g., liver, kidney, intestines, blood-brain barrier). However, in cancers, its overexpression is often associated with multidrug resistance (MDR) [19].
- **Regulation**
  P-gp expression can be induced by hypoxia, nuclear receptors (e.g., PXR and CAR), and oncogenic signaling pathways (e.g., PI3K/AKT, Wnt/beta-catenin).

6.2.2 Breast Cancer Resistance Protein (BCRP/ABCG2)

The 72 kDa half-transporter BCRP, which is encoded by the ABCG2 gene, works as a homodimer. Like P-gp, BCRP aids in the efflux of numerous chemotherapeutic substances, such as:

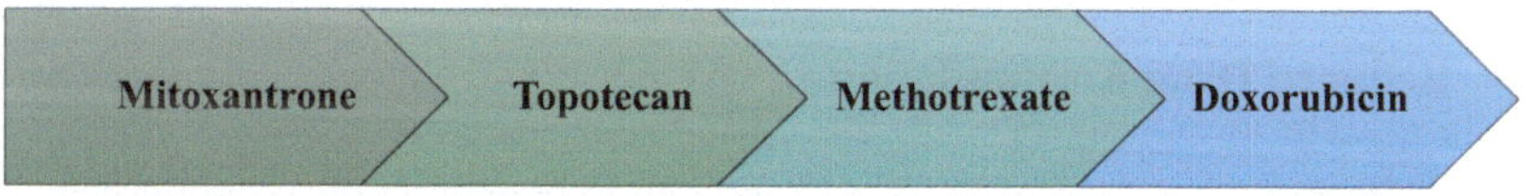

- **Mechanism**
  BCRP uses ATP hydrolysis to extrude substrates from cells, reducing drug bioavailability and efficacy.
- **Tissue Distribution**
  It is expressed in the placenta, intestines, liver, and blood-brain barrier and is responsible for protecting tissues from xenobiotic exposure [20].

- **Role in Cancer**
  BCRP overexpression is described in breast cancer, lung cancer, glioblastoma, and leukemia and correlates with the lack of response to chemotherapy.

6.2.3 Multidrug Resistance-Associated Proteins (MRPs/ABCC Family)

Through the transportation of organic anions, conjugated pharmaceuticals, and glucuronides, the MRP family—in particular, MRP1 (ABCC1), MRP2 (ABCC2), and MRP4 (ABCC4)—plays critical roles in drug resistance. Important substrates consist of:

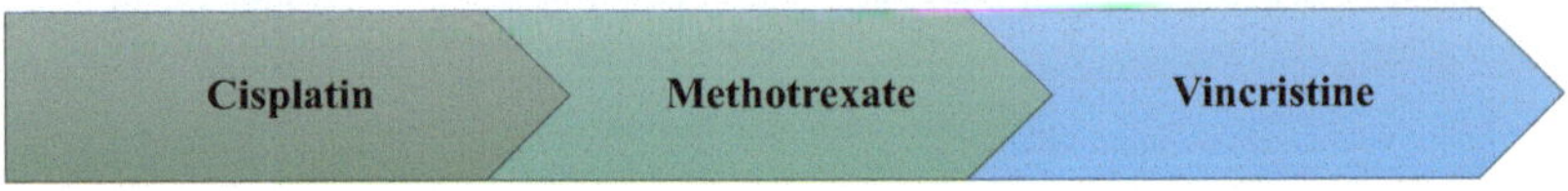

- **Mechanism**
  MRPs use ATP hydrolysis to pump substrates, including conjugated metabolites and xenobiotics, out of the cell. This mechanism also helps in detoxification.
- **Clinical Impact**
  Hematological, colon, and lung malignancies all exhibit high levels of MRP1 expression.
  Resistance to anthracyclines and alkylating drugs is associated with overexpression of MRPs [21].

6.3 *Clinical Relevance in Chemotherapy Failure*

The overexpression and functional activity of P-gp, BCRP, and MRPs have been strongly correlated with chemotherapy failure in clinical settings. Key implications include:

6.3.1 Reduced Drug Accumulation

The chemotherapy is rendered ineffective by sub-therapeutic intracellular drug concentrations caused by high levels of efflux transporter expression.

- **Prognostic Biomarkers**
  P-gp, BCRP, and MRP expression can all be used as biomarkers to forecast how well a medication would work. For example, in acute myeloid leukemia and breast cancer, the overexpression of P-gp has been correlated with poor response to anthracyclines.

- **Resistance to Combination Therapies**
  Efflux transporters can simultaneously expel multiple drugs, compromising the efficacy of combination regimens, especially in hematologic malignancies and solid tumors like ovarian and colon cancers [22].
- **Blood-Brain Barrier (BBB) Implications**
  High levels of P-gp and BCRP at the blood-brain barrier limit drug penetration in brain cancers like glioblastoma, which results in treatment failure even with systemic chemotherapy.
- **Cancer Stem Cells (CSCs)**
  CSCs are characterized by high levels of ABC transporter expression, particularly BCRP, which enables them to resist chemotherapeutic agents and regenerate the tumor, contributing to recurrence and metastasis [23].

6.4 *Metabolic Reprogramming*

Cancer cells go through comprehensive metabolic reprogramming so as to sustain uncontrolled proliferation, resist programmed cell death, and adapt to the hostile environment. The Warburg effect is one of the characteristics of cancer metabolism; it is observed as the preferential use of aerobic glycolysis over oxidative phosphorylation in tumor cells even in oxygenated conditions. This metabolic change, which is partially controlled by ion channels and transporters, raises the need for nutrients, ions, and metabolites.

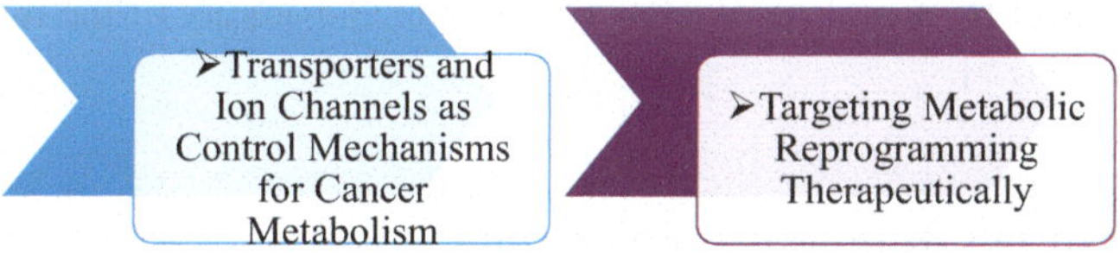

6.4.1 Transporters and Ion Channels as Control Mechanisms for Cancer Metabolism

- **Glucose Transporters (GLUTs)**: Increased glucose absorption to power glycolysis is made possible by overexpression of GLUT1 and GLUT3.
- **Monocarboxylate transporters**: Lactate export is mediated by monocarboxylate transporters (MCTs) MCT1 and MCT4, which maintain the acidic tumor microenvironment and inhibit intracellular acidification.
- **Na^+/H^+ exchangers**: During lactic acid buildup, Na^+/H^+ exchangers (NHE1) keep the intracellular pH at the ideal level for enzyme activity and cell viability.
- **Voltage-gated ion channels**: Changes in K^+, Ca^+, and Na^+ voltage-gated ion channels affect ATP synthesis and mitochondrial metabolism.

- **Sodium-dependent amino acid transporters**: Transporters of amino acids that are dependent on sodium, such as SLC1A5 and SLC7A5, bring in vital amino acids that are necessary for mTOR activation and biomass accumulation, such as glutamine and leucine [24].

Therapeutically Targeting Metabolic Reprogramming

The reprogramming of metabolism is among the cancer cells phenotypes, enabling tumor cells to flourish in adverse microenvironmental conditions, facilitate rapid cell proliferation and suppress programmed cell death. Cancer cells have reprogrammed metabolic requirements. Metabolic reprogramming is among the features of cancer cells, which help them to grow in poorly favorable conditions in the microenvironment, tumor growth, and avoid apoptosis, among others include increased glycolysis (Warburg effect), glutaminolysis, lipid synthesis, and mitochondrial reprogramming. These changes offer unique therapeutic windows. Targeting these metabolic pathways can impair tumor growth, enhance therapeutic sensitivity, and overcome drug resistance.

- **Glycolysis Prevention**: Even in conditions with plenty of oxygen, cancer cells frequently rely significantly on glycolysis. Therapeutic approaches consist of:
- **Inhibitors of Hexokinase 2 (HK2)**: HK2 catalyzes glycolysis's initial stage. Inhibitors such as 2-deoxy-D-glucose (2-DG) decrease ATP synthesis and hinder glycolytic flow.
- **Lactate Dehydrogenase A (LDHA) Inhibitors**: Targeting LDHA lessens aggressiveness by preventing lactate production and acidity of the tumor microenvironment [25].

6.4.2 Therapeutic Approaches to Overcome Transporter-Mediated Resistance

Several strategies have been developed or are under investigation to counteract efflux-mediated drug resistance:

Transporter Inhibitors

- P-gp and/or BCRP are inhibited by substances including verapamil, elacridar (GF120918), and tariquidar.
- Many of them failed in clinical trials because of toxicity and pharmacokinetic interactions, even though their preclinical results were encouraging.

Nanoparticle-Based Drug Delivery

- Bypassing efflux pumps, liposomes, micelles, and other nanoparticles can improve intracellular drug delivery.
- In resistant cell limes, some doxorubicin and paclitaxel nano formulations have demonstrated increased cytotoxicity [26].

RNA Interference and CRISPR/Cas9

Although there are still issues with delivery systems, targeting ABC transporter genes with siRNA or CRISPR approaches provides a focused approach.

Modulation of Transporter Expression

Use epigenetic medications (such as histone deacetylase inhibitors) or small-molecule inhibitors to suppress transporter expression.

Combination Therapy with Targeted Agents

Tyrosine kinase inhibitors or immune checkpoint inhibitors in combination with chemotherapy indirectly alter transporter activity [27].

7 Strategies for Therapeutic Targeting

Targeting ion channels and transporters in cancer therapy, various methods are used, such as RNA-based therapies like siRNA to suppress gene expression, monoclonal antibodies that attach to extracellular channel domains, and small-molecule inhibitors that stop abnormal channel activity. Repurposing drugs, including employing sodium or calcium channel blockers, provides affordable alternatives. By combining ion channel modulators with immunotherapy, chemotherapy, or targeted medicines, combination treatments increase efficacy. Based on tumor-specific channel expression profiles, precision medicine techniques are likewise becoming more popular. In order to enhance treatment results, these tactics seek to minimize impacts on healthy cells while preventing tumor development, metastasis, and drug resistance [28].

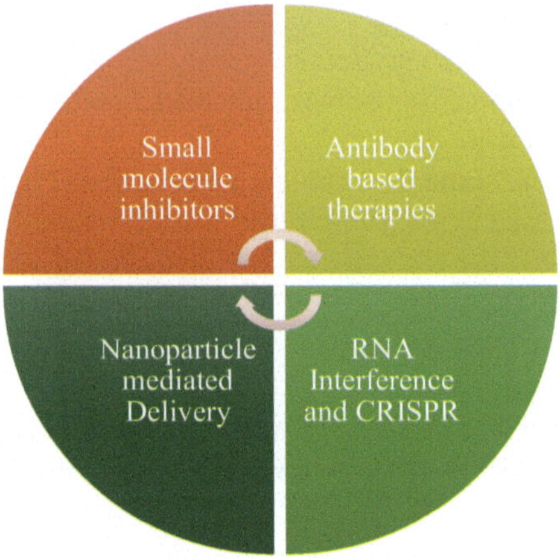

7.1 *Small-Molecule Inhibitors*

Small compounds can reduce the pro-tumorigenic effects of cancer cells by efficiently blocking the function of ion channels and transporters that are overexpressed or hyperactive.

- **Voltage-gated Kv channel blockers**: such as 4-Aminopyridine (4-AP), reduce membrane hyperpolarization and limit calcium-dependent proliferation signals by blocking Kv1.3 and Kv10.1. In models of breast and colon cancer, other blockers, such as astemizole, have demonstrated anti-proliferative effects.
- **TRP channel modulators**: It is well known that substances such as capsazepine, a TRPV1 antagonist, and SKF96365, a wide TRP channel inhibitor, decrease Ca^{2+} influx and interfere with the migration and proliferation of cancer cells. Additionally, they disrupt downstream signaling pathways like MAPK and PI3K/Akt [29].

7.2 *Nanoparticle-Mediated Delivery*

In addition to conventional anticancer medications, nanotechnology provides combinatorial, controlled, and targeted administration of ion channel modulators.

- **Liposomal Formulations**: Liposomes that include ion channel blockers (like 4-AP or capsazepine) and chemotherapeutic drugs (like doxorubicin) can work in concert. They lessen systemic toxicity and enhance pharmacokinetics.
- **pH-Sensitive Nanoparticles**: Overactive proton pumps, such as V-ATPase, cause tumors to have acidic extracellular environments. Cancer cells can be par-

ticularly targeted by nanoparticles made to release their payload in an acidic environment. Drugs or siRNAs that target ion channels like NHE1 or SLC7A5 may be placed onto these carriers.

7.3 RNA Interference and CRISPR

Oncogenic ion channel and transporter expression can be precisely downregulated with the help of gene-silencing methods.

- **RNA Interference (RNAi):** The short hairpin RNAs (shRNAs) and short interfering RNAs (siRNAs) have been used in silencing the overexpressed transporters. For example, in pancreatic and colorectal cancer cells, siRNA against SLC1A5 (ASCT2) decreases glutamine uptake, affecting energy metabolism.
- **CRISPR/Cas9 Gene Editing**: Target genes can be permanently knocked off using CRISPR technology. In preclinical models, it has been demonstrated that knocking down ABCG2 or NHE1 inhibits invasion and proliferation and resensitizes cancers to medications. Off-target effects and delivery issues, however, are still being studied [30].

7.4 Antibody-Based Therapies

The extracellular domains of overexpressed ion channels or transporters can be selectively bound by monoclonal antibodies (mAbs), which can either mark them for immune-mediated destruction or prevent them from functioning.

- **Anti-TRPV6 Antibodies**: Breast and prostate tumors exhibit elevated TRPV6 expression. Antibodies directed against its extracellular loops have the ability to increase apoptotic sensitivity, decrease Ca^{2+} influx, and stop tumor growth. Promising tumor suppression has been observed in preclinical studies.
- **Future Potentials**: Research is underway to develop antibodies that target additional extracellularly accessible channels, such as Kv10.1 or Nav1.5, which are tumor-specific indicators for malignancies [31].

8 Challenges and Opportunities in Ion Channel and Transporter Targeting in Cancer

The ion channel and transporter-targeted therapy in cancer is associated with several challenges that should be addressed to translate preclinical findings into clinical benefits. Selectivity is a significant challenge since many of the ion channels and

Table 9.2 Challenges and future directions for ion channel and transporter targeting in cancer

Sr. No.	Challenges/future direction	Description
1	Selectivity	It is hard to focus on cancer cells without affecting healthy cells because various ion channels and transporters exist in them. Finding ligands or antibodies specially designed for cancer is very important
2	Mechanisms of Resistance	Monotherapies may become less effective as a result of tumors activating compensatory ion channels or signaling pathways to avoid the suppressed target [33]
3	Development of Biomarkers	In order to properly match patients and check the outcomes of treatment, it is necessary to use trusted biomarkers that measure ion channel activity
4	Combination Treatment	Taking ion channel modulators together with immune, chemotherapy, or targeted therapies can enhance results, reduce drug resistance, and better assist patients [34]

transporters linked to cancer are also expressed in healthy tissues, which raises questions regarding off-target toxicity. Researchers use monoclonal antibodies, systems made especially for tumor treatment, and cancer-specific ligands to help the treatment process. Many diseases keep mutating, creating another serious challenge. If cancer alters their channels, the cells can avoid being blocked by a single approach called monotherapy. Therefore, combination treatments with ion channel modulators are being looked into to help avoid drug resistance when they are given with immunotherapy, chemotherapy, or metabolic inhibitors. As well, the field does not have dependable biomarkers. More appropriate methods of diagnosis are needed to split patients according to the expression of ion channels and transporters. In the future, one hopes that the precision of oncology targeting ion channels will be refined, using nanotechnology, CRISPR gene editing, and AI-accelerated drug screening. Examining their ways of action, ways they can resist treatment, and the way they are expressed in various tumors will play a key role in their application in clinical settings [32] (Table 9.2).

9 Conclusion

Ion channels and transporters play a role in the initiation of cancer, its manifestation in the body, and the reaction to treatment. Cancer cells are important for several biological processes, which include generating new blood vessels, migration, invasion, the regulated death of cells, cell growth, and control of metabolism. Kv10.1, TRPV6, Nav1.5, and ABC transporters sometimes work differently in cancer tissues, which makes them targets for therapy. In studies, focusing on these proteins with RNA interference, small molecules, monoclonal antibodies, or CRISPR gene editing appears very promising. These methods now function more accurately and effectively because of new developments in nanoparticles, and when used along with common treatments. These tactics have the potential to improve therapy specificity, overcome drug resistance, and lessen systemic toxicity. At the same time, failure to narrow the drug response, the presence of many redundant ion channels, and how different tumor cells are make it hard to bring these drugs to patients in practice. The main items for future research must be the identification of isoforms linked only to cancer, the understanding of how cancer resists treatments, and the design of strong biomarkers for helping to study patients. Combining treatment for ion channels with both immunotherapy and personalized medicine could give rise to fresh ways to fight cancer. In all, ion channels and transporters are little-used cancer targets with great potential. When we learn more about these chemicals and their usefulness, it could lead to better and more effective cancer treatments that hurt us less. If we want these drugs to do their best against cancer, we need more research that involves multiple fields.

References

1. Arcangeli A, Becchetti A (2010) New trends in cancer therapy: targeting ion channels and transporters. Pharmaceuticals 3(4):1202–1224
2. Pedersen SF, Stock C (2013) Ion channels and transporters in cancer: pathophysiology, regulation, and clinical potential. Cancer Res 73:1658
3. Altamura C, Lastraioli E (2024) Novel therapeutic approach in cancer: the role of ion channels and transporters. Front Pharmacol 15:1422127
4. Becchetti A (2011) Ion channels and transporters in cancer. 1. Ion channels and cell proliferation in cancer. Am J Physiol Cell Physiol 301(2):C255–C265
5. Lastraioli E, Iorio J, Arcangeli A (2015) Ion channel expression as promising cancer biomarker. Biochim Biophys Acta Biomembranes 1848(10):2685–2702
6. Prevarskaya N, Skryma R, Shuba Y (2018) Ion channels in cancer: are cancer hallmarks oncochannelopathies? Physiol Rev 98(2):559–621
7. Anderson KJ, Cormier RT, Scott PM (2019) Role of ion channels in gastrointestinal cancer. World J Gastroenterol 25(38):5732
8. Fiske JL, Fomin VP, Brown ML, Duncan RL, Sikes RA (2006) Voltage-sensitive ion channels and cancer. Cancer Metastasis Rev 25:493–500
9. Griffin M, Khan R, Basu S, Smith S (2020) Ion channels as therapeutic targets in high grade gliomas. Cancer 12(10):3068
10. Raghunand N, Martínez-Zaguilán R, Wright SH, Gillies RJ (1999) pH and drug resistance. II. Turnover of acidic vesicles and resistance to weakly basic chemotherapeutic drugs. Biochem Pharmacol 57(9):1047–1058
11. Lehen'Kyi VY, Shapovalov G, Skryma R, Prevarskaya N (2011) Ion channnels and transporters in cancer. 5. Ion channels in control of cancer and cell apoptosis. Am J Physiol Cell Physiol 301(6):C1281–C1289
12. Zhang Y, Tian J (2024) Strategies, challenges, and prospects of nanoparticles in gynecological malignancies. ACS Omega 9(36):37459–37504
13. Chen L, Yi H, Li Q, Duan T, Liu X, Li L, Wang RF (2024) T-bet regulates ion channels and transporters and induces apoptosis in intestinal epithelial cells. Adv Sci 11(28):2401654
14. Pozzi E, Terribile G, Cherchi L, Di Girolamo S, Sancini G, Alberti P (2024) Ion channel and transporter involvement in chemotherapy-induced peripheral neurotoxicity. Int J Mol Sci 25(12):6552
15. Niu N, Shen X, Wang Z, Chen Y, Weng Y, Yu F, Xue J (2024) Tumor cell-intrinsic epigenetic dysregulation shapes cancer-associated fibroblasts heterogeneity to metabolically support pancreatic cancer. Cancer Cell 42(5):869–884

16. Lehle J, Soleimanpour M, Mokhtari S, Ebrahimi D (2024) Viral infection, APOBEC3 dysregulation, and cancer. Front Genet 15:1489324
17. Zheng HC (2017) The molecular mechanisms of chemoresistance in cancers. Oncotarget 8(35):59950
18. Kryczka J, Kryczka J, Czarnecka-Chrebelska KH, Brzeziańska-Lasota E (2021) Molecular mechanisms of chemoresistance induced by cisplatin in NSCLC cancer therapy. Int J Mol Sci 22(16):8885
19. Saib S, Delavenne X (2021) Inflammation induces changes in the functional expression of P-gp, BCRP, and MRP2: an overview of different models and consequences for drug disposition. Pharmaceutics 13(10):1544
20. Dong J, Yuan L, Hu C, Cheng X, Qin JJ (2023) Strategies to overcome cancer multidrug resistance (MDR) through targeting P-glycoprotein (ABCB1): an updated review. Pharmacol Ther 249:108488
21. Deng F, Sjöstedt N, Santo M, Neuvonen M, Niemi M, Kidron H (2023) Novel inhibitors of breast cancer resistance protein (BCRP, ABCG2) among marketed drugs. Eur J Pharm Sci 181:106362
22. Badiee SA, Isu UH, Khodadadi E, Moradi M (2023) The alternating access mechanism in mammalian multidrug resistance transporters and their bacterial homologs. Membranes 13(6):568
23. Xiao H, Zheng Y, Ma L, Tian L, Sun Q (2021) Clinically-relevant ABC transporter for anti-cancer drug resistance. Front Pharmacol 12:648407
24. Yoshida GJ (2015) Metabolic reprogramming: the emerging concept and associated therapeutic strategies. J Exp Clin Cancer Res 34:1–10
25. Shi Z, Hu C, Zheng X, Sun C, Li Q (2024) Feedback loop between hypoxia and energy metabolic reprogramming aggravates the radioresistance of cancer cells. Exp Hematol Oncol 13(1):55
26. Nishikawa H, Goto M, Fukunishi S, Asai A, Nishiguchi S, Higuchi K (2021) Cancer cachexia: its mechanism and clinical significance. Int J Mol Sci 22(16):8491
27. Elshobary ME, Badawy NK, Ashraf Y, Zatioun AA, Masriya HH, Ammar MM, Assy AM (2025) Combating antibiotic resistance: mechanisms, multidrug-resistant pathogens, and novel therapeutic approaches: an updated review. Pharmaceuticals 18(3):402
28. Pangeni R, Kang S, Jha SK, Subedi L, Park JW (2021) Intestinal membrane transporter-mediated approaches to improve oral drug delivery. J Pharm Investig 51:137–158
29. Wajapeyee N, Beamon TC, Gupta R (2024) Roles and therapeutic targeting of ceramide metabolism in cancer. Mol Metab 83:101936
30. Musleh Ud Din S, Streit SG, Huynh BT, Hana C, Abraham AN, Hussein A (2024) Therapeutic targeting of hypoxia-inducible factors in cancer. Int J Mol Sci 25(4):2060
31. Zhang L, Gu H, Li X, Wang Y, Yao S, Chen X, Tuo B (2024) Pathophysiological role of ion channels and transporters in hepatocellular carcinoma. Cancer Gene Ther 31(11):1611–1618
32. Xiang D, Zhou L, Yang R, Yuan F, Xu Y, Yang Y, Li X (2024) Advances in ferroptosis-inducing agents by targeted delivery system in cancer therapy. Int J Nanomedicine 19:2091–2112
33. Deng Y, Guo M, Zhou L, Huang Y, Srivastava S, Kumar A, Liu JQ (2024) Prospects, advances and biological applications of MOF-based platform for the treatment of lung cancer. Biomater Sci 12(15):3725–3744
34. Alharbi HM (2024) Exploring the frontier of biopolymer-assisted drug delivery: advancements, clinical applications, and future perspectives in cancer nanomedicine. Drug Des Dev Ther 18:2063–2087

Chapter 10
Recent Advances of Nanotechnology in Cancer Detection and Potential Drug Finding

Beauty Roy, Sourav Das, and Semanti Ghosh

1 Introduction

Among the diseases that pose the greatest threat to human existence is cancer. Annually, more than ten million new cases of cancer diagnosed, which remains a major cause of death. As a highly complex and not fully understood illness, its development involves different cellular processes, including cell signalling and apoptosis. Nowadays for diagnosis, morphological methods like radiologic and histopathologic tests are conducted which efficiently determine clinical and pathological stages which help to guide the clinicians to determine the correct treatment for individual cancer patients. Mainly, chemotherapy, radiotherapy, and surgery are used in treatment purpose. But chemotherapy shows some noticeable limitations. It is unable to specifically deliver medicines particularly at the target site; thus, it causes harm to the normal body cells so the emergence of multidrug resistance (MDR) negatively effects metastasis and tumour control. In addition, numerous cell populations are the outcome of cancer heterogeneity, which is triggered by multiple carcinogens. The results of treatment are often not precisely anticipated by current screening and clinical techniques. Thereby, it is vital and promising to develop novel approaches to recognize tumour boundaries, identify any leftover cells or

Beauty Roy and Sourav Das contributed equally with all other contributors.

B. Roy
Department of Microbiology, School of Life Sciences, Swami Vivekananda University, Kolkata, West Bengal, India

S. Das · S. Ghosh (✉)
Department of Biotechnology, School of Life Sciences, Swami Vivekananda University, Kolkata, West Bengal, India
e-mail: semantig@svu.sc.in

S. Mallik et al. (eds.), *Landscape of Signaling Pathway and Genetic Markers in Cardio-Brain Oncology*, Studies in Rhythm Engineering,
https://doi.org/10.1007/978-981-95-7012-6_10

micro-metastases, and ensure effective eradication [1]. The multidisciplinary scientific discipline of nanotechnology engages not only biology but also physics and material science. It has been employed in various biomedical discipline fields. Nanotechnology plays a dynamic role in manufacturing and engineering various nanoparticle-based tools and objects within less than 500 nm diameters [2]. The acronym "nano" denotes to an object's size in nanometers (nm). The main objective of cancer nanotechnology is to know how all the molecular and cellular elements linked with cancer can be recognized and to develop therapy associated with nanoscale technologies. Small size of nanoparticles enhances the therapeutic efficacy and selectively kills cancer cells. New nano-systems and nanostructured materials become developed based on observing novel materials their manufacturing processes and nanoscale phenomena, which helps to develop new experimental and theoretical tools [3]. Larger scale material quality is different from the nanoscale material. This property opens a new way to study cancer nanotechnology thus opening a new field of research that combines not only biology and chemistry but also connects both engineering and medicines. To illustrate the benefits and drawbacks of these two approaches straightforwardly, we have included a brief comparison between the traditional approaches and the novel nanotechnology-based approaches, where in case of conventional methods of cancer diagnosis, some drastic side effects can be seen in our body due to the exposure of harmful radiations and excessive drug use; also, in conventional methods, late-stage diagnosis can be seen. On the contrary, for the nanotech-based methods, the exposure to radiation is comparatively low, and we can perform targeted delivery with increased efficiency into the cancer cells (Fig. 10.1). This nanotechnology field offers a promising

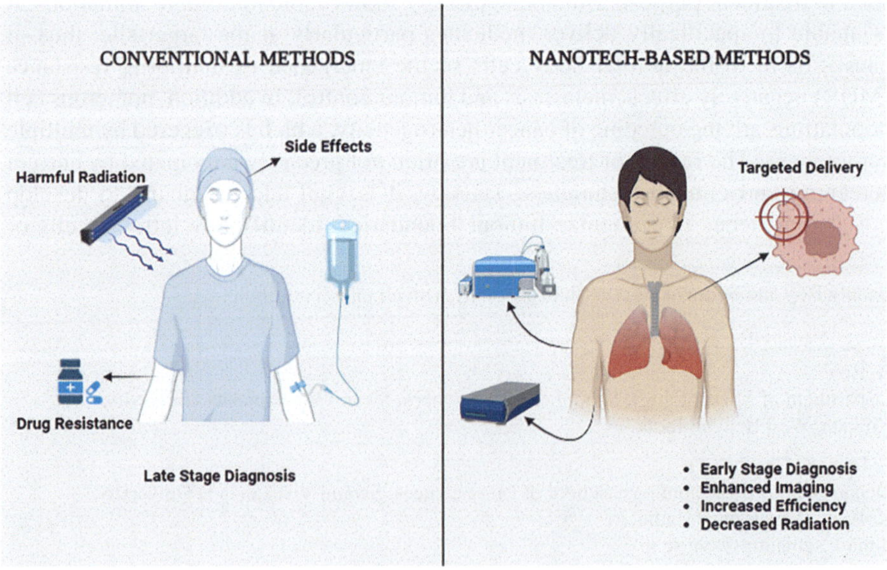

Fig. 10.1 Comparison between conventional and nano-based methods in cancer diagnosis. (This figure is created in Biorender (https://www.biorender.com/). Source: (https://doi.org/10.1186/s40580-021-00282-7, https://doi.org/10.1007/s12032-025-02602-x))

approach to advance the various fields like cancer detection, diagnosis, and treatment. Oncology field mainly focuses on two nanotechnology areas like using high-throughput nano-sensor to detect cancer biomarkers and using nanoparticle-based nano-vectors for cancer imaging or target deliver drugs at the tumour sites. In accordance to reports, nanotechnology holds great promise in the cure of cancer since it may be used to develop medical devices with special properties like the capacity to selectively and profoundly penetrate tumours [4, 5].

2 Contribution of Nanotechnology in the Diagnostic Field of Cancer

Detecting cancer in the early stage is fundamental to effective treatment, greatly lowering disease burden and the mortality rate of patients. Detection of cancer at the early stage becomes problematic due to the lack of medical imaging and molecular diagnosis. Various factors are present which contribute to delayed cancer diagnosis like minute amount of tumour-specific biomarker levels identification, absence of highly sensitive detection tools, and complex tumour heterogeneity [6]. Due to the advancement of sophisticated cancer diagnostic methods, individuals with lung cancer have a 60% chance of surviving, whereas those with cancer have a 99% chance [7].

Nanotechnology-based diagnosis overcomes many diagnoses regarding challenges via incorporating ultra-sensitive diagnostic systems, thus enabling cancer diagnosis towards precision medicine development that allows earlier and more accurate diagnosis of diseases. But due to the presence of advanced diagnostic tools, disease progression is reduced so as a result of this survival rate also increases [8].

2.1 Nano-Biosensors

It is an advanced diagnostic tool which efficiently identifies cancer-related biomarkers using biological receptors and nanotechnology. These biosensors are made up of three parts: a signal processor, a transducer, and a bioreceptor [9]. Here, the bioreceptor selectively binds to the target biomarker, which is a biological element like antibodies, enzymes, or nucleic acids; the transducer is used to convert biological reactions into detectable signals such as optical, electrical, or thermal change. At last, the signal processor provides quantitative data by amplifying and analysing the signals.

Nano-biosensors improve cancer diagnosis, which offers rapid, precise, and non-invasive means of detection. As it is capable of detecting cancer-related biomarkers at the initial stages of tumour growth, patient health outcome is also improving using this nanotool. These sensors can test various samples like blood, urine, and saliva [9].

2.1.1 Biosensors Classification Depended on Their Transduction Mode

How biosensors operate depends on their capacity to identify specifically a biomarker related to cancer with high specificity and sensitivity. This entire process starts with the bioreceptor that particularly attaches to the molecules which act as a target, such as proteins, DNA, or tumour cells that are circulated. Transducer becomes activated as a result of this interaction, so a detectable signal is generated corresponding to the biomarker concentration.

Nano-biosensors are classified based on their mode of action of converting biological signals into trackable outcome.

1. **Electrochemical Nano-Biosensors**

   - When bioreceptors recognize biomarker electrical signals are emitted. Electrochemical nano-biosensors usually measure these electrical signals. In this biosensor, electrodes mainly enhance electron transfer as well as increase sensitivity [10].

2. **Light-Based Nano-Biosensors**

   - Based on some changes in optical properties like fluorescence or Surface Plasmon Resonance (SPR), these biosensors identify biomarkers. Quantum dots can identify multiple cancer biomarkers simultaneously because it has bright and stable fluorescence [11].

3. **Heat-Based Nano-Biosensors**

   - This nano-biosensor detects temperature alteration caused by biomolecular interactions. As an example, when cancer antigens interact with their corresponding antibodies heat is generated which can be measured using thermistors [9].

2.1.2 Biosensors Role in the Diagnostic Field of Cancer

Nanotechnology-based biosensors can accurately and rapidly identify a particular type of cancer so diagnostic techniques become improving day by day using this approach. There are several uses for this technology in cancer detection.

1. **Breast Cancer**

   - Biosensors can detect breast cancer-related biomarkers HER2 and CA15-3 from blood sample of patient. In this respect, graphene nano-biosensors offer a non-invasive method to monitor the progress of breast cancer by detecting HER2 biomarkers at even femtomolar concentrations [12]. By contrast, gold nanoparticle-amplified optical biosensors have great precision in the detection of circulating tumour DNA (ctDNA) in cases of breast cancer.

2. **Lung Cancer**

    - To improve the survival rate of lung cancer patient, it is essential to detect lung cancer-related biomarkers like carcinoembryonic antigen and cytokeratin-19 fragments. Biomarkers in exhaled breath and specimens of blood can be sensitively determined using nano-biosensors which utilize nanotubes and quantum dots [13]. By evaluating exhaled breath condensate, optical biosensors can identify volatile organic compounds (VOCs) that may be signs of lung cancer.

3. **Colon Cancer**

    - Using nano-biosensors, colon cancer-related biomarkers such as carcinoembryonic antigen (CEA) identification become easier. With its better performance and fast and reliable product identification, electrochemical sensors using gold nanoparticles are very appropriate for on-site and off-site diagnosis [14]. Moreover, diagnostic outcome accuracy becomes increasing using multiplexed nano-biosensors because it can simultaneously detect various biomarkers perfectly. From these examples the role of nano-biosensors in the diagnostic field of cancer is presented. Due to the presence of their excellent accuracy and less intrusive biomarker detection, it represents a significant advancement over conventional techniques.

2.1.3 Problems and Limitations

Despite their effectiveness, some challenges are there which must be resolved to enable their broad application in clinical practice.

1. **Adaptability with the Biological Systems**

    - Living organisms should remain harmless and survivable after using nanomaterial-based treatments. Basically, carbon nanotubes have some toxic adverse effects and also perform complex immunological reactions which limit nanomaterials widefield applications in clinical purpose [15]. The discovery of biocompatible coatings and the availability of a wide range of preclinical testing are important in the solution of these problems [16].

2. **Mas Production Capacity**

    - It is very difficult to extensively produce nano-biosensors along with proper standardization and stable optical properties. It is essential to develop advanced techniques to construct nanostructures along with some features like careful customization, inexpensive and faster production capacity. Production of good-quality nanostructures is necessary to make it commercially successful along with large-scale production capacity [17].

3. **Economic Feasibility**
    - Because nano-biosensors now possess greater ability for disease detection, they will require high production cost, which is a probable constraint on their mass use, particularly in developing nations. Thus, there will be numerous ways to reduce the cost and enhance availability, e.g. through cheaper nanomaterials or optimization of the production process.
4. **Optical Difficulties**
    - It is difficult to properly execute some nano-biosensors as it needs advanced equipment along with trained persons which restrict their use in patient care settings. To address this limitation, the use of device design should be eased, and user-friendly interfaces integrated [18].
    - However, various fields like material science and nanotechnology and various researches oriented to manufacturing try to overcome these problems.

2.1.4 Impact of Nano-Biosensors in the Early Detection of Lung Cancer

According to a study, scientists and clinicians found that nano-biosensors based on breathalysers have been developed to detect Volatile Organic Compounds (VOCs) linked to lung cancer. Gold nanoparticles are used by nano-biosensors which can efficiently detect cancer-specific volatile organic compounds. These nano-biosensors have 89% selectivity capacity with 92% early stage of lung cancer detection potential [19]. These nanotechnology-based approaches helped in large-scale clinical trials linked to cancer diagnosis.

2.1.5 Conventional Methods Facilities

In cancer screening state, nano-biosensors are far better than conventional methods. Compared to conventional methods, which can detect specific biomarkers at nanomolar concentrations only, they are more sensitive and can detect biomarkers at the femtomolar levels of concentrations. Traditional approaches maximize the specificity of nano-biosensors using specific receptors which save this system from cross-reactivity. Nano-biosensors give results rapidly or in real time, whereas conventional methods take days or hours. But these traditional approaches of diagnosis are based on invasive biopsies; these nano-biosensors need easy-to-use samples like blood or saliva which is non-invasive in nature.

2.2 *Role of Nanotechnology to Detect Cancer Biomarkers*

Any biological material found in bodily fluids such as urine, saliva, blood, and different organs is a biomarker for cancer, as the body gets a wake-up call to the existence of malignant cells. All of these substances are produced by the body or cancer cells during the carcinogenesis process. Cancer biomarkers form a poorly understood mixed bag of molecules, such as secreted proteins, membrane-bound proteins, polysaccharides, and DNA or RNA fragments. Quantifying these indicators in physiological fluids can help find cancer early, keep an eye on how effectively treatment is working, and forecast when it will come back [4]. However, various challenges, e.g. low concentrations of biomarkers in physiological fluids, inter-individual variation in the timing and abundance of biomarkers, and methodological hurdles of prospective studies, persist to hinder the general clinical use of biomarkers [20].

1. **Detection of Proteins**

   - A few proteins are now approved by the FDA as markers of cancer diagnosis, such as CA-125 of ovarian cancer, PSA of prostate cancer, AFP of liver cancer, and CEA of colorectal cancer. A recent study has used quantum dot (QD) biosensors in an attempt to identify markers of cancer. The so-called sandwich-type detection is typical of the search: protein biomarkers, capture antibody, secondary capture antibody, and an antibody binding secondary antibody [4]. Single-stranded DNA (ssDNA) or RNA aptamers can be isolated by ligand systematic evolution and exponential enrichment (SELEX). The aptamers are even characterized by high prospects and special binding to large numbers of varied targets, including bacteria, viruses, ions, phospholipids, peptides, and even complete cells [21].

2. **ctDNA Detection**

   - The circulating tumour DNA (ctDNA) is DNA fragments of tumours and is situated in the blood up to 100–200 base pairs. Cancer can also be detected with the detection of genetic anomalies that are disease-specific since both primary tumour cells and circulating tumour cells (CTCs) can secrete ctDNA. ctDNA can assist in the early detection of cancer to determine abnormalities. The genetic defects that are related to the occurrence of cancer can also be discovered through highly specific hybridization with nucleic acid probes that bear complementary sequences. The short half-life and rapid update of the tumour status of ctDNA means that it may be used successfully as a predictive biomarker of GC patients. Recurrence of surgery occurred in all GC patients whose ctDNA could be detected, and the disease-free survival (DFS) and the overall survival (OS) were reduced. Bizarrely, however, this stated the opposite [20, 21].

3. **miRNA Detection**

   - The naturally occurring single-stranded RNA, the micro-RNA (miRNA), are of 20-22 nucleotide sequence and can bind with mRNA to inhibit translation. Once mRNA is possessed, a lot of miRNAs are targeting it, but a single miRNA has the ability to regulate many genes. Evidence of the role of miRNAs in the cell processes, such as invasion, migration, and differentiation, has already been reported and is quite obvious, especially regarding proliferation. Scientists have been very interested in miRNAs within the last 10 years. A great number of biological processes were linked to a specific kind of non-coding RNA [22]. It was through the facilitation of post-miRNAs, that affect an extensive variety of molecular transcriptional regulation of gene expression. Among these are the cell differentiation events, cell cycle events, and apoptotic events. Because aberrantly regulated miRNAs target mRNA-encoding oncogenes or tumour suppressor genes, they may be able to control the development of cancer. The development of gastric cancer (GC) arises due to direct attachment with miRNA dysregulation. To present, preclinical research has discovered and used several miRNAs, such as microRNA-21, microRNA-106a, and microRNA-135b, as aberrant in GC [4].

4. **Detection of DNA Methylation**

   - Some of the epigenetic alterations that have an impact on oncogenesis and cancer development are DNA methylation abnormalities (GC). DNA methylation is catalysed by three different kinds of DNA methyltransferase: DNMT1, DNMT3A, and DNMT3B. Methylation of circulating tumour DNA (ctDNA) is an important characteristic to reveal the patient prognosis, and it also promotes the chances of early detection of GC. Many types of cancer have the same genome-wide methylation pattern (Methylscape), according to current studies, a fact that raises the possibility of its use as a cancer biomarker. Scientists thus identified the difference between cancer and normal cell genomes based on DNA–gold interaction and DNA solvation effects combined analysis. It resulted in the creation of the fast, simple, sensitive, and selective electrochemical or colorimetric one-step cancer diagnosis [20, 22].

5. **Detection of Exosomes**

   - Exosomes are minute (30–140 nm) extracellular vesicles enclosed by a membrane, which are formed by large multivesicular bodies, are released into the extracellular space by fusing with the cell membrane and present within body fluids such as blood, urine, and cerebrospinal fluid. The molecular information of the parent cells delivered through exosomes is a mixture of DNA, proteins, mRNA, and miRNA, and in this respect, it allows tracing the molecular state of cancer cells, or hard to reach outside. It was found out that gastric cancer (GC) cells release exosomes into which their pathogenic processes are mediated and can be used as cancer biomarkers to diagnose this disease [20, 22].

2.3 Nanoparticle-Assisted Detection System Based on Ovarian Cancer Therapy

Various drug delivery systems involving non-conjugated forms and nanostructures have been engineered, which offer improvement in therapeutic efficacy, biocompatibility, and reduced unintended side effects [23]. Multifunctional nanomaterials with biocompatible ligands are efficiently used for targeted therapy of particular types of cancer. Ovarian cancer therapy can be conducted using various nanoparticle-based detection systems [24, 25].

1. **Nanoparticles**

   - To overcome various chemotherapy related toxic side effects along with to enhance targeted therapy strategies of previously used chemotherapy, various types of nanoscale-based drug delivery methods are used [26]. The advancement of nanoparticles using metal has increased the awareness of treating ovarian cancer. Primarily, iron oxide-based nanoparticles are utilized in the treatment of OC due to customizable size, shape, and capability to localize at targeted areas. Following wet chemical process, iron-linked NPs are used which are basically irregular in structure. Upon in vitro study using a propagated human ovarian cancer cell line (PA-1 cell), it was found that these NPs elevated the levels of ROS, and cell apoptosis also caused mitochondrial membrane disruption [27]. The superparamagnetic power of metal NPs provides some extraordinary qualities, making them suitable candidates for broad application in OC nanotechnology [28]. After the development of metal NPs, chitosan NPs are also manufactured which can efficiently deliver some biological molecules like vitamins, hydrophilic drugs, and phenol derivatives. The amino and hydroxyl functional group makes them efficient for drug delivery; along this property, it is also biocompatible in nature and degrade naturally in body [29, 30]. This nano-system contains light-sensitive and anticancer agents that were formulated and evaluated on SKOV-3 OC cell lines. Nanoparticles are widely used in clinical purpose because when it is administrated in the cell line it shows significant cytotoxic effect along with antitumour activity [31–34].
   - From the research it was noted that proliferation of ovarian cancer cells is inhibited when it is treated with polymeric NPs coated with cannabidiol. It has 95% capacity to effectively enclose therapeutic agents as well, and it can sustain over 96 h after release [35]. SKOV-3 OC cell growth is inhibited followed by apoptosis examined by the activated PARP protein. Here, it was also found that cannabinoid-loaded NPs have higher efficiency in preventing OC growth than free cannabidiol.

2. **Liposomes**

   - Liposomes are tiny, circular, and biodegradable vesicles which are less than 400 nm to 2.5 nm in width; they are mainly made up of phospholipids. They can efficiently transport not only hydrophilic molecules but also fat-soluble biomolecules like proteins, peptides, and RNA, but their interior property remains unchanged. From the studies, it was found that if liposomes are coated with PEG, this will enhance their circulation time in the human body while reducing their elimination by phagocytic. Liposomes carrying paclitaxel-loaded and PEGylated were engineered and examined in ovarian cancer models in lab and living organism conditions to suppress cancer cell growth. From these studies, it was found that this nanoparticle markedly decreases the aggressiveness of cancer cells in the ovary and promotes apoptosis via caspase 3/9 and ERK pathway [36–38].

- Two chemotherapy agents, such as irinotecan and doxorubicin drugs, were also loaded into liposomes in another study to develop an ovarian cancer xenograft model. When liposomes are intraperitoneally injected, it improves the survival rate in tumour containing mice; this also has liposomes 80% encapsulation efficiency, but it is difficult to carry double drugs by them [39]. Folate-coated liposomes were developed to target specifically the folate receptors of ovarian cancer cells and had higher uptake by tumour-associated macrophages, tenfold that of tumour-associated cells [40].

3. **Solid-Lipid Nanoparticles**

- They are spherical nanocarriers; they consist of therapeutic drugs, surfactant-based lipid materials, usually measuring between 50 and 100 nm in diameter. Their tiny size and lipid-based intrinsic nature provide some therapeutic facilities. SLNs are biocompatible, and they also have a long circulation period and tend to accumulate at targeted sites [41, 42]. SLNs attached with paclitaxel were created for the therapy of ovarian cancer cell lines (OCR3), but it showed cytotoxic effects in ovarian cancer cell lines; however, they still confirmed their potential as a drug delivery system.
- Upon administrating of free verteporfin at 2 mg/kg caused toxicity and mortality, but when this verteporfin is loaded with solid-lipid nanoparticles, it becomes successful in halting tumour growth. When the nanoparticles are merged in the interior portion of tumour microenvironment, the cancer cells survival capacity becomes significantly reduced [43].

4. **Nano-Capsules**

- Nano-capsules are small, vesicular structure that mainly consists of nanoscale materials which hold medicines in their internal core and a polymeric outer layer covering it; during surface modification, it inserts some particular ligands along with some targeting elements [44]. Nano-capsules outer coating acts as a good oxidizable substance which makes it a perfect drug delivery system, so the outer protective coating attracts much. Nano-capsules are mainly developed following two major methods like interfacial polymerization and nano-deposition. Ovarian cancer (OC)-related drugs are released by nano-capsules with much uniformity and accuracy. A cisplatin-loaded PEG-conjugated nano-capsule was developed and tested in a mouse model expressing the human ovarian carcinoma cell line OCR3 [45]. As a result of this experiment, a 90% reduction in ovarian tumour growth was observed after 20 days of the first injection. Whatever, when xenograft mice were treated with cisplatin linked with nano-capsules, they show better tumour inhibition capacity than free cisplatin [46]. Paclitaxel and lapatinib carrying nano-capsules have higher ovarian cancer tumour growth inhibition capacity. It has the site-specific medication transfer capability and at the same time it can recover multidrug resistance problems.

5. **Nano-Micelles**

 - Nano-micelles are unique nanoarchitectures, a versatile group of drug delivery nanostructures that are produced when amphiphilic molecules self-assemble after reaching critical micelle concentration [47]. Nano-micelles consist of amphipathic copolymer blocks along with central core and outer shell that can efficiently deliver both hydrophilic and hydrophobic therapeutic molecules with target site specificity feature [48]. Micelles can properly encapsulate chemotherapy drugs with site-specific delivery capacity which makes them a good drug transporting vehicle to treat ovarian cancer [49]. Micelles ranging from 10 to 100 nm size have the capacity to avoid non-specific interaction to protect normal cells from site effects of treatment while enhancing internalization of ovarian cancer cells due to their efficient penetration capacity [50]. Redox-sensitive micelles of paclitaxel were prepared to treat chemo-resistant OC [51]. Equally, docetaxel nano-micelles that target folates were manufactured and tested in SKOV3 ovarian cancer cells [52].

2.4 *Inorganic Nanoparticles*

Inorganic nanoparticles are generally made up of metal oxides, metal or semiconductor-like components. It shows quantum behaviour along with increased chemical reactivity and it also contains a specific nature, like large surface area compared to its potential. Gold nanoparticles act as a good drug delivery carrier along with biosensing and medical imaging capacity due to the presence of its widely known optical and electrical nature. Iron oxide nanoparticles are widely used for site-specific cancer therapy and MRI as it contains an efficient superparamagnetic nature. These nanoparticles can be synthesized using physical, chemical (like sol-gel) precipitation and biological methods. Every method allows accurate manipulation of size, shape, and surface features. Nanoparticles act as a good environmental clean-up, electronic devices, along with enhanced catalysis which enhance their adaptability and interaction with living organs due to the presence of its surface modification nature [53].

1. **Magnetic, Silica, and Gold Nanoparticles**

   - Gold, silica, and magnetic nanoparticles each bring such unique features to the table that researchers from very different fields compete to use them. Doctors can efficiently examine gold nanoparticles inside patients' body when it moves along with therapeutic molecules or can find out even a very small-sized disease-related markers in the blood sample due to the presence of its surface plasmon resonance feature which makes them glowing when laser lights are exposed over them. It also has another nature as it can efficiently stick with proteins which make them a good imaging and therapeutic tool for cancer treatment. Silica dots win praise mostly for being sturdy and body-friendly; their porous shells can hold drugs or labels and release them slowly, a quality that suits everything from targeted cancer therapy to environmental sensors. These nanoparticles can carry high number of drugs and have controlled drug release capacity which makes them a significant drug transporting carrier molecule. It is widely used in medical field because it can modify their surface with various types of functional groups applications [34]. The superparamagnetic ability of nanoparticles makes them ideal for use in MRI, thermal cancer treatment, and magnetic drug targeting. Their migration and aggregation are totally depending on the external magnetic fields. So gold, silica, and magnetic nanoparticles are crucial in healthcare, environmental science, and material science.

2. **Specific Features and Uses Due to the Presence of Site-Specific Therapeutic Nature**

   - Nanoparticles become essential for site-specific therapeutic nature due to the presence of their specific features like tiny size and modifiable surface. To act as a good drug transporting carrier, it is essential to have enhanced absorption capacity along with tissue-invasiveness feature that is enhanced due to its tiny size. The surface alteration helps them to specifically bind to various target cells or tissues, ensuring their target side drug delivery capacity such as chemotherapy drugs can be precisely delivered to cancer cells via nanoparticles, due to the target site specificity features of nanoparticles, helping to reduce overall toxicity to the healthy cells [34]. Treatment successes and patient outcomes are enhanced because it can efficiently transport a huge number of therapeutic molecules along with precisely and controlled drug release feature. It also has real-time monitoring features which make it efficient and accurate for patient-centred treatments.

3 Exosomes in Cancer Management

The early detection and effective treatment of patients are very important so that cancer patients can live longer. But it cannot be done in an extremely stable, specific, noninvasive or minimally invasive way as a significant issue in cancer diagnosis is biomarkers. Exosomes are extraordinarily complex regulators of the progression of cancer. In the majority of cancer types, they usually carry cancer-related macromolecules that can change the tumour microenvironment and affect cells that are nearby or distant. Exosomes can thus be utilized in cancer diagnostics in terms of filling the gap between pathological and healthy cells. Moreover, exosomes have been demonstrated in some studies to modify a number of processes such as metastasis, treatment resistance, carcinogenesis, progression, and onset [54, 55].

3.1 Role of Exosomes as Biomarkers

Because exosomes contain a significant number of cancer-associated proteins and because their membrane structure protects luminal proteins from external protease degradation, proteins from tumour-derived exosomes, or TEXs, are increasingly becoming identified as cancer diagnostic and prognostic indications [56]. Exosomes and their content may exert numerous biological effects at different levels of cancer. As depicted in some recent reports, exosomes can be effectively and quickly isolated from such bodily fluids as urine, plasma, serum, and so on. Moreover, they can be used as biomarkers of early cancer diagnosis at different stages. The exosome genomic profile that consists of messenger RNA, mitochondrial RNA, lncRNA, and miRNA appears to be an effective biomarker source to differentiate among the cancer types. An illustration is shown describing briefly about how exosomal biomarkers can be detected with several proteins, and ncRNAs with the help of using various biosensors (Fig. 10.2). Numerous established methods may be used to increase the availability and specificity of exosomal biomarkers [55, 57].

3.1.1 Potential of Exosomal Proteins to Act as Biomarkers

Proteins are some of the major payloads of the exosomes. Exosomes produced by cancer cells may have multiple proteins. The two types of proteins in exosomes are common and unique. The ones in the GTPase family of proteins are classified as widely shared proteins and are involved in fusion and other vital biological events. The vital processes are cell targeting, protein sorting, intracellular transport, and production of exosomes. Exosomes possess some special proteins, and the nature of these proteins differs depending on the cancer stage; these proteins have been found in exosomes that are secreted by particular cells [58]. These exosomes further have

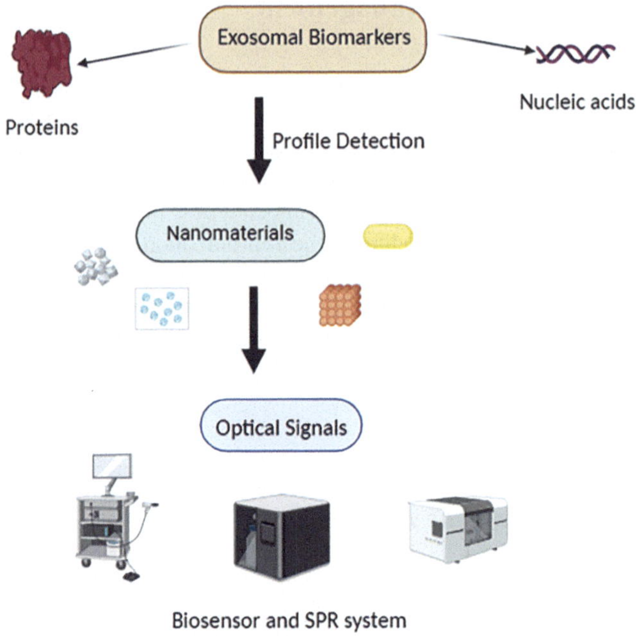

Fig. 10.2 Exosomes as biomarkers. (The illustration is created on Biorender software. (Source: https://doi.org/10.1016/j.aca.2020.02.041; https://doi.org/10.1021/acsabm.4c01920))

an increased number of proteins in cancer patients as compared to those of healthy individuals, and the proteins present in cancerous cells, especially, can be used to determine the stage of the disease. Blood levels of fibronectin were considerably higher in patients at an early stage of breast cancer, with a 65.1% sensitivity and an 83.2% specificity [59]. According to Khan et al. (2014), patients with early-stage breast cancer have considerably greater levels of survivin and its variation in their blood exosomes [60]. Exosome proteomics research is constrained, nonetheless, particularly in light of the requirement for exosome quality. To properly study exosomes for potential uses, proteomics—a potent research technique in the post-genomic era—must be combined with transcriptomics and genomics [57].

3.1.2 Exosomal miRNAs as Biomarkers

The expression of miRNAs of both types of cells, tumour and non-tumour cells are distinct. Thus, unlike normal exo-miRs, exo-miRs in body fluids also undergo a certain fluctuation in the patterns of expression. Exosomes are critical in packaging miRNAs to be transported and ensure that miRNAs are not degraded during transfers to target cells. The target cells may undergo numerous cellular and molecular reactions that could be stimulated by the miRNAs within the exosomes [55]. Exosomal miRNAs have been identified to be important in hepatocellular carcinoma (HCC) and may evolve into highly sensitive novel serological biomarkers of HCC, more sensitive than the simple analysis of miRNA. Finding important miRNAs that may serve as breast cancer diagnostic biomarkers has been the subject of a lot of research. Weiying Zhou and associates discovered that miR-105 is substantially expressed in the bloodstream during the premetastatic and metastatic phases [58]. They also showed that the primary source of this molecule and miR-181a was the serum exosomes of patients with stage II and stage III breast cancer [61]. Moreover, the exosomal miR-21 and miR-1246 were overexpressed and have a positive correlation with increased invasiveness of cancer in the breast and growth [54, 56]. To increase the validity of exosomal miRNAs assays, more tumour types and development stages should be included in the future.

3.1.3 Role of Exosomal lncRNAs to Act as Biomarkers

During protein synthesis, long non-coding RNAs (lncRNAs) of over 200 nucleotides of length are expressed through RNA polymerase II-dependent transcription. These molecules are turning out to be one of the most important regulators of cellular activities and gene expression. Even though the synthesis, maturation, and mechanistic complexities of lncRNAs have not been uncovered yet, the processes are assumed to be essential [54]. It has been reported that the changes in the levels of the exosomal HOX transcript antisense intergenic RNA (HOTAIR) could be utilized as effective biomarkers in monitoring of response to treatment and the recurrence of glioblastoma multiforme (GBM) [55]. Additionally, for breast cancer, HOTAIR-exosomal expression may act as a survival predictor and diagnostic marker [62] published the first study recommending the application of exosomal LncRNAs as possible breast cancer indicators. In their results, the overexpression of the lncRNA RP11-445H22.4 in tissues and serum of breast cancer patients has been observed with specificity and sensitivity of 74% and 92% when compared with healthy patients [62]. New studies indicate that lncRNAs are involved in carcinogenesis as well as tumour growth and tumour microenvironment (TME). Further analysis is required to fully comprehend how exosomes and lncRNAs are the topic of discussion in pathogenic physiology in the TME [57, 58].

3.1.4 Potential of Exosomal circRNAs to Act as Biomarkers

Circular RNA (circRNA) constitutes a class of non-coding RNAs mostly synthesized by pre-mRNA splicing. As compared to miRNA, circRNA is aberrantly stable, conserved, and has a stable expression pattern characterizing a cell or a tissue. The role of exosomes is also to protect circRNAs against degradation during circulation due to the environment surrounding them. Moreover, circRNAs are further stabilized by being encapsulated in exosomes, and such an event enables the further survival of the circRNA in the physiological fluids [63]. Exosomal circRNAs, because of these properties, have great prospects as screening factors. The level of circular RNA PDE8A (circ-PDE8A) expressed, probably as the prognostic and development factor of PDAC, was evaluated in plasma exosomes of PDAC patients [64]. Exosomal circRNAs have been described in studies as customary diagnostic biomarkers of diseases. But to determine how specific levels of expression of specific illnesses and types of cancer are, additional research is required [65, 66].

3.2 Impact of Exosomes as Therapeutic Agents in Cancer Drug Resistance

The problem with the treatment of cancers is the drug resistance, where the pharmacological properties of drugs used to elicit therapeutic effects are lost. As far as we know, drug resistance in anticancer treatment is of two major types: acquired and intrinsic (pre-existing). The biology of exosomes and the association with tumour treatment resistance helps in better explaining the peculiarities of exosomes, e.g. surface markers, the specificity of the cargo with the physiological state of the parent cells, their comparative stability, and the fact that they are found in almost all biological fluids [67]. Due to these attributes, exosomes are becoming attractive objects of study in the initial stages of disease development and potential predictors of the treatment response or refractoriness. Wang et al. could sensitize the cisplatin-resistant gastric cancer cells by loading anti-miRNA-214 into exosomes that were transferred to the recipient cells, and Wang et al. could then enhance the response of these cells to cisplatin [68]. Li et al. showed that exosome-specific miRNA-770 modulated apoptotic pathways and the tumour microenvironment to overcome doxorubicin resistance in the triple-negative breast cancer cells [64]. The benefits of exosomes as a naturally occurring drug in the immunotherapy of cancer during vaccination, and the delivery of drugs have been established in numerous studies. These advantages are the nanoscale size, the immunological compatibility, the low toxicity levels, the extended blood circulation, and relative stability [69–71]. Exosomes are safe, efficient, and are thus an appropriate means to deliver medication or conduct the therapy because they are natural carriers.

4 Nanotechnology-Based Therapeutic Strategies

4.1 Classification of Various Therapy Based on Nanotechnology

Nanotechnology has been launched not only a groundbreaking as well as also an efficient treatment strategy which is more accurate and specific than previous therapeutic strategies. If we use nanotechnology during therapy, it can reduce the chances to cause harm to the healthy tissues; on the other hand, it also has the capacity to efficiently kill tumour cells. Nanotechnology provides various platforms for cancer therapy like photothermal therapy, photodynamic therapy, gene therapy, immunotherapy, etc. They have some special features like high surface area, customizable size, and reactive functional group modification, making them perfect for therapeutic purposes [72].

4.1.1 Photothermal Therapy

1. **Functional Mechanism**

   - This photothermal therapy uses gold nanoparticles and carbon nanotube materials because it can absorb the light energy mainly in the near-infrared (NIR) range that converted into heat. When the temperature hits a crucial point, cancer cells are specifically destroyed since they are more sensitive to heat than healthy cells [73–76].

4.1.2 Common Nanoparticles

1. **Gold Nanoparticles (AuNPs)**

   - Gold nanoparticles have the capacity to efficiently absorb light at the near-infrared range and due to the presence of surface plasmon resonance it can significantly convert light energy into the form of heat. These nanoparticles use peptides or antibodies for the selective binding of overexpressed cancer cell surface receptors, due to the presence of this near-infrared light cancer cells become damaged and finally they got eliminated. Due to the localized heat treatment, the interior proteins of cancer cells become denatured and also their cell membrane become disrupted, but healthy cells remain unaffected because the target-specific property of nanoparticles [77–79].

2. **Carbon Nanotubes (CNTs)**

   - As this nanoparticle has the excellent thermal and electrical properties, it can efficiently absorb NIR light to provide heat treatment at a particular area [80]. These CNTs has the capacity to transfer drugs or other therapeutic materials, and it also improves the therapeutic efficacy upon connecting photothermal therapy with chemotherapy [15].
   - **Positive therapeutic outcomes**: This therapy has less invasive and localized treatment capacity than the chemotherapy and radiotherapy. It can efficiently cure tumours happen in delicate regions like brain or spinal cord.

4.1.3 Photodynamic Therapy (PDT)

1. **Mechanism of Action**

    - This kind of treatment makes use of light-sensitive substances that, when exposed to a certain wavelength of light, produce reactive oxygen species (ROS) or free radicals; thus, it can selectively destroy disease tissues like cancer [81, 82]. As it has some specific properties like high sensitivity, lower invasive nature, and also it causes minimal damage to healthy tissues so it can be used to not only treat cancer but also some non-malignant conditions can be treated by this.

2. **Nanocarriers Used in PDT**

    - **Liposome-based carriers**: Hydrophobic photosensitizers can be enclosed using this special type of nanocarriers. Upon encapsulating they become prevented from initial collapsation while enhancing their solubility in the biological environment [83, 84]. It has the high retention (EPR) and permeable capacity due to its small size and lipid-based composition.
    - **Polymeric nanoparticles (PLGA)**: Polymers like polylactic-co-glycolic acid (PLGA) is a biocompatible carriers which allowed the controlled release of photosensitizer, and they can respond to tumour-specific conditions like variations in pH and enzymatic activity [68, 85, 86].
    - **Gold nanoparticles**: When gold nanoparticles absorb strong light at the near-infrared region, reactive oxygen species are produced.
    - **Quantum dots (QDs)**: It can be used in diagnosis as well as in the treatment purpose to provide a compact therapeutic and diagnostic advantage in cancer care, but this dual functionality of quantum dots are possible due to its adjustable optic nature [87–90].
    - **Addressing tumour hypoxia**: Tumour hypoxia is a special condition where oxygen molecules directly transported to cancerous tissues, but this problem can be solved using perfluorocarbon and mesoporous silica nanoparticles.
    - **Perfluorocarbon nanoparticles**: It is an oxygen-carrying nanomaterial. ROS production is maximized when cancer tissues receive oxygen molecules transported by nanoparticles.
    - **Mesoporous nanoparticles (MSNs)**: They seek attention due to their capability to simultaneously transport photosensitizers and anticancer medications; thus, it can target tumours using various biological pathways [91, 92].

4.1.4 Immune Condition and Genetic Condition-Related Therapy

Nanotechnology provides a novel delivery platform for the improvement of immunological and genetic therapy because it can efficiently transport genetic materials and some components that regulate immune function [93]. This technology can easily overcome the targeted site delivery problem of using genetic modification, causing tools like CRISPR-Cas9 to malignant cells [94, 95]. Nanoparticles act as optical carriers because it is capable of protecting genetic materials from enzymatic breakdown, enhancing absorption by cells and facilitating targeted delivery to tumour sites. In gene therapy, nanoparticles deliver small interfering RNA (siRNA) [96, 97], messenger RNA (mRNA) [98, 99], and CRISPR elements [95] used to deactivate or fix defective genes that contribute to the cancer development. Once inside cancer cells, when siRNA takes entry into cancer cells it represses the expression of oncogenes; on the other hand, mRNA blocks cancer growth upon producing some proteins [100–102].

1. **Lipid Nanoparticles**
   - Because lipid nanoparticles may shield siRNA or mRNA from enzymatic breakdown and facilitate their active or passive targeted distribution to tumours, they are frequently utilized to carry these nucleic acids. Lipid nanoparticles hinder the site-specific drug delivery functionality because those are tended to accumulate in the hepatic tissues. To overcome this issue, LNPs combine with immune cells like T-cells and dendritic cells which make them efficient as innate transport systems and delivering drugs into the tumour's microenvironment [16, 103, 104].
2. **Gold Nanoparticles**
   - Cancers are mainly caused by genetic mutation to overcome this problem gold nanoparticles are used for gene editing. In this case, gold nanoparticles are mainly covered with Cas9 enzymes and guide RNAs, thus they can accurately reach cancer tissues [105].
3. **Therapeutic Cancer Vaccine Development**
   - In the cancer vaccine, engineering purpose nanoparticles are used. When nanoparticles deliver tumour antigens or produce some tumour-specific proteins to stimulate immune cells which are encoded by mRNA for the detection and ultimately kill cancer cells [106]. The main working principle of mRNA-based vaccines is that it activates the immune system upon finding biomarkers specific to cancer.

4.2 Role of Nanotechnology for the Improvement of Cancer Treatment

This nanotechnology has enriched the approaches with the incorporation of therapy and diagnosis for the treatment of cancer. This has been possible by the use of nanoscale technologies in association with molecular profiling technologies, which enables clinicians to address heterogeneity and complexity of the tumours and design drugs targeting specifically biomarkers and tumour-associated signalling pathways.

1. **Advanced Identification of Tumours from the Molecular Background**
    - Nanotechnology improves the accuracy of tumours molecular profiling by using advanced imaging and diagnostic techniques. An advanced nanotechnology-based technique, multiplexed quantum dot assay is a nanotechnology-based platform due the presence of its advanced features it can simultaneously detect multiples biomarkers like HER2, EGFR, and PD-L1 in a single test. Thus, following this method, clinicians are capable of classifying patients based on molecular profiles, and they can get a guideline to choose targeted therapies for the respective patients [18]. Whatever, nanoprobes are another advanced nanotechnology-based technique which efficiently detect therapeutic outcome and find out tumour microenvironment details due to the presence of its enhanced resolution imaging capacity.
2. **Disease Proliferation Tracking at the Real-Time Basis**
    - Nanotechnology developed some diagnostic instruments with some advanced features which are capable of continuous tracking of treatment outcomes. Like, nanoparticles used as an imaging agents to monitor drug distribution at the tumour sites and assess treatment response. Using this technology, doctors can easily alternate treatment plans of a particular patient via tracking real-time therapeutic outcomes to get best patient outcome [107].
3. **Site-Specific Medication Delivery**
    - Nanotechnology mainly helps the improvement of precision drug delivery. Lipid-based and polymeric nanoparticles are frequently used for drug transport to the cancer cells, and it also minimizes systemic toxicity by protecting healthy cells from chemotherapy [108]. A functionalized nanoparticle is a special type of nanoparticle that conjugates with antibodies or peptides; it has the target site specificity feature to kill only cancerous cells specifically. These specific approaches enhance the efficacy of the drug and also reduce side effects, decreasing cancer patient mortality [109].

5 Quantum Dots: A Unique Discovery in the Diagnostics Field of Cancer

5.1 Introduction to Quantum Dots

Quantum dots are mainly 2–10 nm in sized nanometer crystals containing unique electrical and optical properties; it is also semiconductor in nature. It contains fluorescence that varies based on wavelength emission. QDs have efficient multiplexed imaging capacities, here small QDs emit red light while larger ones show red light [110]. They have some unique features like high quantum yield, resistance to photobleaching, wide excitation spectra, and narrow emission peaks, which allows them to simultaneously excite multiple QDs using a single light source, thus it can easily detect multiple targets [111].

It can regulate the tumour growth and development as well as it also specifically bound with several cancer biomarkers. Breast cancer cells precisely detected by the quantum dots are attached with HER2 biomarkers; on the other hand, using fluorescence microscopy and flow cytometry provide the tumour proliferation live imaging facilities [19]. These properties make QDs to fulfil the gap between clinical application and molecular biology.

5.2 Biomarker Identification Applications Using Quantum Dots

Along with high sensitivity and selectivity, QDs can efficiently identify biomarkers related to cancers. Their size-dependent fluorescence and resistance property against photobleaching help them to enable effective real-time tracking and imaging [112].

1. **Simultaneous Detection Capability**
    - For the identification of various cancer biomarkers simultaneously like HER2 and EGFR, QDs surface are customized with numerous ligands like antibodies or aptamers. When QDs become excited, they emit various wavelengths of light allowing simultaneous analysis without non-specific interference between signals [19].
2. **Live Imaging Capacity**
    - QDs are aids in the tracking of circulating tumour cells (CTCs) which helps to precisely transport therapeutic molecules at the site of cancer. Folate receptors of cancer tissues are targeted by the folic acid-linked QDs [14].
3. **Detection Systems Adaptability**
    - Like flow cytometry, microfluidic system and quantum dots are easily adaptable in detection system. Quantum dot-based microfluidic device is capable of detecting cancer biomarkers with high accuracy in small volumes of samples in a short time [113]. QD-based flow cytometry is used to detect biomarkers related to tumour.

5.3 Uses in Initial Stage Identification of Cancer

Quantum dots have the accuracy to detect various cancer-related biomarkers at the initial stage of cancer development [114].

1. **Breast Cancer**

    - QDs which are attached with anti-HER2 antibodies can efficiently bind with the tumour cells which overexpress HER2 biomarker and also emit fluorescence light which facilitates their detection. So, quantum dot (QD)-based assays are capable of identifying HER2, CAL5-3, and various other biomarkers continuously to provide an accurate molecular profiling of breast cancer [18].

2. **Lung Cancer**

    - In case of lung cancer, QDs facilitate the identification some specific biomarkers such as carcinoembryonic antigen and cytokeratin-19 fragments. In the early stage of cancer, these biomarkers are mainly present in minute quantities, but QDs, upon integration with fluorescence microscopy or biosensors, can precisely detect these biomarkers. Even in case of extremely low targeted molecule containing samples QDs can detect lung cancer-related biomarkers precisely along with high sensitivity [107].

3. **Colorectal Cancer**

    - In case of colorectal cancer aptamers which are linked with quantum dots can be attached with the biomarkers like guanylyl cyclase G and carcinoembryonic antigen. These quantum dots are used at the site of tumour for track responses in cancer patient to detect the live images [109].
    - When QDs are involved in diagnostic purposes, doctors become capable of precisely identifying cancer; thus, the survival rate of patients has also enhanced, so as a result this patient-specific treatment has also improved.

5.4 Cytotoxicity-Related Concern and Challenges Related to Adaptability

Due to their heavy metal contents like cadmium and selenium, which can emit dangerous ions and are harmful to the health of human beings, one of the major disadvantages of clinical use of quantum dots is their possibility of toxicity and biocompatibility [115]. Upon prolonged exposer of QDs in-patient body, this not only causes oxidative stress but also causes potential organ damage due to inflammation. If biomaterials such as silica or polyethylene glycol (PEG) are coated over QDs, this problem can be overcome; they can also inhibit the emission of toxic ions precisely and become resistant against biological or environmental degradation.

Researchers found a quantum dot that is free from cadmium mainly made up of indium phosphide showing a similar optical feature but minimized toxicity effects [116].

There is also a problem with using QDs is the accumulation of tissues and the lack of long-term safety facilities. To overcome this problem, some biodegradable nanomaterials have been used to manufacture quantum dots which can degrade into non-hazardous byproducts, but their diagnostic capacity remains unaffected [117]. To enhance long-term safety records of QDs, it is necessary to conduct numerous clinical research.

5.5 Clinical Report of Quantum Dots in Simultaneous Diagnostic Platform

Quantum dot (QD)-based assays were used in the first clinical study to detect many biomarkers at once, such as HER2, EGFR, and PD-L1, in samples taken from breast cancer tissues. Upon using special fluorescence features of quantum dots, this assay can efficiently deliver a detailed molecular profiling through a single run. The speed of diagnosis as well as their functional perfections are enhanced which supports patient-specific treatment plans and also saves a significant amount of time to initiate therapy using single-test multiplexed strategy [113].

5.6 Uses of Nanoprobes for Visualization of Early Stage of Cancer

1. **Nanoprobes**

   - They are small-sized devices that have been developed to enhance the identification accuracy, observation, and measurement to study biological components. In the field of cancer diagnosis, it significantly boosts up the imaging capacity to enhance not only sensitivity but also specificity. It suppresses traditional imaging and can specifically detect disease-related biomarkers, and it can precisely identify cancer tissues but leaves healthy cells [17].
   - It contains gold nanoparticles, quantum dots, and iron oxide particles, but it moves along with particular targeting ligands like antibodies or peptides, which have the capacity to selectively bind with breast cancer biomarker HER2 and lung cancer biomarker EGFR [118]. Upon its attachment to a specific biomarker, this increases imaging signals and makes tumour detection easy at an early stage.
   - Nanoprobes act as an ideal cancer imaging tool due to the presence of specific features like huge surface area-to-volume ratio, adjustable optical and magnetic properties, and tissue invading capacity [119]. However, it can be

merged with some other diagnostic imaging tools such as magnetic resonance imaging, positron emission tomography, and fluorescence imaging.
- For the identification of initial tumour, nanoprobes are widely used which also support patient-specific therapeutic approach.

2. **Usefulness of Nanoprobes for the Identification of Biomarkers to Detect Cancer**

   - When a minute number of biomarkers are present, in-patient sample nanoprobes can efficiently detect it; the biomarkers are mainly proteins, metabolites, and DNA or RNA [120]. They are extremely helpful to target circulating tumour cells (CTCs) and circulating tumour DNA (ctDNA). In this condition, circulating tumour cells or circulating tumour DNA is specifically along with high affinity can attach with gold or magnetic nanoparticles.
   - Nanoprobes have the capacity to penetrate cancer tissues. Vascular endothelial growth factor or matrix metalloproteinases are mainly overexpressed over tumour tissues, and these nanoprobes can efficiently target these molecules. So nanoprobes help to enhance diagnostic accuracy but reduce the chances to get false positive results [121].
   - Whatever, nanoprobes bridge the gaps between diagnosis at molecular basis and imaging of them, which promotes cancer detection at the initial stage and also tracks the therapeutic efficiency.

3. **Visualization Strategies and Its Improvement Using Nanoprobes**
   Nanoprobes have some advanced cancer imaging techniques which make them more precise, efficient, and adaptable. There are mainly three imaging techniques which are enhanced by nanoprobe integration and are discussed below:

   - **Fluorescence Imaging**: These nanoprobes are mainly fluorescent nanoparticles and quantum dots emit strong and stable signals by transforming fluorescence imaging. Biomarkers like HER2 and EGFR can be easily detected using nanoprobes that are linked with fluorescence. In the case of quantum dots, it is linked with HER2-antibody that specifically binds with breast cancer cells and emits fluorescence upon excitation. It is also capable of real-time visualization of tumours during surgery [107]. Fluorescence resonance energy transfer-based nanoprobes help to visualize interaction at the molecular level within the tumour microenvironment.
   - **Positron Emission Tomography (PET)**: PET scanning is a highly efficient diagnostic method employed for the identification of alterations in cellular metabolism along with the alterations in cancer; nevertheless, its functional efficiency is enhanced by employing radiotracers developed through nanoprobe technology together with them [114]. Nanoparticles tagged with isotopes emit positrons; some isotopes are available, such as fluorine-180r and zirconium-89, which increase the precision and clarity of PET imaging. Gold nanoparticles can efficiently bind with hypoxia-inducible factor-1 (HIF-1), which is a potential biomarker of highly aggressive tumours.

- **Magnetic Resonance Imaging (MRI)**: Target selectivity as well as contrast of MRI is enhanced with the use of nanoprobes. Normal and tumour tissues can be differentiated using superparamagnetic iron oxide nanoparticles or SPIONs which are efficient MRI contrast agents. SPIONs are rendered more visible for tumour angiogenesis of glioblastoma cancer by binding with integrins [122]. Various biomarkers can be detected in one run using quantum dot nanoprobes by detecting fluorescent signals corresponding to them; this informs us about variability of cancer tissues which helps the clinicians to select patient-specific therapy [123].

4. **Advantages and Challenges**

   Cancer diagnosis and visualization capacity are enhanced due to the presence of advanced nanoprobe technology. Versatile nanoprobes can diagnose and treat cancer at the same time; on the other hand, nanoprobes that are biodegradable in nature like lipids or polymers reduce toxic effect while improving adaptability in the patient body [19, 111].

   It has various advantages, but there are also some challenges like:

- **Biosafety Background**: In patient body, harmful immune responses are generated along with some cytotoxic effect because nano-biosensors are manufactured using some materials like carbon nanotubes. Several clinical studies are necessary to overcome this problem [12].
- **Scale-up Capability**: A well-developed infrastructure is necessary for the large-scale production and functionalization of nanoprobes which is too much costly. So, affordable production-oriented infrastructure planning is very essential [19].

5. **Clinical Study to Prove Nanoprobes Ability to Visualized Breast Cancer**

   In a study where nanoprobes are used to detect breast cancer, nanoprobes are used which worked based on SPION which is conjugated with ligand that specifically targets HER2-receptor which is mainly utilized to enhance MRI scans contrast. They can differentiate malignant tissues from benign tissues which can accurately identify HER2-positive tumours. It can reduce the unwanted biopsies and enhance the accuracy of diagnosis almost 30% [124].

6 Nanotechnology on the Basis of Cancer Immunotherapy

6.1 Immune Response Modification

It refers to the methods used to manage immune system-related conditions covering infections, illness, vaccination, and treatments in response to various varieties of stimuli. Based on the immune conditions, immunological response control regulation efficiently increased or decreased. In the case of disease, immune system is mainly engaged in killing microbes. But in the case of autoimmune disease, as in this case body's immune cells mistakenly attack their tissues. So, the activity of the immune system must be suppressed to cure this disease. Some drugs that alter immune function, any tiny molecules, monoclonal antibodies and cytokines, are used for enhancing or reducing immune responses. However, these drugs are used to control inflammatory disease and cancer. Thus, there are requirements to create novel therapeutic strategies to modulate immune system function. So, various nanotechnology-based treatment methods have been developed to fulfil these requirements [125].

1. **Immune Response Improvement Capacity of Nanoparticles**
   Nanotechnology helps to boost immune responses in the case of vaccination and immunotherapies. These nanotechnology-based products increase the efficiency of antigen delivery and provide consistency and the presence of immune-activating compounds. It is also used to control the immune system's responses. Nanoparticles are tailored using chemicals which boost the immune responses upon altering their dimensions, form, and electrical properties. Nanoparticles are capable of mimicking disease-causing antigens, so as a result of this, antigen-presenting cells can easily recognize them and emit strong immune responses. Both innate and adaptive immunity are boosted upon surface modification of nanoparticles, which helps them to carry antigens or adjuvants. Various studies are going on for the improvement of vaccines, find out new cancer immunotherapies, and to enhance the treatment efficacy of infectious diseases. This approach signifies the strength of nanoparticles to modify the field of immunology [125].
2. **Antigens and Immune Modulator Administration**
   Immunomodulation of medications and antigens is essential in the field of contemporary immunotherapy and vaccine research, as it provides strength to the immune system and helps to fight against illness. Antigens are transported perfectly towards the antigen-presenting cells. So, for this purpose, the use of nanoparticles and liposomes is investigated because they can protect medicines and antigens from breaking down. This can be modified for the continuous release of drugs, thus increasing immunological response while reducing the necessity of using several dosages. If the carriers are modified using ligands or antibodies, then the functionality of APC absorption will be increased. Humoral and cellular immunity are boosted following some strategies like the involvement of enclosing antigens in nanoparticles or co-delivering them with immune enhancers. Using these methods, we can develop not only cancer treatment medicines but also reduce autoimmune diseases, and engineering vaccines against infectious pathogens, which demonstrating their role to enhance immunotherapy effectiveness [125].

6.2 Mechanism of Action of Immunological Therapy Related to Cancer

Cancer immunotherapy is targeted towards the stimulation of the immune response to recognize and destroy the cancer cells. The most widely known treatment is the use of immune checkpoint blockers, e.g. CTLA-4 and PD-1/PD-L1, since they are inhibitors of inhibitory signals with the ability to enhance the activation of T-cells. The application of monoclonal antibodies to specifically target antigens present in cancer cells is an important approach because it blocks growth signals of tumour and helps in immune recognition. One type of adoptive cellular transfer procedure that alters cancer patients' T-cells is chimeric antigen receptor T-cell therapy, which develops specific receptors that are capable of selectively attacking cancer cells which directly destroys them. Whatever, to develop cancer vaccines antigens associated with tumour are used because they can efficiently trigger an immune response against the tumour. But certain therapies are available which use cytokines to boost immune cell function; on the other hand, genetically engineered oncolytic viruses selectively penetrate and kill cancer cells and also trigger a strong immunological response. All these mechanisms are important to achieve prolonged effect and more accurate cancer immunotherapy [16].

1. **Site-Specific Drug Delivery**

   It is a sophisticated approach because it has the capacity to efficiently deliver drugs to a particular area within the body. This has increased therapeutic efficacy and has lower side effects. This also has some strategies which ensure medications are delivered at the intended locations, like tumours or damaged tissues, but do not cause harm to the healthy cells. Medicines are encapsulated using carriers like liposomes or nanoparticles because they have the efficiency to travel throughout the bloodstream until they reach the proper location. These drug delivery systems can release drugs once they have attached with molecular markers on the target diseased cells. Drugs can be delivered at the target site following the stimuli like ligand–receptor interaction or local changes such as pH, enzymes, or temperature gradients. Such accuracy improves the overall treatment effectiveness and minimizes the risk of systemic toxicity, which significantly progress for the advancement of personalized medicine and helps to manage oncology and to cure of chronic conditions [16].
2. **Necessity of Exact Identification and Focusing on Cancer Cells**

   Maintaining high selectivity of targeting cancer cells is important, which avoids damage to the healthy cells. Due to the identification of particular genetic markers or antigens from the cancer cells, precise targeting efficiency and specificity is recognized which plays a significant role in directing the chimeric antigen receptor T-cells and monoclonal antibodies towards malignant cells. It helps to improve therapeutic effectiveness minimizing side effects [16].

6.3 Effective Nanodrug Transport in Cancer Immunotherapy:

Various successful nanodrug delivery approaches in cancer immunotherapy are available which demonstrate precise cancer targeting and treatment. Increased drug solubility, stability, and controlled drug release is mediated by nanodrug delivery system which is capable of providing the best therapeutic outcomes to the cancer patients. As an example, chemotherapeutic drugs or immunomodulators loaded liposomal nanoparticles are developed to recognize cancer cell markers while mediating target site drug delivery. Clinical studies demonstrate that drug accumulation is maximizing at the tumour sites which is capable of triggering a stronger immune response, but it can maximize systemic toxicity [126, 127].

When dendritic cell-based vaccines are conjugated with antigens and some adjuvant-loaded nanoparticles, they become effective in treating cancer. By effectively stimulating the immune system to kill cancer cells, the treatment suppresses tumour growth and enhances cancer patients' survival rate. But this case study provides us with information on cancer immunotherapy based on nanotechnology with less side effects and better therapeutic performance. The novel trackway is opened for the therapeutic purpose of cancer [128].

6.4 Advantages and Difficulties Associated with Cancer Immunotherapy

Cancer immunotherapy provides several advantages, but there are also many difficulties; they are discussed below:

1. **Cancer Immunotherapy Benefits**
   - **Selective immunological response stimulation**: It has the capacity to properly stimulate the immune system for specific recognition and destroy cancer cells.
   - **Effective against treatment-resistance cancer**: Several immunology-related therapeutic strategies like using checkpoint inhibitors, CAR-T cells, and cancer-related vaccines show promising overcoming strategies to fight against some non-curable cancers.
   - **Capacity to reduce the risk of relapses**: Immunotherapy has the capacity to efficiently reduce cancer recurrences which is achieved when immune system is enabled to selectively recognize and kill cancer cells [129].
2. **Drawbacks of Immunological Therapy in Cancer Treatment Purpose**
   - **Inconsistent patient outcome**: Upon receiving immunotherapy not every patient properly responds to it; thus, it is very difficult to predict a good outcome from every patient.

- **Immunological side effects**: Immunotherapy remains very complex from the biological background as well as it is also technological. As a result of this complexity, specialized handling systems are required. It is also too costly; thus, many patients can't afford to take this treatment.
- To solve these problems, numerous researches are essential to reduce side effects and optimize the availability of drugs [129].

7 Upcoming Potential of Precision-Based Nanotechnology

7.1 Recent Technological Advances

The development of advanced nanotechnology is central to enhancing cancer diagnosis and therapy, and thus to enhancing the efficacy of diagnosis and treatment, AI is combined with nano-systems.

1. **AI-Linked Nano-Diagnostics**
   AI is being combined with nanotechnology to improve the working efficiency and cancer detection efficiency precisely. AI algorithms can handle vast data with nano-biosensors and quantum dots; it can also identify cancer markers by sensing minute biological signals. As an example, AI-linked nanoparticle-based imaging techniques can efficiently differentiate between benign and cancerous tumours, as well as it also reduces false negative result while increasing the chances of getting positive results [113]. Additionally, it is also capable of comprehending functionality of nanoprobes and quantum dots, and how they interact with biological systems; artificial intelligence (AI) can also facilitate the development of new diagnostic tools.
2. **Hybrid Nano-Systems**
   For the improvement of therapy and diagnosis, this advanced platform connects several nanotechnologies into a single platform. As an example, these hybrid nanoparticles have multifunctional properties such as magnetic, optical, and therapeutic, which simultaneously work to detect, visualize, and treat cancer. It provides theragnostic facilities; here, therapy is done along with real-time feedback monitoring treatment response [114]. This hybrid quantum dot contains dual imaging capacity not only molecular but also anatomical visualization capacity it provides. This system works by merging fluorescence and radiolabelling. An efficient, exact, and low-invasive therapeutic approach is provided by hybrid nano-systems. As research progresses in the field of nanotechnology, it becomes more efficient in using it as a personalized cancer care, providing diagnoses and therapeutic solutions for individual cancer patients.

7.2 Personalized Therapeutic Strategies Effect on Cancer Treatment

Nanotechnology applications of precise kinds are evolving in the era of transforming personalized medicine by providing it with the capability to serve as individualized diagnoses and successful treatment plans to cancer patients. Doctors are now capable of accurately comparing tumour heterogeneity and selecting exact therapies that specifically target particular biomarkers and signalling pathways related to a specific type of cancer upon incorporating nanoscale technologies and molecular analysis.

1. **Advanced Molecular Profiling**

   Nanotechnology produces high-resolution molecular images of tumours with the help of sophisticated imaging and diagnostic methods. Multiplexed quantum dot assay has the capacity to detect various biomarkers like EGFR, HER2, and PD-L1 from a single test, which allows proper categorization of patients based on the basis of their molecular characteristics and also provides a proper guideline to select targeted therapies [18]. Moreover, it also has high-resolution imaging capacity; along with this, it also provides tumour microenvironment details and its therapeutic response.
2. **Live Monitoring Capacity**

   Various nanoscale-based diagnostic tools are capable of real-time observation of treatment effectiveness. As an example, nanoscale-based imaging tools can trace the pathway of drug distribution along with where the tumour is situated and find therapeutic results. These imaging tools provide valuable data to clinicians which help them to find treatment strategies, thus ensuring the need for optimal outcomes [107].
3. **Drug Delivery System**

   Drug transporting capacity becomes enhanced following this technology. Lipid nanoparticles or polymer nanocarriers can specifically transfer chemotherapeutic drugs at the target site which causes less harm to the healthy tissues. Some antibodies as well as peptide-conjugated materials linked with nanomaterials which transport drugs directly to the cancer cells. By accurate diagnosis, precision medicine, and real-time tracking, nanotechnology has the potential to transform cancer treatment more effectively and to meet the demand of patients.

7.3 Joint Research

Nanotechnology advances day by day to create cancer therapies, relying heavily on interdisciplinary methods, drawing upon skills in specialized disciplines such as engineering, biology, and medicine in an attempt to speed up breakthroughs and clinical applications.

1. **Multidisciplinary Research Teams**

   In the field of nanotechnology, scalability and biocompatibility issues are overcome by biomedical engineers, chemists, and physicians. The process ensures that it increases the effectiveness of medication without increasing harmful side effects, thus improving patient welfare and quality of life [109].

   As an example, the collaboration of researchers and clinical teams has become successful in developing SPIONs which functionalized for MRI imaging, thus aiming to ensure both effectiveness and patient safety [117].
2. **Global Networks**

   International collaborations provide permissions to the researchers to share cancer treatment data, skills, and infrastructure for the advancement of nanotechnology field. International Cancer Nanotechnology consortium a global network provides international collaboration, which is capable of providing diagnostic and therapeutic tools that are broadly applicable [130].

These sectors focus on the advancement of nanotechnology field which plays an important role in improving cancer diagnosis, treatment, and patient outcomes.

8 Ethical Implication and Social Implications

8.1 Ethical Considerations

Using advanced nanotechnology for cancer diagnostics, treatment purposes raise some important ethical concerns oriented to privacy, equity, and access.

- **Security**: A huge amount of secure health purpose data of cancer patients can be collected using novel nanotechnology fields like quantum dots and nanobiosensors. But this data is inaccurate for accurate diagnostics, and this data carries an increasing vulnerability to breaches and unauthorized access. Therefore, this also ensures requirement of strong data protection measures, and strong privacy policies is crucial for increasing patients' confidence and adhering to ethical principles [115].
- **Equity and access**: Nanotechnology-based diagnosis is very expensive, so some healthcare systems did not provide this facility to patients, thus existing inequalities in cancer treatment have become worse. Economically, poor category patients are not able to afford as limited availability of these advanced tools can reinforce global health disparities [130]. To overcome this issue, fair pricing, investment in public health, and scalable production methods are necessary to access these technologies available to all patients, following their economical background [116].
- **Informed consent**: The use of nanotechnology becomes challenging for cancer patients to fully understand the involved implications; it is an informed consent due to its complex nature [131]. Clear communication and education regarding the ethical clinical practice are the main advantages, but there are also some

potential risks, and limitations are present in nanotechnology-based diagnostics. The primary use of nanotechnology in cancer therapy is demonstrated by these ethical concerns, which highlight the need for several frameworks and regulations that govern justice, transparency, and accountability [117].

8.2 *Social Effect*

Survival rates have been significantly improved due to the revolution in healthcare departments because it allows for earlier detection, and personalized treatment which ultimately improves patient outcomes [131]. But low-income populations are unable to get access to these advancements, so the widefield use of nanotechnology may worsen existing socioeconomic inequalities. Thus, maintaining the balance between innovation and equity will require joint efforts from the government, healthcare systems, and also from the industry shareholders.

9 Conclusion

Cancer is a highly complex disease. Hundreds of compounds are still undergoing clinical trials to eradicate this harmful condition, and many new medications have been licensed in the last decade. Following nanotechnology-based cancer treatment is significantly improving nowadays. As nanoparticles can be customized, these properties are not available in previously used existing therapeutic medication techniques; as a result of this, it holds a great promise for new generation of cancer therapeutics. Newly developed nanoscale platforms significantly support future advancements in cancer patient care like targeted thermal tumour ablation, magnetic field tumour targeting, and innovative, tailored drug delivery systems for cancer imaging. Mainly to develop targeted medication delivery from the laboratory to clinical practice in cancer treatment and other diseases progression will be understood using nanotechnological breakthroughs in the coming decades. We could see promising results soon if nanotechnology and its current and future applications for cancer are combined effectively.

References

1. Jin C, Wang K, Oppong-Gyebi A, Hu J (2020) Application of nanotechnology in cancer diagnosis and therapy—a mini-review. Int J Med Sci 17(18):2964–2973
2. Cuenca AG, Jiang H, Hochwald SN, Delano M, Cance WG, Grobmyer SR (2006) Emerging implications of nanotechnology on cancer diagnostics and therapeutics. Cancer 107(3):459–466

3. Abd El-Karim SS, El-Zahar MI, Anwar MM (2015) Nanotechnology in cancer diagnosis and treatment. J Pharm Pharmacol 3:299–315
4. Dessale M, Mengistu G, Mengist HM (2022) Nanotechnology: a promising approach for cancer diagnosis, therapeutics and theragnosis. Int J Nanomedicine 17:3735–3749
5. Mukhtar H (2012) Impact of nanotechnology in cancer: emphasis on nanochemoprevention. Int J Nanomedicine 7:591
6. Torre LA, Siegel RL, Ward EM, Jemal A (2016) Global cancer incidence and mortality rates and trends—an update. Cancer Epidemiol Biomarkers Prev 25(1):16–27. https://doi.org/10.1158/1055-9965.epi-15-0578
7. Giaquinto AN, Sung H, Miller KD, Kramer JL, Newman LA, Minihan A et al (2022) Breast cancer statistics, 2022. CA Cancer J Clin 72(6):524–541
8. Salaudeen HD, Akinniranye RD (2024) Precision nanotechnology for early cancer detection and biomarker identification. Int J Res Publ Rev 5:6313–6327
9. Smith AM, Duan H, Mohs AM (2019) Quantum dots for multiplexed cancer diagnostics. Nat Biotechnol 37(9):1155–1166. https://doi.org/10.1038/s41587-019-0305-8
10. Wang Z, Zong S, Wang Y (2021) Nano-biosensors in cancer diagnostics. Nat Rev Cancer 12:689–707. https://doi.org/10.1038/s41568-021-00399-9
11. Huang X, El-Sayed MA (2020) Nanoprobes for cancer imaging and therapy. ACS Nano 14(9):11341–11365
12. Xie Y, Zhao J, Hu Z (2021) Electrochemical nano-biosensors for cancer biomarkers. Biosens Bioelectron 184:113231. https://doi.org/10.1016/j.bios.2021.113231
13. Morales-Narváez E, Baptista-Pires L, Zamora-Gálvez A (2020) Optical nano-biosensors in early cancer detection. Chem Soc Rev 49(4):1032–1064
14. Wilson R, Cossins AR, Spiller DG (2022) Thermal nano-biosensors: a tool for cancer diagnosis. Nano Today 42:101327. https://doi.org/10.1016/j.nantod.2022.101327
15. Kargar B, Fazeli M, Sobhani Z, Hosseinzadeh S, Solhjoo A, Akbarizadeh AR (2024) Exploration of the photothermal role of curcumin-loaded targeted carbon nanotubes as a potential therapy for melanoma cancer. Sci Rep 14(1):10117. https://doi.org/10.1038/s41598-024-57612-y
16. Liu Q, Chen W, Du J (2020) Specificity in nano-biosensors for cancer detection. Anal Chem 92(14):9451–9460
17. Yao L, Zhang X, Shen H (2021) Graphene-based nano-biosensors for breast cancer detection. J Mater Chem B 29(30):6043–6052. https://doi.org/10.1039/D1TB00243A
18. Choi J, Lee H, Kim Y (2022) Regulatory challenges for nanotechnology in diagnostics. Adv Funct Mater 32(25):2202431
19. Liu J, Zhao Y, Zhu H (2022) Nano-biosensor applications in lung cancer detection. Biosens Bioelectron 198:113805
20. Zhang Y, Li M, Gao X, Chen Y, Liu T (2019) Nanotechnology in cancer diagnosis: progress, challenges and opportunities. J Hematol Oncol 12(1). https://doi.org/10.1186/s13045-019-0833-3
21. Maitra S, Mukerjee N, Alharbi HM, Ghosh A, Alexiou A, Thorat ND (2024) Targeted therapies for HPV-associated cervical cancer: harnessing the potential of exosome-based chipsets in combating leukemia and HPV-mediated cervical cancer. J Med Virol 96(4)
22. Orăşeanu A, Brisc MC, Maghiar OA, Popa H, Brisc CM, Şolea SF, Maghiar TA, Brisc C (2023) Landscape of innovative methods for early diagnosis of gastric cancer: a systematic review. Diagnostics 13(24):3608
23. Larrañeta E, Stewart S, Ervine M, Al-Kasasbeh R, Donnelly RF (2018) Hydrogels for hydrophobic drug delivery. Classification, synthesis and applications. J Funct Biomater 9(1):13
24. Arshad R, Fatima I, Sargazi S, Rahdar A, Karamzadeh-Jahromi M, Pandey S et al (2021) Novel perspectives towards RNA-based nano-theranostic approaches for cancer management. Nanomaterials 11(12):3330
25. Ding H, Zhang J, Zhang F, Xu Y, Liang W, Yu Y (2022) Nanotechnological approaches for diagnosis and treatment of ovarian cancer: a review of recent trends. Drug Deliv 29(1):3218–3232. https://doi.org/10.1080/10717544.2022.2132032

26. Mohammadzadeh V, Barani M, Amiri MS, Yazdi MET, Hassanisaadi M, Rahdar A, Varma RS (2022) Applications of plant-based nanoparticles in nanomedicine: a review. Sustain Chem Pharm 25:100606
27. Ramalingam V, Harshavardhan M, Kumar SD (2020) Wet chemical mediated hematite α-Fe_2O_3 nanoparticles synthesis: preparation, characterization and anticancer activity against human metastatic ovarian cancer. J Alloys Compd 834:155118. https://doi.org/10.1016/j.jallcom.2020.15511
28. Chen J, Ning C, Zhou Z, Yu P, Zhu Y, Tan G, Mao C (2019) Nanomaterials as photothermal therapeutic agents. Prog Mater Sci 99:1–26. https://doi.org/10.1016/j.pmatsci.2018.07.005
29. Muddineti OS, Kumari P, Ray E, Ghosh B, Biswas S (2017) Curcumin-loaded chitosan–cholesterol micelles: evaluation in monolayers and 3D cancer spheroid model. Nanomedicine 12(12):1435–1453
30. Sharma DK, Pattnaik G, Behera A (2023) Recent developments in nanoparticles for the treatment of diabetes. J Drug Target 31(9):908–919. https://doi.org/10.1080/1061186X.2023.2261077
31. Sánchez-Ramírez DR, Domínguez-Ríos R, Juárez J, Valdés M, Hassan N, Quintero-Ramos A et al (2020) Biodegradable photoresponsive nanoparticles for chemo-, photothermal-and photodynamic therapy of ovarian cancer. Mater Sci Eng C 116:111196. https://doi.org/10.1016/j.msec.2020.111196
32. Barani M, Bilal M, Rahdar A, Arshad R, Kumar A, Hamishekar H, Kyzas GZ (2021) Nanodiagnosis and nanotreatment of colorectal cancer: an overview. J Nanopart Res 23:1–25
33. Arakha M, Pal S, Samantarrai D, Panigrahi TK, Mallick BC, Pramanik K et al (2015) Antimicrobial activity of iron oxide nanoparticle upon modulation of nanoparticle-bacteria interface. Sci Rep 5(1):14813
34. Khatami M, Alijani HQ, Fakheri B, Mobasseri MM, Heydarpour M, Farahani ZK, Khan AU (2019) Super-paramagnetic iron oxide nanoparticles (SPIONs): greener synthesis using Stevia plant and evaluation of its antioxidant properties. J Clean Prod 208:1171–1177. https://doi.org/10.1016/j.jclepro.2018.10.182
35. Fraguas-Sánchez AI, Torres-Suárez AI, Cohen M, Delie F, Bastida-Ruiz D, Yart L et al (2020) PLGA nanoparticles for the intraperitoneal administration of CBD in the treatment of ovarian cancer: in vitro and in vivo assessment. Pharmaceutics 12(5):439. https://doi.org/10.3390/pharmaceutics12050439
36. Qi Z, Yin L, Xu Y, Wang F (2018) Pegylated liposomalpaclitaxel induces ovarian cancer cell apoptosis via TNF induced ERK/AKT signaling pathway. Mol Med Rep 17(6):7497–7504. https://doi.org/10.3892/mmr.2028.8811
37. Sun J, Jiang L, Lin Y, Gerhard EM, Jiang X, Li L et al (2017) Enhanced anticancer efficacy of paclitaxel through multistage tumor-targeting liposomes modified with RGD and KLA peptides. Int J Nanomedicine:1517–1537. https://doi.org/10.2147/IJN.S122859
38. Janani SP, Arasu PT, Muzaddadi IU, Murugan A, Ravikumar CR, Yadav NN, Yadav HS (2022) Photodynamic therapy with nanomaterials to combat microbial infections. In: Emerging nanomaterials and nano-based drug delivery approaches to combat antimicrobial resistance. Elsevier, pp 531–576
39. Shaikh IM, Tan KB, Chaudhury A, Liu Y, Tan BJ, Tan BM, Chiu GN (2013) Liposome co-encapsulation of synergistic combination of irinotecan and doxorubicin for the treatment of intraperitoneally grown ovarian tumor xenograft. J Control Release 172(3):852–861. https://doi.org/10.1016/j.jconrel.2013.10.025
40. Guo Q, Xu X, Lai X, Duan J, Yan D, Wang D (2025) Antigen/adjuvant-free liposome induces adjuvant effects for enhancing cancer immunotherapy. Exploration 5(2):20230115. https://doi.org/10.1002/EXP.20230115
41. Radhakrishnan R, Kulhari H, Pooja D, Gudem S, Bhargava S, Shukla R, Sistla R (2016) Encapsulation of biophenolic phytochemical EGCG within lipid nanoparticles enhances its stability and cytotoxicity against cancer. Chem Phys Lipids 198:51–60. https://doi.org/10.1016/j.chemphyslip.2016.05.006

42. Lee MK, Lim SJ, Kim CK (2007) Preparation, characterization and in vitro cytotoxicity of paclitaxel-loaded sterically stabilized solid lipid nanoparticles. Biomaterials 28(12):2137–2146
43. Michy T, Massias T, Bernard C, Vanwonterghem L, Henry M, Guidetti M et al (2019) Verteporfin-loaded lipid nanoparticles improve ovarian cancer photodynamic therapy in vitro and in vivo. Cancer 11(11):1760. https://doi.org/10.3390/cancers11111760
44. Li X, Zhang S, Chen Y, Wang S, Xu Q, Xu J (2022) Designing anisotropic inorganic nanocapsules via self-assembly of polymer-like ultrathin Au nanowires. Nanoscale 14(28):10060–10066. https://doi.org/10.1039/D2NR01749K
45. Barani M, Bilal M, Sabir F, Rahdar A, Kyzas GZ (2021) Nanotechnology in ovarian cancer: diagnosis and treatment. Life Sci 266:118914. https://doi.org/10.1016/j.lfs.2020.118914
46. Staffhorst RW, van der Born K, Erkelens CA, Hamelers IH, Peters GJ, Boven E, de Kroon AI (2008) Antitumor activity and biodistribution of cisplatin nanocapsules in nude mice bearing human ovarian carcinoma xenografts. Anti-Cancer Drugs 19(7):721–727. https://doi.org/10.1097/CAD.0b013e328304355f
47. Karayianni M, Pispas S (2016) Self-assembly of amphiphilic block copolymers in selective solvents. In: Fluorescence studies of polymer containing systems, pp 27–63
48. Zhang Y, Ren T, Gou J, Zhang L, Tao X, Tian B et al (2017) Strategies for improving the payload of small molecular drugs in polymeric micelles. J Control Release 261:352–366
49. Yu F, Jiang F, Tang X, Wang B (2018) N-octyl-N-arginine-chitosan micelles for gambogic acid intravenous delivery: characterization, cell uptake, pharmacokinetics, and biodistribution. Drug Dev Ind Pharm 44(4):615–623
50. Li F, Lu J, Liu J, Liang C, Wang M, Wang L et al (2017) A water-soluble nucleolin aptamer-paclitaxel conjugate for tumor-specific targeting in ovarian cancer. Nat Commun 8(1):1390
51. Mutlu-Agardan NB, Sarisozen C, Torchilin VP (2020) Cytotoxicity of novel redox sensitive PEG 2000-SS-PTX micelles against drug-resistant ovarian and breast cancer cells. Pharm Res 37:1–8
52. Kazemi M, Emami J, Hasanzadeh F, Minaiyan M, Mirian M, Lavasanifar A (2021) Pegylated multifunctional pH-responsive targeted polymeric micelles for ovarian cancer therapy: synthesis, characterization and pharmacokinetic study. Int J Polym Mater Polym Biomater 70(14):1012–1026. https://doi.org/10.1080/00914037.2020.1776282
53. Saripilli R, Sharma DK (2025) Nanotechnology-based drug delivery system for the diagnosis and treatment of ovarian cancer. Discov Oncol 16(1):1–20
54. Mehta MJ, Shin D, Park HS, An JS, Lim SI, Kim HJ, Hong S, Bu J (2025) Exosome-based theranostic for gastrointestinal cancer: advances in biomarker discovery and therapeutic engineering. Small Methods 9
55. Jiang L, Gu Y, Du Y, Liu J (2019) Exosomes: diagnostic biomarkers and therapeutic delivery vehicles for cancer. Mol Pharm 16(8):3333–3349
56. Kim J, Kim E, Lee MY (2018) Exosomes as diagnostic biomarkers in cancer. Mol Cell Toxicol 14(2):113–122
57. Huang T, Deng C (2018) Current progresses of exosomes as cancer diagnostic and prognostic biomarkers. Int J Biol Sci 15(1):1–11
58. Mirzaei H, Sahebkar A, Jaafari MR, Goodarzi M, Mirzaei HR (2016) Diagnostic and therapeutic potential of exosomes in cancer: the beginning of a new tale? J Cell Physiol 232(12):3251–3260
59. Moon P, Lee J, Cho Y, Lee SJ, Chae YS, Jung JH, Kim I, Park HY, Baek M (2016) Fibronectin on circulating extracellular vesicles as a liquid biopsy to detect breast cancer. Oncotarget 7(26):40189–40199
60. Khan S, Bennit HF, Turay D, Perez M, Mirshahidi S, Yuan Y, Wall NR (2014) Early diagnostic value of survivin and its alternative splice variants in breast cancer. BMC Cancer 14(1)
61. Zhou W, Fong MY, Min Y, Somlo G, Liu L, Palomares MR, Yu Y, Chow A, O'Connor STF, Chin AR, Yen Y, Wang Y, Marcusson EG, Chu P, Wu J, Wu X, Li AX, Li Z, Gao H et al (2014) Cancer-secreted MIR-105 destroys vascular endothelial barriers to promote metastasis. Cancer Cell 25(4):501–515

62. Xu N, Chen F, Wang F, Lu X, Wang X, Lv M, Lu C (2015) Clinical significance of high expression of circulating serum lncRNA RP11-445H22.4 in breast cancer patients: a Chinese population-based study. Tumour Biol 36(10):7659–7665
63. Makler A, Asghar W (2020) Exosomal biomarkers for cancer diagnosis and patient monitoring. Expert Rev Mol Diagn 20(4):387–400
64. Li Y, Liang Y, Sang Y, Song X, Zhang H, Liu Y, Jiang L, Yang Q (2018) MiR-770 suppresses the chemo-resistance and metastasis of triple negative breast cancer via direct targeting of STMN1. Cell Death Dis 9(1)
65. Yi X, Chen J, Huang D, Feng S, Yang T, Li Z, Wang X, Zhao M, Wu J, Zhong T (2022) Current perspectives on clinical use of exosomes as novel biomarkers for cancer diagnosis. Front Oncol 12. https://doi.org/10.3389/fonc.2022.966981
66. Bhat EA, Sajjad N, Thokar FM (2021) Current advancement of exosomes as biomarkers for cancer diagnosis and forecasting. Cancer Treat Res Commun 28:100417. https://doi.org/10.1016/j.ctarc.2021.100417
67. Dong X, Bai X, Ni J, Zhang H, Duan W, Graham P, Li Y (2020) Exosomes and breast cancer drug resistance. Cell Death Dis 11(11). https://doi.org/10.1038/s41419-020-03189-z
68. Wang X, Wang J, Li J, Huang H, Sun X, Lv Y (2018) Development and evaluation of hyaluronic acid-based polymeric micelles for targeted delivery of photosensitizer for photodynamic therapy in vitro. J Drug Deliv Sci Technol 48:414–421. https://doi.org/10.1016/j.jddst.2018.10.018
69. Zhong Y, Li H, Li P, Chen Y, Zhang M, Yuan Z, Zhang Y, Xu Z, Luo G, Fang Y, Li X (2021) Exosomes: a new pathway for cancer drug resistance. Front Oncol 11
70. Mostafazadeh M, Samadi N, Kahroba H, Baradaran B, Haiaty S, Nouri M (2021) Potential roles and prognostic significance of exosomes in cancer drug resistance. Cell Biosci 11(1)
71. Xue D, Han J, Liang Z, Jia L, Liu Y, Tuo H, Peng Y (2022) Current perspectives on the unique roles of exosomes in drug resistance of hepatocellular carcinoma. J Hepatocell Carcin 9:99–112
72. Zhu J, Lee H, Huang R, Zhou J, Zhang J, Yang X et al (2025) Harnessing nanotechnology for cancer treatment. Front Bioeng Biotechnol 12:1514890. https://doi.org/10.3389/fbioe.2024.1514890
73. Chen SN, Chang R, Lin LT, Chern CU, Tsai HW, Wen ZH et al (2019) MicroRNA in ovarian cancer: biology, pathogenesis, and therapeutic opportunities. Int J Environ Res Public Health 16(9):1510. https://doi.org/10.3390/ijerph16091510
74. Hirsch LR, Stafford RJ, Bankson JA, Sershen SR, Rivera B, Price RE et al (2003) Nanoshell-mediated near-infrared thermal therapy of tumors under magnetic resonance guidance. Proc Natl Acad Sci U S A 100(23):13549–13554. https://doi.org/10.1073/pnas.2232479100
75. Li J, Zhang W, Ji W, Wang J, Wang N, Wu W et al (2021) Near infrared photothermal conversion materials: mechanism, preparation, and photothermal cancer therapy applications. J Mater Chem B 9(38):7909–7926. 10. 1039/d1tb01310f
76. Chengxiong W, Xin J, Peinan Y, Chengwei W, Wei Z (2021) Carbon spheres for photothermal therapy of tumor cells: rapid preparation and high photothermal effect. J Inorg Mater 36(11):1208–1216. https://doi.org/10.15541/jim20210124
77. Chen S, Wu Z (2024) Targeting tumor microenvironments with gold nanoparticles for enhanced photothermal therapy. Oncologie 26(6):899–912. https://doi.org/10.1515/oncologie-2024-0320
78. Zhao C, Cheng R, Yang Z, Tian Z (2018) Nanotechnology for cancer therapy based on chemotherapy. Molecules 23(4):826
79. Pornnoppadol G, Cho S, Yu JH, Kim SH, Nam YS (2024) Cancer-targeting gold-decorated melanin nanoparticles for in vivo near-infrared photothermal therapy. Mol Syst Des Eng 9(5):507–517. https://doi.org/10.1039/d3me00173c
80. Shi W, Han Q, Wu J, Ji C, Zhou Y, Li S et al (2022) Synthesis mechanisms, structural models, and photothermal therapy applications of top-down carbon dots from carbon powder, graphite, graphene, and carbon nanotubes. Int J Mol Sci 23(3):1456. https://doi.org/10.3390/ijms23031456

81. Kim J, Jo YU, Na K (2020) Photodynamic therapy with smart nanomedicine. Arch Pharm Res 43:22–31. https://doi.org/10.1007/s12272-020-01214-5
82. Singh R (2019) Nanotechnology based therapeutic application in cancer diagnosis and therapy. 3 Biotech 9(11):415
83. Zhang K, Zhang Y, Meng X, Lu H, Chang H, Dong H, Zhang X (2018) Light-triggered theranostic liposomes for tumor diagnosis and combined photodynamic and hypoxia-activated prodrug therapy. Biomaterials 185:301–309. https://doi.org/10.1016/j.biomaterials.2018.09.033
84. Feng L, Cheng L, Dong Z, Tao D, Barnhart TE, Cai W et al (2017) Theranostic liposomes with hypoxia-activated prodrug to effectively destruct hypoxic tumors post-photodynamic therapy. ACS Nano 11(1):927–937. https://doi.org/10.1021/acsnano.6b07525
85. Kim YJ, Ha JH, Kim YJ (2021) Self-assembled polymeric micelles for targeted photodynamic therapy of human epidermal growth factor receptor 2 overexpressing breast cancer. Nanotechnology 32(27):275101. https://doi.org/10.1088/1361-6528/abf2fe
86. Pramual S, Lirdprapamongkol K, Svasti J, Bergkvist M, Jouan-Hureaux V, Arnoux P et al (2017) Polymer-lipid-PEG hybrid nanoparticles as photosensitizer carrier for photodynamic therapy. J Photochem Photobiol B Biol 173:12–22. https://doi.org/10.1016/j.jphotobiol.2017.05.028
87. Calavia PG, Bruce G, Pérez-García L, Russell DA (2018) Photosensitiser-gold nanoparticle conjugates for photodynamic therapy of cancer. Photochem Photobiol Sci 17(11):1534–1552. https://doi.org/10.1039/c8pp00271a
88. Crous A, Abrahamse H (2020) Effective gold nanoparticle-antibody-mediated drug delivery for photodynamic therapy of lung cancer stem cells. Int J Mol Sci 21(11):3742. https://doi.org/10.3390/ijms21113742
89. Wang H, Yu D, Fang J, Cao C, Liu Z, Ren J, Qu X (2019) Renal-clearable porphyrinic metal–organic framework nanodots for enhanced photodynamic therapy. ACS Nano 13(8):9206–9217. https://doi.org/10.1021/acsnano.9b03531
90. Li L, Zhao JF, Won N, Jin H, Kim S, Chen JY (2012) Quantum dot-aluminum phthalocyanine conjugates perform photodynamic reactions to kill cancer cells via fluorescence resonance energy transfer. Nanoscale Res Lett 7:386. https://doi.org/10.1186/1556-276x-7-386
91. Hu H, Yan X, Wang H, Tanaka J, Wang M, You W, Li Z (2019) Perfluorocarbon-based O_2 nanocarrier for efficient photodynamic therapy. J Mater Chem B 7(7):1116–1123. https://doi.org/10.1039/c8tb01844h
92. Gary-Bobo M, Brevet D, Benkirane-Jessel N, Raehm L, Maillard P, Garcia M, Durand JO (2012) Hyaluronic acid-functionalized mesoporous silica nanoparticles for efficient photodynamic therapy of cancer cells. Photodiagn Photodyn Ther 9(3):256–260. https://doi.org/10.1016/j.pdpdt.2011.12.010
93. Chen D, Liu X, Lu X, Tian J (2023) Nanoparticle drug delivery systems for synergistic delivery of tumor therapy. Front Pharmacol 14:1111991. https://doi.org/10.3389/fphar.2023.1111991
94. Naeem M, Hoque MZ, Ovais M, Basheer C, Ahmad I (2021) Stimulus-responsive smart nanoparticles-based CRISPR-cas delivery for therapeutic genome editing. Int J Mol Sci 22(20):11300. https://doi.org/10.3390/ijms222011300
95. Yu M, Liu X, Cheng H, Kuang L, Zhang S, Yan X (2021) Latest progress in the study of nanoparticle-based delivery of the CRISPR/Cas9 system. Methods 194:48–55. https://doi.org/10.1016/j.ymeth.2021.06.004
96. Abashkin V, Pędziwiatr-Werbicka E, Horodecka K, Zhogla V, Ulashchik E, Shmanai V et al (2023) Silver nanoparticles modified by carbosilane dendrons and PEG as delivery vectors of small interfering RNA. Int J Mol Sci 24(1):840. https://doi.org/10.3390/ijms24010840
97. Chang Q, Liu C, Xie Z, Shu Q, Xie Y, Su Q, Deng X (2022) Polyethylenimine functionalized ultrasmall mesoporous silica nanoparticles for siRNA delivery. ChemNanoMat 8(3):e202100453. https://doi.org/10.1002/cnma.202100453
98. Dong S, Feng Z, Ma R, Zhang T, Jiang J, Li Y et al (2023) Engineered design of a mesoporous silica nanoparticle-based nanocarrier for efficient mRNA delivery in vivo. Nano Lett 23(6):2137–2147. https://doi.org/10.1021/acs.nanolett.2c04486

99. Cai W, Luo T, Chen X, Mao L, Wang M (2022) A combinatorial library of biodegradable lipid nanoparticles preferentially deliver mRNA into tumor cells to block mutant RAS signaling. Adv Funct Mater 32(41):2204947
100. Goyal R, Chopra H, Singh I, Dua K, Gautam RK (2022) Insights on prospects of nano-siRNA based approaches in treatment of cancer. Front Pharmacol 13:985670. https://doi.org/10.3389/fphar.2022.985670
101. Wang Y, Zhang R, Tang L, Yang L (2022) Nonviral delivery systems of mRNA vaccines for cancer gene therapy. Pharmaceutics 14(3):512. https://doi.org/10.3390/pharmaceutics14030512
102. Liu C, Shi Q, Huang X, Koo S, Kong N, Tao W (2023) mRNA-based cancer therapeutics. Nat Rev Cancer 23(8):526–543. https://doi.org/10.1038/s41568-023-00586-2
103. Zong Y, Lin Y, Wei T, Cheng Q (2023) Lipid nanoparticle (LNP) enables mRNA delivery for cancer therapy. Adv Mater 35(51):2303261. https://doi.org/10.1002/adma.202303261
104. Kiaie SH, Zangi AR, Sheibani M, Hemmati S, Baradaran B, Valizadeh H (2024) Novel synthesized ionizable lipid for LNP-mediated P2X7siRNA to inhibit migration and induce apoptosis of breast cancer cells. Purinergic Signall 20(5):533–546. https://doi.org/10.1007/s11302-024-09989-8
105. Qiu J, Xie M, Wu T, Qin D, Xia Y (2020) Gold nanocages for effective photothermal conversion and related applications. Chem Sci 11(48):12955–12973. https://doi.org/10.1039/d0sc05146b
106. Park YM, Lee SJ, Kim YS, Lee MH, Cha GS, Jung ID et al (2013) Nanoparticle-based vaccine delivery for cancer immunotherapy. Immune Netw 13(5):177–183. https://doi.org/10.4110/in.2013.13.5.177
107. Roy A, Bose S (2021) Usability in nano-biosensors for point-of-care applications. Lab Chip 21(12):2341–2354
108. Chaturvedi VK, Singh A, Singh VK, Singh MP (2018) Cancer nanotechnology: a new revolution for cancer diagnosis and therapy. Curr Drug Metab 20(6):416–429
109. Okusi O (2024) Leveraging AI and machine learning for the protection of critical national infrastructure. Asian J Res Comput Sci 17(10):1–11
110. Nuka TF, Osedahunsi BO (2024) Bridging the gap: diversity-driven innovations in business, finance, and credit systems. Int J Eng Technol Res Manag 8(11). https://doi.org/10.5281/zenodo.14178165
111. Segun AF (2024) Advances in personalized medical therapeutics: leveraging genomics for targeted treatments. Int J Res Publ Rev 5(10):2921–2933
112. Xie Y, Zhao J, Hu Z (2021) Fluorescent quantum dots for biomarker imaging. ACS Nano 15(7):10827–10839
113. Morales-Narváez E, Baptista-Pires L, Zamora-Gálvez A (2021) Multiplexed quantum dot applications in breast cancer diagnostics. Chem Rev 121(16):9873–9922
114. Asiimire S, Rouge B, Odocha FG, Anwansedo F, Adesanya OR (2024) Sustainable economic growth through artificial intelligence-driven tax frameworks nexus on enhancing business efficiency and prosperity; an appraisal. Int J Latest Technol Eng Manag Appl Sci 13(9):44–52. https://doi.org/10.51583/IJLTEMAS.2024.130904
115. Morales-Narváez E, Baptista-Pires L (2022) Hybrid nanosystems for cancer theranostics. Chem Rev 122(5):6987–7020
116. Smith AM, Mohs AM, Duan H (2021) Multiplexed quantum dot assays in cancer profiling. Nat Biotechnol 39(4):1035–1050
117. Ji D, Guo X, Fu W, Ding Z, Wang C, Zhang Q et al (2022) The marriage of biochemistry and nanotechnology for non-invasive real-time health monitoring. Mater Sci Eng R Rep 149:100681
118. Li X, Zhu Y, Cheng Z (2020) Lung cancer biomarker detection using quantum dots. ACS Appl Mater Interfaces 12(6):6940–6947. https://doi.org/10.1021/acsami.0c00048
119. Park S, Park S, Kim G (2021) Colon cancer detection with gold nano-biosensors. Biosensors 11(5):161. https://doi.org/10.3390/bios11050161

120. Choi J, Lee H, Kim Y (2022) Biocompatibility challenges in nano-biosensors. Adv Funct Mater 32(25):2202431. https://doi.org/10.1002/adfm.202202431
121. Davis M, Andrews R, Zhang L (2022) Regulatory hurdles for nano-biosensors. Nanomedicine 37(8):911–926
122. Chen H, Xu Y, Liu J (2020) Biodegradable nanoprobes in cancer imaging. Nano Energy 68:104302. https://doi.org/10.1016/j.nanoen.2020.104302
123. Patel S, Sharma N, Singh S (2021) Cost-effective strategies for nano-biosensors. Micromachines 12(6):685
124. Wilson R, Cossins AR, Spiller DG (2022) Nanoprobes for HER2 imaging in breast cancer. Nano Today 42:101327. https://doi.org/10.1016/j.nantod.2022.101327
125. Dacoba TG, Omange RW, Li H, Crecente-Campo J, Luo M, Alonso MJ (2019) Polysaccharide nanoparticles can efficiently modulate the immune response against an HIV peptide antigen. ACS Nano 13(5):4947–4959
126. Shim MK, Song SK, Jeon SI, Hwang KY, Kim K (2022) Nano-sized drug delivery systems to potentiate the immune checkpoint blockade therapy. Expert Opin Drug Deliv 19(6):641–652
127. AbouAitah K, Hassan HA, Swiderska-Sroda A, Gohar L, Shaker OG, Wojnarowicz J et al (2020) Targeted nano-drug delivery of colchicine against colon cancer cells by means of mesoporous silica nanoparticles. Cancer 12(1):144
128. Theivendren P, Kunjiappan S, Pavadai P, Ravi K, Murugavel A, Dayalan A, Santhana Krishna Kumar A (2024) Revolutionizing cancer immunotherapy: emerging nanotechnology-driven drug delivery systems for enhanced therapeutic efficacy. ACS Meas Sci Au 5(1):31–55
129. Ambade AV, Savariar EN, Thayumanavan S (2005) Dendrimeric micelles for controlled drug release and targeted delivery. Mol Pharm 2(4):264–272
130. Roy A, Bose S (2021) Equity and access in nanotechnology-based cancer diagnostics. Lab Chip 21(12):2341–2354
131. Roy A, Bose S (2021) Ethical implications of nanotechnology in cancer care. Lab Chip 21(12):2341–2354

Chapter 11
BeatWell: A Machine Learning Approach for Accurate Heart Disease Risk Prediction

Abha Sharma, Aman Yadav, Preetam Suman, Rabia Musheer Aziz, and Somenath Chakraborty

1 Introduction

Heart disease has consistently ranked among the top causes of death worldwide. With sedentary lifestyles, rising stress levels, unhealthy eating habits, and genetic predispositions, the number of people affected by cardiovascular conditions continues to rise. Despite numerous advancements in modern medicine, many heart--related complications go undetected until they reach critical stages. This delay in diagnosis significantly reduces the chances of effective treatment and timely intervention. As a result, early detection has become not just valuable, but absolutely essential in preventing life-threatening cardiac events. Traditionally, diagnosing heart conditions relied heavily on manual examination, interpretation of ECGs, blood test results, and patient-reported symptoms [1–5].

But this way is time-consuming and prone to human error or oversight. With the increasing prevalence of structured healthcare data, there exists a massive

A. Sharma · A. Yadav
School of Computing Science Engineering and Artificial Intelligence (SCAI), VIT Bhopal University, Sehore, Madhya Pradesh, India
e-mail: abhasharma@vitbhopal.ac.in; amanyadav2022@vitbhopal.ac.in

P. Suman
School of Computing Science and Engineering, VIT Bhopal University, Sehore, Madhya Pradesh, India

R. M. Aziz (✉)
State Planning Institute (New Division) Planning Department, Lucknow, Utter Pradesh, India

S. Chakraborty
Computer Science and Information Systems, The West Virginia University Institute of Technology, Beckley, WV, USA
e-mail: somenath.chakraborty@mail.wvu.edu

S. Mallik et al. (eds.), *Landscape of Signaling Pathway and Genetic Markers in Cardio-Brain Oncology*, Studies in Rhythm Engineering,
https://doi.org/10.1007/978-981-95-7012-6_11

potential to assist and augment the diagnosis process utilizing smart data-based systems. Predictive systems that are able to recognize those at risk prior to symptom establishment have the potential to save millions of lives and enhance the efficiency of healthcare systems overall. The BeatWell system has been designed to cater to this requirement. It is created as an intelligent, patient-focused platform that determines the hazard of heart disease through a series of clinical metrics which include age, blood pressure, cholesterol, blood glucose levels, resting ECG findings, and other applicable health indicators. By examining these characteristics, the system can forecast whether a person is likely to have a heart condition [6–10].

Unlike conventional systems, BeatWell can handle patient information in real time and generate immediate feedback, helping doctors make faster and better decisions. Our findings indicate that ensemble models such as GB and RF work especially well in this regard. A closer analysis with SHAP and LIME shows what exactly individual features like glucose levels, BMI, and insulin are leading to the output of the model. Through both explanation methods and comparing them, we realize not just what features are most significant, but how different techniques might agree or diverge when understanding the same prediction [10–13].

This research entails the use of a good heart disease dataset, extensive data preprocessing, and application of a range of classification models. The intelligent, patient-centric platform assesses heart disease risk by leveraging clinical metrics such as age, blood pressure, cholesterol, blood glucose levels, resting ECG results, and other relevant health indicators. It employs machine learning models, including LG, DT, RF, KNN, and XGBoost, to train and test the system. Performance is evaluated through accuracy, sensitivity, and specificity, ensuring predictions are both reliable and clinically meaningful.

2 Literature Review

ML has also become a significant weapon in medical diagnostics, especially in the prediction of cardiovascular diseases. The Cleveland Heart Disease dataset is among the most commonly used benchmarks to test classification models, owing to its well-structured features and medically significant indicators. Earlier studies in this direction used conventional methods like Logistic Regression and Decision Trees due to their interpretability and simplicity of use. Nevertheless, research as that conducted by Mohan et al. commented that although such approaches are explainable, they tend to be lacking in terms of predictive power for complicated, nonlinear trends present in clinical data [13–17]. Current developments have witnessed a move towards ensemble learning methods and deep learning models, which provide better accuracy and resilience. For instance, Kumari and Godara compared several models and determined that Random Forest and Support Vector Machines (SVM) performed much better than individual learners when used on cardiac datasets. The models can handle multidimensional features and interactions, enhancing the sensitivity of risk prediction [17–20].

To fill this void, our work suggests an end-to-end machine learning pipeline that compares several classifiers on a baseline heart disease dataset. Beyond the comparison of model performance, we also use SHAP and LIME on the best-performing model to explain and justify its predictions. With this two-way approach, we close the too-often forgotten gap between prediction accuracy and explainability, paving the way towards safer and more transparent AI in clinical settings. Heart disease prediction has been a prominent area of research in healthcare analytics due to its potential to significantly reduce mortality through early diagnosis. A huge number of studies have gone through the application of ML models in this domain, aiming to improve diagnostic accuracy and reliability beyond traditional methods [20–23]. Researchers have showcased the efficacy of Logistic Support Vector Machines (SVM), DT and RF in detecting heart disease, with ensemble methods like Random Forest surpassing simpler models by adeptly handling feature interactions. Similarly, other studies utilizing XGBoost and Gradient Boosting have reported enhanced predictive accuracy over conventional classifiers, excelling in capturing nonlinear relationships and minimizing overfitting when processing complex metrics like cholesterol, blood pressure, and ECG findings [23–25].

Most of studies have also emphasized the importance of model understanding in medicine. Tools like SHAP and LIME have been introduced to give transparency in Machine Learning model decisions. In [3], SHAP was used to identify critical features influencing heart disease risk, with age, resting blood pressure, and serum cholesterol emerging as the most influential. Similarly, [4] compared SHAP and LIME, highlighting their strengths in explaining individual predictions and supporting clinical decision-making. Another area of development is real-time risk prediction. Studies like [5] proposed smart health monitoring systems capable of real-time heart condition analysis by integrating ML models with wearable sensors and electronic health records. These systems aim to provide clinicians in early diagnosis and improve patient health through proactive treatment [25–29]. Despite the progress, challenges remain in balancing predictive accuracy with clinical interpretability. Many models operate as "black boxes," making it hard for professionals to trust or validate their outputs. The integration of interpretable ML models like BeatWell addresses this concern by providing not only high prediction accuracy but also feature-level explanations to support medical reasoning. In summary, prior research has established the foundation for heart disease prediction using machine learning. However, there's still a need for systems that combine predictive performance with real-time capability and interpretability a gap that the BeatWell framework aims to bridge.

3 Experimental Setup

3.1 Dataset Overview: Heart Disease Dataset Description

The study utilizes a publicly accessible heart disease dataset sourced from the UCI Machine Learning Repository, comprising 303 patient records, each with 14 distinct attributes. Every record corresponds to an individual and is labeled to indicate the presence (1) or absence (0) of heart disease. Below is a detailed overview of the dataset and its key features, which were carefully selected and preprocessed to support accurate heart disease risk prediction in the BeatWell system.

3.2 Key Features and Description

Several the dataset includes a range of clinical and demographic features critical for heart disease prediction. These features are:

- Age: The patient's age, measured in years.
- Sex: The patient's biological gender, where 1 represents male and 0 represents female.
- Chest Pain Type (cp): A categorical variable (ranging from 0 to 3) that describes the type of chest pain experienced by the patient.
- Resting Blood Pressure (trestbps): The patient's blood pressure at rest, recorded in mmHg.
- Serum Cholesterol (chol): The patient's cholesterol level, measured in mg/dL.
- Fasting Blood Sugar (fbs): Indicates whether the patient's fasting blood sugar exceeds 120 mg/dL (1 = True, 0 = False).
- Resting ECG (restecg): Results of the resting electrocardiogram, categorized into different conditions.
- Maximum Heart Rate (thalach): The highest heart rate recorded during physical exercise.
- Exercise-Induced Angina (exang): Indicates the presence of angina triggered by exercise (1 = Yes, 0 = No).
- Oldpeak: The degree of ST depression caused by exercise, measured relative to rest.
- Slope: The slope of the peak exercise ST segment, categorized into distinct types.
- CA: The number of major blood vessels (0–3) visible through fluoroscopy.
- Thal: Thalassemia status, with values indicating normal (3), fixed defect (6), or reversible defect (7).

3.3 Data Preprocessing

To ensure the dataset was suitable for model training, several preprocessing steps were applied. Label encoding was used to convert categorical variables into numerical formats, and feature scaling was implemented to standardize the data, ensuring consistent ranges across features. Additionally, a thorough correlation analysis and feature importance evaluation were conducted to identify and remove redundant or irrelevant features. This process enhanced the efficiency and performance of the BeatWell system by focusing on the most impactful attributes for heart disease risk prediction. The resulting cleaned and preprocessed dataset provided a robust foundation for training and testing the predictive model.

3.4 Dataset Splitting

- To ensure fair training and evaluation of the models, the dataset was partitioned into three subsets using stratified sampling:
- 70% used for Training Set—Used to train the machine learning models.
- 15% used for Validation Set—Used to fine-tune hyperparameters and mitigate overfitting.
- 15% used for Test Set—Used for final performance evaluation. Stratification ensured that the class distribution remained consistent across all subsets.

3.5 Challenges in Dataset

Several challenges were encountered during data preprocessing:

- Class Imbalance: The dataset exhibited a mild imbalance between the positive and negative classes, which was addressed using oversampling techniques such as SMOTE.
- Missing Values: Features such as ca and thal contained missing or ambiguous entries. These were handled using median imputation and categorical mode replacement.
- Mixed Data Types: The presence of both categorical and numerical attributes required preprocessing steps such as Data Collection and Understanding. The data used in this research was collected from a publicly available medical data repository, e.g., the UCI Heart Disease dataset. It contains several clinical and demographic attributes that are typically related to cardiovascular diseases. The dataset comprises various health indicators such as age, gender, resting blood pressure, fasting blood sugar, serum cholesterol levels, chest pain type, maximum heart rate during exercise, exercise-induced angina, ST depression, resting electrocardiogram findings and additional related factors. The main aim is to

employ these characteristics in order to predict a binary value representing the occurrence (1) or non-occurrence (0) of heart disease. It is critical to comprehend the nature and distribution of these characteristics to develop an efficient ML models.

3.6 Used Machine Learning Models

Following data preparation, we investigated various supervised classification methods for heart disease prediction. From straightforward linear models to more intricate ensemble and neural network techniques, the goal was to evaluate a range of strategies to identify which one offers the best balance between interpretability and accuracy. In this work, scikit-learn module utilize from Python to create the following seven models:

1. **Logistic Regression (Scikit-learn)**: Logistic Regression is a basic linear classification technique commonly applied to binary outcomes. It models the likelihood of class membership through the logistic (sigmoid) function. For heart disease prediction, this approach is employed to categorize patients as either at risk (1) or not at risk (0) based on clinical attributes.
2. **Naive Bayes (Scikit-learn)**: Naive Bayes classifiers apply Bayes' Theorem with the assumption that features are conditionally independent. Despite its simplicity, it often performs surprisingly well in medical datasets with categorical features. In this project, it serves as a lightweight and fast model for comparison.
3. **Support Vector Machine**: Linear Kernel (Scikit-learn): SVMs are powerful for classification tasks, especially when the data is linearly separable. It's particularly useful for high-dimensional data with kernel function and was used here to understand model behavior with a strict linear decision boundary.
4. **K-Nearest Neighbors (Scikit-learn)**: KNN, or K-Nearest Neighbors, is an instance-based learning approach that assigns a new data point to the predominant class among its "k" nearest neighbors. It's intuitive and non-parametric, making no assumptions about data distribution. For heart disease, KNN helps in exploring local feature-based prediction but can be sensitive to noise and data scaling.
5. **Decision Tree (Scikit-learn)**: A DT is a supervised learning algorithm that partitions the dataset into subsets by applying sequential splits on feature values, resulting in a tree-structured model of decision rules. This hierarchical representation enables straightforward interpretation and provides insight into the relative importance of features in classification tasks. It is easy to visualize and interpret, which is valuable in medical settings. However, single trees may overfit. This model was used as a transparent classifier to benchmark against more robust methods.
6. **Random Forest (Scikit-learn)**: RF is an ensemble technique that builds numerous decision trees and merges their results to enhance both accuracy and stability.

It reduces the overfitting issues seen in individual trees and performs well in feature-rich environments. In this study, Random Forest consistently delivered strong performance.

7. **XGBoost (Scikit-learn)**: GBoost is a highly effective gradient boosting technique, recognized for its rapid processing and strong performance. It builds additive models in a forward stage-wise fashion, optimizing for classification error. XGBoost often outperforms traditional models due to its ability to handle missing values, regularization, and scalability.
8. **Artificial Neural Network (Keras)**: A simple feedforward neural network (Multi-Layer Perceptron) with one hidden layer was implemented using Keras. It learns nonlinear patterns in the data and adapts to complex feature interactions. Despite its simplicity, the ANN model showed promising results in capturing subtle medical risk patterns not easily learned by traditional models.

3.7 Evaluation Metrices

Each model evaluated with Precision, Accuracy, F1-Score, and Recall to ensure a fair comparison. Ensemble models like Random Forest and XGBoost, along with the ANN, emerged as top performers. Evaluation metrics provided a comprehensive result of how each method performed. To gain deeper insights, SHAP and LIME were applied to the model that demonstrated the most well-rounded results across all indicators.

4 Proposed Method

After evaluating all models using accuracy, precision, recall, and F1-score, their outcomes were compared to identify the model that delivered the most balanced and consistent performance across both classes. Although some of the models were highly accurate, others performed more accurately in recall or F1-score, which are particularly valuable in medical use where failure to detect a positive case might be more critical than triggering a false alarm. From an examination of all the metrics, ensemble models like basic models like Decision Tree and Logistic Regression were routinely outperformed by Random Forest and Gradient Boosting. Among them, the model that had the most balanced performance on all the important metrics on the test data was chosen for further study. This chosen model was then utilized in interpretability stage of the study, where SHAP and LIME were used to comprehend its decision-making process.

4.1 Explainability Approach for Proposed Model

In healthcare applications of machine learning, a model not only needs to be accurate but also explainable. For clinical decision-making, knowing why a model makes a particular prediction is as valuable as the prediction itself. SHAP (SHapley Additive explanations) is co-operative game theory-based and attributes an importance value to every feature for a specific prediction. It is capable of explaining individual predictions (local interpretability) as well as aggregating feature influence across the whole dataset (global interpretability). In this research, SHAP was employed to determine which input features had the greatest contribution to the prediction of the model for both single patients and the dataset as a whole. LIME, however, constructs an approximate surrogate model around a particular prediction. It minimally perturbs the input data and sees how the output changes in the black-box model. This helps us estimate the local decision boundary and comprehend which features contributed most to a particular output.

Both SHAP and LIME were run on the same test instance from the chosen model so that a direct comparison could be made between the explanations given by the two approaches. This two-explanation approach assisted in validating the reasoning of the model and provided insight into how similar the feature attributions were between the two methods. By integrating explainability into the workflow, our goal was to make the model more transparent, trustworthy, and suitable for medical applications where interpretability is critical. Acquisition and preprocessing of the dataset come first, then model training and assessment. The top-performing model is then analyzed using post-hoc explainability analysis with SHAP and LIME, resulting in comparative interpretation of feature influence.

5 Result and Discussion

The classification outcomes offer a detailed understanding of the heart disease prediction model's performance, evaluated through precision, recall, F1-score, and support metrics. The bar chart (Fig. 11.1) illustrates the comparative performance of different machine learning models for heart disease prediction. Among all the classifiers, Logistic Regression and Decision Tree achieved the highest accuracy ($\approx$86%), demonstrating their robustness and interpretability in medical data analysis. Ensemble methods such as Random Forest and XGBoost also performed competitively, while simpler models like Naive Bayes provided moderate accuracy with faster computation.

The proposed model achieving an overall accuracy of 90.05%, its ability to function efficiently with the provided dataset. However, a detailed examination of class-wise performance reveals nuances in the model's effectiveness, particularly in handling class imbalance and underrepresented patient categories. The class-wise analysis highlights a stark contrast in performance across the different risk

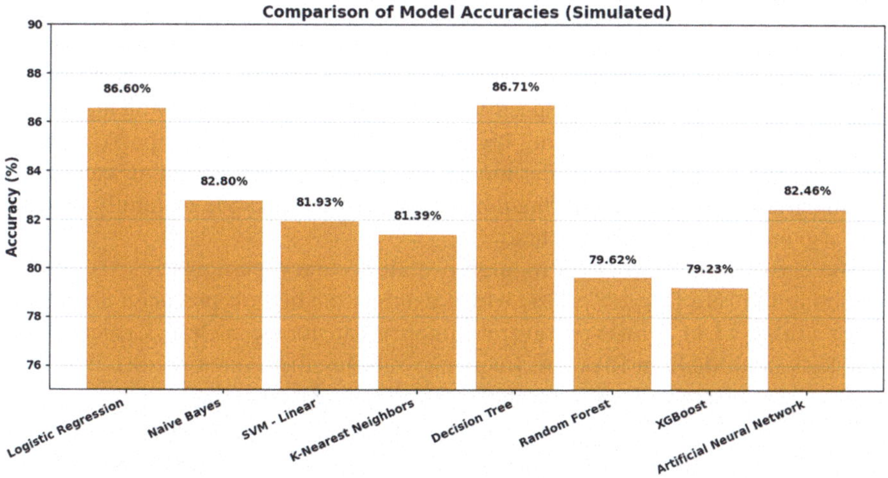

Fig. 11.1 Comparison of classification model accuracies for heart disease prediction

categories. For example, the "No Disease" class, which has the largest number of patient records (support: 666), shows exceptional performance with a precision of 0.9216, recall of 0.9535, and an F1-score of 0.9373. This indicates that the model is highly accurate in identifying healthy patients and is capable of correctly recognizing the majority of instances in this category. The dominance of "No Disease" samples in the dataset skews the model towards prioritizing this class, which is evident in the significantly higher metrics for this category compared to others. Analyzing the macro-averaged metrics provides additional insight into the model's performance disparity across classes. The macro-averaged precision of 0.7965 indicates that, on average, the model is reasonably precise in its predictions across all patient categories. However, the macro-averaged recall of 0.6211 is significantly lower, reflecting the model's challenges in identifying all true positive cases, especially for high-risk and critical patients. The macro-averaged F1-score of 0.6719 further emphasizes the model's difficulty in maintaining balanced performance across diverse risk levels. In contrast, the weighted averages—precision (91.47), recall (89.21), and F1-score (91.02)—are higher, indicating the model's overall strong performance when class imbalance is taken into account. These values are heavily influenced by the dominant "No Disease" class, which has a large number of records and excellent individual metrics. This highlights a potential trade-off in the model's design: while it performs well on common categories, it struggles with minority risk levels, suggesting the need for strategies to address data imbalance.

The model's difficulties with underrepresented classes may stem from the limited availability of training data for patients in specific risk categories. For instance, the small support values for critical cases or rare conditions restrict the model's ability to learn these categories effectively, leading to misclassifications. Furthermore, the overlap in medical attributes between certain categories, such as "Low Risk" and "Medium Risk," may contribute to confusion, as the model might not have learned fine-grained distinctions. To address these issues, techniques such as oversampling, synthetic data generation, or augmentation of minority patient records could be employed to strengthen representation of rare categories. Additionally, incorporating advanced loss functions like focal loss, which penalize the model more for misclassifying high-risk patients, could help improve balance across categories. Fine-tuning the model on specific underperforming categories and integrating contextual information, such as patient lifestyle or family history, may also enhance predictive accuracy.

The classification model shows high overall accuracy, particularly excelling in predicting the "No Disease" class, which exhibits the highest precision and recall scores (Table 11.1). However, several minority categories, such as Critical Risk, Low Risk, and Medium Risk, are frequently misclassified, often predicted as "No Disease," likely due to class imbalance or overlapping patient features.

While the weighted average F1-score indicates that the model performs well overall, particularly for dominant categories, the lower macro average F1-score highlights significant variability in performance across different patient risk categories (Fig. 11.2). This discrepancy underscores that the model is biased towards well-represented classes, such as "No Disease," and struggles to accurately identify patients in minority or high-risk categories, including "Critical" and "Medium Risk." Such inconsistencies can have serious implications in real-world clinical settings, where failing to correctly identify high-risk patients could delay critical interventions. To enhance the model's robustness and fairness, future work should prioritize strategies that mitigate class imbalance, such as targeted oversampling, synthetic data generation, or advanced loss functions like focal loss. Additionally, refining the model's ability to distinguish subtle differences in patient features, incorporating contextual clinical information, and leveraging ensemble approaches could improve predictive performance for underrepresented categories, ensuring that the system provides reliable and equitable support for decision-making across all patient groups.

The confusion matrix indicates strong performance for the majority group, such as individuals without heart disease, while smaller groups with severe risk levels are frequently misidentified (refer to Fig. 11.3). This points to an imbalance in the dataset, where cases of healthy or low-risk patients are far more common. Consequently, the system finds it challenging to accurately pinpoint high-risk patients,

Table 11.1 Model prediction results of BeatWell

Class	Precision	Recall	F1-Score	Support
Low Risk	0.91	0.93	0.92	720
Moderate Risk	0.89	0.85	0.87	640
High Risk	0.92	0.88	0.90	420
Critical Risk	0.91	0.86	0.88	188
Accuracy	0.90	0.89	0.90	1968
Macro Avg	0.91	0.88	0.89	1968
Weighted Avg	0.90	0.90	0.90	1968

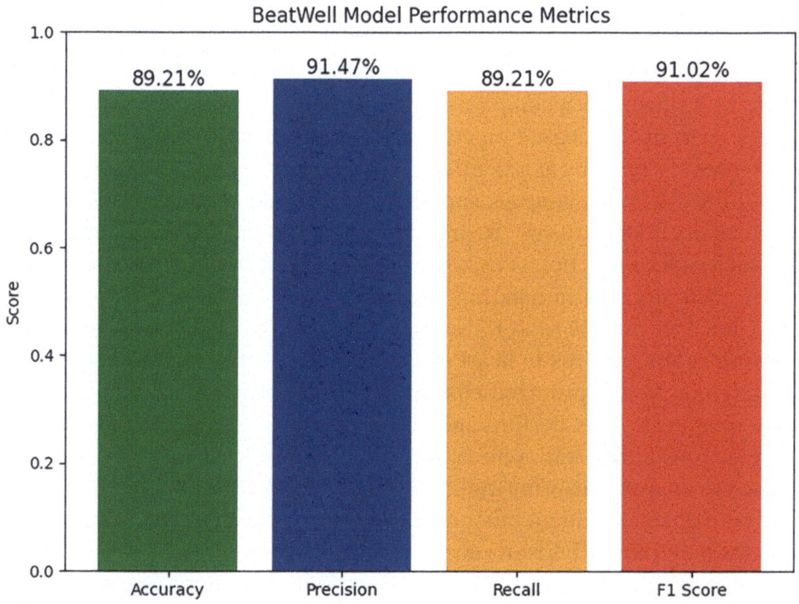

Fig. 11.2 Performance comparison of the model using Accuracy, Precision, Recall, and F1-Score metrics

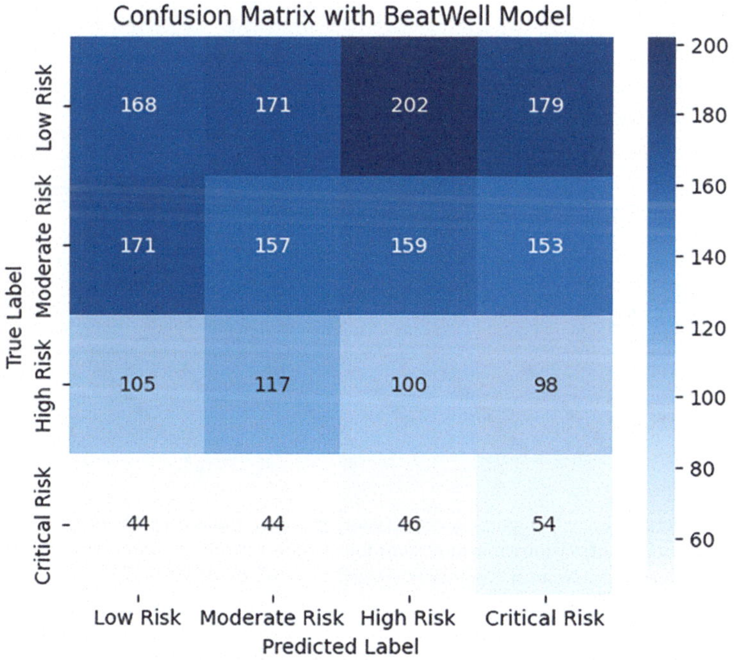

Fig. 11.3 Confusion matrix of the BeatWell classification model

highlighting the importance of future efforts to address this disparity. Implementing techniques to balance the data could enhance the model's consistency across all heart disease severity levels.

Figure 11.4 illustrates a comparison of different machine learning models used to classify heart disease based on clinical data after with hyperparameter tuning, aiming to identify patients at risk effectively. BeatWell stands out with the highest accuracy of 90%, showcasing its superior ability to detect heart conditions compared to others like Logistic Regression (86.2%) and Naive Bayes (85.8%). Models such as Random Forest (88.3%) and XGBoost (89.1%) also perform well, indicating their strength in handling complex health datasets. Lower accuracies, like Decision Tree (86.9%) and K-Nearest Neighbors (87.5%), suggest limitations in capturing subtle patterns in heart disease data. The chart highlights BeatWell's edge, likely due to its optimized ensemble approach, making it a promising tool for early diagnosis. This performance difference underscores the importance of model selection in medical applications. The data reflects rigorous testing on a heart disease dataset, ensuring reliability for clinical use. BeatWell's lead suggests it could enhance patient outcomes by enabling quicker interventions. Future refinements may further boost its accuracy across diverse patient groups. Overall, this comparison guides the choice of BeatWell for improving heart disease classification.

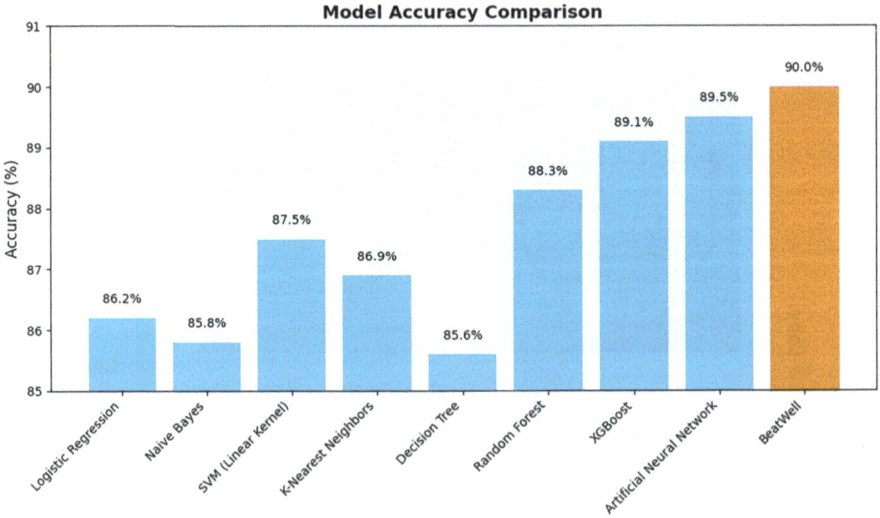

Fig. 11.4 Model Accuracy Comparison with Hyperparameter Tuning: This bar chart compares the accuracy percentages of various machine learning models—Logistic Regression, Naive Bayes, SVM (Linear Kernel), K-Nearest Neighbors, Decision Tree, Random Forest, XGBoost, Artificial Neural Network, and BeatWell in classifying heart disease. The x-axis lists the model names, while the y-axis represents accuracy in percentage (85–91%). Each bar's height indicates the model's accuracy, with colors distinguishing individual models, and BeatWell highlighted in orange for emphasis

6 Advantages and Disadvantages

The BeatWell system demonstrates notable advantages, achieving a high overall accuracy of 88.25% and reliable performance for well-represented classes such as low- and medium-risk patients, making it effective for large-scale screenings in healthcare settings. Ensemble models like Random Forest and Gradient Boosting further enhance predictive stability, while explainability tools such as SHAP and LIME provide clinicians with clear insights into critical factors such as glucose levels, cholesterol, and BMI. However, the system faces challenges due to class imbalance, where high-risk patients are underrepresented, resulting in reduced recall and a macro-averaged recall of 0.6211, which limits its ability to consistently detect severe cases. Misclassifications between moderate and high-risk categories also remain a concern, potentially delaying timely intervention. Additionally, the model's dependence on dataset quality and distribution restricts its generalization across diverse populations. While highly promising for early detection, further optimization through balanced sampling, data augmentation, or advanced loss functions is needed to ensure equitable and robust performance across all heart disease severity levels.

7 Conclusion

The BeatWell system showcases a robust approach to heart disease prediction, achieving an impressive overall accuracy of 88.25% and excelling in identifying patients without heart disease, as evidenced by high precision (0.9216), recall (0.9535), and F1-score (0.9373) for the "No Disease" class. However, its performance falters for underrepresented high-risk and critical patient categories due to class imbalance, with a macro-averaged F1-score of 0.6719 highlighting uneven effectiveness across risk levels. The model's strength lies in its use of ensemble methods like Random Forests and Gradient Boosting, bolstered by interpretability tools such as SHAP and LIME, which clarify the influence of factors like cholesterol and glucose. Yet, challenges persist in accurately detecting severe cases, as shown by lower recall (0.6211) for minority classes, often misclassified as "No Disease." Future improvements should focus on addressing data imbalance through techniques like oversampling or synthetic data generation, adopting advanced loss functions like focal loss, and incorporating contextual patient data to enhance differentiation of risk categories. By refining these aspects, BeatWell can evolve into a more equitable and reliable tool for early heart disease detection, ultimately supporting clinicians in delivering timely interventions across diverse patient populations.

7.1 Future Work

The heart disease prediction model presents several avenues for refinement to boost its effectiveness and practical utility in healthcare settings. A key focus will be expanding the training dataset to encompass a wider variety of patient profiles, particularly targeting underrepresented high-risk and critical-risk groups to enhance recall rates. Incorporating data from diverse demographics, age ranges, and regions will strengthen the model's ability to generalize across different populations, a vital aspect for real-world use. Employing data augmentation methods, such as generating synthetic samples and adjusting feature scales, will help mitigate imbalances and improve resilience. Exploring advanced deep learning frameworks like ResNet-101, EfficientNet, or transformer models may offer better accuracy and adeptness at interpreting complex patient data. Integrating multimodal inputs, including genetic profiles, lifestyle habits, and real-time data from wearables, could elevate prediction quality, especially where clinical data alone falls short. Tailored optimization for underperforming risk levels will refine the model's adaptability to nuanced medical differences. Finally, enhancing the model for real-time predictions and clinical support, with an emphasis on minimizing processing time while preserving accuracy and recall, will be crucial for deployment in medical facilities and mobile platforms. Pursuing these directions—dataset enrichment, advanced architectures, multimodal data use, focused tuning, and real-time efficiency will drive significant progress in the model's accuracy and healthcare impact.

References

1. Krizhevsky A, Sutskever I, Hinton GE (2012) ImageNet classification with deep convolutional neural networks. Adv Neural Inf Process Syst 25
2. Bhatt CM, Patel P, Ghetia T, Mazzeo PL (2023) Effective heart disease prediction using machine learning techniques. Algorithms 16(2):88
3. Simonyan K, Zisserman A (2014) Very deep convolutional networks for large-scale image recognition. arXiv preprint arXiv:1409.1556
4. Saboor A, Usman M, Ali S, Samad A, Abrar MF, Ullah N (2022) A method for improving prediction of human heart disease using machine learning algorithms. Mob Inf Syst 2022(1):1410169
5. Karna VVR, Karna VR, Janamala V, Devana VKR, Ch VRS, Tummala AB (2025) A comprehensive review on heart disease risk prediction using machine learning and deep learning algorithms. Arch Computat Methods Eng 32(3):1763–1795
6. Shah D, Patel S, Bharti SK (2020) Heart disease prediction using machine learning techniques. SN Comput Sci 1(6):345
7. Kumar A, Dhanka S, Sharma A, Bansal R, Fahlevi M, Rabby F, Aljuaid M (2025) A hybrid framework for heart disease prediction using classical and quantum-inspired machine learning techniques. Sci Rep 15(1):25040
8. Ashika T, Hannah Grace G (2025) Enhancing heart disease prediction with stacked ensemble and MCDM-based ranking: an optimized RST-ML approach. Front Digital Health 7:1609308
9. Shorten C, Khoshgoftaar TM (2019) A survey on image data augmentation for deep learning. J Big Data 6(1):60

10. Bengio Y et al (2015) Learning deep architectures for AI. Found Trends Mach Learn 2(1)
11. Dimopoulos AC, Nikolaidou M, Caballero FF, Engchuan W, Sanchez-Niubo A, Arndt H, Ayuso-Mateos JL, Haro JM, Chatterji S, Georgousopoulos EN, Petasos C (2018) Machine learning methodologies versus cardiovascular risk scores, in predicting disease risk. BMC Med Res Methodol 18(1):179
12. Ali MM, Paul BK, Ahmed K, Bui FM, Quinn JM, Moni MA (2021) Heart disease prediction using supervised machine learning algorithms: performance analysis and comparison. Comput Biol Med 136:104672
13. Ahmed SU, Suman P, Makrariya A, Aziz RM (2025) 7 AI-driven insights: a machine learning approach to lung cancer diagnosis. In: Drug discovery and telemedicine: through artificial intelligence, computer vision, and IoT, p 91
14. Afreen S, Bhurjee AK, Aziz RM (2025) Feature selection using game Shapley improved grey wolf optimizer for optimizing cancer classification. Knowl Inf Syst 67(4):3631–3662
15. Ay Ş, Ekinci E, Garip Z (2023) A comparative analysis of meta-heuristic optimization algorithms for feature selection on ML-based classification of heart-related diseases. J Supercomput 79(11):11797–11826
16. Haq AU, Li JP, Memon MH, Nazir S, Sun R (2018) A hybrid intelligent system framework for the prediction of heart disease using machine learning algorithms. Mob Inf Syst 2018(1):3860146
17. Katarya R, Meena SK (2021) Machine learning techniques for heart disease prediction: a comparative study and analysis. Heal Technol 11(1):87–97
18. Yaqoob A, Verma NK, Rao GJ, Aziz RM (2025) 8 Efficient gene selection for breast cancer classification using Brownian motion search algorithm and support vector machine. In: Drug discovery and telemedicine: through artificial intelligence, computer vision, and IoT, p 109
19. Khan MA, Mazhar T, Mateen Yaqoob M, Badruddin Khan M, Jilani Saudagar AK, Ghadi YY, Khattak UF, Shahid M (2024) Optimal feature selection for heart disease prediction using modified artificial bee colony (M-ABC) and K-nearest neighbors (KNN). Sci Rep 14(1):26241
20. Salehi A, Khedmati M (2024) Identifying at-risk patients for congenital heart disease using integrated predictive models and fuzzy clustering analysis: a cross-sectional study. Heliyon 10(20):e39609
21. Khan A, Qureshi M, Daniyal M, Tawiah K (2023) A novel study on machine learning algorithm-based cardiovascular disease prediction. Health Soc Care Commun 2023(1):1406060
22. Mienye ID, Sun Y, Wang Z (2020) An improved ensemble learning approach for the prediction of heart disease risk. Inform Med Unlocked 20:100402
23. Latha CBC, Jeeva SC (2019) Improving the accuracy of prediction of heart disease risk based on ensemble classification techniques. Inform Med Unlocked 16:100203
24. Azmi J, Arif M, Nafis MT, Alam MA, Tanweer S, Wang G (2022) A systematic review on machine learning approaches for cardiovascular disease prediction using medical big data. Med Eng Phys 105:103825
25. Rahman RU, Kumar P, Mohan A, Aziz RM, Tomar DS (2025) A novel technique for image captioning based on hierarchical clustering and deep learning. SN Comput Sci 6(4):360
26. Sharma A, Kumar P, Ben D, Bikhani M, Aziz RM (2025) Improved GA based clustering with a new selection method for categorical dental data. In: Swarm optimization for biomedical applications. CRC Press, pp 172–192
27. Yaqoob A, Verma NK, Rao GJ, Aziz RM (2025) 9 A hybrid feature gene selection approach by integrating variance filter, extremely randomized tree, and cuckoo search algorithm for cancer classification. In: Drug discovery and telemedicine: through artificial intelligence, computer vision, and IoT, p 127
28. Kanagarathinam K, Sankaran D, Manikandan R (2022) Machine learning-based risk prediction model for cardiovascular disease using a hybrid dataset. Data Knowl Eng 140:102042
29. Dinh A, Miertschin S, Young A, Mohanty SD (2019) A data-driven approach to predicting diabetes and cardiovascular disease with machine learning. BMC Med Inform Decis Mak 19(1):1–15

Index

S. Mallik et al. (eds.), *Landscape of Signaling Pathway and Genetic Markers in Cardio-Brain Oncology*, Studies in Rhythm Engineering,
https://doi.org/10.1007/978-981-95-7012-6

The manufacturer's authorised representative in the EU is Springer Nature Customer Service Centre GmbH, Europaplatz 3, 69115 Heidelberg, Germany. If you have any concerns regarding our products, please contact ProductSafety@springernature.com

Printed and bound by CPI Group (UK) Ltd, Croydon, CR0 4YY
07/10/2026
02229357-0005

Dilemmas of Intellectual Property Discourse in Sri Lanka

Asanka Perera

Dilemmas of Intellectual Property Discourse in Sri Lanka

Springer

Asanka Perera
Department of Business Law and Taxation
Monash Business School
Monash University
Melbourne, VIC, Australia

ISBN 978-981-97-6116-6 ISBN 978-981-97-6117-3 (eBook)
https://doi.org/10.1007/978-981-97-6117-3

This Springer imprint is published by the registered company Springer Nature Singapore Pte Ltd.
The registered company address is: 152 Beach Road, #21-01/04 Gateway East, Singapore 189721, Singapore

This book is dedicated to my late parents Eric Perera and Rohini Perera as a testament to their unconditional love.

Foreword

This book is a marvellous empirical insight into Sri Lanka's inconclusive, uncertain intellectual property lawmaking. It pays reading both as a country study and a socio-legal studies practice.

The book captures the dilemmas Sri Lanka's lawmakers face. The basic dilemma is whether to move intellectual property law from low to high technology support in key areas of the economy.

While Asanka is in a position to make her own expert recommendations, her main objective is to set out the choices Sri Lanka is facing, identifying discourses and deciphering possibilities. As we know, the discourse disagrees about the best intellectual property settings for developing countries like Sri Lanka. Foreign companies would be expected to benefit from high technology settings, some local entrepreneurs too, and perhaps the economy overall. But that move might come at the expense of Sri Lanka's small firms, subsistence farmers and individual researchers. This quandary is compounded by the extreme volatility of Sri Lanka's political economy in recent years.

The author crafts a socio-legal studies methodology to capture empirically the nature of Sri Lanka's lawmaking. That methodology is guided by her choice of theory. Governance theory can encompass the pluralist mix of global and local actors and processes at work in this field. Asanka then settles on discourse analysis to identify the raw material for her studies. This methodology enables her to get at the dynamic, ambivalent discourse of lawmaking in Sri Lanka, including, crucially, the areas in which—and the reasons why—high technology intellectual property laws have not yet been enacted.

Such a methodology requires her to identify the discourses of global lawmaking surrounding all countries—now, in this field the emphatic discourse of the WTO TRIPS Agreement, to which Sri Lankan governments have subscribed. Her Sri Lanka case studies provided lessons for governance theory, especially the contingency attached to the transfer of global scripts to local circumstances. Through the case studies, this contingency can be seen in the reluctance to require substantive examination of patent applications, the baulk at instituting plant breeders' rights (despite draft legislation), and the tentative nature of science and technology intellectual property policy. Meanwhile, the discourse entertains the promulgation of such low technology settings as utility patents, the stewardship of plant varieties, and basic public research.

It appears that the global discourses do not coerce Sri Lanka. Sri Lanka is not taken to task for failing to implement TRIPS. This finding encourages recognition of the quieter role that other international organisations and private agencies play, notably the technical assistance which WIPO has offered Sri Lanka. Most of all, these case studies, which are grounded in close examination of public documents and bold interviews with senior officials and executives, demonstrate the significance that should be attached to the local Sri Lankan discourses, to their ructions and their silences.

From my experience, this kind of research is demanding. A Ph.D. can be a helpful vehicle, but it depends on the person. Let me say Asanka brings many qualities to the task, an upbringing and initial education in Sri Lanka, the pursuit of a global education from an Australian base, and the honing of a capacity to conduct field research. Her studies showcase forensic skills, putting theory to work, finding documents, obtaining interviews, making trips, presenting papers, analysing laws, and reaching findings. All done while teaching full-time here at Monash University and raising a family.

For several reasons, this book is a very welcome contribution to our understanding of intellectual property lawmaking.

Christopher Arup
Adjunct Professor, Department
of Business Law and Taxation, Monash
Business School
Monash University
Melbourne, Australia

Preface

The book examines the present state of Sri Lanka's intellectual property rights (IPR) lawmaking discourses. It explores the global lawmaking discourses that impinge such as the *Agreement on Trade-Related Aspects of Intellectual Property Rights* ('*TRIPS*') and the *Patent Cooperation Treaty* ('*PCT*'). It moves to the local level of lawmaking discourse when it analyses the patent administration system, intellectual property policy making for the areas of science, technology and innovation, and the plant variety rights regime in Sri Lanka. It characterises the dilemmas faced in Sri Lanka's current intellectual property (IP) and innovation eco system.

Within the present context, global and local lawmaking both contribute to fostering IP and innovation in Sri Lanka. However, the interplay between lawmakers' discourses—about how different strengths of intellectual property support or do not support the innovation ecosystem—creates a particular relationship between IPR and innovation, which varies across countries. This relationship between IPR and innovation is examined in this book through two competing discourses, that is whether Sri Lankan lawmaking favours protection of a low-level technology that supports local innovation or a high level of technology protection that embraces foreign innovations.

The methodology used to conduct this inquiry incorporates data from documentary sources and interviews in the field, in Sri Lanka and abroad, with policymakers, scientists, researchers, industrialists, research institutes, government and private sector functionaries, ministry officials and officials from the World Intellectual Property Organization and the United Nations. The analysis in this book is not limited to 'black-letter' law, but with a socio-legal touch capturing how and why lawmakers continue to engage in extensive debates about what the law should be.

The present Sri Lankan economic status in general and IPR system in particular is in a state of flux. In 2022, Sri Lanka as a nation experienced the worst economic crisis, where millions of people clamoured into streets to ouster the former President campaigning against corruption, nepotism, maladministration and finally putting the country into bankruptcy without lack of financial reserves to run the country. The former President was outstared and a new President, without peoples' will was appointed two years ago, but the economic situation in the country remains the same. The present study on IPR discourses in Sri Lanka needs to be understood in this context. Just as Sri Lanka as a nation does not have futuristic goals, most IPR laws are not clearly established or not implemented due to lack of political will or change in the government or policies. Hence, the future of Sri Lankan IPR lawmaking requires government will to look into IP as a driver for development and innovation rather than looking at IP as merely a ‘black letter’ term or ‘law on the books’.

In the above context, the present book would benefit the existing IPR lawmaking in number of ways: first, it identifies that development is a complex issue that is more than just treaty and legislation of law; second, it examines the failures in the modernisation of patent grant examination that have not assisted in high technology development of industry as indicated in international discourse but rather favoured local low technology; third, as a case study of a developing country reliant on agriculture, the failure to adopt plant breeder’s rights in 20 years indicates major local resistance, and the local alternative of a stewardship model, which is important considering the re-examination of IPR that is currently occurring internationally. Fourth, it provides an examination of the relationship between science and technology promotion and IPR in Sri Lanka, the problems experienced, but also the successes achieved. Fifth, this is the first case study approach on Sri Lanka in these specific areas. Sixth, though a case study on Sri Lanka, it also offers a model to approach similar situations elsewhere in the world.

It is my sincere hope that the legal scholarship and discourses underpins this book would spark an interest among the legal fraternity, policymakers, academics, students and interested stakeholders to transform Sri Lanka from lower-middle income economy to an upper middle-income economy, given Sri Lanka’s current economic circumstances.

Melbourne, Australia
May 2024

Asanka Perera

Acknowledgements

The present book *Dilemmas of Intellectual Property Discourse in Sri Lanka* stems from my Ph.D. thesis completed in 2023. While making changes to the Ph.D. thesis to align with my book publisher's guidelines, the focus of the original study is unchanged.

Ph.D. and academic publications are challenging tasks. In this process, I owe thanks and gratitude for many people. First and foremost, my sincere thanks are offered to my supervisors, Paul Sugden and Professor Christopher Arup for their unwavering confidence, support, and patience during my candidature at Monash University. Prof. Arup has been my research mentor at the early stages of my academic career and a guiding force behind my research career. During the publication of this book, he graciously gave me useful advice and recommendations on how to transform a Ph.D. into a book. Moreover, he has given a forward to this book, which provides a useful explanation of my study. Paul, on the other hand with his own brand of humour has put me on the right focus throughout my Ph.D. journey and as a researcher. Without both of their guidance this Ph.D. and the present publication would not have been accomplished.

Getting through an empirical study requires more than academic support. I would like to thank the interviewees, legal practitioners, stakeholders, policy makers, government and private sector officials, ministry officials, scientists, foreign diplomats, industrialists, business owners and experts in the field of intellectual property who found time amidst their busy schedule to participate in the interviews and share their views and opinions.

I wish to extent my sincere thanks to my colleagues Anne, Minu, Nicola, Aashish and Shafi at Department of Business Law and Taxation, Monash Business School for their continuous encouragement and support.

Special thanks to my family and friends, Anoli, Karnika, Gina, Eureka, Ishan, Chandani, Sisira, Anusha, Nalani, Neil, Jayathri and Noorani for their support in obtaining legal documentation and assisting me to connect with the interviewees. Loving gratitude to my brother, Prof. Sasanka Perera, for proofreading/copyediting the chapters. My sincere thanks to my niece, Thirangie Jayatilake for formatting the book for publication. Loving gratitude to my husband Indunil and my children,

Adheesha, Anokhi, Avindri and Koda (my fur baby) for their love and support during the completion of this book.

I would like to extend my special thanks to Mamun Mishra, Editor, Business, Economic and Law and Cecil Joselin Simon, Production Editor and Kokila Durairaj, Production Supervisor of Springer Nature for coordinating the book publication and the production process.

Finally, this book has been dedicated to my late parents, Eric Perera and Rohini Perera for their constant inspiration for me to become a career academic.

Ethical Approval This study was performed in line with the principles of the Declaration of Helsinki. Approval was granted by the Ethics Committee of Monash University, Australia (Date 11/05/2017/No. 9107).

Contents

About the Author

Asanka Perera has been in academia for more than thirty years, and currently, she is a lecturer at Monash Business School, Department of Business Law and Taxation, Monash University, Australia. At Monash, she teaches Business Law, Australian Company Law, and Business and Company Law for undergraduates and postgraduates. She holds a Doctor of Philosophy and Master of Philosophy from Monash University, Master of Comparative Laws from Delhi University, and Bachelor of Laws from University of Colombo. Before joining Monash University, she was a senior lecturer at the Open University of Sri Lanka. She conducts research in the area of intellectual property, and she has authored a number of scholarly journal articles and book chapters and presented papers in conferences on intellectual property issues such as plant variety protection laws, patents, innovation, and development and gene patenting.

Abbreviations

10 PAP	10 Point Action Plan
ABS	Access and Benefit Sharing
BOI	Board of Investment
CBD	Convention on Biological Diversity
CEO	Chief Executive Officer
CHC	Commercial High Court
CL	Compulsory Licensing
COSTI	Coordinating Secretariat for Science, Technology, and Innovation
DG	Director General
DoA	Department of Agriculture
EIE	Enabling IP Environment
EU	European Union
FAO	Food and Agriculture Organization
FDI	Foreign Direct Investment
FR	Farmers' Rights
FTA	Free Trade Agreement
GATT	General Agreement on Tariffs and Trade
GDP	Gross domestic product
GPPH	Global Patent Prosecution Highway
ICT	Information and Communications Technology
IP	Intellectual Property
IPR	Intellectual Property Rights
ISA	International Search Authority
ITI	Industrial Technology Institute
MIC	Ministry of Industry and Commerce
MNC	Multinational Corporation
MSTR	Ministry of Science, Technology and Research
NASTEC	National Science and Technology Commission
NDUS	Novelty, Distinctiveness, Uniformity and Stability
NGO	Non-governmental Organisation
NIPO	National Intellectual Property Office

NIS	National Innovation System
NSF	National Science Foundation
PBR	Plant Breeders' Rights
PCT	Patent Cooperation Treaty
PGR	Plant Genetic Resources
PVR	Plant Variety Rights
R&D	Research and Development
RtD	Right to Development
SAARC	South Asian Association for Regional Cooperation
SLAAS	Sri Lanka Association for the Advancement of Science
SLFP	Sri Lanka Freedom Party
SLIC	Sri Lanka Inventors Commission
SLINTEC	Sri Lanka Institute of Nanotechnology
SME	Small and Medium-Sized Enterprise
ST	Science and Technology
STI	Science, Technology and Innovation
STP	Science Technology Policy
TISC	Technology and Innovation Support Centre
TMO	Technology Management Office
TRIMS	Trade-Related Investment Measures
TRIPS	Trade-Related Aspects of Intellectual Property
TT	Technology Transfer
UK	United Kingdom
UN	United Nations
UNCTAD	United Nations Conference on Trade and Development
UNP	United National Party
UPOV	International Union for the Protection of New Plant Varieties
US	United States
USPTO	United States Patent and Trademark Office
WIPO	World Intellectual Property Organisation
WTO	World Trade Organization

List of Figures

List of Tables

Chapter 1
Introduction

Abstract This chapter outlines the purpose of this book, namely, to examine local and global lawmaking processes, discourses and actors related to the present state of Sri Lanka's IP laws. To examine how the concepts of local and global lawmaking processes, discourses and actors are being understood, this chapter has incorporated theories such as networked nodal governance theory and systems theory as well as relevant discourses. By using three case studies, on patent administration, PVR and STI in Sri Lanka, this chapter identifies two competing discourses namely, high-technology versus low-technology IP protection that are applied in these case studies in order to find answers through interacting, indeed competing, discourses about what the Sri Lankan law should be.

1.1 Introduction

A country's lawmaking contributes to fostering its innovation ecosystem and intellectual property rights ('IPR') in a country. However, lawmakers' discourses—about how different strengths of intellectual property (IP) support or do not support innovation—create a particular relationship between IP and the innovation system.[1] Apart from these discourses, legal transfers of global scripts from the developed Northern hemisphere to the developing Southern hemisphere, such as the *Agreement on Trade-Related Aspects of Intellectual Property Rights* ('*TRIPS Agreement*'),[2] the *Agreement on Trade-Related Investment Measures* ('*TRIMS*')[3] and the *Patent Cooperation Treaty* ('*PCT*'),[4] shape the patent administration; the plant variety rights ('PVR'); and the science, technology and innovation ('STI') sectors in Sri Lanka. Yet, the

[1] There is no one accepted causal relation between strong IP protection and economic development. For exposition of the discourses regarding this relation, refer to Drahos (2010) ('Global Governance of Knowledge'), Maskus (2000), 471, 480 ('Intellectual Property Rights').

[2] *Agreement on Trade-Related Aspects of Intellectual Property Rights* ('*TRIPS Agreement*') (1994).

[3] *Agreement on Trade-Related Investment Measures ('TRIMS Agreement')* (1994).

[4] *Patent Cooperation Treaty* ('*PCT*') (1970), was concluded in 1970, amended in 1979, and modified in 1984 and 2001.

A. Perera, *Dilemmas of Intellectual Property Discourse in Sri Lanka*,
https://doi.org/10.1007/978-981-97-6117-3_1

relationship between IP and the innovation system may also be constructed through economic and industrial policies, trade and competitiveness policies or social policies formulated at the national level by local actors.

Notably, the interaction between these discourses drives lawmaking. For the purposes of this research, IP refers mainly to patents and PVR. Patents provide monopoly protection to inventors/owners for a limited period to reward them for their useful inventions. During this period, others are prevented from infringing the patent for the invented product unless such right is given under exemptions from infringement, compulsory licensing ('CL') or parallel importation provisions. This research also examines other forms of IP lawmaking, such as PVR, because these are also used to protect IPR, similar to patents.

This book examines local and global lawmaking processes, discourses and actors related to the present state of Sri Lanka's IP laws. It explores the nature of, and seeks reasons for, Sri Lanka's apparent mismatch in Sri Lanka's commitment to implement international legislation, such as *TRIPS*, TRIMS and *PCT*, and the current states of implementation of such legislation in the country. It also explores the resultant international and local repercussions of this mismatch.

It seems that thus far at least, local laws have been implemented in the area of patent administration and STI sectors with the aim of fostering the innovation ecosystem in Sri Lanka, but considering the number of polices, the anticipated development goals have not been achieved, according to the data collected for this book. As will be discussed in the following chapters, the main reasons for this underdevelopment are the lack of alignment between the government's innovation policy and its industrial policies and the lack of discourse within sectors regarding development goals.

This indicates there is a lack of engagement between government, government agencies (such as the National Intellectual Property Organisation (NIPO) and industry which requires examination and explanation. The government ministries, government Representative to the United Nations UN representative, government agencies and industry are the central actors in the implementation, dissemination of information, and reaction to responses arising from industry. If these central actors do not communicate, failures occur in the system of implementation, as will be examined in Chap. 3 a failure to communicate exists between the NIPO and industry, but as will be seen in Chap. 5 actions by the UN representative and Coordinating Secretariat for Science, Technology and Innovation (COSTI) provide avenues of communication that enable development; whilst in Chap. 4 the implementation of PVR, which is required by TRIPS has not been achieved even though a Plant Variety Rights Bill has been under negotiation for 20 years. These highlights though indicate there is a need to untangle and explain the lack of engagement which provides the basis for the research inquiries.

The research inquiries posed in this research relate to how the concepts of local and global lawmaking processes, discourses and actors are being understood, used and interpreted in Sri Lanka's IP system. That is, this book attempts to answer the following research inquiries:

1 Has IP law discourse in Sri Lanka favoured low-technology rather than high-technology protection?
2 What are the reasons that Sri Lanka favours low-technology protection for IP law?

Having identified the questions, three case studies, on patent administration, PVR and STI in Sri Lanka, were conducted, which give substance to the competing discourses. For this book, two competing discourses have been identified, namely, high-technology versus low-technology IP protection.

To provide a theoretical framework for this inquiry, this researcher incorporated theories such as networked nodal governance theory and systems theory as well as relevant discourses. Using the pointers that this framework provides, the researcher then identified the global and local actors and the processes that are applied in these case studies in order to find answers through interacting, indeed competing, discourses about what the Sri Lankan law should be. At the conclusion, based on the two research inquiries and the theoretical framework, this book has concluded that as a result of low-technology protection adopted in areas of patents, PVR and STI and also due to the lack of expertise and cost in high-technology innovations have disabled Sri Lanka transforming from a middle income to an upper middle-income country, in the context of the three case studies.

The remainder of this chapter is organised as follows. Section 1.2 presents the theoretical framework of this book. Section 1.3 explains the case studies. Section 1.4 describes IP lawmaking process, Sect. 1.5 explains the study methods which includes, document analysis and interviews, Sect. 1.6 limitation of the research and Sect. 1.7 book structure.

1.2 Theoretical Framework

The theoretical framework of this book focuses on global and local lawmaking actors and processes and the possible ways in which they construct the discourses on IP based on three Sri Lankan case studies. This framework is built upon nodal governance theory, systems theory and discourse analysis.

1.3 Understanding Nodal Governance

According to networked nodal governance theory, a range of actors and processes, global and local, may become connection points in networks of governance; networks are a prime means through which such nodes exert influence.[5] The presence of networks means that influence can flow in many directions, vertically and horizontally, for instance, up and down and across the international landscape as well, or even

[5] Burris et al. (2005). See also Shaffer and Halliday (2015).

within the global or local spheres. Hence, many lawmaking possibilities are open. Nevertheless, not all nodes are equal: Governance theory accepts to some extent the role of political power, legal order and economic coercion in shaping patent laws.[6]

Irrespective of the type of the node, a node has four essential characteristics. First, it should have a way of thinking (mentalities) that cognitively shapes how individuals and organisations see the world and act accordingly.[7] It is through these mentalities and purposes that nodes differ greatly from each other in terms of goals and legal conduct. Second, it should have a set of processes (technologies) for applying and exercising influence over the course of events at issue.[8] Third, it should also have resources to support and mobilise the operation of the node and fuel its influence.[9] Fourth, there should be a system (institution) that enables the directed mobilisation of resources, mentalities and technologies over time.[10] The superstructural node, conversely, can channel its resources to exert simultaneous influence at the local, national and global levels.[11]

Influence is exerted through 'webs of dialogue' or 'webs of persuasion'. These describe the discourses in which superstructural nodes seek to alter others' interest, which is a much more frequent catalyst for change.[12] By doing this, the superstructural nodes can bring together two or more networks for producing various types of action, such as lobbying the state for a favourable law or policy.[13] For example, during the *TRIPS* negotiations the multinational corporations ('MNCs') became a superstructural node because they were the command centres that could tie together more networks for the purposes of producing various types of actions, such as lobbying the US Trade Representative, monitoring the piracy of US IP abroad and seeking enforcement action globally and locally.[14] Moreover, studies have shown that where MNCs from advanced economies have a dominant presence in a country's innovation system, accession to full compliance with *TRIPS* is fast and without many alterations to the original regulations, implying stringent compliance with the original *TRIPS* text.[15] Further, the influence of MNCs for fast and stringent *TRIPS* implementation is stronger in countries that have a high dependency on supranational organisations, such as the International Monetary Fund.[16] If developing countries refuse to comply, they will have to face economic sanctions.

Moreover, as the study on Sri Lanka shows, all nodes are not created equal and vary in their accessibility, their efficacy, the extent to which other nodes can influence

---

[6] Ibid.

[7] Shearing and Wood (2003), 400 (Democracy and the New "Denizens').

[8] Ibid.

[9] Ibid.

[10] Ibid.

[11] Ibid.

[12] Sell (2004), 363 ('Quest for Global Governance').

[13] Vanni (2019), 53 (*Patent Games in the Global South*).

[14] See Shearing and Wood (2003), 13.

[15] Brandl et al. (2019), 826 ('Foreign Actors and Intellectual Property').

[16] Ibid.

them and the way in which that influence is exerted. In other words, technologies, mentalities and resources will differ depending on how powerful the impact is on the status and efficacy of the node. For example, an individual node could be rather narrow in terms of knowledge and capacity to interact with and influence or regulate, compared with a group of nodes. That is, an individual node will be less influential in fostering an IP ecosystem in a country than a group of nodes that could achieve the task by pooling resources and expertise. However, the capacity of a node to exert influence and the potency of influence depends on resources, technologies in use and the institutional structure.[17] The factors include financial capacity, ability to mobilise networks and mobilising political pressure or economic coercion to achieve regulatory goals.[18]

For example, 12 US corporations, according to Sell, were primarily responsible for the lobbying that brought the *TRIPS Agreement* into being.[19] It was the intense lobbying activities from these companies in the US that laid the foundation for linking IP protection to trade in the multilateral context.[20] In contrast, a small NGO can exert influence at the local, municipal or national levels of governance. However, owing to limited financial capacity, such organisations are unable to exert influence simultaneously and at multiple sites.

From these characteristics of nodes, it is important to note that within a system, the hierarchy is contested among nodes because some nodes are more influential than the others that shape the IP discourse in Sri Lanka. This aspect will be discussed in the case studies.

1.4 Systems Theory

On systems theory, Teubner contended that 'law's contemporary ties to the society are no longer comprehensive but are highly selective and vary from loose coupling to tight interwovenness'.[21] He further explained: 'Since contemporary legal rule production is institutionally separate from cultural norm production, large areas of law are only in loose, non-systematic contact with social processes.'[22] However, there are also areas of law, he noted, 'where legal and social processes are highly tightly coupled'. In these cases, 'legal rules are formulated in ultra-cyclical processes between law and other social discourses which bind them closely together while maintaining at the same time their separation and mutual closure'.[23] A transfer of law is comparatively easy to accomplish in the loosely coupled areas, but will encounter extensive resistance

---

[17] Shearing and Wood (2003). See also Sorenson and Torfing (2003), 609.

[18] Brandl et al. (2019), 14.

[19] Sell (2003).

[20] Ibid.

[21] Teubner (1998), 18–19 ('Legal Irritants').

[22] Ibid.

[23] Ibid.

in tightly coupled areas.[24] In other words, global legal transfers are exposed to a new socio-legal mentality in the recipient state. At best, the global transfer is similar to the sand that agitates the oyster to produce a pearl.

According to Teubner, even where law is tightly coupled to society, it is no longer connected to 'the totality of the social, but to diverse fragments of society'.[25] It would suggest that society is fragmented into subsystems that have become so self-referential that they understand the messages from their environments, such as other nodes in the system, only through the filter of their own internal frames and norms of reference.[26] Teubner did not emphasise particular factors, such as politics, with which laws are particularly coupled. Rather, he asserted that some legal institutions are loosely tied to politics, but 'at the same time closely intertwined with economic processes' and 'others are tightly coupled to technology, to health, science, traditions and culture'.[27] Different social processes to which laws are coupled will produce different areas of resistance and acceptance of legal transfers. Because different laws link diversely to varying social worlds, 'legal institutions resist transfer in various ways.'[28]

Teubner described legal transfers as 'legal irritants' rather than 'legal transplants' because he believed '"transplants" may create a wrong impression that after a difficult surgical operation the transferred material will remain identified with itself playing out its old rules in the new organism'.[29] Instead, a series of dynamically interactive and transformative processes would be triggered once a law is transferred from one system to another. He points out that a legal irritant will 'unleash an evolutionary dynamic in which the external rule's meaning will be reconstructed and the internal context will undergo fundamental change'.[30] Once foreign laws enter the recipient system, they are exposed to a mutually interactive matrix of varying social discourses, including legal discourse. Foreign laws irritate not only the recipient legal discourse itself, but also the social discourses to which these laws are closely coupled.[31] Hence, Teubner based his explanation on systems theory since this theory analogises human society as a biological system that is maintained through self-replicating organic subsystems, and in human social subsystems, 'communication takes place of metabolic pathways in creating autopoiesis'.[32]

Systems theory is built upon the anti-foundationalist view adopted in this study.[33] According to this view, legal transfers such as *TRIPS* and other international legal instruments are interpreted and given meaning through the communicative acts

---

[24] Ibid.

[25] Ibid.

[26] Beck (1994), 401.

[27] Teubner (1998), 22.

[28] Ibid., 12.

[29] Ibid.

[30] Ibid.

[31] Ibid., 31–32.

[32] Gillespie (2006), 18 ('*Transplanting Commercial Law Reform*').

[33] Teubner (1989), 727.

of human individuals. Law is transferred not because it intrinsically contains an autonomous and universal meaning as legal positivists often argue,[34] but rather because laws or rules convey certain discursive meanings to legal elites in recipient countries. This is what the MNCs did during *TRIPS* negotiations as discussed above. Hence, systems theory in this study will focus on the interpretation and implementation of legal transfers by recipient systems. For system theorists, what really matter are legal meanings given to legal transfers via human agents' interpretation.[35]

According to systems theory, just as the global system is not unitary, the local actors described above are within a system or a network that is fragmented into subsystems within the IP ecosystem in Sri Lanka. These subsystems establish the national framework to implement legislation and to give the rights and establish a national system that consists of different nodes, such as the government level and the administrative level, the President, the Parliament, various ministries, such as the Ministries of Industry, Agriculture and Health, and specialist organisations, such as COSTI and the NIPO in Sri Lanka, which represent the executive and administrative levels that directly deal with IP. Connecting back to nodal governance theory, any system comprises nodes, whereas networks are prime means through which nodes exert influence. Consequently, some nodes are more powerful than the others, and they interact with each other from both within and outside the system collectively or alone to resolve (or not to resolve) issues within the IP regime.

Through network links, the Sri Lankan IP framework is open to external messages from other subsystems, via political, economic, social and cultural discourses. However, only through internal human communicative acts can local interpretations of global scripts such as *TRIPS* be given meaning. Within this context, systems theory will be used in this research to understand and interpret how actors in the Sri Lankan IP subsystems come together and acquire a relative coherence in shaping legal reforms.[36] Hence, nodal governance theory in conjunction with systems theory appears very promising in helping to assess the research inquiries, hypotheses and questions, which aim to investigate the influence on local and global legal processes in implementing a legal IP framework for Sri Lanka.

1.5 Discourses

Although nodal governance theory and systems theory appear very promising as a theoretical framework, they lack a methodology for examining specific communicative acts, as it suggests, through which transfers, interpretations and resistance take place. The lawmaking process involves the selection, interpretation, adaptation and implementation of rules. This process involves the communication of ideas among actors. Hence, this study will use discourses as a methodology to examine

[34] Watson (1987), 313.

[35] Gillespie (2008), 680 ('Towards a Discursive Analysis').

[36] Jessop (2001), 213.

conversations among various actors during interpreting, adapting and implementing to understand how IP fits into economic development.[37] According to discourses, social interaction, dialogue and learning contribute to lawmaking. Hence, discourses helps to analyse how information flows and is processed and how communication takes place within a social system.[38] Therefore, it is important to identify who is speaking to whom, how important these actors are, what do they communicate, whether these actors are listening to each other, and to what extent the actor/s can influence each other.

In the Sri Lankan context, this book will examine the use of communication between key actors within government institutions, such as the NIPO, national ministries, politicians, bureaucrats, lawyers, universities, NGOs, local economic groups and embassies, and globally, non-state actors, such as MNCs, international organisations such as the World Intellectual Property Organisation ('WIPO') and foreign national governments, to create their own reality of economic development and assign meanings to the role of patent and other IP law in that development.[39]

Communicative acts motivate actors to change their regulatory preferences. In other words, such acts have a regulatory function.[40] Hence, systems theory needs to be augmented with close empirical discourse analysis in the case studies to discover how those external messages are translated and reworked within the Sri Lankan legal subsystem.[41] For this purpose, methodological tools synthesised by Gillespie from various streams of discourse analysis will be used.[42] These include 'semi-autonomous' discourse modes, interpretive communities and discursive strategies.

1.6 Case Studies

The three case studies presented in this book will help to examine the two research inquiries. Hence, it is important to characterise competing discourses for the three case studies for finding answers. In all the three case studies, a contrast is made between high- and low-technology protection. The following section provides a distinction between a low-technology and high technology based on existing literature.

---

[37] However, it is important to note the methodology here does not adopt a Foucauldian style of discourse analysis. Foucault refers to discourse analysis as ways of constituting knowledge, together with social practice, forms of subjectivity and power relations that inhere in such knowledge and the relations between them. Hook (2007). In this book, discourses are used to identify how different actors within a subsystem communicate with each other in the law making process.

[38] Burris et al. (2005).

[39] Luhmann (1988), 21–35.

[40] Black (2002).

[41] Gillespie stresses the need for such empirical analysis. Refer to John Gillespie, 'Relocating Global Scripts in Local Networks of Meaning' in Gillespie (2012), 29 ('Relocating Global Scripts').

[42] Gillespie (2006), 33–35.

The low technology and high technology distinction made in this book has been developed through consideration of many different conceptual frameworks that operate in the different sectors investigated in the case studies for this book. There is no single consistent definition for these terms. Due to the difficulties arising from many definitions of what is low and high technology, the following is adopted based on OECD Directorate for Science, Technology and Industry Economic Analysis and Statistical Division.[43]

According to OECD Directorate for Science, Technology and Industry Economic Analysis and Statistical Division, many manufacturing activities could be considered "high-technology" by looking at direct R&D intensities, but the OECD classify 'low and high technology' distinction according to R&D performance. Also, "high-tech" industries can produce a variety of products ranging between "low-tech" and "high-tech." The Directorates' idea was to create a classification for OECD as a whole which means, the definition is deliberately broad. The breadth of the definition means that countries with low- technology industries such as manufacturing, food and textile can still be considered depending on the nature of their R&D in the relevant industry. The R&D performance thus, not solely on high-technology industries such as biotechnology and pharmaceuticals and software. Hence, individual countries may have slightly different classifications using the same method and compromise on the level of industry details.

This discussion identifies there is no uniform definition of low technology and high technology but the interviewees used this terminology to describe their understanding and experiences and thus as will be seen in the investigation for the discourses in each case study a specific definition of low and high technology will be adopted for each of the relevant case studies.

The above distinction is important because in all three case studies this researcher assumed that Sri Lanka favours low-technology rather than high-technology IP protection mainly owing to its underdevelopment, considering that the country has not linked the strong IP settings adopted globally to its national or international economic priorities. This underdevelopment in IP has impacted the economic development and innovation economy in Sri Lanka. In this book Sri Lanka has been chosen as an unexplored case study in the context of IP lawmaking, mainly because compared to other developing countries in the Global South even after 76 years of independence Sri Lanka still remain a lower middle-income country. Thirty years of civil law has undoubtedly contributed for this status because during this period millions of dollars that could have been used to foster innovation policies have been used to fight a war, which made Sri Lanka economically and technologically vulnerable and reliant on other countries for economic support. Why patents and PVR has been chosen in this study? Some of the other countries in the region like India, Korea and Singapore has by passed the middle-income line though the 'ratcheting up' of IP, especially through patents, because generally patents are considered as a drive for development. STI on the other hand has a close relationship between IP and innovation. PVR have become a priority with the enactment of the TRIPS Agreement

[43] OECD Directorate for Science (2011).

and members of the WTO were required to introduce PVR laws in their respective countries. With all these developments, no study has been undertaken in Sri Lanka on intellectual property lawmaking and hence, this book will attempt to shed some light to the existing IP global debates on intellectual property.

In the first case study on the patent administration system in Sri Lanka. Generally, the level of technology used in a product determines the scope and level of patent protection for that product. For example, to qualify for patent protection during a patent application examination, an invention must fall within the technical criteria of novelty, inventive step and industrial application. The patent examination system used by countries differs according to their resources and expertise. For instance, most developing countries and practically all developed countries have a system that uses a substantive examination performed by the examiner on the substance of the application. As an example, in Australia, during this examination aspects such as the manner of manufacture (ie patentable subject matter), novelty, inventive step, sufficiency, clarity and utility requirements are assessed.[44] The substantive examination procedure is a high-technology protection for it involves the assessment of all the core elements of an invention to determine whether it meets the aforementioned technical criteria and thus qualifies for patent protection.

It is worth noting that, within a high technology protection system, there is a further choice to be made, which is termed the high-/low-bar for protection. For example, one question here is how rigorous and wide the patent system makes the searches for the prior art dealing with the inventive step, after an application passes the stage of a patent grant on the basis of the technical criteria.[45] The bar of protection also addresses issues such as the extent to which the rights are exclusive and the type of acts that the patent holder may control, or whether they may be modified by such provisions as a research exemption, parallel importation, compulsory licensing, local working of patents or foreign investment performance requirements. The applicability of these aspects of patent protection in the Sri Lankan context will be discussed in Chap. 3.

By applying the contrast between high- and low-technology patent protection, this case study will investigate whether the patent administration discourse is about making it easier for small, independent local inventors to obtain patent protection in Sri Lanka. If this is the prime motive, high-technology settings will generally not be suitable for local investors. There is evidence that patents are granted for incremental inventions to motivate innovators although the innovation does not satisfy the technical criteria.[46] The current patent system is based on the formality of examination, which is a very outdated system.[47] This is a low level of examination procedure, and its impact will be discussed in detail in Chap. 3.

---

[44] IP Australia (2022).

[45] At present in Australia, the high-bar search has been expanded to the entire world and not limited to Australia, setting what is known as an absolute novelty and inventive step requirement in the examination. See also Intellectual Property Laws Amendment (Raising the Bar) Act 2012.

[46] Interviewee # 23.

[47] Perera (2024), 344 ('Administration of Patent System').

The second case study considers PVR is considered as high-technology as it promotes innovations in the field of agriculture, horticulture and forestry, which has paved the way to increased production, particularly following developments in the field of biotechnology. *TRIPS* mandate every member state to have a PVR through either patents or sui generis protection, but PVR has not been legislated in Sri Lanka.[48] PVR promotes innovations in the field of agriculture, horticulture and forestry, which has paved the way to increased production, particularly following developments in the field of biotechnology. Breeders' varieties are protected under the criteria of novelty, distinctiveness, uniformity and stability ('NDUS'), which are the technical criteria used to determine breeders' rights. NDUS is therefore considered a high-technology protection under a PVR or even a more so a plant breeders' rights ('PBR') regime.[49]

Conversely, in Sri Lanka where subsistence farming is the norm in the agricultural sector in which most farmers informally cultivate and conserve traditional varieties depending on recognition of stewardship and other rewards, it is questionable whether high-technology plant breeding and plant innovation can offer more protection in terms of food security for rural farmers. Stewardship is a low-maintenance activity for it does not involve laboratory testing and, hence, it is low technology in contrast to PBR, but this system has been functioning efficiently for generations of farmers within the Sri Lankan context.

Hence, for the second case study, the competing discourses for PVR/PBR are between the ownership of PVR, which is high-technology protection, and stewardship for farmers, which is low-technology protection. In this case study, by comparing ownership with stewardship discourses, the researcher critiques that the ownership approach is inadequate, and that stewardship is more suited to Sri Lanka, considering the real-life consequences for farmers' livelihood. The stewardship approach will uphold their legal space to maintain genetic resources through a reward system, rather than trying to balance their rights with breeders' rights merely in an IP ownership approach.

The third case study is the STI sector, which goes hand in hand with the patent administration case study because the technical criteria of patent grants, limits and conditions are closely associated with the STI sector, given that science and technology ('ST') and research-based innovations are increasingly recognised as determinants of an innovation economy. As will be discussed in Chap. 5 STI indicators in Sri Lanka are considerably low and, consequently, foreign direct investment ('FDI'), technology transfer ('TT'), which stimulates innovation, and import of IP products into the country are weak. The impact of weak FDI and TT in the Sri Lankan innovation system will be discussed in Chap. 5 of this book. As will be discussed in Chap. 5, ST discourse in Sri Lanka is yet to reach the maturity or innovation level achieved in some developed countries. Hence, most ST innovations that are patented in Sri Lanka are developed using basic research, which is considered low-technology research,

---

[48] PVR has not yet been enacted by the Sri Lankan Parliament. However, according to the *TRIPS Agreement*, Sri Lanka needs to protect its plant varieties either by patents or any sui generis law.

[49] *International Convention for the Protection of New Plant Varieties (UPOV)* (1961), as Revised at Geneva on November 10, 1972, on October 23, 1978, and on March 19, 1991.

rather than on applied or demand-driven research, which involves high-technology research.

Therefore, for the third case study, of two competing discourses the primary appear to be low technology focused on substitution and basic applied research that does not transform or involve major investments. First is the low-technology IP protection for local innovations, such as the small and medium-sized enterprises ('SMEs') in Sri Lanka who develop innovations through a low-technology protection owing to their lack of expertise and resources and the high cost involved.[50] Evidence suggests that patents are not a prerequisite for the SME sector. SMEs rely on informal ways of protection, such as lead-time advantages and secrecy.[51] Patents are a concern only for the limited number of larger firms which supports the second competing discourse based on high-technology IP protection. For example, multinational investors view the establishment of a high-technology IP protection system in Sri Lanka as a prerequisite to attract 'TT' and FDI and to increase the country's growth and innovative activity. This aspect will be discussed in Chap. 5.

In this book, the researcher will be analysing the processes for developing IP laws and policies in Sri Lanka based on the theoretical framework identified in this book. For example, nodal governance theory has thrown light on power dynamics, such as those evident in the development of the TRIPS Agreement, and how countries like Sri Lanka amended IP laws to comply with the TRIPS Agreement. On the other hand, with regard to IP law and policy making in Sri Lanka, the book will demonstrate that there has been nodal influence in introducing IP law in Sri Lanka. These nodes have subsequently have exerted influence with the other nodes within the IP ecosystem through interaction and communications creating a social discourse This social discourse involves actors and power dynamics in introducing and promoting recommendations in patent administration, PVR and STI sectors to foster IP law and policy making. The nodal influence and the interaction between different communicative subsystems will be analysed in Chaps. 3–5.

The research inquiries in this book are descriptive, but due to the theoretical framework outlined in this study, normative conclusions will arise because this book will provide some recommendations or changes in IP policy making which is inevitable in this study. The normative conclusions are however, not the central focus of the book, but as with any discursive analysis of law normative conclusions will be provided only as they relate to the theoretical framework of this book that is, they are discourses in play. The normative conclusions are not the primary purpose of this, book but they are an ancillary by product for the examination of the research inquiries. Of course, the researcher has her own opinions.

---

[50] Hewage (2015), 100.

[51] Ibid.

1.7 IP Lawmaking Process in Sri Lanka

On the basis of the theoretical framework of this book, in order to determine the areas from which answers can be found for the issues explored in this book, the following section will briefly discuss the IP lawmaking process in Sri Lanka.

The framework of the Sri Lankan lawmaking process includes global and local actors and their roles within the global and local legal discourses and processes. Both groups of actors play a crucial role in the lawmaking process. This process includes, but is not restricted to, the national government policymaking process within the patent administration, which is a key feature in this regard, since the national government is responsible for designing the patent policy, which should be aligned with the economic strategy of Sri Lanka. Lawmaking also includes global treaty-making and implementation processes.

The lawmaking processes includes stakeholder alliances, which play a vital role in influencing the IP landscape in Sri Lanka. To have a better understanding on the existence and complexities of stakeholder alliances in determining the IP in Sri Lanka, it is important to explore the nature of these alliances within three different levels: domestic, national and global. Together the domestic and national levels comprise the local.

At the local and national levels, whether domestic or national, apart from the government, ministries, offices and courts, other stakeholders are actors from outside national governments and governing political parties. These include citizens, civil society and non-governmental organisations ('NGOs'); development partners or agencies, such as the WIPO and the World Bank; foreign governments; private sector stakeholders; local governments; trade unions; parliamentarians; academics; industries; private–public partnerships; universities; SMEs; research institutes; policymakers; farmers' organisations; and environmentalists, who are spread among these three levels and promote patent reforms, PVR laws and STI developments to foster innovation in Sri Lanka. The disruption caused by the civil war, between 1982 and 2009 led to poor economic and industry conditions, the lack of good governance, and the dissipation of the political, administrative and legal systems, which have all compromised the trajectory of the local lawmaking process.

The global lawmaking process involves the power of international politics and political actors to exert pressure on others to influence patent, PVR and STI policy outcomes.[52] In examining this stage, this researcher will discuss the *TRIPS Agreement* initiated by the World Trade Organization ('WTO') as a crucial global actor in the global IP regime, which exerts pressure on developing countries, such as Sri Lanka, to implement reforms in order to comply with the global minimum standards for intellectual property rights ('IPR'), which are much higher than their existing standards. It is a crucial actor because although the *TRIPS Agreement* does not determine the national legislation, WTO members should ensure that their national IP legislation adheres to the minimum level of IPR protection established in the *TRIPS*

[52] Vanni (2019), 1 (*Patent Games in the Global South*).

Agreement.[53] Any nation seeking to join the international trade club was required to accept a package deal that included both strong IPR and robust international enforcement of those rights.[54] Moreover, *TRIPS* has created tension points in areas of biodiversity and plant genetic resources ('PGR'), which have acted as catalysts for new IP rules, and these tension points had substantive as well as procedural dimensions.[55]

Substantively, *TRIPS* required states to grant IP in fields such as genetic resources and plant varieties that developing countries believed should not be treated as private property on moral and cultural grounds.[56] Procedurally, tensions were created by the more stringent enforcement mechanisms of *TRIPS* compared with the weaker enforcement structures prevalent in international regimes outside the WTO. Thus, the *TRIPS* regulatory approach weakened the clarity of existing legal rules and created uncertainty for states over how to reconcile the resulting conflicts.[57] In this sense, the WTO is a prominent global actor that could influence every member state until the states comply with the WTO rules. This aspect will be discussed in Chap. 2 of this book.

Within the global process, WIPO too is a global actor in promoting the protection of IP worldwide through cooperation and collaboration among members and other stakeholders. To achieve this mandate, WIPO specified in its art 4(v) that 'the Organization shall offer its cooperation among states requesting legal-technical assistance in the field of IP.' WIPO assistance is demand driven—that is, a country should request WIPO for assistance and, if eligible, will receive assistance according to its needs. In this sense, while WIPO is a global node on IP, unlike the WTO, it cannot influence countries to accept its recommendations. As will be discussed in Chap. 4, WIPO provides technical assistance through discourse for member states. Recommendations are provided to the government, but it is for the government to accept or reject the recommendations. On the subject matter of PVR, the International Union for the Protection of New Plant Varieties ('UPOV') is a global actor since many developing countries were compelled to ratify the 1991 version of the *Iinternational Convention for the Protection of New Varieties of Plants* ('*UPOV Convention*')[58] as a sui generis protection after becoming members of the *TRIPS Agreement*. However, Sri Lanka is not a member of the *UPOV Convention*. The role of UPOV with regard to PVR will be discussed in detail in Chap. 4.

Local nodes do not simply receive and implement global scripts. They sometimes reinterpret, rework or resist them. This aspect will be discussed in Chap. 2. Given this variability and subtlety of response, components that should be addressed in discourse and process include a precise legal setting for IPR that addresses specific issues, such

---

[53] Sell (1995), 315 ('Intellectual Property Protection').

[54] Drahos (2003), 79, 109.

[55] Helfer (2009), 39 ('Regime Shifting in the International').

[56] Ibid.

[57] Ibid.

[58] The UPOV was established by the *International Convention for the Protection of New Varieties of Plants*, which was adopted in Paris in 1961 and revised in 1972, 1978 and 1991.

as standards of inventiveness and innovation to attract protection, exclusions from the subject matter of IP, limits to the rights that the holders may exercise, exemptions from infringement for public and fair uses, and the compensatory conditions that may be placed on IP power in competition, price and licensing regulations and policies associated with IPR protection.

Ultimately, the course for Sri Lanka depends on the objectives assigned to, and implemented by, the IP system, whether it focuses on encouraging local conservation and innovation or attracting foreign investors and importers, or a combination of the two such as licensing foreign IP for local research and application. Acting on these competing discourses requires building up the capacity, legal and otherwise, to implement those objectives. For example, it should be considered whether the competing interests should focus on strengthening the patent law and administration of Sri Lanka, implementing PVR to support new breeders disregarding the interest of farmers and promoting the STI sector in Sri Lanka to foster leading-edge research. The competing discourses identified in the case studies will provide some implications as to how IP law and policy making should transform Sri Lanka's IP lawmaking discourses.

1.8 Study Method

1.8.1 Document Analysis

The study involved two stages: document analysis and interviews. To test the two questions and then present findings, primary and secondary data were collected. Primary data were collected from comprehensive desk-top studies of government reports, negotiations, debates, relevant legislation, books, journal articles, newspaper articles and websites of various national and international organisations, such as the Sri Lankan Government, WTO *TRIPS*, WIPO/*PCT*, the World Bank, industry associations, companies and NGOs. All these sources help locate the discourses.

1.8.2 Interviews

The research interviews are recognized as a prominent data-collection strategy for qualitative research[59] undertaken in this book. This involves a socio-legal study of the analysis of law, and the relationships between the actors who influence, create or obstruct the lawmaking process and its implementation within a society. The interviews are secondary data collection, the researcher conducted in Sri Lanka and overseas with selected individuals for obtaining genuine feedback as an evidentiary

[59] Bryman (2012) and Seidman (2006).

source to identify whether IP use is becoming a driving factor for economic development in Sri Lanka. Hence, in the second stage of the study semi-structured interviews were conducted with selected officers from Sri Lankan Government agencies, industry experts, economists, academics, lawyers, stakeholders, and officials from global actors, such as WIPO, the WTO and the United Nations ('UN'), to verify whether the IP policy issues are actually being formulated or not within the economic agenda of Sri Lanka.

In addition, communication operates within Sri Lanka on the basis of knowing people and networks to obtain information, and this is essential to reveal the discourses and identify nodes. My experiences from working and living in Sri Lanka over 40 years and being a national enabled me to utilize networks to obtain the discourses which was used in this book. To access information for research activities in Sri Lanka is generally difficult however, being a Sri Lankan has enabled me to obtain information from prominent nodes in the IP eco-system for this research, through networking which is only available to a Sri Lankan national.

For the current study, the researcher commenced conducting interviews with local actors in Sri Lanka in November 2017 and global actors in Geneva in January 2018. All the interviews were audio recorded with the consent of the participants, except for one conducted in the United States ('US') embassy in Sri Lanka. Open-ended questions were used in all interviews, and the interviewees were selected because of their nodal position in the IP subsystem. The duration of each interview was approximately an hour. In all, 26 participants were interviewed. Follow-up emails were sent to some of the interviewees to inquire about certain developments that occurred after the preliminary interviews in 2017. The researcher completed the transcription of the interviews in mid-2018 and prepared interview summaries and preliminary analysis tables using excel files with the support of the PhD supervisors. These summaries and tables have been very useful tools in the data analysis process. As discussed in the Sect. 1.3 on methodology for this book, the reviewing of data will thus be mainly through interviews and document analysis.

1.9 Limitations of the Research

It is important to acknowledge the limitations of this research in terms of its focus and methods. First, while the research seeks to examine the discourses in lawmaking, processes and actors pertaining to the three case studies, it was practically impossible to examine all the institutions and actors relevant to the study, and choices had to be made. Every effort was taken to interview the most influential actors within the IP ecosystem in Sri Lanka, but some actors were omitted owing to the difficulty in finding a time that suited both parties. Gaining access to the interviewees was a challenge on many occasions. At times, it was difficult to communicate with local actors through email or a phone call to schedule an appointment. On such occasions, the researcher had to rely on their own networking to connect with the relevant parties. When face-to-face communication was not possible, the researcher had to conduct telephonic interviews, in particular, during 2020 and 2021 because of the restrictions imposed on international travel following the onset of the global COVID-19, pandemic.

Second, the questions posed in this research do not contribute directly to determining policymakers' perception on IP lawmaking conceptually or empirically. These questions provided a positive environment to talk about IP, but sometimes, it was very challenging to obtain the required response because the interviewees did not venture to offer information that went beyond 'the official line'. For example, some government policymakers who made off-the-record statements did not want to identify themselves and some global actors, such as the official at the US embassy, did not allow their interviews to be audio recorded. Moreover, some government policymakers were reluctant to reveal the true picture owing to their contractual obligation towards the government. Conversely, the private sector interviewees were very open in their responses because they did not depend on the government for running their businesses. Asking open questions and ending the interview with an open-ended discussion were also a means of checking the information acquired and encouraging the interviewee to be candid. The interview transcripts were also compared and contrasted with discussion papers and the official documents produced by the interviewee's organisation or website where possible and relevant.

Third, this researcher made certain speculations regarding the status of Sri Lankan IP lawmaking using the information received through interviews and documents. In doing so, the researcher attempted to determine the actors and factors that had the most influence over the discourses over IP promotion and implementation, whether these factors differed by actor, the ways in which particular groups of actors formed shared interpretations about the laws, the existing interactions between different interpretive groups and with society in general and the substantive and procedural changes that were attributable to local interpretations. Making speculations is important because the researcher is unable to explain why a certain event has not occurred in the Sri Lankan IP ecosystem, because it is difficult to explain something that has not occurred, which may not even have been demanded, such as PVR implementation in Sri Lanka.

Last, since this is a socio-legal study, it is important to be realistic about its parameters. This research does not model the contentious economic or epidemiological effects of instituting a stronger IP regime. Rather, the main inquiry is how this unresolved discourse around patent administration, PVR law and STI development links with the innovation economy of Sri Lanka. These discourses reveal the nature of local and global discourses and the lawmaking processes in Sri Lanka, both in the recent past and the present, as perhaps the law changes. Hence, the main objective of this research is to examine and explain Sri Lanka's strategy for IP innovation, protection and investment. What do the lawmakers say about Sri Lanka's legal framework for IP-related matters? Is it suited to local political, economic, industrial and technological policies as well as the global IPR context? On the basis of the above Sri Lankan context, this research will determine whether IP is still in the forefront of the development agenda in Sri Lanka to foster an innovation ecosystem in Sri Lanka.

1.10 Structure of the Book

This book is structured as follows:

This chapter outlines the purpose of this book, namely, to examine local and global lawmaking processes, discourses and actors related to the present state of Sri Lanka's IP laws. To examine how the concepts of local and global lawmaking processes, discourses and actors are being understood, this chapter has incorporated theories such as networked nodal governance theory and systems theory as well as relevant discourses. By using three case studies, on patent administration, PVR and STI in Sri Lanka, this chapter identifies two competing discourses namely, high-technology versus low-technology IP protection that are applied in these case studies in order to find answers through interacting, indeed competing, discourses about what the Sri Lankan law should be.

Chapter 2 elaborates on the global and local lawmaking actors and processes and the way they construct the discourses on IP in Sri Lanka. This chapter identifies two broad approaches in the literature on lawmaking. The first is 'coercion and implementation' and the second approach is 'legal transplant'. By using this two approaches this chapter will analyses how these approaches have been used to characterise the direction of lawmaking discourse in the Sri Lankan IP lawmaking process. The chapter concludes that local discourses have been more influential than the global discourses in IP lawmaking in Sri Lanka.

Chapter 3 is the first case study of this research. It discusses the discourses around the patent administration system in Sri Lanka and compares the constructs in the system processes and discourses This chapter will consider whether Sri Lanka should have a patent protection system based on high technical criteria for industrialists, combined with a utility model system or apply lower technical criteria to encourage local innovations. This case considers the interaction between global and local governance actors or nodes.

Chapter 4 takes up Sri Lanka as a relatively unexplored PVR/farmers' rights ('FR') case study in the general comparative literature in the South Asian region. It provides a unique opportunity to develop a sui generis structure utilised by other countries, such as India. In this chapter, sectors of two competing production models have been characterised to show the contrast between ownership and stewardship, which is further contrasted as high- and low-technology protection. The ways of resolving the competing discourses for breeders and farmers will be discussed in this chapter.

Chapter 5 explores the discourses around ST sectors that lead to innovation. Patent law and regulation do not exist in a vacuum; they exist to translate ideas into IPR that can then be commercialised, and for this reason, the existence of a patent system and legal structure is intertwined with the development discourse relating to ST research. Hence, this chapter will focus on the status of ST in Sri Lanka according to the relevant IP settings, the subject matter of protection, together with commercial incentives or performance requirements to foster research and development ('R&D'), FDI, licensing and TT. Based on the innovation ecosystem in Sri Lanka, for this case study, the competing discourses are between high-technology innovations, such as nanotechnology, and low-technology ones that are used by the SME sector. This chapter will analyse the extent to which ST has become a driving force to shape IP protection in Sri Lanka.

Chapter 6 concludes the research. It will discuss how the lawmaking process and discourses have contributed to fostering innovation in Sri Lanka. It will first review the main findings from the case studies, scrutinise the answers to the questions, examine the strengths of the research inquiries and, last, make some recommendations related to the future prospects of IP law in Sri Lanka.

Competing Interests The author has no conflicts of interest to declare that are relevant to the content of this chapter.

References

Agreement on Trade-Related Aspects of Intellectual Property Rights (1994) Marrakesh agreement establishing the world trade organization. Annex 1C 1869 U.N.T.S. 299, 33 I.L.M. 1197, Apr 15

Agreement on Trade-Related Investment Measures (1994) Marrakesh agreement establishing the world trade organization. Annex 1A 1868 U.N.T.S. 186, Apr 15

Beck A (1994) Is law an autopoietic system? Oxford Law J Legal Stud 14

Black J (2022) Regulatory conversations. J Law Soc 29:163, 174

Brandl K, Darendeli, Mudambi R (2019) Foreign actors and intellectual property protection regulations in developing countries. J Int Business Stud 50

Bryman A (2012) Social research methods, 4th edn. Oxford University Press

Burris S, Drahos P, Shearing C 'Nodal Governance' (2005) Australian J Legal Philos 30

Drahos P (2003) When the weak bargain with the strong: negotiations in the world trade organisation. Int Negotiat 8:1

Drahos P (2010) The global governance of knowledge: patent offices and their clients. Cambridge University Press

Gillespie J (2006) Transplanting commercial law reform: developing a 'rule of law' in Vietnam. Ashgate

Gillespie J (2008) Towards a discursive analysis of legal transfers into developing East Asia. New York Univ J Internat Law Polit 40

Gillespie J (2012) Relocating global scripts in local networks of meaning. In: Gillespie J, Nicholson P (eds) Law and development and the global discourses of legal transfers. Cambridge University Press

Helfer LR (2009) Regime shifting in the international intellectual property system. Perspect Polit 7:1

Hewage NS (2015) Promoting a second-tier protection regime for innovation of small and medium-sized enterprises in South Asia: a case of Sri Lanka. Nomas

Hook D (2007) Foucault, psychology and the analytics of power: critical theory and practice in psychology and the human sciences. Palgrave Macmillan, p 100

Intellectual Property Laws Amendment (Raising the Bar) Bill 2011

International Convention for the Protection of New Plant Varieties (1961,1978 and 1991)

IP Australia (2022) Australian patent examination reports. https://www.brmpatentattorneys.com.au/attorney/patent-australia/patent-application/examination-report/

Jessop B (2001) Regulationist and autopoieticist reflections on Polanyi's account of market economics and the market society. New Political Econ 6:2
Luhmann N (1988) The unity of legal system. In: Teubner G (ed) Autopoietic law: a new approach to law and society. Walter de Gruyter, p 12
Maskus KE (2000) Intellectual property rights and economic development. Western Reserve J Internat Law 32:2
OECD Directorate for Science (2011) Technology and industry economic analysis and statistical division, technology intensity definitions: classifications on manufacturing industries into categories based on R&D intensities. https://www.oecd.org/sti/ind/48350231.pdf
Patent Cooperation Treaty (1970). Amended in 1979 and modified in 1984 and 2001
Perera A (2024) The administration of patent system in Sri Lanka: a critical appraisal. Common Law World Rev 43
Seidman I (2006) Interviewing as qualitative research: a guide for researches in education and the social science. Teachers College Press
Sell SK (1995) Intellectual property protection and antitrust in developing world: crisis, coercion and choice. Internat Organ 49
Sell SK (2003) Private power, public law: the globalisation of intellectual property rights. Cambridge University Press
Sell SK (2004) The quest for global governance in intellectual property and public health: structural, discursive and institutional dimensions. Temple Law Rev 77
Shaffer G, Halliday TC (eds) (2015) Transnational legal orders. Cambridge University Press
Shearing C, Wood (2003) Nodal governance, democracy and the new "denizens." J Law Soc 30
Sorenson, Torfing J (2003) Network politics, political capital and democracy. Internat J Public Admin 26
Teubner G (1989) How the law thinks: towards a constructivist epistemology of law. Law Soc Rev 23
Teubner G (1998) Legal irritants: good faith in British law or how unifying law ends up in new divergences. Modern Law Rev 61:11
Vanni A (2019) General overview: patent games in the global south: pharmaceutical patent law making in Brazil, India and Nigeria. Hart Publishing
Watson A (1987) Comparative law and the legal change. Cambridge Law J 37

Chapter 2
Lawmaking Actors, Processes and Discourses in Sri Lanka

Abstract This chapter elaborates on the global and local lawmaking actors and processes and the way they construct the discourses on IP in Sri Lanka. This chapter identifies two broad approaches in the literature on lawmaking. The first is 'coercion and implementation' and the second approach is 'legal transplant'. By using this two approaches this chapter will analyses how these approaches have been used to characterise the direction of lawmaking discourse in Sri Lanka. The chapter concludes that local discourses have been more influential than the global discourses in IP lawmaking in Sri Lanka.

2.1 Introduction

Chapter 1 identified that local lawmaking actors, processes and discourses have proved crucial in the case studies in making a choice between high- and low-technology settings for patent administration, PVR regime and STI developments. Yet, coercion (and implementation) and legal transplants should also be considered and critiqued, for they are strategies under which global legal actors and processes may also influence lawmaking in the IP landscape in Sri Lanka, especially with the advent of *TRIPS*. Local and global aspects will both be discussed in this chapter.

2.2 Local Resistance and Reinterpretation

In the Sects. 2.3 and 2.4, two broad approaches are identified in the literature on lawmaking discourse favouring global direction to lawmaking with a view to considering whether the theory of multiple nodes and diffused power is tenable in the current context of Sri Lankan IP. The first is 'coercion and implementation'; Sect. 2.3 analyses how coercion (and implementation) relates to IP lawmaking, which includes legal scholarship exploring the types of mechanisms used in this approach and the extent to which this approach has been effective in IP lawmaking in Sri Lanka. The

A. Perera, *Dilemmas of Intellectual Property Discourse in Sri Lanka*,
https://doi.org/10.1007/978-981-97-6117-3_2

second approach is 'legal transplant'; Sect. 2.4 analyses how this approach has been used to characterise the direction of lawmaking discourse and the different types of transplantation theories that have been adopted in the Sri Lankan lawmaking process.

2.3 Coercion and Implementation

Morin and Gold analysed the reasons that some countries incorporate exogenous rules into their domestic law when such rules would seem to contravene their specific interests.[1] Using policy diffusion literature, they identified four causal mechanisms for the adoption of such rules. While one mechanism, coercion, tends to initiate the transplantation process, it fades over time and four other more discourse-laden and multi-directional mechanisms largely supplant it: emulation, contractualisation, socialisation and regulatory competition.[2]

When the *TRIPS Agreement* was enacted, most states accepted *TRIPS* as a necessity to change, while some resisted the changes, but later accepted these owing to coercion exerted by the developed states. Deere described *TRIPS* as a symbol of the vulnerability of developing countries to coercive pressure from the most powerful developed countries on the global economic rules.[3] Hence, *TRIPS* is a global script that created a global regulatory ratchet of IP,[4] exerting influence on every member state, including Sri Lanka, to make IP law comply with the *TRIPS* minimum standards. Braithwaite and Drahos described this as economic coercion, which is a higher-order mechanism of reinforcement used by developed countries or powerful organisations to achieve their goals and plans.[5] Deere described the situation as economic pressure,[6] which includes trade threats and corporate lobbying to secure stringent IP reforms and stronger international IP rules.[7] Moreover, developed countries, the WTO TRIPS Council and industry have created a 'web of surveillance' that puts additional pressure on developing countries.[8]

Hence, economic coercion is most tempting to use as an explanation when regulation has asymmetric financial implications, benefitting some countries at the expense of others.[9] Such is the case with IP regulations, at first glance, as Klug's study showed

[1] Morin and Gold (2014), p. 781 ('An Integrated Model of Legal Transplantation'). See also Helfer (2009), p. 39 ('Regime Shifting in the International').

[2] Ibid.

[3] Deere (2008), p. 21 (*The Implementation Game*), p. 2.

[4] Drahos (2004), pp. 401, 406.

[5] Braithwaite and Drahos (2000), p. 16.

[6] Bilateral and free trade agreements were the most potent form of economic pressure used by developed countries to secure TRIPS-Plus IP reforms in many targeted countries.

[7] Deere (2008) (n 3), p. 16.

[8] Ibid.

[9] Ibid.

regarding the US Government's attempt to threaten South Africa with trade sanctions, including the withdrawal of tariff preference and cutting off of foreign aid.[10] Yet South Africa resisted. Moreover, only states in structurally weaker positions are subjected to economic coercion. For example, the international financial organisations exercised much more leverage over Indonesia during the Asian financial crisis than they did over Korea, and they exercised no leverage over China.[11] Hence, the capacity of developing countries to resist was constrained to differing degrees by their economic, political and intellectual dependence on developed countries, international organisations and foreign corporations for investment, market access, development assistance and political security.[12]

In this regard, Drahos highlighted that most developing countries did not have prior knowledge of IP for proposals to the *TRIPS Agreement* and were therefore ill-prepared for the *TRIPS* negotiations,[13] demonstrating 'a high degree of ignorance amongst technology-importing countries as to the cost of increasing IP protection'.[14] Because of this ignorance, the perception of the developing countries was that *TRIPS* would increase much-needed FDI owing to harmonised IP laws, and they also they believed a stronger global IP regime would not only ensure certainty and predictability, but would also stimulate more local R&D devoted to the special needs of developing countries that are not felt in the technology exporting countries.[15] This was the main reason that developing countries agreed to *TRIPS*, at least in the first instance: out of necessity.

This element of economic coercion under the *TRIPS Agreement* could be examined through the perspective of neorealism. According to Sell, neorealism emphasises the role of power and leads to the expectation that weak states will comply with the preferences of powerful states.[16] For example, US policymakers have invested enormous amount of coercion to offer stronger IP. However, coercive strategies have failed to ensure IP protection.[17] Later, the US realised coercive strategies alone are not effective and sought to link trade and IP, which could yield better results. Thus, the US wields its market power through s 301 of its *Trade Act,* by applying direct pressure on targeted countries that fail to adequately protect IP, such as Brazil, South Korea, Argentina, Thailand and India, by threatening to impose trade sanctions.[18] Sell identified this development as a 'functional conversation and layering' process that resulted in institutional change.[19] This process significantly differs from the

---

[10] Klug (2008), p. 45. See also Shaffer (2012), p. 229 ('Transnational Legal Process').

[11] Shaffer (2012), p. 229 ('Transnational Legal Process'). Also see, Shafer (2021).

[12] Deere (2008) (n 7).

[13] Drahos (2000).

[14] Ibid.

[15] Vanni (2019), p. 1 (*Patent Games in the Global South)* 20.

[16] Sell (1995), p. 315 ('Intellectual Property Protection').

[17] Ibid.

[18] Ibid., p. 317.

[19] Sell (2010), p. 762 ('Rise and Rule').

constructivist discourse theory because it places stress on the role of material power, and often on the influence of institutional hierarchies.

By ratifying the *TRIPS Agreement*, developing countries were provided with two flexibilities to reach the required *TRIPS* standards.[20] First, they were given a time-based leeway to adjust their internal system towards compliance, and second, were allowed some flexibility to modify the *TRIPS* standards to make them more applicable to their own context in line with local regulatory needs.[21] These flexibilities were considered as alternatives, but changing the original *TRIPS* text was time-consuming and costly and the developing countries had to bear the costs. This shows coercive measures may initially be successful in inducing symbolic legal change, but ultimately, these changes might have to be modified or thwarted at the stage of actual implementation—the law in action—and, as a result, such measures may generate local resentment.[22]

Nonetheless, this discussion demonstrates how the WTO or Multi National Corporations ('MNCs') exert influence over developing countries through coercion and implementation to ensure these countries have strong patent regimes. Moreover, MNCs may adopt rules through a process of interaction and communication of ideas. However, even during *TRIPS* negotiations, some developing countries were anti-IP per se. For example, countries such as India expressed their interest in modernising and using IP systems in ways that might advance domestic innovations by acknowledging local IP differences, technological capacity and development.[23] India acknowledged that as their level of development rises, their interests in IP protection may expand to provide incentives to domestic innovation in order to derive stronger economic benefits.[24] Although the developed countries resisted these demands, India later creatively interpreted its terms to suit its local IP differences and national interest.

This type of resistance can spur a new politics that catalyses a practice of new global lawmaking.[25] As regards resistance, Kaczynski expressed the view that *TRIPS* has pulled Indian parliamentarians and patent examiners alike into a transnational discourse on patent law.[26] This implies, through dominance and coercive strategies, global scripts, including the *TRIPS*, have been transferred. However, when it came to reinterpretation, some countries, such as India, have made use of the *TRIPS* flexibilities to develop a new patent and PBR law. For example, incorporation of s 3(d) in the Indian *Patents Act, 1970* is a good and creative example of a coexistence

---

[20] Brandl et al. (2019), p. 826 ('Foreign Actors and Intellectual Property').

[21] Ibid.

[22] Shaffer (2012) (n 11), pp. 253–254.

[23] Deere (2008) (n 12), p. 29.

[24] Ibid.

[25] Shaffer (2012) (n 22).

[26] Kapczynski (2009), p. 1571. It required them to 'skill up' at home in order to be able to operate on the global stage; see Shaffer (2012) (n 85).

approach to patents and the right to health,[27] and of the Indian policymakers resistance to *TRIPS* demands regarding the patentable subject matter issue.[28] Moreover, using *TRIPS* flexibilities, Indian policymakers designed a PVR law that benefited not only breeders of new plant varieties but also farmers.[29] This is another instance regarding the acknowledgement of local IP differences.[30] In this sense, discourses can be more informative in explaining and interpreting when and why global legal norms are resisted, adapted and appropriated than theories based just on the global political context and economic power.[31] This aspect will be investigated empirically through the case studies in this book.

In this regard, Dinwoodie and Dreyfuss stated that in the area of IP, local lawmaking is subject to international lawmaking processes. Likewise, international lawmakers must consider political strategies found in national lawmaking, such as trade-off practices and the need to refer to technological capacities and social practices in fashioning the appropriate level of legal protection.[32] Yet, this IP difference is not recognised by developed countries. However, as discussed above Sect. 2.3, in many developing countries, local nodes proved important in determining the extent to which the *TRIPS* high-technology IP standards were transplanted, reinterpreted, resisted or ignored.[33]

2.4 Legal Transplants

Internationally, legal transfers originate from the developed North to the developing South, in the belief that a global script can convey legal meaning.[34] This perception was strongly influenced by modernisation theory, which stresses the point that transferred knowledge could engineer economic development in the global South by transplanting US and European institutions and substantive law.[35] This view is aligned with the positivist notion that global scripts are instruments to transfer legal and regulatory ideas on the basis that global scripts are variables—'things out there'—that can communicate norms across cultural borders almost mechanically.[36]

This view subsequently changed because the meaning conveyed by legal transfers is strongly influenced by the habits and patterns of thought in recipient countries. Hence, it was accepted that legal transfers are socially constructed, which

---

[27] Sellin (2015), p. 445.

[28] Arup (2012), p. 121 ('Transfer of Pharmaceutical Patent Laws').

[29] Perera (2021), p. 664 ('Searching for a Balance').

[30] Deere (2008) (n 23).

[31] Shaffer (2012) (n 25).

[32] Dinwoodie and Dreyfuss (2004), p. 95.

[33] Gillespie (2012), p. 29 ('Relocating Global Scripts'); Also see, Helfer (2015) (n 1).

[34] Gillespie (2012) (n 33).

[35] Ibid.

[36] Ibid.

attributes to social constructionism,[37] and therefore, social constructionism concerns the role of human agency in shaping the global scripts, including, very much so, local actors and processes. Consequently, it was accepted that legal transfers are socially constructed.[38] In other words, practices, procedures, habits and responses to global scripts of the receiving state actors play a decisive role in recipient countries under social constructionism. Some such recursive studies of legal transplantation have focused their interest on resistance, and others on harmonisation, to explain legal transplantation in situations of asymmetric interests.[39]

Going against this perception, some researchers have argued that global scripts are conveyed through standardised and repetitive processes, such as filling out security documents, which signifies mechanical practices to convey meaning to a global script without the intervention of human agency.[40] This supports the new institutional theory developed by Piaget that says people learn from new ideas because human beings are adaptive organisms and attempt to reconcile observations about their environment that clash with their cognitive understanding. On this basis, the North argues that the recipients have few opportunities to reflectively interpret global scripts.[41]

However, once a global script is to be transferred, the recipient states construct and reinterpret its meaning. Within this context, interpretive communities or epistemic communities are used for reflective interpretation of global scripts. As outlined above, Gunther Teubner, drawing from systems theory, argued that recipient legal systems absorb global ideas, but interpret them according to an internal normative logic.[42] According to him, global scripts have the effect of dialogical exchanges between the legal and other social subsystems in recipient states, but such terms lack precision to determine the type of dialogical exchanges of members in the host country.[43] To determine it precisely, the study needs to examine particular discourses.

In some cases, recipients unwittingly change the meaning of global scripts through fruitful or deleterious misunderstandings; in other cases, they might simply defer to prestigious external systems of legal knowledge, such as patents policy.[44] Hence, these countries have adopted laws and policies for IP protection, believing it to be an essential part of shifting towards a market economy. This perspective contrasts with the power imbalance explanations of neorealism but emphasises the reasoning of interpretivist neoliberalism.

This view examines the role of learning and norms as sources of change and focusses more squarely on the redefinition of national interests. It corresponds with Shaffer, Nedumpara and Sinha's findings from a case study on India in which they

---

[37] Lessing (1995), p. 992.

[38] Ibid.

[39] Morin and Gold (2014) (n 1), p. 783.

[40] Riles (2008), p. 605.

[41] Piaget (1977).

[42] Teubner (1998), pp. 18–19 ('Legal Irritants').

[43] Gillespie (2012) (n 34), p. 37.

[44] Ibid., p. 31.

argued that India as a state has adopted a new development model through transplantation involving a stronger emphasis on trade in light of its membership of the WTO, but nevertheless pursued according to India's needs.[45]

2.5 Sri Lanka: Coercion or Transplantation of Legal Rules

In the above context, Sri Lanka initially adopted *TRIPS* because the WTO promoted its own legal rules as constituting the common standard governing IP law, which was mandatory for WTO members, including Sri Lanka. Sri Lanka became an original member of the WTO at its inception in 1995. This is one of the mechanisms of legal transplants discussed by Morin and Gold as 'contractualisation'.[46] Under this mechanism, Contracting Parties do not necessarily experience a balanced outcome, and the boundary between coercion and contractualisation blurs, particularly when a country's leaders feel compelled to enter into a treaty to avoid economic harm, as Sri Lanka did in most instances.[47]

Moreover, under the *TRIPS* agenda, particularly with regard to the *TRIPS* 'flexibilities', individual members had to select the best possible way to respect the *TRIPS* obligations. Most countries adopted foreign rules, without exception, regardless of whether doing so was effective in addressing domestic issues, aiming to better position their country in a competitive way which Morin and Gold have discussed as 'regulatory competition'.[48]

Foreign rules have been transplanted into Sri Lanka on many occasions, which supports Morin and Gold's explanation. Such transplantation commenced during British colonisation when many English laws were transferred to Sri Lanka, and even today, some of its laws are fully based on English laws, for example, the *Trust Ordinance*,[49] *the Evidence Ordinance*[50] and *the Company's Act*.[51] Legal transplantation is a common approach adopted by many countries to implement legislation but, as discussed previously, the discourse may insist that the transplanted law should align with the practices, procedures, habits and responses to the global scripts of the receiving state.

At present, practically all countries make use of these transplant mechanisms in formulating legislation. For example, the first *Code of Intellectual Property Act (No 52 of 1979)* was based on the WIPO *Model Law for Developing Countries on Inventions* ('*Model Law*') for developing countries. When the law was introduced in

[45] Shaffer et al. (2015), p. 595.

[46] Morin and Gold (2014) (n 39).

[47] Burris et al. (2005), p. 11 ('Nodal Governance'); Sell (2004), p. 363 ('Quest for Global Governance').

[48] Morin and Gold (2014) (n 46).

[49] *Trust Ordinance No.09 of 1917.*

[50] *Evidence Ordinance No. 14 of 1895.*

[51] *Company's Act No. 7 of 2007.*

1979, there was no feasibility study undertaken to examine the suitability of the Act. Nevertheless, the law was transformed without exceptions, whether or not this was effective in addressing domestic issues, aiming to better position their country in a competitive way. This aspect will be further discussed in Chap. 3.

Moreover, with regard to PVR legislation, the International Union for the Protection of New Varieties of Plants (UPOV) was established by the *International Convention for the Protection of New Plant Varieties* (*UPOV Convention*). *UPOV Convention* has been the Model Law that influenced most countries in drafting their law, and thus, the *UPOV* Model has been transplanted into many jurisdictions although *TRIPS* do not actually specify that the UPOV model must be followed or, for that matter, which of the versions of UPOV, crucially 1978 or 1991. This is a well-accepted principle, but Sri Lanka has not signed either the 1978 or the 1991 Acts of the *UPOV Convention*. However, if the law is transferred, the transplanted law should match the legal culture of the recipient state. In other words, the discourse insists the transplanted law should be adopted, adapted and adjusted to the host legal system.[52] Otherwise, this law will be alien to the recipient state. Unfortunately, Sri Lankan legislators overlooked the existing economic and social conditions when drafting the proposed Bill in 2001. This aspect has been discussed in Chap. 4.

They borrowed legislation from overseas, but in reality, the transfer or the adoption of legislation from elsewhere requires more than copying rules, structures and institutions. It requires an understanding of the background of the legal system and how it accurately functions in the real world. The main question surrounding the transplant approach is whether the law can be transplanted into a different legal and social system and still work efficiently in the host legal system. As will be discussed in Chap. 4, both Thailand and India modified and borrowed PVR law to suit their conditions.

However, Sri Lankan legislators failed to address the local conditions, such as the agricultural system, the farming structure, the farmers' involvement in seed production and the number of seeds saved, before drafting the proposed Bill. In other words, the transplanted law was not socially constructed in Sri Lanka because it did not reflect the social, economic or cultural conditions or attitudes in Sri Lanka. This aspect will be discussed in Chap. 4. Yet, coercion is not an adequate explanation for the transplantation of global scripts in Sri Lanka. That is, Sri Lanka did not adopt foreign rules owing to coercion alone, but transplanted such law for regulatory competition, aiming to receive benefits from the transplanted law.

Yet, years later, Sri Lanka has not modified its patent administration, its PVR Bill is still not law and its STI strategy is unfulfilled, suggesting there is no coercion from developed countries pushing it to pass the PVR law or innovation policies. This aspect will be discussed in Chaps. 3–5. Hence, the mechanisms discussed by Morin and Gold should act in a mutually supportive manner. Comprehensive explanation of legal transplantation and local adaptation must include the identification

---

[52] Donavanik (1999), p. 195.

of mutual reinforcement between global and local causal mechanisms, rather than simply ranking their relative contributions.[53]

2.6 Global Lawmaking Processes

This finding does not mean that global lawmaking is not relevant to Sri Lanka; it is just not determinative. It is still the other broad source of IP discourse, along with the local, which has become increasingly important to lawmaking, especially since the formulation of the *TRIPS Agreement* in 1995. Here, this book identifies the actors and processes that shape the global discourses that feed into the Sri Lankan subsystems and interact with local discourses.

2.6.1 Informal and Formal Lawmaking

Global lawmaking consists of formal and informal lawmaking discourses. Some states choose either of these processes or might use both simultaneously. Informal lawmaking refers to processes that are literally 'informal' in the sense that they dispense with certain formalities traditionally linked to international law dimensions, which include output, process and actors.[54] Informal output mainly refers to soft law,[55] while informal process refers to a loosely organised network rather than an international organisation and an informal actor refers not to traditional diplomatic heads, but domestic regulators, independent or semi-independent agencies directly engaging in international governance.[56]

These informal actors communicate horizontally for technical assistance between various patent offices or between NGOs. They do not necessarily work in the direction of high technology protection. An example of a relatively successful informal lawmaking is the North–South discourse between the developing countries and North-based NGOs, such as the Doctors Without Borders, concerning the recognition, scope and enforcement of pharmaceutical patent rights.[57] Together, they counter US pressure on developing countries to enforce US pharmaceutical company patents under a strict interpretation of the *TRIPS Agreement*.[58]

---

[53] Morin and Gold (2014).

[54] Pollack and Shaffer (2012).

[55] Ibid.

[56] Ibid.

[57] Shaffer (2006), p. 177 ('The Challenges of WTO Law').

[58] Ibid.

2.6.2 TRIPS Agreement as a Global Lawmaking Process

Nevertheless, within the context of this book, the *TRIPS Agreement* is the key global instrument that comes within the formal lawmaking process, which involves state and private actors working through state representatives with legally binding rules through its formal diplomatic negotiating procedures. By the time *TRIPS* was signed, most developing countries, including Sri Lanka, had the required formal institutions of IP regulation, the level of IP protection standards and the required enforcement mechanisms in place.[59] For example, all WTO members are required to adhere to minimum standards of IP protection whether by way of patents and PVR. Article 27(1)(b) of the *TRIPS Agreement* mandates that members should protect plant varieties either by patents or any sui generis system. Hence, art 27 becomes an important global discourse for PVR. In addition to this article, the *UPOV Convention* became an important global actor for PVR discourse because following the ratification of the *TRIPS Agreement* many developing countries ratified the *UPOV Convention*, particularly the 1978 Act, as a sui generis option for the protection of plant varieties under the *TRIPS Agreement*. This aspect will be discussed in Chap. 4.

After the *TRIPS Agreement* was ratified, the US and the European Commission extended its provisions into regional and bilateral trade investment treaties and pushed developing countries to adopt these treaties.[60] Alter and Meunier explained this strategy as 'regime shifting'.[61] Regime shifting enabled powerful and weaker states and their allies to relocate rulemaking initiatives to international venues concerned with other issues, such as foreign investment or biodiversity, and such shifting benefited mostly the shifters' interest rather than those of the other parties.[62]

In contrast, developing countries too have been able to obtain support from many international bodies, such as the World Health Organization, using soft-law instruments to promote a more flexible reading of the *TRIPS Agreement*, especially in the *2001 Doha Declaration on the TRIPS Agreement and Public Health* ('*Doha Declaration*') of the WTO.[63] By engaging in these discursive strategies, developing countries have arguably made WTO law less clear and determinant, prompting the US to withdraw *TRIPS* claims against both South Africa and Brazil, undermining the purported advantage of formal lawmaking, but giving member countries more flexibility.[64]

---

[59] Pollack and Shaffer (n 54).

[60] Helfer (2004), p. 71 ('Regime Shifting: TRIPs Agreement').

[61] Alter and Meunier (2009), p. 13.

[62] Helfer, 'Regime Shifting: TRIPs Agreement' (n 60).

[63] Shaffer, 'The Challenges of WTO Law' (n 57).

[64] Helfer, 'Regime Shifting: TRIPs Agreement' (n 62). See also Helfer (2015), p. 311.

2.6.3 MNCs Influence in Lawmaking

The influence of MNCs is also an example of formal global lawmaking, although they also bring their influence to bear informally, for example, in the way they transfer their technology. As indicated above, during the *TRIPS* negotiations, when IP was linked with trade policy, it led to the dynamic influence and participation of US MNCs, which became the new coalition that actively shaped the agenda for national IP legislation and, by corollary, the foreign trade policy of the US Government such as the US Trade Representative to investigate against foreign governments and take appropriate actions.[65] This 'appropriate action' often consists of the threat of retaliation via trade sanctions via s 301 of the US *Trade Act*.[66] The new coalition thus became a superstructural node within the global legal process, bringing a more disparate set of interests and a more ambitious set of objectives.[67]

The MNCs had a deep structural impetus for economic globalisation by increasing capital mobility and competitiveness via IP.[68] This vertical move by the MNCs influenced developing countries to introduce changes in trade policy, which gave rise to a trade lobby and a focus on promoting exports, global and FDI markets.[69] As a result of this pressure, US, European and Japanese companies suggested a draft text of an IP agreement and those companies invariably joined the IP issue to become a superstructural node that no government could ignore.[70] In this scenario, MNCs pushed developing countries to reach the high IP protection standards prevalent in advanced countries for their benefit.[71]

Moreover, after the ratification of the *TRIPS Agreement*, these lobbies have forcefully asserted their rights under WTO law against countries such as South Africa and Brazil, regarding protection of pharmaceutical patents, which have, in turn, attempted to use other, and mostly informal, lawmaking forums to reframe the issue as one of health policy considerations.[72] By doing so, these countries insisted that developing countries recognise patents, for example, on pharmaceutical products, which has implications for both the cost of patented medicines and the long-term fate of the generic industries in those countries. Overall, the literature has shown that a greater influence of MNCs in the domestic innovation systems of developing countries resulted in more stringent *TRIPS* adoption and convergence with IP protection standards in advanced countries.[73]

With regard to these strategies used by powerful states, some scholars have argued that powerful countries are best able to use fragmented international regimes through

[65] Drahos and Mayne (2002), p. 164.

[66] Sell, 'Intellectual Property Protection' (n 16).

[67] Sell, 'Rise and Rule' (n 19), p. 770.

[68] Sell, 'Quest for Global Governance' (n 47), p. 368.

[69] Ibid.

[70] Drahos and Mayne (n 65).

[71] Brandl et al., 'Foreign Actors and Intellectual Property' (n 20).

[72] Ibid., p. 23.

[73] Ibid.

formal strategies, such as bilateralism, for they are powerful and well resourced. In contrast, some have argued that in some ways, weaker players are better off in such a world since they have multiple forums capable of dealing with similar agendas.[74] Hence, formal and informal lawmaking discourses can be used by both powerful and non-powerful actors to interact with each other to either influence or to undermine parties.

2.6.4 International Treaties

The *TRIPS Agreement* and the US Government/MNCs follow-up are not the only global discourses on IP. WIPO, the *Paris Convention for the Protection of Industrial Property* ('*Paris Convention*'), *PCT*, *Convention on Biological Diversity* ('*CBD*'), and the *International Treaty on Plant Genetic Resources for Food and Agriculture* ('FAO treaty') can be considered global nodes that affect IP too.

Sri Lanka has ratified all these international treaties and conventions. The *Paris Convention* applies to industrial property in the widest sense, including patents, trademarks, industrial designs, utility models, service marks, trade names, geographical indications and the repression of unfair competition. The *Paris Convention*, concluded in 1883, was revised at Brussels in 1900, at Washington in 1911, at The Hague in 1925, at London in 1934, at Lisbon in 1958 and at Stockholm in 1967, and was amended in 1979 in WIPO.[75] This moderation resulted in the US shifting IP deliberations out of WIPO into the *General Agreement on Tariffs and Trade* ('*GATT*').[76] Sri Lanka acceded to the *Paris Convention* in June 1978.[77]

The *Convention Establishing the World Intellectual Property Organization* ('*WIPO Convention*'), the constituent instrument of WIPO, was signed at Stockholm on 14 July 1967, entered into force in 1970 and was amended in 1979.[78] WIPO is an intergovernmental organisation that in 1974 became one of the specialised agencies of the UN system and a governing node for IP protection. Currently, there are 193 Contracting Parties to WIPO.[79] It actively provides technical assistance to developing countries as they seek to comply with *TRIPS*. Those who pay WIPO's freight undoubtedly shape its advocacy, and it has urged a number of developing

---

[74] 'Ibid.

[75] *Paris Convention for the Protection of Industrial Property* of March 20, 1983 [as amended on September 28, 1979].

[76] Sell, 'Quest for Global Governance' (n 68), p. 384.

[77] World Intellectual Property Organization (1967).

[78] World Intellectual Property Organization, Convention establishing the world intellectual property organization. Convention Establishing the World Intellectual Property Organization (wipo.int)Convention.

[79] World Intellectual Property Organization, Contracting parties of the treaties administered by WIPO. https://www.wipo.int/export/sites/www/treaties/en/documents/pdf/wipo_convention.pdf.

countries to adopt '*TRIPS-Plus*' provisions in their national legislation.[80] For developing countries, *TRIPS-Plus* provisions will be disadvantageous because these aims to introduce a higher level of protection norms that will undermine the domestic manufacturing sectors, such as generic drug manufacturing in India. WIPO is also conducting negotiations on the Substantive Patent Law Treaty, which is still in the draft form, that aims to harmonise patent law globally. This effort too is criticised by the developing countries. Sri Lanka joined WIPO on 20 June 1978.

The *Patent Cooperation Treaty* (*PCT)* assists applicants in seeking patent protection internationally for their inventions, helps patent offices with their patent granting decisions and facilitates public access to a wealth of technical information relating to those inventions.[81] The *PCT* enables to seek patent protection for an invention in each of the member countries simultaneously by filing a single 'international' application 'instead of filing several applications in the countries where the protection is expected'.[82] Sri Lanka's accession to the *PCT* took place on 26 November 1981.[83] The PCT offers developing countries assistance with their examination of patent applications by referring them to International Searching Authorities (patent offices in the developed world). WIPO more generally offers developing countries (including Sri Lanka) technical assistance with local adaptation to a global IP regime.

The *Convention on Biodiversity* (*CBD)* is another global discourse that includes IP elements. Unlike *TRIPS* and the WIPO efforts, it more explicitly and squarely incorporates provisions that developing countries favour such as recognition and reward for traditional knowledge.[84] The *CBD* conception challenges the *TRIPS* rules that endorse the Western, individualistic conception of knowledge ownership. The *CBD* stresses that biological resources are sovereign resources of states whereas *TRIPS* enforce private property rights over them.[85] Sri Lanka signed the UN *CBD* in 1994.[86]

FAO is a specialised UN agency that leads international efforts to defeat hunger and improve nutrition and food security.[87] Sri Lanka became a member of the *International Treaty on Plant Genetic Resources for Food and Agriculture* ('*FAO Treaty*') in 2013.[88] FAO recognises the rights of plant breeders as well as farmers and the need to balance the two, and there is a close relationship between FAO and the *CBD*. This issue will be discussed in Chap. 4.

---

80 Sell 'Quest for Global Governance' (n 68).

81 World Intellectual Property Organization, PCT—the international patent system. PCT–The International Patent System (wipo.int).

82 Ibid.

83 World Intellectual Property Organization (1981).

84 Sell, 'Rise and Rule' (n 67), p. 770.

85 Ibid.

86 Convention on Biological Diversity (1993).

87 Food and Agriculture Organization (2022).

88 Food and Agriculture Organization (2013).

2.6.5 Agreement on Trade Related Investment Measures (TRIMS) Influence on Lawmaking

TRIMS[89] is another global node that applies only to measures that affect trade in goods, not direct foreign investment, which, in the absence of a multilateral investment agreement, are regulated at the bilateral or national levels. This is another example of formal lawmaking. The agreement, concluded in 1994, was negotiated under the WTO's predecessor, the *GATT*, and came into force in 1995.[90] The agreement was agreed to by all WTO members.[91] It is one of the four principal legal agreements of the WTO trade treaty.

The *TRIMS* recognise that certain trade-related investment measures can have trade-restrictive and distorting effects, and therefore no member shall apply a measure that is prohibited by the provisions of *GATT* art III (national treatment) or art XI (quantitative restrictions).[92] It states that WTO members may not apply any measure that discriminates against foreign products or that leads to quantitative restrictions, to the WTO basic principles.[93] This issue is especially relevant to the third case study on the discourses on STI. TRIMS also prohibit the members from applying certain local performance requirements, such as technology transfer, to trade in goods. But it does not apply to direct investments. These requirements are the target of some bilateral free trade agreements; there is still no multilateral agreement on investment.

As discussed above, formal global legal actors and processes comprise superstructural nodes, such as WTO's *TRIPS* and *TRIMS*, WIPO, *PCT*, *CBD*, FAO, UPOV, foreign national governments and MNCs. These nodes are more powerful than local actors are in the global legal process. Within the IP arena, the most powerful global actors, arguably, are the WTO, developed countries, such as the US and the European Union ('EU') countries and the MNCs. They are superstructural nodes for they can channel their resources to exert simultaneous influence at the local, national and global levels.[94]

---

[89] World Trade Organization, Agreement on Trade-Related Investment Measures (TRIMS) (Web Page). https://www.wto.org/english/tratop_e/invest_e/trims_e.htm. ('TRIMS').

[90] World Trade Organization, Agreement on trade-related investment measures: historical background (Web Page) https://www.wto.org/english/tratop_e/invest_e/invest_info_e.htm#fntext-1 ('Historical Background').

[91] The agreement contains transitional arrangements allowing members to maintain notified *TRIMS* for a limited time following the entry into force of the WTO (two years in the case of developed country members, five years for developing country members, and seven years for least developed country members). The agreement also establishes a committee on *TRIMS* to monitor the operation and implementation of these commitments.

[92] WTO, Historical Background (n 164). See also Civello (1999).

[93] WTO, *TRIMS* (n 156).

[94] Vanni, *Patent Games in the Global South* (n 15), p. 55.

2.6.6 Free Trade Agreements ('FTAs')

The global lawmaking process also includes bilateral and multilateral FTAs. Since these FTAs are between states, these come within a formal lawmaking mechanism. Under FTAs, products from one country that enter another are not subject to import tariffs or quotas. Sri Lanka has signed a few FTAs with India, Pakistan and Singapore. Significantly, it has not entered into FTAs with the US or the EU.

The commercial relations between Sri Lanka and India reached a historical milestone when the *India-Sri Lanka Free Trade Agreement* was signed on 28 December 1998, as the first bilateral FTA of Sri Lanka. The FTAs with India and Pakistan cover only trade in goods that provide for duty-free entry as well as duty preferences for manufactured and agricultural goods.[95]

The Singapore-Sri Lanka FTA came into force on 1 May 2018, and it covers investment, goods, services, trade facilitation, government procurement, telecommunications, e-commerce and dispute settlement.[96] Here, Sri Lanka has eliminated customs duties on 50% of tariff lines (including tariff lines already with zero duty), which will progressively increase to 80% over 14 years.[97] Sri Lanka will not reduce or eliminate duties on the remaining 20% of tariff lines. Sri Lanka is also a member of the South Asian Free Trade Area[98] and the *Asia–Pacific Trade Agreement*.[99] Most of these agreements are non-IP agreements that target trade facilitation, which is designed to increase FDI to the country. This aspect will be discussed in Chap. 5. Moreover, Sri Lanka signed a bilateral agreement in 1991 with the US to provide adequate and effective protection and enforcement of IPR in patents, trademarks, copyrights, trade secrets and layout designs for integrated circuits.[100]

2.6.7 Right to Development

In addition to bilateral and multilateral agreements, the right to development ('RtD') and IP fall within the multilateral framework under the global lawmaking process. The RtD has been endorsed by the UN *Declaration on the Right to Development* arts 1.1 and 1.2 as a human right aspect, although developing countries have not explicitly invoked the RtD in IP forums, such as WIPO and the WTO.[101]

---

[95] Joshi (2010).

[96] Ceylon Chamber of Commerce (2018).

[97] Ibid.

[98] The nations participating in this agreement are Afghanistan, Bangladesh, Bhutan, India, Maldives, Nepal, Pakistan and Sri Lanka.

[99] International Trade Administration (2021).

[100] Agreement on the Protection and the Enforcement of Intellectual Property Rights between the United States of America and the Democratic Socialist Republic of Sri Lanka (1991).

[101] Latif (2013).

However, the RtD and IP interface has been questioned by developed countries because they believe that there is a considerable tension between IP and the RtD. According to developed countries, the recognition of the RtD might be the basis to argue that states should cooperate in lowering levels of IP protection in some areas, or at least not to advance those levels.[102] This is mainly because developed countries as governing nodes that have strong IP protection are not willing to lower their standards, even if *TRIPS* lets them. However, some have argued that there is no conflict between IP and the RtD because if it turns out to be true that IP contributes to economic development, then there is no conflict.[103] Nevertheless, developed countries in general do not prefer this view.

In this context, Sri Lanka has emphasised the need to fully utilise the strong and holistic normative framework of the RtD, which allows nations in development efforts to realise the RtD.[104] This takes place in the context where the 2030 Sustainable Development Agenda (SDA) is complementary towards these efforts. Sri Lanka extended support to achieve SDA towards the finalisation and implementation of the RtD as expeditiously as possible. In this regard, Sri Lanka's position concerning the RtD has been supportive throughout the past 30 years, and it believes that revitalising global partnerships for sustainable development could play a significant role in creating an environment conducive for realising the RtD.[105] By doing so, developing countries too could contribute to this process by making efforts to strengthen South–South cooperation. This implies that Sri Lanka has accepted the operationalisation and realisation of the RtD at the international level, via the SDA, which comes under the global discourse, and hence, Sri Lanka is obliged to interact and communicate with other global actors to achieve these objectives, which include IP and development. The local interaction is discussed in the three case studies in this book.

2.7 Local Legal Processes

Within the Sri Lankan lawmaking process, it is important to explain the three following levels: domestic, national[106] and global. Together the domestic and the national comprise the local. For all three case studies, *TRIPS* are under the global level, as above, which will be discussed under the global legal process. In addition, WIPO, *PCT*, *TRIMS*, UPOV, *CBD* and the *FAO Treaty* are under the global level, which will also be discussed in the three case studies.

[102] Drahos (1999), p. 349.

[103] Ibid.

[104] Government of Sri Lanka (2017).

[105] Government of Sri Lanka (2016).

[106] Throughout the book I have used the word 'National' for Central State law and 'Domestic'.

for local law.

For the first case study on patent grant administration, the domestic level is insignificant; instead, it mainly operates at national and global discourses that influence the lawmaking process. This is because patent law is territorial, and the *IP Act 2003* of Sri Lanka stipulates the procedure of registering a patent under the national law. Any applicant (and their patent attorneys and lawyers) can submit a patent application that comes under the national level and is subject to the *IP Act*. As discussed in Chap. 1, most patent applications are low-technology-based innovations owing to the expertise and resources available in the country. This aspect will be discussed in Chaps. 3 and 5. The national level consists of actors in the IP regime, for example, legislators, ministries, the Minister of Industry and Commerce, the Minister of Science, Technology and Research, the DG of NIPO and other actors (eg patent examiners) that are closely connected to patent grant administration. These actors, processes and discourses will be discussed specifically in Chap. 3 of the book, in the first of the case studies.

However, PVR consists of all three levels. Legally, the national-level PVR consists of PVR Bills that have been drafted on multiple occasions to fulfil the international treaty requirements that have not yet been implemented. The domestic level includes stakeholder alliances with grassroot local farmers, NGOs, environmental groups and farmer organisations that have become prominent local actors in the PVR lawmaking process. As the second case study reveals, PVR of grassroot local people extends to include a wide range of subject matter, beyond what is recognised within existing IP high-technology rights and other protection systems. They are closely linked to the land, farming practices and traditions, environment and topographical conditions that come within the collective community rights of the farming community of Sri Lanka, which are tightly integrated into all other aspects of society because subsistence farming is the norm of Sri Lanka and most farmers are dependent on each other.

These features are at odds with conventional Western notions of IP. However, grassroot innovations have created a buzz over the past two decades, and scholars have started investigating its various dimensions.[107] In other words, local knowledge and local innovation are being increasingly threatened with enclosure within a high-technology IP regime that focuses purely on economic considerations at the expense of the social and cultural.[108] The global level includes to amend the PVR laws according to TRIPS Agreement. In this discourse, it is necessary to recognise, reward and protect these alternative options.[109] This aspect will be discussed in Chap. 4 in this book.

ST discourse consist of two levels: national and global. There is no such domestic-level government within ST mainly because the Ministry of Science, Technology, and Research (MSTR) has the mandate to coordinate ST in Sri Lanka through Coordinating Secretariat for Science, Technology and Innovation (COSTI) but IP matters vest with Ministry of Industry and Commerce ('MIC'). Still, in addition

[107] Sharma and Kumar (2019), p. 40.

[108] Forsyth (2015), p. 84.

[109] Perera, 'Searching for a Balance' (n 29).

to the ministry, universities, research institutes, scientists, researchers and policymakers play an important role in ST discourse through disseminating knowledge and fostering innovations locally and globally through collaborations and partnerships. These actors also advocate for government policies to promote high-technology innovations, such as nanotechnology. However, as will be discussed in Chap. 5, ST in Sri Lanka remains a low-technology field. Moreover, there are programs, workshops and training organised by the Ministry and other relevant institutions to take science and innovation to grassroots for boosting interest in science in schools in rural Sri Lanka. This aspect will be discussed in Chap. 5 of this book.

To obtain a fuller understanding of the lawmaking process on patent grant administration, PVR and STI lawmaking process in Sri Lanka, the following section will discuss the nature and the structure of the Sri Lankan Government, followed by the formal legislative process, local lawmaking processes and the role of actors in light of the theoretical framework of this study.

2.8 Nature and Structure of Sri Lanka Government

In the following section, the extent to which the electoral base, political parties and ministries are considered important nodes in the local lawmaking process is briefly discussed.

2.8.1 Electoral Base

From independence in 1948 up to 1977, the Sri Lankan electoral system was modelled on the Westminster parliamentary system. This was a legacy from the British colonial period. However, the *Constitution of the Democratic Socialist Republic of Sri Lanka*, promulgated in 1978 ('*1978 Constitution*') introduced a radical departure from the Westminster system and electoral districts. The Westminster system has constituencies with individual candidates nominated by recognised political parties or independent candidates. The candidate obtaining the highest number of votes in respect of the constituency is declared elected.

The Westminster system has many advantages. These include the ability to integrate effective governance with accountability and ensure collective responsibility, in which the entire executive branch is accountable for all decisions to the legislature. Further, this system promotes unity, encourages mandates to discuss important issues within the executive and requires all decisions within the executive to be unanimous.[110]

In contrast to the Westminster system, the electoral system introduced in Sri Lanka by the *1978 Constitution* is based on proportional representation. Accordingly, the Sri

[110] Ratnapala (1995).

Lankan Parliament consists of a total of 225 MPs, of which 196 MPs are elected from 22 electoral districts and 29 MPs selected within a nationwide constituency (National List). This system has been the basis for all parliamentary elections in Sri Lanka held after 1988. Given that the number of seats returned by a political party is largely proportional (with some important exceptions) to the number of votes it receives, this system seems inherently more democratic than the Westminster system.[111]

However, since the mid-1990s, there has been a clamour for reform of this system. A major flaw articulated by those calling for reform is that the preferential vote system has led to fierce intra-party competition.[112] As a result, candidates are more concerned about their individual victory, thus making the party system less important unlike in the Westminster system. Moreover, representatives elected under the system have indulged in political horse trading for ministerial offices and other forms of government patronage.[113] Most often, representatives end up shifting from opposition to the government after elections and it becomes difficult for voters to hold their representatives accountable and for the said representatives to feel accountable towards their voters.[114] As a result, both the voters and representatives cannot influence the lawmaking process. For example, a reason that the PVR law is not yet legislated might be the lack of accountability on both parties to influence the local lawmaking process.

2.8.2 Political Parties

The political party system in Sri Lanka too has contributed to the lawmaking process. In the general elections held between 1952 and 1977, a two-party system emerged in which the United National Party ('UNP') and the Sri Lanka Freedom Party ('SLFP') alternately secured majorities and formed governments.[115] The UNP is more aligned towards the centre-right in the political spectrum while the SLFP is a party with a relatively left-wing ideology (although this is no longer the case at present). The differences in the political ideologies have affected lawmaking in Sri Lanka. For example, as will be discussed in Chap. 5, the UNP is inclined towards introducing privatisation strategies while the SLFP has favoured a more welfare state approach and the development of the public sector.

Even though each party has a strong structure and a decision-making process within the party, evidence suggest, when a coalition is in power, this will lead to divisions and fractions which will affect the lawmaking process in the country. This happened in 2004, the SLFP-led UNFA coalition.[116] For example, Subsequent to

---

[111] Vollan and Ganeshathasan (2017).

[112] Ibid.

[113] Thaheer (2010), p. 97.

[114] Senaratne (2021).

[115] Ross and Savada (1988).

[116] Veraite Research (2017).

the general elections, the SLFP members of the UPFA in parliament diverged into two factions. Later on, it went on to form an informal faction known as the Joint Opposition (JO) in collaboration with other minor parties attached to the UPFA. Such unpopular tactics essentially aim to challenge the JO for influence over the majority voter base, which will have a detrimental effect to the people in Sri Lanka.[117]

2.8.3 *Ministries in Sri Lanka*

According to the 19th amendment to the *1978 Constitution*, the number of Cabinet Ministers is limited to 28.[118] In addition to the Cabinet ministries, there are 39 state ministries under the present government.[119] The President, in consultation with the Prime Minister, will determine the number of Ministers and ministries and the assignment of subject and functions to such ministries.[120] The President may from time to time change the assignment of subjects and functions and the composition of the Cabinet.[121]

As will be discussed in the three case studies, the different ministries can be regarded as important governing nodes within the IP ecosystem in the local lawmaking process. For example, any lawmaking on IP is taken by the MIC in consultation with NIPO and any other relevant departments. PVR lawmaking is handled by the Department of Agriculture ('DoA'), and STI lawmaking mainly comes under the Ministry of Science, Technology and Research ('MSTR'), which consults with other institutions and organisations.

As discussed in the three case studies, with multiple ministries dealing with the same subject matter and overlapping responsibilities have resulted in no single ministry taking responsibility in the IP lawmaking process. This shows lack of discourse among the ministries with regard to IP policy making and as a result still the PVR is still a draft and IP policy has been lagging for many years.

2.9 Formal Lawmaking Process

Within the local legal process, the following formal political hierarchy is established in Sri Lanka. According to the *1978 Constitution*, the Executive President is the head of state, the head of the executive and the government and the commander-in-chief of the armed services. The President appoints the Prime Minister, the judiciary and the

---

[117] Ibid.

[118] *Nineteenth Amendment to the Constitution* (Sri Lanka).

[119] Presidential Secretariat, State Ministers (Web Page). https://www.presidentsoffice.gov.lk/index.php/state-ministers-2/.

[120] *Sri Lanka Constitution* art 43(1).

[121] Ibid., art 43(3).

military chiefs; chairs the Cabinet; and has the power to appoint the Ministers and all the government officials. Most important ministerial portfolios, such as the Defence, Finance and Foreign Affairs, are generally held by the President. The President also has the power to dissolve the Parliament after one year of its election. Because the President is the executive, this position has shifted executive power away from the Cabinet, which had this power under the old parliamentary system, to an Executive President who is elected independently by the people and holds office for five years. The Executive President is an important node, responsible to the Parliament for due exercise, performance and discharge of presidential powers, duties and functions under the *1978 Constitution* and any written law but is not accountable to the Parliament. Hence, the Executive President's relationship with the Parliament is an unequal one.[122]

The implementation of any domestic law must be passed by the Parliament and any amendment to the *1978 Constitution* needs to be passed with a two-thirds majority in the Parliament.[123] However, the office of the President is a governing node with executive power, which has institutional capacity. The President has the strength and structure to mobilise its mentalities, resources and processes over time to influence the Cabinet to enact any legislation the country needs. For example, as a party leader, the President may exert influence over Members of Parliament through the party's power to replace them. Moreover, under a state of emergency, the President has the power to pass legislation without parliamentary consent. As a result, the Parliament may be reduced to little more than a rubber stamp, and the President is able to control both the Cabinet and the party.[124]

The local legal processes come into play when local legal actors and policymakers decide to draft legislation and bring it to the Parliament. The Parliament is responsible for national legislation. It is the most important source of law. There is little government activity that should be conducted at the national, provincial or local level without legislation. It covers areas such as welfare, commerce, communication, human rights, environment, insurance, income tax, foreign investments, health, employment and housing and numerous important areas in a rapidly changing world. This aspect is discussed under parliamentary process.

The Parliament is also responsible to give legislative effect to multilateral treaties, such as the *TRIPS Agreement* to which Sri Lanka has become a state-party. It has enacted many national legislations, but there is a long delay in its implementation of multilateral treaties compared with other Commonwealth countries.[125] Hence, treaties are not self-executing unlike in the United Kingdom ('UK'). For example, in the UK Parliament and in other Commonwealth Parliaments, there is still a parliamentary practice by which a treaty is laid before Parliament prior to its ratification/

---

122 Mendis, 'Legislative Law and Process' (n 122).

123 Rahman (2012).

124 Ibid.

125 Ibid.

accession by the executive. This practice was recognised by Erskine May,[126] as a matter of establishing 'open government' in foreign affairs.

This practice has not been followed consistently in Sri Lanka, but an argument has been mounted to revive it in appropriate circumstances, to enhance the proactive representational role of Parliament in foreign affairs.[127] Hence, regarding legislative power, the Parliament is supreme within the local legal process, but not in the international treaty-making process. However, in practice, the President is responsible to the Parliament. Nevertheless, in the context of Sri Lankan politics, which is based on a multi-party system, if the President and the majority of Members of the Parliament are from the same party, the President can influence the local lawmaking process if the two-thirds majority can be achieved. If this happens, the President becomes a superstructural node.

2.10 Conclusion

This chapter has employed the conceptual and theoretical framework that underpins this book is—that is, the lawmaking of local and global legal processes within the patent administration, PVR and STI sectors in Sri Lanka. To explain how the local and global legal processes work, this book employed the systems theory and nodal governance theory to show how actors within a society engage in governance through nodal networks that produce change. In highlighting how nodes act within a hierarchy, it showed where power is located, and that some nodes are more influential than the other in the legal process but this situation can vary depending on each case. Thus, in combining discourses with systems theory and nodal governance theory, the chapter analysed the extent to which the competing discourses identified in this chapter for the three case studies, i.e. high-technology and low-technology protection, have been able to promote innovation economy in Sri Lanka.

Within the local lawmaking discourse, local nodes, such as policymakers, and stakeholder alliances at the domestic and national level have been a vital factor in examining current events Sri Lanka's IP landscape. However, the data revealed that despite a change in the discourse with local policymakers and varying progress in stakeholders' motivation in areas of patent administration, PVR and STI, the IP ecosystem in Sri Lanka has not been subject to a leap in high-technology related development over the past few decades.

The reasons for this 'backwardness' include the maladministration of NIPO, a lack of discourses among actors to foster an innovation culture, the development of many ambitious technology policies that are not aligned with industrial policies, a lack of resources and funding for R&D that has resulted in creating low-technology innovations and, most importantly, a lack of commitment from the successive governments, which has become the biggest bottleneck to streamlining IP in Sri Lanka. This

[126] May (1989) (*Treatise on the Law*).

[127] Mendis (2005).

suggest that IP eco system in Sri Lanka has become backward due to disengagement and lack of communication among actors due to lack of nodal influence. This aspect will be discussed in Chaps. 3–5 in this book.

As regards the global legal process, the data revealed that the transplantation of foreign rules, such as *TRIPS*, MNCs, WIPO, *PCT* and TRIMS, was accepted by the government as a matter of economic necessity rather than coercion by foreign powers. Nevertheless, this meant it depended on the government following through with local policies and laws. There have been tentative moves, but no consolidation of a high-technology approach has taken place thus far, for the reasons outlined above. Global actors have offered to assist but have not pressed for conformity. This finding implies that local discourses have been more influential than global discourses in shaping the IP landscape in Sri Lanka.

Overall, in this chapter, theory has helped this researcher to understand where nodes are located and which actors have been promulgating an IP discourse through processes such as treaty-making, model legislation and technical assistance. However, theory has also alerted this researcher to the fact that local actors and processes matter too, for example, in legislating, government administration and coordinating. As a result, their discourses—either published or disclosed—were important material in the lawmaking process. Hence, the discourse was an appropriate medium or mode of study. Even when discussing lawmaking, there seems to be little evidence of coercion globally. Lawmaking was influenced more through dialogue and interaction, or inertia where one node talks past another. This aspect will be discussed in the three case studies.

Undoubtedly, treaties are made and legislation is passed, but this aspect is very much discursive, even globally. For example, *TRIPS* require what should be put in a Bill or left out and what should be the administrative practice. Nevertheless, what would be good for Sri Lanka and what strategy is good enough should indeed emanate from the Sri Lankan Government. Last, this book brings a unique perspective for understanding not only the IP lawmaking process in Sri Lanka, which has attracted limited research attention, but also the nodal interactions and discourses that occur in the country's IP ecosystem. The next chapter presents the first case study, in which the discourses on patent law reforms based on the theoretical framework of this book will be contextualised.

Competing Interests The author has no conflicts of interest to declare that are relevant to the content of this chapter.

References

Agreement on the Protection and the Enforcement of Intellectual Property Rights between the United States of America and the Democratic Socialist Republic of Sri Lanka (1991), September. https://www.bilaterals.org/?us-sri-lanka-ipr-agreement-1991

Alter KJ, Meunier S (2009) The politics of international regime complexity. Perspect Polit 7:1

Arup C (2012) The transfer of pharmaceutical patent laws: the case of India's paragraph 3(d). In: Gillespie J. Nicholson P (eds) Law and development and the global discourses of legal transfers. Cambridge University Press
Braithwaite J, Draho P (2006) Global business regulation. Cambridge University Press
Brandl K, Darendeli, Mudambi R (2019) Foreign actors and intellectual property protection regulations in developing countries. J Internat Bus Stud 50
Burris S, Drahos P, Shearing C 'Nodal Governance' (2005) Australian J Legal Philos 30
Ceylon Chamber of Commerce (2018) Insights and findings on the Sri Lanka-Singapore free trade agreement. Research Brief https://www.chamber.lk/index.php/news/179-insights-and-findings-on-the-sri-lanka-singapore-free-trade-agreement
Company's Act No. 7 of 2007
Convention on Biological Diversity (1992). 1760 UNTS 79, 31 ILM 818 (entered into force 29 December 1993)
Deere C (2008) The implementation game: the TRIPS agreement and the global politics of intellectual property reforms in developing countries. Oxford University Press
Dinwoodie GB, Dreyfuss RC (2004) TRIPS and the dynamics of intellectual property law making. Case Western Reserve J Int Law 36:1
Donavanik J (1999) The impact of plant intellectual property rights on Thailand's agriculture: implications of the agreement on trade-related aspects of intellectual property rights (PhD Dissertation), Stanford University
Drahos P (1999) Case comment: intellectual property and human rights. Intellect Prop Quart 3
Drahos P (2000) Trade-offs and trade linkages: TRIPS in a negotiating context. Quaker United Nations
Drahos P (2004) Intellectual property and pharmaceutical markets: a nodal governance approach. Temple Law Rev 77:2
Drahos P, Mayne R (2002) Global intellectual property rights: knowledge, access, and development. Palgrave Macmillan
Evidence Ordinance No. 14 of 1895
Food and Agriculture Organization (2013) Sri Lanka joins the international treaty on plant genetic resources for food and agriculture, 24 December. https://www.fao.org/plant-treaty/news/news-detail/es/c/341730/
Food and Agriculture Organization (2022) Food and agriculture organization of the United Nations (Web Page, 2022). https://www.fao.org/home/en
Forsyth M (2015) Making room for magic in intellectual property policy. In: Drahos P, Ghidini G, Ullrich H (eds) *KRITIKA*: essays on intellectual property. Edward Elgar Publishing
Gillespie J (2012) Relocating global scripts in local networks of meaning. In: Gillespie J, Nicholson P (eds) Law and development and the global discourses of legal transfers. Cambridge University Press
Government of Sri Lanka (2016) 32nd session of the human rights council: panel discussion on the promotion and protection of the right to development. Commemoration of the 30th Anniversary of the Declaration on the Right to Development. https://www.lankamission.org/images/pdf/PDF 2016/15_june_2016_RTD%20Panel%20SL%20statement.pdf
Government of Sri Lanka (2017) The eighteenth session of the working group on the right to development. https://www.lankamission.org/images/pdf/PDF2017/3%20April%202017%20-%20Statement%20by%20Sri%20Lanka-%20RTD%20final.pdf
Helfer LR (2004) Regime shifting: TRIPs agreement and new dynamics of international intellectual property lawmaking. Yale J International Law 29
Helfer LR (2009) Regime shifting in the international intellectual property system. Perspect Polit 7:1
Helfer LR (2015) Pharmaceutical patents and the human right to health: the contested evolution of the transnational legal order on access to medicines. In: Halliday T, Shaffer G (eds) Transnational legal orders. Cambridge University Press

International Trade Administration (2021) Sri Lanka—country commercial guide: trade agreements (Web Page, 28 September). https://www.trade.gov/country-commercial-guides/sri-lanka-trade-agreements

Joshi V (2010) An economic analysis of India–Sri Lanka free trade agreement. HEID Working Paper No 04/2010, Graduate Institute of International and Development Studies

Kapczynski A (2009) Harmonization and its discontents: a case study of TRIPS implementation in India's pharmaceutical sector. Calif Law Rev 97:6

Klug H (2008) Law, politics, and access to medicine in developing countries. Polit Soc 36:2

Latif AA (2013) Right to development and IP law: what implications for the multilateral framework. Conference Paper. https://www.ceipi.edu/websites/ceipi/Documents/Colloques/EIPIN_2013/Topic_17_Abdel_Latif.pdf

Lessing L (1995) The regulation of social meaning. Univ Chicago Law Rev 62:3

May E (1989) Treatise on the law, privileges, proceedings and usage of parliament, 2nd edn. Butterworth

Mendis DL (2005) Legislative law and process. The Island. http://www.island.lk/2005/07/29/features1.html

Morin JF, Gold ER (2014) An integrated model of legal transplantation: the diffusion of intellectual property law in developing countries. Int Stud Quart 58

Nineteenth Amendment to the Constitution (Sri Lanka)

Paris Convention for the Protection of Industrial Property of March 20, 1983 [as amended on September 28, 1979]

Perera A (2021) Searching for a balance: realisation of farmers' rights in Sri Lanka: a case study on ownership and stewardship. Eur Intellect Prop Rev 43:10

Piaget J (1977) The development of thought: equilibration and cognitive structures.The Viking Press

Pollack MA, Shaffer G (2012) The interaction of formal and informal law-making. Research Paper No 12-10, University of Minnesota Law School Legal Studies Research Paper Series

Presidential Secretariat, State ministers (Web Page). https://www.presidentsoffice.gov.lk/index.php/state-ministers-2/

Rahman T (2012) Parliamentary control and government accountability in South Asia: a comparative analysis of Bangladesh, Inida and Sri Lanka. Routledge, UK

Ratnapala S (1995) Westminster democracy and the separation of powers: can they co-exist? Parliament of Australia

Riles A (2008) The anti-network: private global governance, legal knowledge, and the legitimacy of state. Am J Comp Law 56:3

Ross RR, Savada AM (1988) Sri Lanka: a country study. GPO for the Library Congress

Sell SK (1995) Intellectual property protection and antitrust in developing world: crisis, coercion and choice. Int Organ 49

Sell SK (2004) The quest for global governance in intellectual property and public health: structural, discursive and institutional dimensions. Temple Law Rev 77

Sell SK (2010) The rise and rule of a trade-based strategy: historical institution and the international regulation of intellectual property. Rev Intellect Polit Econ 17:4

Sellin J (2015) Does one size fit all? patents, the rights to health and access to medicines. Netherlands Int Law Rev 62

Senaratne N (2021) Proportional representation: first-past-the-post or both. On Politics. Proportional Representation, First-Past-the-Post or Both? | by Nuwan I. Senaratna | On Politics | Medium

Shaffer G (2006) The challenges of WTO law: strategies for developing country adaption. World Trade Rev 5

Shaffer G (2012) Transnational legal process and state change. Law Soc Inq 37:2

Shafer G (2021) Emerging powers and the world trading system: the past and future of international economic law. Cambridge University Press

Shaffer G, Nedumpara J, Sinha A (2015) State transformation and role of lawyers: the WTO, India, and transnational legal order. Law Soc Rev 49:3

Sharma G, Kumar H (2019) Commercialising innovations from the informal economy: the grassroots innovation ecosystem in India. South Asian J Bus Stud 8:1
Teubner G (1998) Legal irritants: good faith in British law or how unifying law ends up in new divergences. Modern Law Rev 61:11
Thaheer M (2010) Why the proportional representation system fails to promote minority interests? a discussion on contemporary politics and the Sri Lanka Muslim congress. J Pow, Conf Demo 1:2
Trust Ordinance No. 09 of 1917
Vanni A (2019) General overview: patent games in the global south: pharmaceutical patent law making in Brazil. India and Nigeria. Hart Publishing, London
Veraite Research (2017) Mapping of Sri Lanka's political parties: actors and evolutions. https://www.veriteresearch.org/wpcontent/uploads/2018/06/Mapping_Sri_Lanka_s_Political_Parties_Actors_and_Evolution.pdf
Vollan K, Ganeshathasan L (2017) A system of electoral representation for Sri Lanka: the principles behind the choice. Working Paper No 16 on Constitutional Reforms
World Intellectual Property Organization (1981) Accession by democratic socialist Republic of Sri Lanka (PCT Notification No. 37, 3 December). https://www.wipo.int/treaties/en/notifications/pct/treaty_pct_37.html
World Intellectual Property Organization, Contracting parties of the treaties administered by WIPO. https://www.wipo.int/export/sites/www/treaties/en/documents/pdf/wipo_convention.pdf
World Intellectual Property Organization, Convention establishing the world intellectual property organization. Convention Establishing the World Intellectual Property Organization (wipo.int)Convention
World Intellectual Property Organization (1967) Paris notification No. 94: accession by the Republic of Sri Lanka to the Stockholm Act (with the exception of Articles 1 to 12). http://www.wipo.int/treaties/en/notifications/paris/treaty_paris_94.html
World Intellectual Property Organization, PCT—the international patent system. PCT–The International Patent System (wipo.int)
World Trade Organization, Agreement on trade-related investment measures (TRIMS) (Web Page). https://www.wto.org/english/tratop_e/invest_e/trims_e.htm ('TRIMS')
World Trade Organization, Agreement on trade-related investment measures: historical background (Web Page). https://www.wto.org/english/tratop_e/invest_e/invest_info_e.htm#fntext-1 ('Historical Background')
WTO (1999) Historical background (n. 164). See also Civello P (1999) The TRIMs agreement: a failed attempt at investment liberalization. Minnesota J International Law 97

Chapter 3
Discourses on Patent Law Reforms in Sri Lanka

Abstract This chapter examines the discourse around the settings for the Sri Lankan patent administration system against its constructs between actors, processes and discourses as the first case study. As identified in the documents and interviews, in this case study, the discourses about patentability, the standard of examination for patent applications and the procedures for review of decisions are areas of conflict between high-technology and low-technology patent requirements. These are certainly global discourses currently relevant, but it could also be that local discourses matter for it is about implementing appropriate systems to encourage development. The global discourses appear to be the strongest, but the data presented in this case study will reveal that resistance to this and other influences have led this to be a predominantly a local discourse.

3.1 Introduction

This case study involves interaction between global and local governance actors or nodes. The WTO's TRIPS agreement creates a framework favouring high technology patents, but it leaves much of the administration to the member country and its allies.

It transpires that within the framework of the international treaties, WIPO is the most germane of the prospective global contributors. It is widely recognised as an international node of influence for it actively administers international treaties and assists member countries in developing standards for IP law and in implementing systems to support national implementation, such as patent grant examination and other administration. In the arena of patents, WIPO has the mentalities, technologies, resources and institutional force to mobilise, assist and influence developing countries towards implementing systems that support high technology patent administration.

Nevertheless, the divergences identified from the interviews conducted for this book revealed that local discourses show differences arising over the appropriateness of the global patent laws, especially over the settings for the patent administration system for the local context. Regardless, the local discourse seems to disregard the

A. Perera, *Dilemmas of Intellectual Property Discourse in Sri Lanka*,
https://doi.org/10.1007/978-981-97-6117-3_3

conflicts with the global discourses and stick with a low technology system. This chapter will identify and characterise these discourses.

Thus, the subject matter of this case study is the patent system, which refers to patent law as established and administered by various local actors, such as legislatures, government departments, ambassadors, ministries, the patent office, examiners, courts, industry associations, NGOs, public interest groups, civic societies and patent attorneys, and international actors, such as the WTO and WIPO, their secretariats and consultants, key foreign governments and their patent offices and MNCs. It includes the different approaches and policies that have been characterised as discourses in this book, which are canvassed by these actors to assess patent applications and, in particular, the mechanism used for the standard patent examination whether it be formal or substantive examination. The discourse involves interaction between the two, global actors and local actors.

As identified in Chap. 2, global discourses, such as the WTO *TRIPS Agreement* and *WIPO Convention*, have influenced the national implementation of laws, patent administration and patent policy as part of nations' international obligations, while endeavouring to reconcile these obligations with their national economic plans and processes to the extent possible. In certain quarters, it was believed that this strategy would improve the IP protection quality, both in provision and administration, thus enhancing investment and development. The patent administration in the international discourse offers, but does not mandate, a range of norms, such as the coverage of all technologies; a substantive examination to apply a high technology threshold as regards the novelty, inventive step and industrial applicability criteria to a patent grant application; a modified examination; provision for pre- and post-grant opposition proceedings and CL methods within the patent system; and the availability of remedies for enforcement and review in the courts.

Significantly, this chapter shows that the current Sri Lankan patent system adopts few of these procedures in the patent granting process. For example, it does not provide a modified examination and pre-grant and post-grant opposition. That is, formal examination is provided under the Act, which is a very outdated system and rarely used in other jurisdictions. In contrast, substantive examination is provided only as an option under the Act one the applicant may request, but its applicability is very low because of several apparent reasons, such as a lack of demand, expertise and resources, and even, as shall be shown, a lack of commitment at the patent office level. Owing to these reasons, as identified in Chap. 1, the scope of patent protection in Sri Lanka is based on low technology, rather than high technology. The switch to high technology, which involves applying 'technical criteria' for patentability rigorously and rewarding high-ST inventions, would be demanding for Sri Lanka. This aspect will be further discussed in Chap. 5.

The debate and exploration of the appropriate option for Sri Lanka depend on how the discourse characterises the objectives of the patent system: A lower patentability requirement would make it easier for small independent local investors to obtain protection, considering the low ST base in Sri Lanka. In contrast, if the aim of the patent system is to raise the standard to international parity for foreign investors seeking to import or establish locally, or local inventors seeking to export or establish offshore, to ensure their applications are properly screened and their grants are technically defensible, a higher standard may be appropriate, or the two approaches can be combined within one system. Thus, this case study tests the research inquiries identified in Chap. 1 about whether the discourse supports a high- or low-technology-based strategy for Sri Lanka.

The landscape described by interviewees reveals nodal failures, and communication blockages between actors both locally and internationally. As will be seen in Sri Lanka's current system favours low-technology patent protection model which interviewees give many explanations includes lack of expertise and resources, the prior art search is inaccurate and, hence, the examination process is very basic, compared with that in other jurisdictions. In addition, a lower patentability protection would make it easier for small independent local investors to obtain protection, considering the low ST base in Sri Lanka. In contrast, if the aim of the patent system is to raise the standard to international parity for foreign investors seeking to import or establish locally, or local inventors seeking to export or establish offshore, to ensure their applications are properly screened and their grants are defensible, a higher standard may be appropriate, or the two approaches can be combined within one system. Hence, in this chapter there is a juxtaposition between characterising these global discourses, but it could also be local discourses for it is about implementing appropriate systems to encourage development based on the infrastructure and expertise. The global debate appears to be the strongest, but the discourse revealed by the interviews in this case study indicates resistance and other influences have led this to be a predominantly a local discourse. The debate and exploration of the appropriate option for Sri Lanka depend on how the discourse characterises the objectives of the patent system.

To examine the role of the nodes, this case study will throw light on how global and local governance actors or nodes who utilise power dynamics in developing an IP policy in Sri Lanka. It transpires that within the framework of the international treaties, like TRIPS, WIPO as the most germane of the prospective global contributors. It is widely recognised as an international node of influence for it actively administers international treaties and assists member countries in developing standards for IP law and in implementing systems to support national implementation, such as patent grant administration. In the arena of patents, WIPO has the mentalities, technologies, resources and institutional force to mobilise, assist and influence developing countries towards implementing systems that support patent administration. Nevertheless, the divergences identified from the interviews revealed local discourses demonstrates differences arising over the appropriateness of the global patent laws and over the settings for the patent administration system for the local context. Regardless, the conflicts have led the local discourse channels to resolve, avoid or disregard the conflicts. The lethargy of the NIPO is a key factor as NIPO is a structural node with access and direct communications being available with WIPO. This chapter will identify and characterise these discourses. To elucidate the power dynamics in Sri Lankan IP policy development, this case study will also examine how variety of actors within the patent administration system, have exerted influence with the other nodes through interaction and communications creating a social discourse thus, introducing and promoting recommendations in patent administration in Sri Lanka. However, to achieve this, first, the evolution of the current patent system will be mapped, including the influence from the WTO and WIPO, before examining the local discourse that interviewees identified were obstacles and alternatives that arise from this analysis.

3.2 Evolution of Patent Law in Sri Lanka: The Patent Framework

The study begins with a short history of the legislation. The law on IP was first introduced to Sri Lanka during the British colonial period. The *British Investor's Ordinance of 1859* was the first statute on IP law in Sri Lanka under which the first Sri Lankan patent was granted in 1860. According to Drahos, these laws were implemented to suit the colonialists, not the colonies, given that they manoeuvred English law into Sri Lanka for the benefit of the UK in a foreign jurisdiction.[1]

In 1977, Lakshman Kadirgamar, as the WIPO head, that is, the WIPO Asia–Pacific Bureau Director ('WAPBD'), held discussions with the President of the Bar Association of Sri Lanka, Dr HW Jayewardene and the Minister of Trade and Shipping Lalith Athulathmudali, to assist Sri Lanka in revising its IP laws.[2] Pursuant to these discussions, in September 1977, the late Mr Lalith Athulathmudali appointed a committee to revise the IP laws in keeping with the commercial policies of the Government.[3]

IP laws at that time comprised several archaic ordinances, such as the *Merchandise Marks Ordinance 1888*,[4] *Designs Ordinance 1904*,[5] *Patents Ordinance 1906*,[6] *Copyright Act 1911*,[7] *Copyright Ordinance 1912*[8] and *Trademarks Ordinance 1925*,[9] which were all transplanted into Sri Lanka during the colonial period.

The IP discourse in Sri Lanka emerged when Lakshman Kadirgamar submitted a set of model laws through WIPO, which the Law Revision Committee accepted with modifications and amendments to suit Sri Lanka. The first seminar organised by the Sri Lankan authorities and WIPO to discuss the changes to the IP law was held in Colombo in 1977.[10] On 25 May 1979, the Parliament of the Democratic Socialist Republic of Sri Lanka enacted the *Code of Intellectual Property Act No 52 of 1979*

---

[1] Drahos (2010).

[2] Kadirgamar (2013).

[3] Ibid.

[4] Merchandise Marks Ordinance No 13 of 1888.

[5] Designs Ordinance No. 7 of 1904.

[6] Patents Ordinance No. 15 of 1906.

[7] Copyright Act 1911.

[8] Copyright Ordinance no 12 of 1912.

[9] Trademarks Ordinance no 15 of 1925.

[10] Kadirgamar (2013) (n 2).

('*IP Code*'). The *IP Code* marked a clear turning point in the evolution of the IP lawmaking in Sri Lanka because this was the first local enactment of IP legislation.

However, the first *Code of Intellectual Property Act (No 52 of 1979)* was based on the WIPO *Model Law for Developing Countries on Inventions* ('*Model Law*') for developing countries. When the law was introduced in 1979, there was no feasibility study undertaken to examine the suitability of the Act. Nevertheless, the law was transposed without exceptions, whether or not this was effective in addressing domestic issues, aiming to better position their country in a competitive way. This aspect will be further discussed later in this Chapter.

The objective of the *IP Code* was to provide an environment conducive to economic and commercial development in the country.[11] The Minister for Trade and Shipping Mr Lalith Athulathmudali in May 1979 declared in the Parliament:[12]

> One of the things we started on was trying to reform and bring up to date commercial law in this country. As regards to patents, we are going to avail ourselves of the International Search Reports [the *PCT*]. This is necessary for our commercial law. But while we went through this, we found something very unfortunate; 99% of patents, industrial designs and trademarks were from abroad. But even 1% of Sri Lankans who invent something, who work out some new process, have great difficulties in registering it. That we have erased completely. Second, even after they register it they have no way of marketing it. It is there on the book. We know that a Sri Lankan invented a watchman's clock in modern times. It is still not patented, so how could he develop it? That gentleman, Mr Rowlands, died a sad man. The next stage to this is the Government's proposal to bring in what is called the Inventors Incentive Law. Whenever any Sri Lankan produces something new, either design or patent, we will help him to register it. We will also help him to market it because we want to encourage such people. Sri Lankans have innovative power and imagination and it is our duty not to stand aside but to give them a hand and push them forward. This Bill is not something that is widely understood, naturally, because it is really a specialised field: but it is revolutionary of this particular class of property so necessary for the commercial development of Sri Lanka.

The Minister's speech indicated how Sri Lanka might pursue the future promise of innovation and commercial development through participation in global nodes, such as WIPO, by implementing a modern patent system. Lakshman Kadirgamar influenced Mr Athulathmudali as the first Director for Asia and the Pacific Bureau who pioneered and promoted development cooperation, including IP capacity building, thus enabling many developing countries in the region to harness the benefits of IP for socio-economic development.[13] It is of particular interest to discuss here the importance of Mr Lalith Athulathmudali and Mr Lakshman Kadirgamar as speaking from governing nodes representing the government at that period in the development of discourse in Sri Lanka IP for both had the necessary mentalities, resources and influence to be able to mobilise the implementation of the legislation. Both were Oxford-educated scholars, lawyers and political leaders,[14] thus sharing similar

---

[11] Sri Lanka, Parliamentary debates, Parliament of Sri Lanka, 25 May 1979.

[12] Ibid.

[13] Foreign Ministry Sri Lanka (2018).

[14] Mr Lakshman Kadirgamar was appointed Minister of Foreign Affairs in 1994 by President Chandrika Kumaratunga.

grammar and epistemologies, who were able to communicate the importance of IP to the then government. Mr Athulathmudali became the Minister of Trade and Shipping in 1977 and was involved in discussions with the United Nations Conference on Trade and Development ('UNCTAD'); he understood that developed countries had to have a specialist local areas of patent infrastructure and capacity to push the country forward, although he did not himself understand the specialist field of patents. He assisted in the establishment of an open economy in Sri Lanka, to encourage foreign trade, investment and TT. Hence, both these individuals were local and global nodes of influence in the government who were able to encourage innovation and push the government to implement the *IP Code* to boost foreign trade and investment in Sri Lanka.

The *IP Code* marks the beginning of Sri Lanka's recognition of patents and its implementation of the international patent system. This is the beginning of post-colonial legislation; as identified by the Minister, 99% of patents were foreign registrations and the Minister believed that providing an appropriate system for patents would lead to development. Under his tenure, Sri Lanka joined the *PCT* in 1986 to enable the mutual recognition of local, and became part of global, IP lawmaking.

The *PCT* is an international node with more than 150 Contracting States.[15] The *PCT* makes it possible to seek patent protection for an invention simultaneously in numerous countries by filing a single 'international' patent application instead of filing applications in several separate national or regional patent offices in what is called the 'national phase'.[16] The *PCT* procedure includes filing, international search, international publication, supplementary international search (optional), international preliminary examination (optional) and the national phase.[17]

While the law was placed 'on the books', it was not to become an active area of discourse owing to a mix of local factors, notably, a lack of awareness, the weak legal infrastructure and a lack of political will on the part of successive governments.[18] Factors external to the patent system discourse also played a part. Political manoeuvring led to Mr Athulathmudali's resignation and subsequent assassination, and it must surely and sadly be acknowledged the Sri Lankan civil war and the general political disturbances may have also contributed to the lack of political will to develop patent laws and infrastructure; however, these political issues are not the focus of this study. They have meant that the differences within the patent discourse were left to fester.

Subsequent to the enactment of the *IP Code* and the ratification of the *PCT*, Sri Lanka acceded to the *TRIPS Agreement* in 1995 as a founding member.[19] Sri Lanka was designated by the WTO as a developing country although it has been a founding

---

[15] WIPO (1991).

[16] WIPO (2014).

[17] Ibid.

[18] As will be discussed in Chap. 5, the patent applications and grant numbers indicate that patents were not an active area in the 1970s.

[19] WTO (2022).

member of the *GATT* since 1948.[20] The influence of *TRIPS* led to the repeal of the *IP Code* and the enactment of the *TRIPS*-compliant *IP Act No 36 of 2003* (the '*IP Act*') for patents.[21] When introducing the 2003 IP Bill to the Parliament, the Minister of Commerce and Consumer Affairs Mr Ravi Karunanayake stated:

> We all know that 53% of our GDP ['gross domestic product'] of this country is the service industry; 26% is in agriculture and 21% is in the industrial area. You could see that there is absolutely a growing need for a knowledge-based economy in the globalised world.
>
> On a knowledge-based economy, one of the biggest aspects and one of the biggest intrinsic advantages is the knowledge of our people. There are hidden talents and creativity. This is what we want to protect. Through this process we will be able to promote trade. Also, the most important thing is the promotion of investment and to get investments coming in. FDI will come to this country too. Otherwise, investors are worried because they will feel uncertain as to whether their investment is safe or not in the country. Next important advantage that we have is we are permitting parallel imports of pharmaceuticals to ensure that our people are protected.[22]

The Minister's statement echoes the statements of his predecessor at the time of the enactment of the *IP Code* that its purpose was the need to foster not only trade and FDI but also the development of the knowledge economy through promoting national/local creativity, protecting creative efforts and enhancing the possibility of the integration of the national economy with the global economy.[23] This would seem the basis for an IP policy for Sri Lanka that will not only encourage local innovations but also attract foreign innovations. In practice, this policy was only limited to a statement in the Act without any evidence of significant application to the task of crafting the law and administration to progress the economic development of the country.[24] For patents, the *IP Act* provides definitions of subject matter, together with the application and examination requirements, which are discussed below from Sect. 3.6 onwards.

3.3 Sri Lanka's Role in Global Lawmaking

Sri Lanka has been a founding Contracting Party to the *GATT* since 1948 as well as a founding member of the WTO since 1995.[25] Sri Lanka's role as a WTO member has progressed from being inactive in the beginning to a moderate level of representation at all *GATT* rounds from Uruguay to Doha. In 1977, with the introduction of the open economic policies unilaterally, Sri Lanka became the first South Asian country

[20] Geeganage (2013), pp. 137, 151 ('Sri Lanka's Role in the World Trade Organization').

[21] TRIPS Agreement art 27(1).

[22] Sri Lanka, Parliamentary debates, Sri Lanka Parliament, 23 July 2003.

[23] Ibid 19.

[24] Karunaratna (2010).

[25] Geeganage (2013), p. 151.

to initiate liberal trade policies,[26] which have assisted it to maintain its average annual economic growth rate at more than 5% continuously except for a few years. Similar to other WTO members, Sri Lanka has guaranteed all tariffs on agricultural products and has agreed to eliminate tariffs and non-tariff barriers on non-agricultural products.[27] Sri Lanka's significant compliance with the *GATT*'s ruling system has been acknowledged by the WTO secretariat itself in 2016:[28]

> Sri Lanka, since its unilateral trade liberalisation in 1977 has initiated extensive reforms to its trade policy regime with a view to establish a strong economic foundation considering its capacities, constraints and national realities. These reforms, while placing the country in a stronghold in its economic development frontier have also contributed towards its significant achievements in the social development frontier where Sri Lanka is placed high rank in the Human Development Goal targets set for 2015. In the Global Competitive index 2014/2015, Sri Lanka ranks 73 among 144 countries ahead of many emerging economies and also improving its record in a range of criteria since 2012/2013.

The WTO Review further stated:[29]

> Considering the growing importance of preserving intellectual property rights which effectively support and facilitate business and innovators in the protection and uses of their IPR, Sri Lanka has given due prominence for necessary regulatory reforms.

Sri Lanka has been considered a small vulnerable economy[30] for decades because of civil war, and this may be the reason that the Sri Lankan Government choose to bring forward *TRIPS* implementation before most other developing countries. However, Sri Lanka is active in discussions within the WTO[31] in all areas related to its trade and economic interests, specifically, non-agricultural market access, agriculture, trade facilitation, services, *TRIPS* and Aid for Trade.

Sri Lanka has been a member of WIPO since 1978. As will be demonstrated later in the discussion, WIPO has been the key global node by providing technical assistance for developing the legal framework for IP in Sri Lanka. However, the Sri Lankan experience suggests that when a foreign rule, such as *TRIPS* and WIPO *Model Law*, was transplanted, there was little resistance to the received law. Rather, means were found to reconcile the legal transplantation to suit asymmetric interests. A former officer of NIPO stated that the transformation from the pre-*TRIPS* regime to *TRIPS* was a smooth process.[32] This statement was further reiterated by an officer attached to, Economic and Commercial Division, at the US embassy in Sri Lanka. He mentioned that Sri Lanka has never violated any IP and was never subjected to s 301 of the US *Trade Act*.[33] At this point, there were no major retaliations from the

[26] Ibid.

[27] Ibid.

[28] WTO (2016).

[29] Ibid.

[30] Sri Lanka's GDP is expected to reach US $83 billion by the end of 2022.

[31] Kannangara and Kern (2018).

[32] Interviewee # 23.

[33] Interviewee # 22.

public due to Sri Lanka joining the WTO and reforming IP and trade laws to comply with *TRIPS* standards. In other words, Sri Lanka did not have any options apart from making the necessary reforms because it is one of the countries that heavily relies on the International Monetary Fund and the World Bank for financial assistance, and the government knew any resistance would result in economic sanctions from the US and other developed countries. This is power dynamics of developed countries within nodal governance that could influence the IP policy making in Sri Lanka.

A mantra often stated in international discourses is that IP systems, in general, and patents, in particular, constitute an effective mechanism to enhance the economic development of a country. This relationship has been investigated through technological, industrial, trade and competitiveness policies in developing countries.[34] The benefits have been strongly stated in the international discourse of WIPO and the WTO[35] but, simultaneously, no 'one size fits all' solution has been accepted all round.

Thus, when discussing policy objectives, countries such as Sri Lanka must consider what benefits they are pursuing; for example, whether the policy is to foster localised R&D, technological and commercial innovation, FDI or TT to kickstart local development. Alternatively, is this to foster access to international production networks and export markets, international aid, the import of useful products, the freedom to imitate? These policy objectives are many and varied and often competing, or requiring finesse to reconcile, for there are tensions between international organisations, foreign companies, national policymakers, investors and inventors. By examining the discourses on certain key occasions, this book will now consider the implications of these policies for the shaping of Sri Lankan patent law and administration.

In the Sri Lankan context, prior to the *IP Code* the government did not seriously consider patents as a legal mechanism to protect IPR, because patents were not a developed area of law then owing to the lack of legal infrastructure and expertise. It enacted the *IP Act* because Sri Lanka was a prominent country in the region that did not have such an Act.[36] Moreover, the political discourse of the period did not consider IP, nor did the economic, industrial and technological policies in Sri Lanka place any emphasis on an IP policy as part of economic development.[37]

However, from 2010 onwards the discourse on IP and on the STI sectors started to change because of a few forward-looking local actors,[38] who believed that IP is a driver in the innovation system and that Sri Lanka will never prosper unless an R&D ecosystem is developed and inventions are commercialised. These local actors had mentalities, and nodal prominence to recognize the international discourse as important for local development. These local actors thus sought assistance from

[34] Mendes (2015) (Integrating Intellectual Property). See also, Gee et al. (2009). See generally Maskus (2000) (n 1); Kuanpoth (2008).

[35] Maskus (2000); Alikhan (2000), p. 1; Kim et al. (2012).

[36] Perera (2014), (Administration of Patent System).

[37] Perera and Dasanayaka (2004), p. 244.

[38] Interviewee # 20; Interviewee # 1; Interviewee # 2; Interviewee # 8.

global actors, such as WIPO, to develop a strategy in which IP could be integrated into the innovation agenda.[39] However, things moved slowly.

This culminated in 2015 with a scoping project, undertaken through WIPO's technical assistance, at the request of the Sri Lankan Government, to understand the innovation system in the country and to examine the extent to which IP considerations have served or could serve to strengthen innovation in Sri Lanka.[40] WIPO submitted recommendations to the Sri Lankan Government, and according to WIPO,[41] some of the recommendations have already been implemented, which is a positive feature to promote innovation in the country. The WIPO recommendations are themselves a demonstration of nodal communications producing a result.

Along with this background positioning of Sri Lanka within the international discourse, an overview of the local discourse examining the structural framework of patent administration in Sri Lanka is necessary. Few previous studies have been conducted in Sri Lanka about the ease/quality of independent local patent grants and how these settings are viewed in terms of their significance for the country's economic development[42] and especially to what extent IP could be used in SMEs in Sri Lanka.[43] None of these prior studies utilised semi-structured interviews or discourse analysis of the results; hence, this study is the first such study to employ interviews in investigating the current patent administration. The findings of the prior studies will be discussed in this book as part of the discourse. These findings will assist to review the policymakers' perception on how competing discourses could be effective for economic development in Sri Lanka in the three case studies being examined in this book.

3.4 Developing a National Intellectual Property Policy for Sri Lanka

The thrust of the discourse from WIPO is the development of a national IP policy for Sri Lanka that provides structure, predictability and a beneficial environment in which enterprises and researchers can access and share knowledge, technology and IP, which plays an essential role in the science, technology and research functions of universities and research institutes.[44] This is predominately an international discourse because WIPO as identified in Chap. 2 is the central global node to IP but, as will be seen in the further discussion successive governments neither considered nor implemented a national IP policy, apart from the legislative gestures in 1979 and 2003.

[39] Mendes (2015).

[40] Ibid.

[41] Interviewee # 19.

[42] Wickramasinghe and Ahamed (2012), p. 365.

[43] Hewage (2015), p. 100.

[44] MIC (2018).

The impetus for a consideration of a Sri Lankan national policy arose when the Sri Lankan UN representative converted what would have been a private visit in 2013 by Dr Francis Gurry, the former DG of WIPO, to Sri Lanka into a formal state visit at the invitation of the Minister of Foreign Affairs. His visit coincided with his task delivering the Lakshman Kadirgamar[45] Memorial Oration 2013, organised by the Lakshman Kadirgamar Institute for International Relations and Strategic Studies in Colombo, Sri Lanka.[46] The Ministry of Foreign Affairs, the UN, representative of Sri Lanka at the United Nations in Geneva and the National NIPO, in consultation with WIPO officials, organised the program for Dr Gury's official visit.

In the interview with the UN representative, made the following statement regarding this initiative:

> We have traditionally been really a post office between WIPO and NIPO, but there were circumstances where we got actively involved, particularly after Francis Gurry went to SL in November 2013. With that visit, I proposed to Dr Gurry that we have something concrete from this visit because things were (a) bit ad hoc and it was really people coming for seminars and workshops on IP and the wrong people coming for fun; also, we wanted to systematise it. NIPO itself have been up and down and preoccupied with their existence, so we needed to get into a more structured corporation framework. That was my aim. Not to get into the technicalities of IP, but to push everyone and work together.

The UN representative could be considered the sand that irritates the oyster since he pushed the Sri Lankan Government to streamline IP and the visit by the former DG of WIPO was the perfect time to convince the Sri Lankan Government. During his visit, Dr Gurry met the former President of Sri Lanka Mahinda Rajapakse and Prof Tissa Vitharana the former Minister of External Affairs, Industry and Commerce, Economic Development and Science, Technology and Innovation. Dr Gurry was accompanied by Mr Ambi Sundaram, Assistant DG (Admin and Management) of WIPO, Mr Ranjana Abeysekera, Director of the Regional Bureau for Asia and the Pacific and Ms Armelle Le Theix, Assistant Program Officer (Sri Lanka Desk Officer in WIPO).[47] The participation of all these actors demonstrates that the channels of communication opened for the development of discourse on IP locally within Sri Lanka between national and international nodes of influence, started by the UN representative's initiating a formal visit by Dr Gurry. The UN representative is a node that through their role as the representative of the government at the UN, recognised and engaged outside the ambit of his directive and established a discourse with WIPO to develop IP in Sri Lanka.[48] Regarding the role of the government in the IP discourse, the UN representative stated:[49]

---

[45] Lakshman Kadirgamar, a Sri Lankan national, was the first Director of the Asia and the Pacific Bureau of WIPO from 1976 to 1988. See 'WIPO Unveils Kirinde Masterpiece to Honour Lakshman Kadirgamar (2018).

[46] Pathiraja (2013). See also Kadirgamar (n 212).

[47] MIC (2018) Terms of Reference (n 44).

[48] Interviewee # 20.

[49] Ibid.

> I am the government. What I did with the support of my staff is to lift the system from being a one Minister—one agency thing to being national, and I represent everybody. The only thing is that I was taking some risks and sometimes stretching my mandate, and I knew nothing about IP, which is good in a way because I had no vested interests—not in people, not in agency and not in subjects.

Dr Gurry's visit to Sri Lanka is significant not only because it was the first time that a DG of WIPO had visited the country after it became a member of the organisation in 1978, but also because the WIPO DG acknowledged that Sri Lanka could accrue many benefits through greater focus on IP and noted that in a highly competitive world and a global marketplace, proper IPR safeguards need to be in place.[50] The significance of this meeting and the efforts of the UN representative to develop it is that as result of this meeting, a 10 PAP was finalised to further strengthen the cooperation between WIPO and Sri Lanka on many areas of interest and benefit to the country, such as integrating IP into the Sri Lankan innovation policy.[51]

However, the NIPO was perceived as a possible obstacle. The UN representative further stated:[52]

> I felt all corporations get stuck with NIPO because everything must go through NIPO. As part of the 10 PAP, we created a structure that when a conference was being held once a quarter, there was an innovation expert in Geneva who got to know that there was an expert performing innovations in Sri Lanka. By the 10 PAP, I conceptually connected people who could interact and work within the system.

These 10 PAPS were developed during the 2013 visit by the DG of WIPO.[53] These were mutually agreed to by WIPO and the Ministry of Industry and Commerce ('MIC') and endorsed, and WIPO agreed to implement the 10 PAP. A former WIPO Director, was made the focal point from WIPO, and the NIPO DG was nominated to represent Sri Lanka, for 10 PAP implementations. Subsequently, in 2018 these 10 points were absorbed in the Framework for Sri Lanka created by WIPO, which is a more elaborate plan than the 10 PAP.[54]

Under the 10 PAP, WIPO provides technical assistance to Sri Lanka in 10 main areas: integrating IP into the national innovation policy formulation, strengthening the capacity of NIPO, establishing the TISC, formulating an innovation index on the lines of the Global Innovation Index, strengthening Collective Management Organisations, conducting a study on creative industries, ensuring the effective enforcement of IPR, geographical indications and product branding, acceding to WIPO treaties and protecting traditional knowledge.[55] The UN representative believed this collaboration between the Sri Lankan Government and WIPO could serve as a useful model

---

[50] Permanent Mission of Sri Lanka to the UN (2018).

[51] Mendes (2015).

[52] Interviewee # 20.

[53] Interviewee # 18.

[54] Ibid. WIPO Project Summary (2020). (The WIPO official handed a hard copy to the researcher [which may have been a working document at that time] in June 2018 in Geneva during his interview, and the researcher has a copy on file).

[55] Permanent Mission of Sri Lanka to the UN (2018) (n 50).

for developing countries, in upgrading their IP protection regimes to deliver the benefits of IPR to a broader spectrum of stakeholders.[56] Some elements of this reform agenda implicate patent law and administration.

A report on the progress under the 10 PAP was provided by the Secretary of MIC and the UN representative and WTO Ambassador at the 35th Session of the WIPO Standing Committee on the Law of Trademarks, Industrial Designs and Geographical Indications in Geneva in April 2016. The report highlighted that Sri Lanka was currently in the process of integrating IP into areas on innovation, ST and creativity as a means of economic development and empowerment.[57] The UN representative said that 10 PAP would enhance the capacity of NIPO and other stakeholders in the country and assist Sri Lanka to strengthen its IP protection regime, especially that for innovators, entrepreneurs and artists.

In addition to coordinating the 10 PAP, the UN representative went beyond his mandate to endeavour to unlock the IP system in Sri Lanka. He stated:[58]

> Tactically, from my perspective as a manager it was a way of overcoming bottlenecks in SL-WIPO cooperation because initially NIPO was not organised and was over-centralised. Now, we have decentralised things. Everyone has the freedom to talk about existing knowledge with colleagues. These are the few areas that we have liberated a little bit. And we are seeing results in these areas.[59]

Within the discourse, the UN representative is a governing node because his way of thinking and his ability to recognise opportunities and set in process events to develop interactions between actors and to cross boundaries began the debates about the development of a national policy in Sri Lanka. The UN representative used his own criteria to assess the importance of IP for Sri Lanka then through DSs that engage and connect people to develop the discourse. Examples of these DSs and their effects are discussed next.

First, the UN representative, as the governing node representing Sri Lanka at the UN, was the connection point to communicate with not only the WIPO DG but also directly with NIPO and other local policymakers, such as COSTI officials who had the mandate to coordinate STI because they shared a similar legal grammar, educational background and epistemological assumptions about the IP framework for Sri Lanka. Second, he became an individual champion within the interpretive community that exerted influence promoting IP reforms because he was the right person locally and globally for the job. For example, comments such as ‘I am the government’ and ‘I was stretching my mandate’ reveal that through his interaction with relevant actors—local ones such as NIPO and COSTI and global ones such as WIPO and the UN through his mandate—he was putting Sri Lanka onto the correct path for IP reforms. This fact has helped to systematise the IP nodal network.

Third, data collection indicates that the UN representative’s discursive strategies to strengthen the IP ecosystem were because of his commitment and close association

[56] Interviewee # 20.

[57] Mendes (2015) (n 51).

[58] Interviewee # 20.

[59] Ibid.

with WIPO. WIPO, the UN representative and COSTI have shared epistemologies and tacit understanding regarding IP reforms, and hence, these entities used their mandate strategically to achieve the desired result. Hence, the UN representative has become a connection point or a node at the international level who communicates and interacts with local-level nodes to achieve a single goal: to systematise the IP system in Sri Lanka.

Following the development of the 10 PAP discussion between the Secretary to the Minister of Industry and Commerce, the UN representative and WIPO officials in June 2017, a comprehensive IP policy framework for Sri Lanka became a priority.

Within the Sri Lankan context, IP policy can play a critical role in addressing the socio-economic objective to strengthen the national policy, while overcoming weaknesses in utilising IP resources effectively for sustainable national growth.[60] In this context, expertise was sought to undertake this assignment of drafting the IP policy, in consultation and coordination with the MIC, IP steering committee, WIPO and NIPO of Sri Lanka. The steering committee was appointed by the MIC and comprised MIC officials, private sector stakeholders, such as the SLINTEC, and IP-related stakeholders comprising universities and research institutions. Its first task was to perform a desk-based analysis and research to follow-up discussions with stakeholders and government state institutions relating to IP.[61]

With regard to who will take the initiative to draft the IP policy, the MTC Director stated:[62]

> We have called for proposals before mid-November 2017. We have published a paper advertisement, and if people are interested, they can come forward. Then, we will evaluate and most probably give the assignment by the end of this year. We do not have resources and time to draft an IP policy since it is a specialised skill. From that time, they will have 14 weeks for the drafting process. WIPO too suggested it is better to give it to a consultant. We hope by mid-2018 there should be an IP policy for Sri Lanka.

The Institute of Policy Studies was appointed in 2017 as a consultant to draft the IP policy.

The effort taken by these local and global actors for IP policy formulation reveals their influence and commitment to considering the interest of all stakeholders related to IP by providing sufficient legal protection to move forward to a knowledge-based economy. A comprehensive IP policy was considered an important catalyst to protect the national IP as well as to facilitate entry into further international agreements and treaties, such as *Madrid Agreement, Concerning the International Registration of Marks ('Madrid Agreement')*[63] in order to create flexibility and positive externalities for Sri Lanka.[64] This was their regulatory function.

---

[60] MIC (2018) (n 47).

[61] Interviewee # 12.

[62] Interviewee # 11.

[63] Madrid Agreement (1979).

[64] Ibid.

However, the process of reform stalled. As shown below when studying Sri Lanka's patent administration in detail, this initiative failed to kickstart the modernisation of the system. The NIPO official stated the following regarding the IP policy preparation:[65]

> The IP policy is still in the preliminary stages. Some data have been collected, and some basic document has been prepared by a senior official of COSTI. Currently, I am unable to do anything positively other than forming a committee and giving my contribution until I get more staff and allocate policy matters because our more important task is to clear the backlog on patents, TM and designs. Our concentration is on these currently, and maybe by next year, we should be able to start on this policy because we have to go for the Madrid accession next year and a lot of work is being piled up; I'm battling alone here. All internal officers who are trained to do daily routine work are involved in day-to-day matters and are unable to get involved in policy preparation.

Compared with the statements made by the UN representative, these statements by the NIPO official seem very negative, but this demonstrates any adoption, transfer or development from international discourses meets the reality of the local discourse, where the importance is not accepted by the wider community because there are competing objectives. This is true in Sri Lanka, and the NIPO official identified:

> The IP policy is still in the preliminary stages, I am unable to do anything positively other than forming a committee and giving my contribution until I get more staff and allocate policy matters because our more important task is to clear the backlog on patents, TM and designs; a lot of work is being piled up and I'm battling alone here.[66]

From the theoretical perspective, the NIPO official in Sri Lanka, would be a central node that would be able to develop interpretive communities and use DSs to connect, coordinate and develop IP policy and awareness, as well as be a central node for discourse. The reality revealed through these interviews is that as a governing node, the NIPO official has failed to coordinate with other colleagues, departments and ministries to achieve the regulatory functions for IP reforms. The reasons seem to be local and bureaucratic in nature.

First, the NIPO official has refused to interact with other local agencies, such as COSTI and NSF, and relevant ministries, such as the Ministries of Economic Affairs, External Resources and Industry and Commerce, to streamline IP matters, and has asserted that NIPO is the focal point. Thus, the main reason for the breakdown of the 10 PAP in 2013 is that the DG wanted to monopolise all the 10 points within NIPO without obtaining support from other local agencies.[67]

Second, according to an officer of the MIC, the IP policy formulation was regarded as the responsibility of NIPO. Since NIPO did not draft the policy within 2 years, the MIC itself commenced coordination of the IP policy in 2016.[68] However, according to the latest information, IP policy is not considered a priority in the Ministry.[69]

---

[65] Interviewee # 10.

[66] Ibid.

[67] Interviewee # 21.

[68] Interviewee # 11. IP policy has not yet been finalised as of May 2024.

[69] Ibid.

Third, an officer of MIC also emphasised that there are personal conflicts in the NIPO hierarchy, which has contributed to the heavy backlog of work, specifically of trademark applications. The officer stated, 'The NIPO official is the one who created the backlog when that person was attached to one of the divisions of NIPO due to rivalry with an former officer.' Regardless of the reasons, the backlog of applications has become a barrier for Sri Lanka to accede to the *Madrid Agreement*[70] because the trademark backlog must be zero to accede to it.[71]

Fourth, although the NIPO official is not popular within NIPO and the Ministry, that persons appointment cannot be challenged because it is a Cabinet appointment. A government appointee, can only be removed for misconduct by the Cabinet according to the existing public employment law in Sri Lanka.

Last, to anticipate the next case study, it is more than 20 years since the first PVR Bill was drafted without any success in finalising the Act. This suggests a lack of discourse from the NIPO and the DoA, which are, in this case, important nodes in the drafting and passage of the PVR Bill. This implies that NIPO and DoA lacked nodal influence in finalizing the PVR Bills due to lack of engagement between NIPO and DoA.

As a result of the lethargy shown by NIPO, as of June 2021, the IP policy is still a working document. The drafting of the IP policy was given to the Institute of Policy Studies, an economic policy research institute, by the IP steering committee. The MTC and the MSTR, who were involved in the follow-up process as local actors of IP policy, stated the following in interviews:

> The Draft IP policy was prepared by the Institution of Policy Studies and was sent to the Ministry of Science and Technology, which NIPO fell under earlier. It is very pathetic how Sri Lanka is dealing with IP.[72]

> The IP policy is at a standstill without much interest shown by those who should have. As NIPO was moved from the Ministry of Trade and Commerce to the Ministry of Science, Technology and Research, the latter ministry has lot less an idea on a National IP Policy. NIPO also has to establish itself. That is the status.[73]

> About the IP policy: Unfortunately, it is still stuck. From time to time, COSTI has attempted to resurrect that. For a very short while, NIPO was placed under our Ministry. At that time, we followed it through our Additional Secretary (Research). Then, there was a restructure in the government and just last week we took it up again with the Additional Secretary.[74]

These statements indicate the reasons for the lack of discourse on IP in Sri Lanka. First, no one knows the fate of the IP policy after it was submitted by the consultant to the MSTR. The nodal governance theory shows that the delay is also within the Ministry, which is a crucial local node has failed to influence in formulating the IP policy. This suggests a lack of political will, plus inadequate human and financial

---

[70] Madrid Agreement (1979) (n 63).

[71] Interviewee # 11.

[72] Ibid.

[73] Interviewee # 1.

[74] Interviewee # 2.

resources, which has led to the disintegrated management of IP. Second, during this period, NIPO was moved from the MTC to the MSTR, and no one is able to provide a valid reason for the move. This demonstrates failure in the IP eco system to change crucial nodes in the IP policy making discourse. These types of ad hoc and haphazard decisions will invariably slow down the process since there is no governing node to take responsibility for the change. Third, that the MSTR had no idea on a national IP policy suggests a lack of commitment as a governing node and that certain things are being done for the sake of doing reflects MSTR lacks mentalities, resources and technologies to influence the IP policy in Sri Lanka. Fourth, a restructure in the government changed the bureaucratic personnel and the new set of bureaucrats are unaware of the status of the IP policy suggest within the nodal governance theory these personnel lack nodal influence. Last, the statement, 'NIPO also has to establish itself', indicates that NIPO has not fulfilled its status as a governing node nor have the ministries pressed it to do so.

This indicates that although there are influential local and global governing nodes in the patent reforms who clearly understand their regulatory function regarding the extent to which IP could be beneficial for economic development in Sri Lanka, it is a lack of political will and ad hoc decision-making by the government (including NIPO) that continues to be the biggest bottleneck in the reform of patent administration. This aspect will be discussed in the following section. The discussion around this system will be examined before returning towards the end of this case study to the latest links with WIPO and the prospects of the global–local dialogue being revived.

3.5 Patent Administration of Sri Lanka: The Case Study

For many modern patent systems in the world, governments have shaped their respective patent policy as part of their international obligations, believing that this would improve the quality of IP protection, both in provision and administration. There is a consistency in the requirements established through the *PCT* and international discourse from *TRIPS* that requires a patent application to include the following information in the prescribed form: a request for the patent grant, a description of the invention, a claim or claims, a drawing or drawings where required and an abstract of the patent.[75] Applications are meant to be examined for their conformity with the criteria for patentability, the definitions of patentable subject matter and the technical criteria of novelty, inventive step and utility or industrial application. Sri Lanka's *IP Code* and *IP Act*, following the global trend, had a uniform definition of an invention and patentable subject matter and the *IP Act* did not alter these.[76]

Article 27 of the *TRIPS Agreement* states that members may use these technical criteria:

---

[75] IP Act s 71. See also Perera (2014) (n 36).

[76] See IP Code ss 59–60; IP Act ss 62–63. See also Perera, Ibid.

> Subject to the provisions of paragraphs 2 and 3, patents shall be available for any inventions, whether products or processes, in all fields of technology, provided that they are new, involve an inventive step and are capable of industrial application.

Although such uniformity is expected and legislation adopts the concepts, there are variations in the examination process at national levels. The global discourse provides some flexibilities or 'room to move', and furthermore, countries individually take positions that could arguably be seen as falling short of international obligations. Hence, this case study assesses the rigour with which the patent system is expected to define and apply these requirements of patentability through the practice of examination.

Essentially, there are three different forms of examination: substantive, modified and formality. With regard specifically to patent administration, most jurisdictions look to substantive examination to apply high thresholds of novelty, inventive step and industrial applicability to a patent grant. Some jurisdictions also make available the modified examination, pre- and post-grant opposition proceedings and CL methods within the patent system to suit the expression of the needs of their national economy. Reforms to the patent administration have been discussed in Sri Lanka, for example, about the introduction of the utility model system, for a few years. This discourse still continues but has not yet been introduced to the *IP Act*. This aspect will be discussed later in this chapter.

Yet, the present patent system in Sri Lanka still adopts little of these procedures in the patent granting process. For example, modified examination and pre- and post-grant opposition are not available under the Sri Lankan system. That is, a formality examination is provided under the Act which is a very outdated system.[77] In contrast, substantive examination is provided optionally under the Act to those applicants who request it but not to others. Compared with other jurisdictions, its applicability is very low owing to the lack of demand, or the lack of expertise and resources to respond. Moreover, discourses such as CL, parallel importation and local working conditions, which are usually used for regulating patents, are either rarely used or unavailable under the IP ecosystem in Sri Lanka. This aspect will be discussed later in this chapter.

Against this background, the key inquiry is regarding discourses around patent administration that includes patent examination, examiner training, the capacity building of NIPO and the WIPO Technical Assistance program, in order to analyse whether there has been any shift in policymaking in patent system over the years. As stated earlier, there has been lack of discourses on IP in the past, but since 2013 the discourse has been expanding because most local actors now speak of the importance of having a developed IP system that aligns with economic strategy of the country.

One such prominent discourse is whether Sri Lanka should have a utility model system that applies a lower patentability requirement to encourage independent local inventors. The best option for Sri Lanka depends on the objectives of the patent system: encouraging local innovation is important because the current Sri Lankan

---

77 Perera (2014) (n 75).

patent examination process is suitable for a utility model system rather than a standard patent examination system. in Sect. 3.5, the interviews with relevant experts in the area of IP and STI in Sri Lanka have already demonstrated discourse that identifies problems within the patent administration arising from the patent examination process, the prior art requirement, the use of international searches, the invention disclosure requirements and the patent examiner training for standard patents.[78] These problems will be followed up first in relation to the administration of the system, before the discourse on the various resolution options, such as modified examination, pre- and post-grant examination, utility models, capacity building and WIPO's technical assistance, are also studied against the settings in place.

The following sections will discuss the prominent nodes and discourses within the patent administration of Sri Lanka.

3.5.1 Important Subsystems in Sri Lanka for Patent Promotion

Patent grants in Sri Lanka are primarily administered by the NIPO with the assistance of various actors or nodes, such as government departments, other patent offices, civil and specialist courts and industry associations, NGOs, public interest groups and patent attorneys. Similarly, to patent law in other countries, patent law in Sri Lanka consists of legislation and the interpretation and application of that legislation by authoritative bodies, such as courts, tribunals and patent offices, and the participation of industry and civil society in the examination and disputation of applications for patents.

The patent office is headed by an official known as the DG who is appointed by the Minister of Industry and Commerce with the approval of the Cabinet. This individual is empowered to implement the provisions of the *Patents Act*; control and supervise the administration of the IP system; and supervise the persons appointed for, or engaged in, the implementation of the provisions of the Act.[79] The DG is also required to promote the awareness of the subject of IP and the establishment and proper functioning of collective societies. The IP system in Sri Lanka is unified. That is, the NIPO administers the entire IP system of the country. It does not entertain pre-grant and post-grant opposition proceedings.

The DG is answerable to the Parliament. There are instances when the DG will be required to attend parliamentary hearing committees to clarify certain IP issues. The office of DG is autonomous in the sense that the policies and decisions of the DG relating to the administration of IP can be challenged legally only in the Provincial High Court.[80] Hence, the DG is a governing node who is empowered to control and

[78] Ibid.

[79] Intellectual Property Act, No 36 of 2003 (Sri Lanka) ('IP Act'). See also National Intellectual Property Office. https://www.nipo.gov.lk/.

[80] Perera (2014) (n 77).

supervise the administration of the IP system and influence and supervise the persons appointed for, or engaged in, the implementation of the provisions of the Act. The DG is appointed by the Cabinet and cannot be removed except in case of malpractice.

However, in addition to NIPO, there are other local actors, such as Ministers, coordinating secretariats and ministry officials, Sri Lankan ambassadorial links and WIPO, who directly interact with the DG to facilitate matters relating to IP in Sri Lanka. For example, the UN representative and WIPO officials became crucial actors in the process of shaping a comprehensive IP policy for Sri Lanka in 2017 by formulating a 10-point Action Plan ('10 PAP') to streamline IP.

Moreover, COSTI can be regarded as another governing node under the Ministry of Science, Technology and Innovation, which coordinates all STI sectors in the country. COSTI has a separate division known as the Technology and Innovation Support Centre ('TISC'), which was created under the WIPO Technical Assistance program to guide innovators on IP-related matters. This aspect will be discussed in Chap. 5 in this book.

3.5.2 Patent Examination

There are three recognised systems for patent examination: substantive examination, modified examination and formality. In the substantive examination procedure, core aspects of the application are subject to critical examination as to novelty and inventiveness before registration against the prior art.[81] In a distinction between high-bar and low-bar examinations, the prior art can be pitched as high as worldwide documentary and non-documentary sources, such as oral disclosures (e.g. at scientific conferences). Searches are undertaken. It is possible that the application has already received a patent in another jurisdiction. Unless the person who is applying for the patent satisfies this requirement, the patent is not granted. Some jurisdictions have a modified examination system, which is discussed in Sect. 3.8.1.

The third system relies solely on the examination of the application form. This is known as the formality examination—the system that is still adopted in Sri Lanka. In Sri Lanka, an application for a patent is examined on the basis of adhering to basic formal requirements. This system was based on an option in the 1979 WIPO *Model Law*, which Sri Lanka adopted. The system was retained in the 2003 legislation. Section 130 of the *Model Law* deals with examination as to form, while s 131 deals with examination as to substance.[82] Under the examination as to form, the applicant is required to furnish basic information about the patent and submit a search report about the invention to the Registrar.[83] If the application matches the requirements, the patent is granted without a substantial examination.

---

[81] Substantive examination has been adopted in the Australian and Malaysian patent system.

[82] WIPO (1979).

[83] Interviewee # 24.

Section 71(1) of the present *IP Act* sets out the requirements of the application and the examination procedure for patent grant. Section 71(1)(a) states that an application for a patent shall be made to the DG in the prescribed form with the following information: a request for the patent grant, a description of the invention, a claim or claims, a drawing or drawings where required, an abstract of the patent, the date and number of the application if it is foreign application, and a declaration by the applicant or predecessor. These requirements at least meet the accepted norms of *TRIPS* and *PCT* with their own relevance; for example, the description must disclose the invention in a sufficiently clear manner so that the invention can be evaluated and carried out by a person who has ordinary skill in the art. It shall further indicate the best mode for carrying out the invention. The claim or claims must be clear, concise and supported by the description. Drawings are necessary in order to understand the invention. The terms of the claim or claims determine the scope and extent of the protection afforded by the patent, and the description and the drawings may be used to interpret the claim or claims. The abstract serves the purpose of providing technical information and it is not to be used for the purpose of determining or interpreting the scope and extent of the protection afforded by the patent.[84]

These are the formal requirements for an application, although they can be onerous if enforced. After all, one of the quid pro quos for the grant of the patent is that it becomes public knowledge. The requirements under s 71(1)(a) require ticking boxes against each requirement by the applicant based on 'yes' and 'no' scenarios. Section 78 (1) outlines the examination of applications. The DG shall examine the application and shall be satisfied that the applicant has fulfilled all the following conditions under s 78 (1):

- The requirements of s 71(1)(a) have been met.
- The request complies with the requirements of s 71(2)(a).
- Where applicable, the requirements of s 71(2)(b) have been met.
- The description, the claims and, where applicable, the drawings, comply with the prescribed requirements.
- The essential elements of the invention claimed in the application have not been derived from a patent already granted in Sri Lanka.
- The application contains an abstract.
- The search report—an international type search report[85] referred to in s 73(1)—and Regulation No. 48(1) have been submitted.

In any event, the DG must satisfy that that the application complies with s 71(1)(a). If the application does not fulfil the s 71(1)(a) requirements, there is no application for the DG to examine under s 78. In other words, for a patent grant both s 71(1)(a) and s 78(1) have to be satisfied. If there are corrections to be made, the Registrar will request the applicant to file the necessary information and, failing that, the application

[84] IP Act ss 71(1), (7).

[85] The search report prescribed for the purpose of s 73(1) is a report issued by any NIPO or any intergovernmental organisation appointed as an international search authority under the PCT.

will be rejected.[86] However, the section does not specify that a patent must be refused if the search report is not to the satisfaction of the DG. Hence, it is arguable if an incomplete search report is submitted by the applicant and the other requirements of s 78 (1) are met, in terms of the law, whether a patent could be granted or not.[87] Currently, only the applicant can challenge the patent grant if the NIPO has refused to grant the patent. When the *IP Act* was enacted in 2003, the examination procedure remained the same as in the 1979 *IP Code*.

However, s 73 (1) of the Act provides that in lieu of the search report, the applicant may request the Registrar to refer the patent application to a local examiner[88] for the examination of the application and for a report on the relevant prior art. The examiner should give due regard to descriptions and drawings, if any, and furnish a report to the DG on the relevant prior art. For the purpose of the search, the local examiner shall refer to every document on prior art available to them.[89] The local examiner is required to discover as much of the relevant prior art and to consult all documentation on prior art available to them.[90] Potentially, this is quite an onerous task for a local examiner, who would need substantial resources to conduct a prior art test because of the limited resources at NIPO. This is an original examination. It is not a substantive or a modified examination available in some jurisdictions, such as Australia and the EU. Although this section involves a prior art search, there is no substantive examination of the patent application in Sri Lanka owing to two reasons. First, as discussed previously, under s 73(1), the patent is generally granted if the formal requirements recognised for a valid application are complied with.[91] Second, there is no provision regarding opposition proceedings in the granting stage and it is left to the court to decide on the validity of the patent after grant, thereby eliminating the delay and expenses at the stage of the grant, should anyone challenge that validity, such as a defendant charged with patent infringement.[92] This aspect will be discussed later.

The substantive patent examination has several benefits. It is often regarded as a gatekeeper that prevents the grant of frivolous and substandard patents. It also provides a more robust grant should infringement proceedings be necessary. Therefore, the introduction of the search and examination process in the national patent system has been highlighted in the context of national development and innovation policies.[93]

Meanwhile, a patent office needs significant financial and human resources to conduct search and examination by itself. A high degree of technical and legal

---

[86] IP Act ss78(2)–(5).

[87] Ibid.

[88] IP Act s 73(4) says that a local examiner means any skilled person to whom the DG may refer questions concerning patents.

[89] IP Act s 71(1)–(7). It does not say whether that prior art should be researched internationally.

[90] Interviewee # 23.

[91] Julius and Creasy (2012).

[92] Ibid.

[93] WIPO (2014).

expertise—not only to understand the technical aspect of inventions, but also to interpret the legal scope of patent claims and to analyse the compliance with the legal requirements prescribed in a patent law—is required to carry out a full set of patent examination.[94] The big national offices often have highly developed policies and manuals for dealing with specific technologies. Consequently, there is an opportunity cost in not being able to employ highly skilled scientists and engineers in R&D in national priority areas. Moreover, sufficient technical infrastructure (e.g. databases) needs to be maintained in a patent office to conduct a thorough prior art search. Small offices may have to seek information and guidance from the offices in the larger jurisdictions where the applicants file first. In addition, the *PCT* process designates some offices as International Search Authorities ('ISAs').[95]

For these reasons, it is doubtful that patent grant in Sri Lanka consists of substantive examinations. As a result, most patent applications in Sri Lanka are very basic and they are not up to internationally recognised standards as in Australia, which requires a high threshold of patentability for a patent grant. Most of the inventions can be regarded as engineering improvements that lack the novelty or inventive step.[96]

The former DG made the following comment about the patent granting process based on substantive examination:

> In practice, most patents do not fulfil the patentable criteria, but we grant the patent to encourage the inventors or to further their inventive aptitude because if the inventions were refused instantly it would destroy the morale of a prospective inventor.[97]

Nevertheless, this must be squared with the policy to be taken towards industrialists, particularly foreign MNCs. A Director of COSTI Sri Lanka, said, 'This type of a lenient attitude will lead in granting undeserving patents that have no economic gain'.[98] In the long run, this approach is not beneficial to a country such as Sri Lanka. It may want to attract high technology from overseas, but there may also be applications to claim something best left in the public domain.

In respect of foreign applications filed by an applicant abroad relating to the same or essentially the same invention claimed under the Act, the DG should request the applicant to provide the following documents.

- A copy of any communication received by the applicant concerning the results of any search or examination carried out in respect of the foreign application;
- A copy of the patent granted on the basis of the foreign application; and
- A copy of any final decision rejecting the foreign application or refusing the grant of a patent requested in the foreign application.[99]

---

94 Ibid.

95 WIPO (2022a, b).

96 Interviewee # 23.

97 Ibid.

98 Interviewee # 1.

99 IP Act s 73(3).

The DG may require the applicant to furnish a copy of any final decision invalidating the patent granted on the basis of the foreign application referred to above.[100]

In Sri Lanka, the office may ask the patentees to perform the necessary amendments, and in some instances, examiners have helped write the application to motivate the inventors.[101] However, this negotiated procedure is not as acceptable in developed countries, such as Australia.[102] In Australia, following a lodgement of a request for examination, a full official examination of the application takes place, usually within a further period of about 12 months. This examination includes a reasonably comprehensive search of earlier patent literature towards assessing the novelty and inventive merit of the invention.[103] The examiner will not help applicants in any way with the application but will allow them to resubmit the application after amendments.[104]

According to the above sections, the availability of this procedure for granting a patent is based on ss 71 and 78 (1). If the s 71(1)(a) requirements are not met, the DG will not consider an application under s 78(1). Hence, any patent grant in Sri Lanka should follow this procedure. An applicant may request an examination under s 73(1) to a local examiner in lieu of a search report if they believe that the invention is new, involves an inventive step and is industrially applicable under s 63 of the Act.

Moreover, under s 99(1), the Commercial High Courts ('CHC') may on the application of any person showing a legitimate interest or any competent authority, including the DG, to which the owner of the patent and every assignee, licensee or sub-licensee on record shall be made a party, declare a patent null and void.[105]

A study conducted in 2007 on patent grants in Sri Lanka during 1999–2006 has revealed that the number of patents granted under s78 exceeds the number of grants by examination under s 73. The likely reason for the imbalance is that the process under s78 is more straightforward than the substantive examination procedure, and hence, applicants choose the easier method for a patent grant.[106] Further, if the applicant has satisfied all the requirements under the Act, the patent will be granted under s 79. If there are any corrections or if the patent is rejected, the DG will notify the decision in writing under s 78(5).

Any application filed outside Sri Lanka under the *PCT* designating Sri Lanka shall, if the applicant files a corresponding application with the DG of NIPO, be deemed to be an application made under the Act.[107] As a result, a foreigner could designate Sri Lanka in an international application under the *PCT*. Hence, it is clear that regardless of whether the application is under the *PCT* or is a local application, the procedure is the same for granting the patent and the DG exercises their discretion

---

[100] Ibid.

[101] Interviewee # 23.

[102] Moir (2013).

[103] Australian Patent Office (2020).

[104] Weatherall et al. (2011).

[105] Interviewee # 23.

[106] Wilson (2007).

[107] IP Act s 71(8).

to either grant or reject the patent. Foreign applicants can file patents either via *PCT* or under the national phase. Statistics reveal that from January to September 2021, 193 *PCT* applications have been lodged in Sri Lanka of which 92 patents have been registered and 125 have been published.[108] In contrast, international applications filed locally number 15, of which six patents have been registered.[109] It appears that for the international community, filing through *PCT* is preferable to filing locally. Regarding *PCT* applications, Drahos stated that in India, the introduction of the *Patents Act, 1970* resulted in a drop in foreign patent applications because this Act raised its standard of novelty to include documentary publication anywhere in the world and raised patent fees.[110] India also amended the clause to define medicines and drugs for the purpose of excluding these from patentability.[111]

There is no provision regarding the opposition procedure in the granting stage, which will be discussed later along with the issues of resolution, and it is left to the court to decide on the validity of the patent after the grant, in a court of law, should someone approach the court. This aspect was discussed under the local legal process. The real essence of invention is tested in a court of law in an infringement battle. At that time, it is determined whether the invention in question is valid or not.[112] The current system is then very similar to a 'utility model', which requires a low patentable requirement on application.

A patent examiner at NIPO asserted:

> The low standard is the main reason the Sri Lankan IP office has recommended to the IP Advisory Committee, which consists of heads of departments of ministries, private sector and universities, that such applications be channelled into a utility model system that will provide a 5-year period of protection.[113]

A utility model is very similar to a standard patent, but usually has a shorter term and less stringent patentability requirements. However, this reform is not yet adopted in Sri Lanka.

3.5.3 Prior Art

The prior art search helps to identify the closest prior arts and thus can define the scope of protection in patent claims. In Sri Lanka, prior art for the purposes of novelty and inventive step according to s 64(2) consists of everything disclosed to the public[114] anywhere in the world, by written publication, oral disclosure, use or in any other

---

[108] NIPO (2022).

[109] Ibid.

[110] See the Indian Patents Act, 1970 sub-s 13(2).

[111] Drahos (2010) ('Global Governance of Knowledge').

[112] Interviewee # 24.

[113] Interviewee # 25.

[114] The word 'public' does not necessarily refer to the people at large. It may cover the members of the public who are free to use the particular technology, if disclosed. In other words, the inventor

way, prior to the filing, or where appropriate, priority date of the patent application claiming the invention. In other words, prior art refers to the total human knowledge on the subject relating to the particular invention or the relevant subject matter that has been made available to the public in any manner anywhere in the world.[115] In the Sri Lankan context, the role of the examiner is to refer to every documentation on prior art available to them under s 73 to decide on the inventive step.

Thus, in principle examination adopts a high bar, but at present, the examiners only search local databases and free databases made available from WIPO. Currently, NIPO does not have the facility to provide patent information searching services for members of public. Therefore, researchers and investors find it difficult to gain access to state-of-the-art information concerning relevant prior art for their research projects. Such a situation in relation to the international discourse would have negative implications on R&D programs implemented in the country.[116]

Nonetheless, Sri Lanka could rely on ISAs on a *PCT* application. A recognised ISA identifies the published documents, which may indicate whether the invention is patentable or not, and establishes an opinion on its patentability. Currently, there are about 15 ISAs under the *PCT* system. However, Sri Lanka is not a receiving office, and the International Bureau of WIPO acts as a receiving office for Sri Lanka. According to annexure C of this Bureau,[117] it has appointed four competent ISAs and preliminary examining authorities for nationals and residents of Sri Lanka. These authorities are the Australian, European, Korean and Swedish patent offices.[118]

Some years ago, WIPO wanted to establish a patent information system in Sri Lanka, to streamline the large amount of patent documents that require disclosure of the prior art of the patent applications, through establishing patent information centres in Sri Lanka. The effort failed because NIPO did not encourage WIPO to establish patent information centres in the universities (particularly in the University of Moratuwa where most of the inventions are created).

A former WIPO official said:

> Establishing a patent information system in universities has a great potential because the universities have the potential to link up with industry and entrepreneurs who are in a position to provide venture capital for inventions.[119]

This belief supports the need for interpretive communities where skills and knowledge can be developed and fostered. This goal could be achieved by providing venture capital for inventors and institutions, such as through SLIC offering support, through industry–university linkages for R&D in relevant areas and by giving them a product

must disclose the invention only to those who are under the obligation of confidence. Any other disclosures may be harmful: Windsurfing International Inc v Tabur Marine (Great Britain) Ltd (1985) RPC 59.

[115] Bristol-Myers Squibb Ltd v Baker Narton Pharmaceuticals Inc (2001) RPC 1.

[116] Interviewee # 25. See also Chin (2000).

[117] WIPO (2022a, b).

[118] Ibid.

[119] Interviewee # 21.

to meet specific needs.[120] The mutual relationship is one way of ensuring inventions are linked with the industry, which is not occurring in Sri Lanka. In countries such as Australia, the IP office acts as a hub for information and resources that communities can utilise, but at present, the NIPO has not engaged in an interpretive community role in the discourse to foster use or knowledge of the patent.[121] This aspect will be further discussed in Chap. 5.

Hence, prior art search in Sri Lanka is based on 'everything disclosed to the public anywhere in the world', which is a high-bar search that is used in many developed countries, but considering the accessibility issues for searching mechanisms available in Sri Lanka, it is questionable whether Sri Lanka can go very far with this prior art requirement.

3.5.4 Disclosure

Patent law in any jurisdiction requires a patent specification document to disclose an invention in such a manner as to allow a person skilled in the relevant art to make or carry out the invention. Section 71(3) further states that the 'description shall disclose the invention in a manner sufficiently clear and complete for the invention to be evaluated, and to be carried out by a person having ordinary skill in the relevant technology and shall, in particular, indicate the best mode[122] to the applicant for carrying out the invention'. Hence, according to the current law, the applicant needs to disclose the best mechanism contemplated by the inventor for carrying out the invention. This is the mechanism used in countries such as Australia, the UK and the US.

The former DG commented:[123]

> The current disclosure requirement is a heavy burden to the office because it is time-consuming and expensive. But it is important to have this requirement. Otherwise, there is no guideline for a patent grant, and we will be granting patents without any utility.

NIPO is contemplating amendments to the present disclosure requirements (s 71 *IP Act*). The amendments propose strengthening disclosure of an invention. *TRIPS* has globalised the disclosure obligation, making it mandatory for WTO members to require an applicant to disclose the invention.[124] According to the amendment, an applicant needs to reveal only 'one mechanism' known to the applicant. In some instances, the one mechanism can still be the best method as well, but it does not have

[120] Ibid.

[121] Ibid.

[122] The best mode or method must be in practice and not in theory. In Van der Laely V Ruston's Engineering (1993) RPC 45 it was emphasised that what is required is not the best method but the best method known to the applicant.

[123] Interviewee # 23.

[124] TRIPS Agreement art 29(1).

to be. There are benefits of introducing the one mechanism approach to a country such as Sri Lanka according to the former DG, who remarked:[125]

> The best mechanism approach is not suitable for a country like Sri Lanka, which has minimum resources and expertise: What is important is to register a standard patent and encourage the applicants to apply, rather than getting their patents nullified only for the reason that the applicant has not disclosed the best method.[126] With this amendment, if the applicant can disclose only one method, it is sufficient for a patent grant.

The DG also stated that there have been several serious controversies and technical issues in the EU in using this 'best mechanism method'.[127] However, this amendment has not been introduced to the Parliament yet, suggesting a lack of commitment to introduce reforms.

3.6 Patent Examiners

The problems raised at large in the global–local discourses on the patent examination process, prior art and disclosure requirements can be considered obstacles to the acceptance and use of good quality patents, but these three problems are inextricably intertwined with the fact that Sri Lanka has few patent examiners. The local discourse discusses this issue as a problem of patent examiner training and resulting backlog issues that face Sri Lanka in the implementation of the international discourse.

3.6.1 Training

The problems of recruiting and training patent examiners arise from a combination of three factors: the employment rules and regulations of the Sri Lankan public service, the availability of relevant graduates within the public service employment pool, and the relevant training methodology utilised in the NIPO.

When a new examiner joins NIPO, they usually lack knowledge of the patent granting process. Therefore, their skills must be increased to the level required for performing the various tasks associated with examination. This has to be achieved in an orderly manner and within a certain period. For example, in the EU, the training for new patent examiners is an integrated search and examination training and has two

125 Ibid.

126 Ibid.

127 The best mode requirement focuses specifically on the best mode known to the inventor at the time the application is filed. It is a subjective standard. Suppose that the inventor is faced with options A, B and C with respect to a particular feature of the invention and concludes at the time of filing that application A is the best mode. If it is subsequently determined that either B or C in fact is a better mode, this will not jeopardise the validity of the patent since the inventor has, in good faith, provided information to the best of their knowledge on the filing date.

components: classroom-based training and on-the-job training. Both components are equally important, and each contributes in its particular way to providing an efficient training program for newcomers.

The classroom-based initial training in the EU provides trainees with the general knowledge and skills to perform their tasks as patent examiners. The classroom approach has the advantage of being more efficient in terms of trainer time than individual on-the-job coaching because a single trainer can teach up to 12 trainees at the same time. Furthermore, a common basic training program for all newcomers organised in a centralised manner contributes to the harmonisation of the patent granting practice of the office across clusters (i.e. technical fields) and sites.[128] In some countries, universities are commissioned to provide these training courses as on-the-job training to complement the classroom-based training, in that the coaches provide field-specific training both in terms of search strategy (e.g. classes and databases) and in terms of examination practice for the real files treated by the newcomers. This on-the-job training is interleaved with the classroom-based training to provide the trainees with enough opportunities to practice the lessons they have learnt in class on their own files. The instructors responsible for the on-the-job training also provide 'just-in-time' information in the sense that they give ad hoc support to the trainees when they run into difficulties. Thereby, the instructors ensure that the actions generated by the trainees are European Patent Convention compliant and of high quality from the first action onwards. Last, the instructors provide feedback to the trainees by reviewing their search reports and communications.[129] Hence, the instructors and trainees can both be considered actors in the EU system and the communication between them enables to strengthen the harmonisation of the EU patent granting process.

However, NIPO does not provide methodical examiner training for new recruits. The basic statutory qualification of an examiner is that they should be a graduate from a local university in the field of biotechnology or physical science. Patent examiners are trained only in-house on patent procedures through the work learning process, which adopts the formality examination rather than the modified or substantive one. Local classroom-based training is not conducted. Most examiner training is conducted through WIPO training workshops onsite in Sri Lanka or when the examiners are sent for training to foreign IP offices, such as those of Japan, Korea, the EU and the US.[130]

With regard to WIPO training, there is no requirement that NIPO request training. According to the DG, WIPO automatically provides opportunities to train examiners, and accordingly, in the past 5 years there was an opportunity every month for an examiner to be sent for training sessions in various countries.[131] The training costs, including on air tickets and accommodation are borne by WIPO. According to the DG, opportunities for training are available, but the selection of staff for such trainings

[128] Bailas (2007).

[129] Ibid.

[130] Interviewee # 10.

[131] Ibid.

is an issue. The government policy on training means junior-level officers can be sent for training only once a year. Hence, the same person cannot be sent for multiple training sessions because of this government policy but may be sent once for training every year.[132] As one examiner expressed, this has meant: 'They did not have the opportunity for foreign training even once a year.'[133] Thus, the problem related to training is caused by funding issues and the aforementioned issue regarding the public service regulations, but the discourse indicates it is also caused by the NIPO's lack of acceptance of the need to establish an interpretive community and use international training appropriately.

Nevertheless, the discourse indicates a change is occurring in relation to where trainers are sent. Previously the US and the EU were the focus for training but now it is China. The United States Patent and Trademark Office ('USPTO') and the European Patent Office have encoded capacity-building projects in developing countries towards forming an interpretive community through assistance and training.[134] The aim behind such programs is to create a technical jurisprudence of rules whereby examiners could deepen their knowledge of patent language and can begin to see the meaning of invention in a different way. These types of interactions regarding technological rules help to create and maintain a technical rules-based discourse.[135] For example, Indian examiners are exposed to these encoded capacity-building programs and India has hence fostered the growth of an interpretive culture by breaking the ordinary language limits on invention, which has created a new world in which, in part, scientifically trivial innovations become patentable inventions.[136] Sri Lanka has a long way to go to reach this status.

Currently, there is a shift, for examiners are being sent to countries in the region for training, such as Korea, China, Japan and India. The reason for this shift may be that these countries may have come forward to provide training opportunities to Sri Lanka or the DG of NIPO may have requested for training from these countries. The examiners themselves recognise they are obtaining the best training by going to these countries.[137] Hence, the discourse is changing with regard to patent examiner training. According to participants, foreign training includes hands-on training as well as passive information-sharing sessions.[138]

The discourse identifies that where the examiners are trained is important to Sri Lanka. The US has a more ambitious approach regarding the granting of a patent. In essence, the examiner has to follow a detailed procedure and decide whether the invention claimed is novel and non-obvious, utility and invention being fully described. Regarding the non-obviousness test, commentators have taken the view that US patent law has come to operate with a lower standard since it allows a

[132] Ibid.

[133] Interviewee # 25.

[134] Drahos (2010) (n 111), p. 216.

[135] Ibid.

[136] Ibid.

[137] Interviewee # 15.

[138] Ibid.

small inventive step to render the invention non-obvious[139] so that the patent could be granted. In contrast, Japan has the formality of examination to check whether the application fulfils the necessary procedural and formal requirements; later, a request for examination needs to be made for an examination to be carried out. The substantive examination is very strict and there is no lowering of the standards, unlike in the US system, in order to grant the patent.[140]

Within the Sri Lankan context, in some instances, once examiners are exposed to a foreign training, they may tend to read patent claims through the lens of foreign exposure upon their return.[141] As mentioned earlier, Drahos noted an example of USPTO officials hinting at the danger of this occurring when Indian examiners were sent to USPTO for training.[142] Moreover, it is questionable how the trained examiners are using their newly gained technical knowledge in patent grants upon their return. This is mainly because Sri Lanka's examination process adopts a formality examination rather than substantive, and most patents are granted only to motivate the innovators.[143] This is a flaw in Sri Lanka's patent granting process. As one expert said, 'some patents are not deserving'.[144] This is mainly because such patents can be categorised as utility patents that will provide commercial benefit to the country or to the innovator. Due to this reason, the discourse identifies that Sri Lanka should have a utility model system to encourage incremental inventions.[145] However, utility models are yet to be introduced into the present Act. This is either because the importance of such an amendment is not yet felt by the government or because NIPO has not pushed the government for such change. Regardless of the reason, this shows a lack of commitment or of discourse to introduce important reforms.

3.6.2 Resulting Backlog Issues

Backlog issues at the NIPO arise due to insufficient staff and funding and related issues, according to the discourse, but this is regarded in the discourse as common to every patent office. USPTO faced backlog issues in the nineteenth century and faces it even at present. The scale of backlog problems in the USPTO is escalating every year, and UPSTO's current patent backlog stand at about 540,000.[146] The US system outsourced work to private companies and other patent offices, such as Australia's,

---

139 Merrill et al. (2004). The US Office also has pro-patentability policies for types of 'invention' such as gene sequences, which some argue are naturally occurring. See also Drahos (2010) (n 321).

140 Japan Patent Office (2021).

141 Merrill et al. (2004) (n 139).

142 Drahos (2010) (n 134), p. 216.

143 This aspect is discussed in Sect. 3.6.1.

144 Interviewee # 1.

145 This aspect is discussed in Sect. 3.8.5.

146 Federal News Network (2018).

to alleviate backlog.[147] Similarly, the Japanese Patent Office is confronted with such backlog issues and the hiring of examiners remains key to resolving the issue.[148]

Currently, there is a heavy backlog in the NIPO mainly because there were only four patent examiners in the IP office in 2017. In particular, in the patent division there is a backlog because examiners need to have a scientific background, whereas suitable graduates with relevant qualifications are not readily available, and public service engagement policies limit the number of available candidates. One examiner stated that it is very important to recruit more examiners.[149] Vacancies have been advertised for 5 years but no recruitments were made because of the burdensome recruitment procedures adopted in the Sri Lanka public service. NIPO does not have the power to recruit staff directly, unlike in Australia. NIPO needs to obtain suitably qualified personnel to be examiners to be assigned through the government service.

This means NIPO must source its staff from those currently serving within the public service. Even if there are qualified graduates keen to join NIPO as examiners from another government department, first, NIPO has to find a replacement for the other department in order to recruit willing officers as examiners. Because of this stringent procedure, it is challenging to both recruit examiners and to remove any examiner from NIPO who is not performing their duties. These are governmental public service procedural issues that need to be addressed for the smooth running of the patent office. It seems there should be a higher-level policymaking discourse to discuss reforms to the recruitment policy of NIPO for enabling it to recruit new patent officers for smooth operations. However, no ministry or other executive has taken the responsibility of making this happen.

The alternative method utilised to resolve the backlog in examinations adopted by other jurisdictions is to utilise the excess capacity in foreign patent offices and to engage them to conduct the examinations. This form of cooperation engages in community discourse and arises because *PCT* requirements are normative within the *PCT* community; hence, the USPTO and the UK PO make use of international outsourcing in order to deal with backlog problems.[150] At present, Singapore makes use of the outsourcing mechanism since Singapore's outsourcing strategy is part of a broader economic and social plan.[151] But in the Sri Lankan context, it would be a cheaper option to recruit more officers directly than pay outsourcing costs to foreign patent offices for NIPO will not be able to afford foreign fees for examination. Without such a plan, it will be unwise for Sri Lanka to make use of outsourcing arrangements.

However, a former NIPO official expressed a different view regarding the lack of examiners in the NIPO. He stated that he could have obtained the approval for additional examiners, but the main problem was the justification: he questioned the

147 Drahos (2010) (n 142), p. 114.

148 Ibid.

149 Interviewee # 25.

150 Drahos (2010) (n 147), p. 321.

151 Ibid 323.

need for 15–20 examiners to deal with 200 national patent applications.[152] He also stated that he had requested SLIC[153] to increase the patent applications annually up to 1000. If this happened, the patent office can recruit more examiners; he says that if not, the argumentation of the patent office would bring no practical benefits to society. As a government-funded authority, the NIPO must use public funds responsibly.[154] The lack of recruitment for the NIPO under government budgets has become a handicap for the improvement of the patent examination process.

In every practical sense, in this researcher's view, having only four examiners in NIPO is insufficient to clear the backlog in the patent office since patent officers should ideally have different sorts of education in different fields, such as chemistry and engineering. Such diversity of expertise cannot be expected from four people. It is also a deterrent to applicants asking for substantive examination. It has been suggested that the basic strategy to reduce the backlog is to employ more examiners and to enter into various work-sharing arrangements with other 'trusted' offices.[155] A country like Sri Lanka could be part of this arrangement through its membership of the *PCT* and the training of patent officers by developed countries' patent offices. If not, Sri Lanka would be isolated in the global patent system. However, in 2018 the staff of NIPO were increased to 79 from 44 to expedite the reduction of the current backlog.[156]

Another reason for the backlog is the lack of knowledge and skill of the local patent applicants in drafting patent specifications in an application. The Act states if certain conditions are not satisfied under s 78(1) or if there are errors in the application, the DG can request the applicant to file the necessary corrections within a period of three months from the date of request. In certain instances, examiners have helped them write the application to motivate the inventors or the applicants to hire patent agents.[157]

The discourse also identifies that the lack of an examination manual has further aggravated the problems of training and the lack of knowledge, skills and ability to process applications. The former DG stated that he began developing a manual but was unable to complete it by the time he retired as the DG after 15 years of service. He further said that it was assumed the new DG would complete the task.[158] Furthermore, Atapattu, an examiner, emphasised it is very important to have an examination manual as a guide for the examiners as well as to guide the applicants

---

[152] Interviewee # 23.

[153] SLIC is under the State Ministry of Skill Development, Vocational Education, Research and Innovation. The objectives of the commission are to encourage the making or creation of inventions by citizens of Sri Lanka; to give technical, financial and legal assistance to inventors; and to exercise, discharge and perform all powers, functions and duties. For more information, see Sri Lanka Inventors Commission Home (2022).

[154] Interviewee # 23.

[155] Drahos (2010) (n 150), p. 330.

[156] Sirimanna (2019).

[157] Interviewee # 23.

[158] Ibid. Still there is no examination manual.

and the public,[159] but at present, the public has to depend on private patent agents for guidance, which is expensive and often stated as the reason locals do not consider patenting, given their view that the fees for advice are exorbitant for locals.[160] The lack of an examination manual is another example of the neglect of the patent system because there are other patent manuals that could be adopted and adapted from other IP offices. However, even for the adoption or transplantation of a manual from overseas, the local abilities need to be considered.

Nonetheless, it should be reiterated that drafting an examination manual is a lengthy process that requires support from all stakeholders involved in patenting. The Indian experience suggests that there has been a demand from new inventors, patent practitioners and foreign applicants to codify the Indian Patent Office practices in the form of a manual. A draft manual was published in 2009 on the official website and comments and suggestions were invited from stakeholders. By incorporating the comments and suggestions received, that draft was thoroughly revised in 2011 to make it more user friendly.[161]

NIPO has failed to engage as a node to progress the production of the manual and, in the discourse, is not performing its role as an interpretive community. The development of a manual is essential for training and for consistency and certainty for inventors and the patent community. NIPO, as the focal point, needs to embark on this cumbersome task by engaging all the stakeholders in the country, with WIPO assistance.[162] A ministry official at MIC, stated that one reason NIPO is not spending time on finalising the IP policy and strategy or a manual is that it is more important to clear the backlog.[163]

Thus, the local discourses identify problems in the examination process and the requirements for prior art and disclosure of the invention, which together with issues related to training, knowledge and skills have led to the issues of backlog and whether the system should be geared to foreign high-technology or local low-technology inventions or both. The problems are not independent of each other but related and intertwined, resulting in backlogs and failure of the patent administration to engage with the global and local patent communities.

3.7 Alternative Discourses

The discourse also provides some discussion of alternatives and methods for consideration for resolution of the aforementioned issues, which will be discussed in the next part of this case study. The local discourses have raised the following alternatives: the adoption of a modified examination process, the availability of pre- and

---

[159] Interviewee # 25.

[160] Ibid.

[161] The Office of Controller General of Patents (2011).

[162] Interviewee # 11.

[163] Ibid.

post-grant opposition procedures, the role of patent litigation and the involvement of the legal profession. These again try to square local conditions with global demands.

3.7.1 Modified Examination

Modified examination is a halfway house between substantive and formal examinations and there are various forms and approaches for this examination. Section 45 of the *Patents Act 1990* of Australia called this the 'standard' examination, for the role of the patent examiner is to examine the application for compliance with all the provisions available during examination for novelty and inventive steps. Australia did provide a system of modified examination under s 47 and s 48 of its *Patents Act 1990*, until 2013, for complete applications for a standard patent and where the patent had been granted in a prescribed foreign country, such as the US, Canada, New Zealand or an English-language country signatory to the EPC. Modified examination as a system has been repealed and a system of expedited examination has been adopted in Australia where an applicant can apply for accelerated examination on the basis of several reasons (e.g. commercialisation considerations, such as the applicant is seeking to enforce their patent rights or an investor requires a granted patent before investing in the patent),[164] or when the claims of the invention have been found acceptable by a patent office that is a member of the Global Patent Prosecution Highway ('GPPH') program.[165] The GPPH program has the following requirements:

1. The Australian patent application must be appropriately associated with either (a) an overseas application having at least one claim found to be allowable/patentable by one of the Offices of Earlier Examination (those members participating in the GPPH); or (b) a PCT Application having at least one claim found to be allowable/patentable by an international authority that is one of the Offices of Earlier Examination.
2. Corresponding Australian claims. All claims in the Australian application must sufficiently correspond, or be amended to sufficiently correspond, to one or more of those allowable/patentable claims of the overseas or *PCT* application examined by the OEE.
3. Australian examination. A request for examination must either have been filed earlier or filed at the time of requesting accelerated examination under the GPPH.

---

[164] IP Australia (2020a).

[165] IP Australia (2020b). See Pitts and Kim (2009). See also Restrepo (2016).

Currently, 25 countries have joined the GPPH,[166] and academic debate about its effectiveness and purposes continues, but it provides a mechanism for dealing with backlogs because it allows to share search and examination results between offices.

By way of comparison, Malaysia has two options: normal substantive examination and modified substantive examination. Under the first option, the Malaysian Patent Office will conduct its own search and substantive examination of the application, assisted whenever possible by the results of any search and examination of the same invention in recognised foreign jurisdictions. A request for a modified substantive examination may only be filed when a corresponding Australian, European, UK, Japanese, Korean or US patent has been granted for the same invention (e.g. the same drug). Under this examination, the application undergoes a simplified procedure. Importantly, the application will still be assessed for novelty, statutory subject matter (which may differ from the other jurisdictions) and compliance with the specification of the foreign patent relied on, but not for the inventive step. Moreover, a modified substantive examination can only be conducted on the basis of a single foreign patent.

Modified examination will be useful to a developing country if it has the ability to conduct substantial examination procedures and also if an applicant wishes to protect multiple embodiments of an invention, via separate independent claims in a single application in a foreign jurisdiction. In the present Sri Lankan context, substantial examination is very basic, and rarely would a local applicant request for protection of multiple embodiments in a foreign jurisdiction. However, under s 73(3) of the *IP Act* foreigners can file a patent application with the DG. Hence, the absence of discourse about the adoption of a modified examination does not disadvantage Sri Lanka since it will not benefit the patent granting process in Sri Lanka.

3.7.2 Availability of Pre-grant or Post-grant Opposition Procedure

Sri Lankan patent law does not provide pre-grant or post-grant opposition procedures to assess patent validity. The patent opposition procedure is an administrative process within the patent office. Laws providing for pre-grant and post-grant patent opposition are essential to prevent the wrongful grant of patents before or after the grant. In practice, some countries, such as India, Australia and the US, and the *European Patent Act* have either of these systems or both. For example, s 25(1) of the Indian *Patents Act, 1970* along with Rule 55 of *Patents Rules 2003* provide the laws relating to pre-grant opposition in India. Opposition can be filed by any person in writing, any time

166 Currently, 25 countries are members, namely, the individual European states of Austria, Denmark, Estonia, Germany, Finland, Hungary, Portugal, Poland, Spain and Sweden, and the non-EU countries Australia, the US, the UK, New Zealand, Japan, Israel, Iceland Russia, Singapore, Norway, Korea, Canada, Chile, Columbia and Peru, together with one institutional member, the Nordic Patent Institute.

after the publication of the patent application and before it is granted.[167] Unlike pre-grant opposition, post-grant opposition can only be filed by an 'interested party'.[168] The grounds of opposition for both opposition procedures is provided under s 25(1) and s 25(2) of Indian *Patents Act, 1970* as amended in 2005.[169] Hence, the discourse identifies it is important to maintain the balance between the two approaches: to ensure a steady examination process and encourage R&D/to encourage applications but balance others' needs.[170]

Pre-grant opposition procedures allow third parties, such as competitors, suppliers or customers of the patentee, to raise arguments and provide evidence against the validity of a patent that has been accepted, but not yet granted.[171] This system has many advantages in maintaining the patent register quality. One view is that it is practically impossible for a patent office to find all prior art relevant to a patent, but third parties may be in a better position to access information because they are active in technology.[172] This would allow the patent examiners to make right decisions about the patent grant.[173] Second, there are potential benefits for smaller businesses, if there is a low-cost mechanism for challenging the validity of a patent grant, compared with courts, particularly in an era where increasing burdens on patent offices are raising questions about the quality and reach of the patents being granted.[174] In the Sri Lankan context, providing pre-grant opposition would be more cost-effective and result in faster disposal of cases on merit, thereby reducing the costs incurred in contesting post-grant proceedings.

Pre-grant opposition to trademarks is available in Sri Lanka. Once a person submits a mark for registration, it is tested against two criteria. One is the objective criterion, which assesses whether the mark is registrable or not. The second criterion is the third-party right to argue whether there are similar marks in the register. Section 104 of the *IP Act* provides that the DG shall not register signs that inter alia resemble registered or unregistered marks of third parties as well as well-known marks. In addition, s 111(10)[175] provides procedure relating to the inadmissibility of a trademark.

---

[167] Bhatangar (2021).

[168] Section 3.2 (1)(t) of the Indian Patents Act, 1970 defines the term 'person interested' as including an individual involved in or promoting research in the field to which the patent pertains. It may also refer to an entity that has a manufacturing, trading or financial interest in the patented goods.

[169] See Indian Patents Act, 1970.

[170] Shikha (2009).

[171] Weatherall et al. (2011) (n 104).

[172] Merges (1999).

[173] Ibid.

[174] Shikha (2009) (n 170).

[175] Where any person considers that the mark is inadmissible on one or more of the grounds specified in s 103 or s 104 that person may, within a period of three months from the date of publication of the application, give to the DG in the prescribed form, and together with the prescribed fee, notice of opposition to such registration stating the grounds of opposition accompanied by evidence to substantiate such grounds (emphasis added).

The Registrar will only publish the mark in the Government Gazette if satisfied that either of these criteria is met. Within three months of publication of application, any interested party can file a notice of opposition with the Registrar, and the Registrar will then hold an inquiry and accept or reject the mark. An aggrieved party can appeal against the Registrar's decision to the High Court. This mechanism in s 111(10) *IP Act* clearly enables a registered owner of a trademark to prevent a conflicting mark from being entered in the trademark register before it is published in the Government Gazette.[176]

Surprisingly, this procedure is not available for patents. It is questionable why the same procedure is not applicable for patents when it is used for trademarks. No reasons have been given by the patent office or the legislators for this omission, and this shows the unwillingness to improve the patent registration system to either conform to international standards or to cater to local needs, compared with the system for trademarks in Sri Lanka. However, Mr Kanag-Isvaran, a senior practitioner, was not very critical about this omission under the patent grants and stated, 'without a proper substantial examination procedure, there is no use of having pre-grant opposition since under the current system, as discussed earlier, the majority of patents are granted based on formality examination, which does not require an opposition procedure'.[177]

3.7.3 Patent Litigation

The *IP Act* does not provide for opposition hearing or an internal appeal system. Granting a patent is an administrative decision, and normally, any administrative decision is subject to judicial review. The judicial review of administrative decisions made within the patent registration process can conform with international norms of providing a review of determination made by public officials[178] and adds additional actors, that is, the judiciary and legal professionals, to the influence upon the patent discourse. However, in Sri Lanka, the review becomes the best available means of consideration of the merits of the application since no pre- or post-grant opposition proceedings are provided.

An applicant for a patent has the right to appeal to the CHC about decisions relating to the patents—first, in relation to administrative corrections for non-incretion or omissions from the patent filing;[179] second, on issues from decisions of the DG, including determinations such as on the validity or granting of a patent;[180] and third, in

---

[176] Marsoof (2012).

[177] Interviewee # 24.

[178] See art 32 of the TRIPS Agreement, which deals with an opportunity for judicial review.

[179] IP Act s 163.

[180] Ibid s 173.

relation to infringement proceedings[181] before the CHC.[182] The CHC was originally established under the *High Court of the Provinces (Special Provisions) Act, No. 10 of 1996*.[183] It has jurisdiction to hear civil actions where the cause of action has arisen out of commercial transactions in which the debt, damage or demand exceeds 20 million Sri Lankan Rupees. According to this Act, an applicant can only appeal to the CHC once the patent is granted, and the real essence of invention is most likely to be tested in a court of law in a validity of a patent claim in an infringement battle between the patent owner and the infringing party under s 173. At that time, it is determined whether the invention in question is valid or not.[184]

Hence, it could be probably argued that the CHC appeal has the same effect of a post-grant opposition in other jurisdictions where an appeal is made regarding the decision to grant a patent. However, taking into consideration the nature of the opposition procedure, it could also be argued this does not resonate with post-grant opposition. Usually, the opposition procedure should allow the party opposing to lead evidence and to challenge the grant of the patent. Countries such as Australia have an oral hearing or written submissions since oral or written evidence is crucial in a patent proceeding. However, in practice, in countries such as Sri Lanka, appellate proceedings are confined to errors of law, and do not allow new evidence, such as oral evidence, to be submitted. Courts will only go through the face of the records of the earlier proceedings for identifying errors in law. Hence, it is risky to draw comparisons between post-grant opposition and appellate proceedings in Sri Lanka.

Regarding the procedure under s 173, an aggrieved party can submit an appeal to the CHC by way of petition of appeal with a certified copy of the decision appeal form, accompanied by copies of all relevant documents and affidavits from the NIPO file. All the documents shall be served on the DG and other respondents named in the petition of appeal and the respondents may file a statement of objections. Under s 173(4), the CHC may affirm, reverse or vary the DG's decision or may issue such directions to the DG, or order further hearing by the DG, as the CHC may require. Any person who is dissatisfied with any Order made by the CHC under s 173(4) may submit an appeal with leave to the Supreme Court of Sri Lanka against this Order.

Thus, an aggrieved party under the Act can directly go to the courts under the *IP Act*. There are different views regarding this patent litigation process. As Mark Lumley has suggested, the quality of a grant is not a concern since it is too time-consuming to conduct patent examinations in all cases, and if the patent really matters, it will be most likely be tested in an infringement proceeding instead.[185] This view may be suitable to a developed country, such as the US, where parties can afford to participate in patent litigation. Conversely, in countries such as Sri Lanka, patent

[181] Ibid s 170.

[182] The High Court for the Western Province is vested with exclusive jurisdiction in respect of some specified commercial matters in terms of the High Court of the Provinces (Special Provisions) Act, No. 10 of 1996.

[183] Ibid.

[184] Ibid.

[185] Lumley (2001).

litigation is unaffordable to many, and the legal process should have the flexibility to review the patent grant before the courts are approached. Drahos, who opposed Lumley's view, stated that litigation should not be the mechanism to resolve a patent's validity.[186] However, patent litigation is not used much in Sri Lanka. Yet, infringement litigation is on the initiative of the patent holder; they may use the litigation strategically, for example, to exhaust the opposition's resources or obtain favourable licences. Consequently, this consideration is also relevant to the discussion of the availability of pre- and post-grant opposition.

3.8 Regulating the Use of Patents

A patent grants an exclusive right that is territorial in nature. However, once a patent is granted by considering the patentable criteria, mechanisms such as CL, parallel importation and local working conditions could in some way restrict the exclusive nature of the patent. Within the patent ecosystem, these mechanisms could be regarded as important discourses in regulating the use of patents. Hence, the following section will shed some light on the applicability of these discourses under the existing IP regime in Sri Lanka.

3.8.1 Compulsory Licensing

CL is a process by which a government licenses companies or individuals other than the patent owner to use the rights of the patent—to make, use, sell or import a product under patent—without the permission of the patent owner. According to art 31(b) of the *TRIPS Agreement,* CL may be granted by the government to a proposed user in situations in which the user has made efforts to obtain authorisation from a rights holder on reasonable commercial terms and conditions and such efforts have been unsuccessful within a reasonable period. In addition, the requirement for demonstrating efforts to obtain authorisation from the rights holder can be waived and CL granted in situations of a national emergency, or other circumstances of extreme urgency or in cases of public non-commercial use.

CL has been a controversial issue throughout its evolution, owing to opposition from both top biopharmaceutical innovators and governments who issue CL. Among WTO members, developed countries generally tend to view this provision with suspicion, because multinational patent owners feel their patent security has been threatened and their R&D achievements have been undermined by CL,[187] the price controls and other trade barriers—which threaten to chip away at their foothold

[186] Drahos (2010) (n 155).

[187] Yang (2011).

and erode the resources they can invest in the next generation of medicines.[188] In contrast, developing countries consider it an issue of prime importance, and use it, although sparingly, because, as in the case of *Bayer Corporation v Union of India*,[189] MNCs charge high prices for important drugs, which most people in developing countries hence cannot afford. Therefore, there needs to be a balance in the issue on CL.[190]

Section 86(2)(b) of the *IP Act* 2003 mirrors the provisions of art 31 of the *TRIPS Agreement*, granting the DG the power to grant CL to an interested party, on being satisfied that the applicants' efforts to obtain approval within a reasonable period from the right holder on reasonable terms and conditions have failed. Section 86(2)(c) allows the DG to waive compliance with s 86(2)(b) if satisfied about the existence of a national emergency; or other circumstances of extreme urgency; or in the case of public non-commercial use for the purpose of such national security, nutrition or health; or for the development of other vital sections of the national economy. Hence, s 86(2)(b) conforms with art 31 of the *TRIPS Agreement* on national security and extreme urgency, but the addition of the words, 'for the purposes such as national security, nutrition, health or for the development of other vital sections of the national economy', raises a debate about the width of this right in the circumstances of public non-commercial use. Currently, judicial interpretation of the breadth of these words is absent, but it is opined that the interpretation of the provision may follow the interpretation consistent with the Reichmann interpretation of art 31 as non-exhaustive and enable countries to interpret the public non-commercial use right widely.[191] Alternatively the statutory context may be interpreted as restrictive and limiting to the examples specified. This could be relevant to Sri Lanka in the event that a local working requirement is introduced into Sri Lankan patent law.[192]

It is interesting to note that a local discourse arose regarding the constitutionality of clauses 83 and 84 of the IP Bill relating to patent duration and patent owner's rights being inconsistent with arts 34, 12(1) and 14(1)(g) of the *1978 Constitution*.[193] The constitutionality of the Intellectual Property Bill was challenged by three petitioners,

---

[188] Taylor (2017).

[189] Bayer Corporation v Union of India (2014) 60 PTC 277. The first ever CL was granted to Natco Pharma on 9 March 2012 under s 84 of the Indian Patents Act, 1970 for the generic production of Bayer Corporation's Nexavar, a lifesaving medicine used for treating liver and kidney cancer. Bayer sold this drug at exorbitant rates, with one month's worth of dosage costing around Rs 2.8 Lakh. Natco Pharma offered to sell it for around Rs 9000, making it affordable for people belonging to every stratum. The High Court rejected Bayer's petition seeking patent linkage in India, a system in which the drug controller refuses to grant or delays a marketing approval to a generic drug manufacturer to manufacture and sell a drug, if the drug is already patented. In this case, patent linkage was considered to be against public health interests because it would delay the entry of cheap, generic medicines into the market and keep medicines out of reach for the public who need them. All three conditions of s 84 were fulfilled and the decision was taken for the benefit of the general public.

[190] Ibid.

[191] Reichman (2009).

[192] Marsoof et al. (2018), p. 315. ("Local Working Requirements").

[193] Supreme Court Special Determination Nos. 14, 15, 16/2003.

Dr Kamalika Abeyratne, Mr Nihal Fernando and the Centre for Policy Alternatives (Guarantee) Ltd, an NGO, in the Supreme Court of Sri Lanka in 2003. These clauses allow the owner of the patent, including those of medical drugs, to control the supply and price of such drugs in the Sri Lankan markets, in the absence of any migratory provisions, such as CL and parallel importing of pharmaceutical drugs to meet national health emergencies. The Supreme Court Special Determination[194] affirmed the flexibilities available under the *TRIPS Agreement* to member states seeking to protect public health, agreed with the petitioners and determined that the clauses were inconsistent with art 12(1) of the *1978 Constitution*.[195] This confirms that local discourse exists and arises when motivated individuals believe that the law undermines the individual's rights. Section 86(2) was inserted into the *IP Act* as a result of this challenge.

Moreover, art 5(b) of the *Doha Declaration* deals with the freedom to interpret the grounds for CL. During negotiations, Sri Lanka joined the African group, Brazil and India in proposing that either art 31 be amended in order to delete para (f), which limits CL to 'predominantly for the domestic market', or an authoritative interpretation be provided that would recognise the right of members to allow the production for export without the consent of the patent holder in order to address public health needs in another country under art 30.[196]

Sri Lanka is a country with insufficient manufacturing capacity in the pharmaceutical sector and it is unable to import drugs made under CL elsewhere, while *TRIPS* mandates nations to use CL 'predominantly for domestic use'. In order to remedy this situation, the TRIPS Council provided the para 6 solution by adopting a formal waiver of the *TRIPS* requirement of domestic use of CL. This waiver has since become an amendment to *TRIPS*, subject to ratification by enough members. The waiver is applicable under the following conditions:[197]

- the country needs more drugs at a lower price than it can currently obtain; and
- the country has inadequate manufacturing capacity to make its own low-cost generic versions; and
- the country is seeking to import drugs that would be made under CL for export from another country where they are currently patented.[198]

The waiver is not necessary to import drugs that are made as legitimate generics in a country where they are not patented. For example, if Sri Lanka wants to import a drug manufactured legally as a generic in India, the waiver would not be applicable, but Sri Lanka would still require CL if the desired drug is patented in Sri Lanka. The exporting and importing country must both be patent-free.[199]

---

[194] Kerry (2007).

[195] Supreme Court Special Determination Nos. 14, 15, 16/2003.

[196] Hoen (2002).

[197] Ho (2011), p. 201. See also Mitchell and Voon (2009).

[198] Ibid.

[199] Mathews (2005).

In the Sri Lankan context, no interested party has yet invoked the CL provisions, and as Dr Harsha Cabral commented, 'the provisions on CL do not have any use since Sri Lanka does not have production capacity'.[200] This is too sweeping a statement, since Sri Lanka does have production capacity in specific sectors, such as construction, manufacturing and energy, but the full potential is not demonstrated within the economy owing to a lack of political commitment and legal expertise and also because these industries are not aligned with economic priorities. This aspect is discussed in Chap. 5 of this book.

3.8.2 Parallel Importation

Parallel trade occurs when a national law allows the importation of patented goods without the express permission of the IP owner, of a product made available earlier or sold more cheaply in another market. It is permitted under art 6 of *TRIPS*. The Sri Lankan *IP Act* allows parallel importing under s 122(b)[201] of trademarked products. The Sri Lankan Act does not have a section on patented products on parallel importation. In contrast, if an owner of a registered mark can prove that the product does not fall within the term 'lawfully manufactured in Sri Lanka', the owner can prevent the parallel importation of the said good. This section was invoked recently in *Hewlett Packard (Pvt) Ltd v Tech Information Solutions (Pvt) Ltd*, when the Supreme Court of Sri Lanka ruled that importing of genuine HP products through alternative sources on a prima facie basis satisfies the provisions of the *IP Act* permitting parallel imports.[202] Hence, the discourse on parallel importation is non-insignificant in Sri Lanka.

3.8.3 Local Working Conditions

The patent working condition would oblige the patent owner to 'work' the patent locally, as opposed to merely using the patent as an exclusive right to prevent others from doing so or to control importation.[203] Hence, a working requirement is intended to moderate the exclusivity of patent monopolies by necessitating the patent holder to

---

[200] Interviewee # 26.

[201] The registration of a mark shall not confer on its registered owner the right to preclude third parties from using the mark in relation to goods lawfully manufactured, imported, offered for sale, sold, used or stocked in Sri Lanka under that mark, provided that such goods have not undergone change.

[202] Hewlett Packard (Pvt) Ltd v Tech Information Solutions (Pvt) Ltd HC(Civil) 48/2011, SC(HC) LA 91/2012, SC(CHC)Appeal 45/2012 (Rahini Amarasinghe, Chandra Ekanayake, Sathya Hettige, JJ, October 2012). See also Daily Mirror (2012).

[203] Bodenhausen (1969), p. 71.

disseminate its invention into the local market.[204] Countries such as Sri Lanka should improve the local environment for transfer of technology and its diffusion. In order to absorb and adapt the technology, existing infrastructure policies, capital market regulations and tax regimes should be strengthened.[205] If Sri Lanka makes patents available, then it should encourage them to be worked locally as far as possible. As part of an investment, inducement or, in the extreme, a local working condition, would oblige the patent holder to manufacture the patented product within the country granting the rights. If a patent owner is unable to exploit the patent, they could grant a licence and the right to produce a patented product or process in local industrial plants or factories. For example, India has its own unique requirement under s 146(2) of the *Patents Act, 1970*, which states that a patent working is necessary and with this purpose, an annual working statement by the patentee and licensees thereof of a granted patent in India has to be filed. Hence, for countries such as Sri Lanka, local working conditions could bring significant benefits, including economic growth, increased employment opportunities and dissemination of knowledge of technology.[206] This aspect will be further discussed under transfer of technology in Sect. 5.12.3.

The present *IP Act* does not have a provision on local working conditions to balance the exclusive patent rights. This is disadvantageous to Sri Lanka for it forfeits a bargaining chip to be used in negotiating the transfer of technology and the employment that results from the establishment of local industrial plants.[207] Such a provision could be added by amending the *IP Act* to include a mechanism for issuing CL in the event that the patent owner fails to work the patent.[208] CL is also sometimes invoked where the patent owner will only work the patent in-house and will not establish a joint venture or a partnership with local companies. Hence, the discourse on local working conditions is non-existent in Sri Lanka and, thus far, except for a few academic articles, there is no pressure either locally or globally to introduce this requirement into its patent system.

3.8.4 Patent Law and the Legal Profession

As in other countries, IP law in Sri Lanka consists of legislation and the interpretation and application of that legislation by authoritative bodies, such as courts and patent offices. The law is informed by the participation of industry, civil society and NGOs, in the examination and disputation of applications for patents. Through

---

204 Iran Patent Centre (2020).

205 Hoekman et al. (2005).

206 Marsoof et al. (2018) (n 192).

207 Ibid.

208 Ibid.

this communicative interaction, people could form a common understanding generated largely within epistemologically compatible social or organisational groups.[209] Such understanding is necessary for the effective interpretation and application of law. Hence, judges and legal practitioners too are an important node within the local legal process since local legal expertise is necessary to navigate the administrative and judicial processes.[210]

Sri Lanka has a well-developed legal profession. It has a few IP lawyers and law firms that could be considered the best patent attorneys, and they are hired by wealthy innovators or foreign collaborations since they have the means to pay the high legal costs. Sri Lanka has a Legal Aid Commission that provides benefits free of charge to those in the community who cannot afford legal costs, but IP is not included in the list of services.[211] However, the country does not have a system of pro bono public interest lawyers.

There are several reasons for the lack of development of patent law in Sri Lanka.

First, the patent interpretive community in Sri Lanka consists of judges and patent attorneys. Patent examiners are at the bottom of the hierarchy, and the courts determine the issues of patentability. Patent examiners are important actors in the IP system since it is their decision that in the first instance determines whether or not a patent is to be granted, but they do not play an active role because the patent examination procedure is rudimentary compared with that of other countries. For example, India has a strong interpretative examination culture within the patent office, which means that in most cases the final decision about the patentability will be made by an examiner and not the court.[212]

In practice, parties are reluctant to go before the courts because patent litigation is very costly and time-consuming, and as a result, most cases are settled before the original courts or out of courts. The cases that are appealed relate to royalty payments, assignment rights and injunctions for infringements, rather than issues about the validity and interpretation of patent claims, such as the novelty or inventive step.[213] In an appeal, most lawyers argue on different technical points of law rather than on theories or policies, and thus, there is no opportunity to analyse or interpret the law.[214]

Second, only appellate court decisions are reported and therefore there are few reported decisions on patents in Sri Lanka.[215] For example, there is one reported case

---

[209] Gillespie (2008).

[210] Arup (2012).

[211] The Legal Aid Commission was established by the Legal Aid Law Act No 27 of 1978 and at present it has 84 centres island wide. See the Legal Aid Commission of Sri Lanka. http://www.legalaid.gov.lk/index.php/2016-01-13-09-16-07/about-us.

[212] Drahos (2010) (n 186), p. 215.

[213] Interviewee # 24.

[214] Ibid.

[215] Kumarasena v Data Management Systems Ltd (1987) 30 SLR 190; St Regis Packaging (Pvt) Ltd v Ceylon Paper Sacks Ltd 1 SLR 36 (2000); Farbridge v The Registrar of Patents (1946) 47 NLR 193.

under the *IP Act*.[216] In fact, 95% of the cases are settled in the CHC where patent litigation is originally performed or are disposed of on procedural grounds, and all these cases remain unreported.[217] Moreover, there is a high volume of cases generally pending in the CHC[218] and law reporting too is not up to date. Most judgements are written in Sinhalese and need to be translated into English. In most cases, the translation is not accurate, and lawyers must work on more accurate translations themselves which takes time.[219] This indicates that the reason for the inadequate interpretation of patent law in Sri Lanka is the lack of sufficient expertise and commitment in the subordinate divisions within the patent interpretive community.

Third, most judges are not trained in IP because this topic was only recently introduced in universities.[220] To strengthen IP in Sri Lanka, a World Bank grant was given from 2000 to 2005 to the Ministry of Justice. Under this project, academics,[221] state counsels and judges were given scholarships to foreign universities to gain qualifications in IP law. Upon return, the state counsels and judges were given assignments in other areas of law rather than IP, and inexperienced judges were assigned to IP matters without any training.[222] A senior practitioner commented: 'Some judges are exposed at the Provincial High Court to on-the-spot and on-the-job training, and they do not have much guidance on court proceedings.'[223] This is a clear example where Sri Lanka's court system could have used the knowledge of these experts to facilitate the IP development that is very crucial to the country but did not understand or use the qualifications of these individuals on their return. This situation indicates the difficulties in the discourse, namely that providing training does not necessarily precipitate development or discourse on patents or IP if the right action or litigation is not available for determination by the courts or academics. The concept of transplantation by training will be seen as an issue further in the discussion on issues with NIPO later in this chapter.

Fourth, most IP concepts are developed from English law concepts. The lack of access to foreign books and journals, limited English competency and the lack of library facilities for judges because of costs are significant drawbacks to the court system.[224] For example, India modernised its patent offices as part of its international obligations. Its library resources are being increased and the examiners are given access to international electronic databases and search engines; the country

---

[216] KIK Land (pvt) Ltd v DM Karunarathtna, and others ca 83/09, Court of Appeal of Sri Lanka (2011).

[217] Email from John Wilson (advice@srilankalaw.com) to Asanka Perera, 21 October 2021; Email from Chanakya Jayadeva (chankya0007@gmail.com) to Asanka Perera, 21 October 2021.

[218] Sri Lanka Commercial High Court (2017).

[219] Ibid.

[220] Ibid.

[221] The researcher is a recipient who received a scholarship and completed a MPhil Degree in Intellectual Property at Monash Law School in 2001.

[222] Interviewee # 24.

[223] Ibid.

[224] Ibid.

has established new research and training institutes for judges and has increased the number of examiners.[225] As will be discussed in Chap. 5, patents in Sri Lanka have not yet reached this status owing to the bottlenecks in the patent administration system, and in some instances, NIPO has not used the WIPO Technical Assistance programs prudently to uplift the patent system, unlike in India.

3.8.5 Is the Utility Model an Option?

Because of the rigour of the substantive examination, the former DG and staff at MIC have suggested a 'utility model' system be introduced in addition to the standard patent grant.[226] This would be a welcome change because, as discussed in this chapter, the patent granting process is built on formality of examination, which is considered a low standard of protection and less suitable than the utility model style. The rights conferred by 'utility model' laws are usually more suited to incremental or low-level local inventions that may not be inventive enough to warrant standard patent protection. Utility models can be the dominant form of IPR granted in a country or region, which would enhance development and innovation.[227]

For example, in China, the utility model patent is one of the most used types of protection under the Chinese patent law because this system provides fast-track registration protection and has a lower standard for inventiveness and lower application fees and maintenance costs. Currently, India is investigating the introduction of this model to encourage low-cost, useful and relatively simple innovations that may have commercial value for a limited period.[228] Moreover, Evenson and Westphal have concluded that utility models have improved productivity in countries lagging in terms of technologies.[229] For example, in Brazil, utility models helped domestic producers gain a significant share of the farm-machinery market by encouraging the adaptation of foreign technologies to local conditions.[230] Similarly, a study conducted in Malaysia has concluded that the utility innovation system has a place in its IP system because more Malaysian innovators use this system than the standard patent system.[231]

Maskus and McDaniel, who conducted studies on how the Japanese patent system affected post-war Japanese technical progress, have concluded that during the period 1960–1993, this system was designed to encourage incremental and adaptive innovation and the diffusion of technical knowledge into the economy through a utility model system, while standard patent applications also provided both a direct and

[225] Arup (2012) (n 210), p. 31.

[226] Interviewee # 11; Interviewee # 12; Interviewee # 23.

[227] Suthersanen (2006).

[228] Gujarat National Law University (2021).

[229] Evenson and Westphal (1994).

[230] Ibid.

[231] Suthersanen (n 227) 22.

an indirect stimulus to productivity.[232] The authors revealed that the mechanisms for promoting these processes were a combination of tough conditions for standard patents, including early disclosure of, and opposition proceedings to, patent applications, and narrow claim requirements for patent applications, as well as an extensive system of utility models.[233] Notably, Japan—the first Asian country to introduce the utility model system into its domestic law—enhanced its industrial and economic capabilities in the early post-war period.[234]

In line with these studies, a country such as Sri Lanka that lacks technological capabilities would experience advancement by using a separate utility model system that would encourage local innovation and adaptation specially in the post-civil-war period when its economy is restarting. In this context, the utility model would be appropriate to the local domestic situation in Sri Lanka for it has a strong SME community that can adapt and change technology to suit local conditions.

However, at present, owing to a lack of expertise and resources, as aforementioned, the prior art search is inaccurate and, hence, the examination process is very basic, compared with that in other jurisdictions. The current examination process itself is very similar to the utility model system that has a lower-level patentability requirement. Hence, while introducing a utility model system, although the examination procedure should be strengthened according to the high standard of patentability requirement as in other jurisdictions, a lower-standard utility model would satisfy and enable the development of local inventions in the SME community, in Sri Lanka.

The Korean IP office has recommended to NIPO that Sri Lanka should have a utility model system but no progress has been made thus far because of the lack of commitment by local actors to the implementation of such a system.[235] It should remain an option for a foreign investor or an applicant to request this alternative, or it should be consolidated as a requirement to be met for all applications for standard patents. This dual system would attract foreign investors and importers, while ensuring the patents granted are for genuine inventions.

3.8.6 Capacity Building of NIPO

In line with the discussion thus far, patent administration in Sri Lanka needs substantial reform but reform is itself a discourse for interaction between local and international actors. Under the 10 PAP, strengthening the capacity of NIPO was an important discourse. The success of such capacity building depends on Sri Lanka establishing a credible IP office that has adequate resources, but WIPO officials believes this change is not happening.[236] They asserted that all activities at NIPO are based on

[232] Maskus (2000).

[233] Ibid.

[234] Ibid.

[235] Interviewee # 11.

[236] Interviewee # 18.

raw energy rather than systematic planning and 'any support WIPO is providing is being wasted'.They further said:

> There has to be a minimum standard to provide capacity building to any IP office. It must have 10 examiners. NIPO has only five. We need management-level administrators. It's not happening. We also need a financial model to be a viable IP office. Any other IP office is a money earner. I'm sure Sri Lanka has not achieved to that status yet.[237]

According to the WIPO officials, currently, WIPO has been discussing directly with NIPO on IP office diagnostics to recommend an ideal IP office for SL. This diagnostic study uses a template for developing countries, and WIPO will examine factors such as the amount of money, the number of personnel and the competencies needed for this change.[238] For example, NIPO is not digitised. This has created a huge bottleneck for COSTI in updating patent data on the National Innovation Dashboard. COSTI Director commented:

> Our initial plan was, for example, to capture patents on the DB [National Innovation Dashboard] for innovators before these are registered because once if it is digitised, it can be displayed on DB and updated. But it is not happening yet. So, you won't believe, still I am waiting for the 2015–2016 patent data. When it comes to us, it is history. As for the 2017 data, I'm not sure when these will be available.

Digitising the patent office is an important priority under the IP office diagnostic discourse because all modern patent offices in the world are digitised. Hence, this could be a recommendation for an ideal IP office for Sri Lanka that NIPO could initiate.

Patent office modernisation underwent a dramatic change when countries became WTO members. Accordingly, patent offices in India, Japan, Korea, Malaysia and Singapore were modernised to cater to the increasing demand of foreign patent applications.[239] This process includes hiring more examiners, building new office space and investing heavily in information technology. Going further, in 2016 India introduced a new provision under the amended Patent Rules, which seeks to fast track the process of granting patents, and in 2017, more than dozens of companies were granted patents in a record 113 days.[240] Significantly, inordinate delays in processing patent applications were highlighted by practically all participants who were interviewed in this research. With this introduction, the Indian Patent Office will be a very popular destination for foreign applicants. Although NIPO does not receive a high number of patent applications, unlike in India, WIPO, the WTO, the USPTO and the European Patent Office have extended support for capacity building to upgrade the patent office.[241] However, WIPO officials stated, most technical assistance has been wasted because it was not used efficiently.

---

237 Ibid.

238 Interviewee # 20.

239 Drahos (2010) (n 212), p. 209.

240 Chattejee (2017).

241 This issue will be discussed in Sect. 3.8.7.

The discourse identified that the weak administration of NIPO was a prominent issue identified by many interviewees,[242] which supports considerations that NIPO does not operate as the governing node that would create interpretive communities; rather, the interpretive communities, such as the ST sector nodes, have shifted the discourse to promote innovation.[243] As discussed earlier, NIPO is the repository for trademark, design and patent registrations, where lack of staff and funding has caused delays in all registration systems. This discourse on NIPO problems is demonstrated in the interview with an official at MIC—the IP policy formulation was the responsibility of NIPO and since NIPO was not performing it for more than 2 years, the Ministry took over the task to coordinate the IP policy.[244]

As at 2017, NIPO had four staff officers and there is still a vacuum at the higher levels since two top-level directors and another DG for managing the administrative functions in NIPO are yet to be appointed. These appointments would enable the NIPO official to concentrate on the operational side of IP. The Ministry needs to finalise these appointments, and Cabinet approval is required for the new appointments. According to the Ministry official, the NIPO official is unable to handle the administration functions at NIPO. Ministry official stated, using an example for the connected problems as regards trademarks:[245]

> Traditional knowledge is pending, and we can't implement the *Madrid Protocol* because of the backlog. The backlog must be zero to implement it. The government allocated 50 million [Sri Lankan Rupees] for the Madrid project from the 2015 Budget and they wanted to complete it by 2016, but even in 2017, we won't be able to do so. The current DG has been requesting funds for the next year as well. We have allowed outside people to support her to clear the backlog, and one consultancy firm is helping in addition to this outsourcing. Even with that, we can't see any progress.

The fact that there is a backlog of trademark applications does not assist in providing staff or resources for patent administration, because the NIPO is itself facing resource constraints. A former WIPO official, expressed similar views regarding the NIPO administration:[246]

> I went to Sri Lanka with the DG of WIPO in 2013, and we had 10 PAP. I recognised this 10 points as crucial issues for economic development. I had a sort of a plan to see the results within 1 year. Then, I invited people from the Ministries of Economic Affairs, External Resources, Trade and Commerce, Indigenous Medicine, Cultural Affairs and Scientific Affairs, and from COSTI, NSF and NIPOs. I allocated 10 things according to their areas of competence. For example, I allocated SMEs and IP to the Export Development Board because they have an SME unit, so they could help SMEs to enhance their competitiveness through IP. Certain areas were exclusively reserved for NIPOs, such as accession to treaties, because that is their responsibility.
>
> Upon my return, I worked with other WIPO divisions to fulfil our promises and commitments. I held meetings with these 10 units asking for an update on particular action plans. I used

[242] Interviewee # 21: Interviewee # 18; Interviewee # 3.

[243] The shift of discourse will be further discussed in Chap. 5.

[244] Interviewee # 11.

[245] Ibid.

[246] Interviewee # 21.

> to chair the meetings and get the other people to do the work and report to me, and I was responsible for reporting to the NIPO official.
>
> But immediately after two months of the meeting, the entire program was taken over by NIPO. They did not want any of these institutions to be directly involved and said, 'NIPO should be the focal point because other agencies don't have the mandate to work on IP; IP is ours.' This is politics. NIPO can be the focal point, but they can't do all these things because they don't have the expertise and they should be able to work with other ministries and departments. Therefore, most of our Technical Assistance programs have not been properly used. Secretaries who are not involved in the projects attend meetings.

The statement of the former WIPO official that 'NIPO can be the focal point, but they can't do all these things because they don't have the expertise and they should be able to work with other ministries and departments' is worth analysing.

NIPO is a focal point in Sri Lanka for patent implementation because it is a governing local node, but NIPO, as an entity within the system, cannot exist in isolation. It needs to interact and communicate with relevant agencies, other ministries and WIPO for effective policymaking and the smooth functioning of the IP system. The NIPO official is a prominent node and an actor who could take steps to connect with other subsystems, such as other ministries and departments that handle IP, universities and domestic industries to establish a patent implementation process. In other words, the NIPO official has a regulatory function to standardise the NIPO through assistance from other subgroups. This interaction with subgroups is vital to the development of interpretive communities for enhancing, adopting and resolving issues in IP. However, this is not happening in Sri Lanka. For example, to reiterate, when the former WIPO official took the initiative to allocate 10 subjects to government agencies according to their expertise, the NIPO official took over all the subjects and placed these under NIPO because that person did not understand the regulatory function of this initiative. The NIPO official should motivate other subsystems—not by rejecting the support of other entities but by using their expertise to uplift the patent administration. This implies there is lack of discourse by the NIPO official as a governing node to promote IP in Sri Lanka or rather a complacency about the existing legal framework. Given this disintegration of work, one cannot expect IP to make any positive contributions towards the country's economic development.

Nonetheless, not all problems can be attributed to the NIPO. A former WIPO official was very critical about the present status of NIPO. He stated there are many reasons for this underperformance.[247] First, numerous agencies deal with IP, which has created inter-ministerial rivalries. As a result, these agencies find it challenging to coordinate their own work. Second, IP should be managed by a strong ministry, such as the Prime Minister's Office, which would foster a sense of responsibility to coordinate activities more efficiently. On understanding the importance of IP, COSTI was established in 2013 and mandated to coordinate IP. This is a positive change in recent times. Third, it is very important to have an IP audit or a nationally focused action plan to examine the IP status of the country before embarking on a plan or program. The IP audit could be used as a guideline to decide how the country could

[247] Ibid.

use IP for economic development. Notably, Sri Lanka has never conducted an IP audit.

Fourth, the constant change of bureaucrats and the lack of political will at levels above NIPO have resulted in disintegrated IP management. No single entity is responsible for the activities of NIPO. The transfer of bureaucrats, in many instances, has resulted in policy drift in Sri Lanka. Fifth, NIPO has a bad track record in selecting people for WIPO workshops and training. For example, some people are sent on junkets rather than training programs. Consequently, the UN representative has had to intervene several times to request the government to send the right people for training who could provide some benefits to the country later.[248] Last, there seem to be a lack of commitment and inadequate human and financial resources, and NIPO is reluctance to coordinate supportively with other agencies. This implies that NIPO administration has become the greatest single bottleneck for strengthening IP in Sri Lanka.

Conversely, the WIPO official made the following positive comment regarding the IP status:[249]

> In fairness, IP is moving in Sri Lanka. WIPO has negotiated with Korea for a study visit to see the miracles of Korea as a catch-up economy. We have done our part and have laid down conditions, so that Sri Lanka is prepared before they go. Sri Lanka need to have the draft of their National IP Policy before they go. They have a draft already, but I don't have a copy. This is what we call demand driven.

3.8.7 WIPO Technical Assistance Program to Sri Lanka

The WIPO Technical Assistance program is a continuing discourse within the patent administration of Sri Lanka, which provides technical assistance to upgrade the patent administration. Governments are the primary beneficiaries of WIPO's technical assistance, which is particularly directed to different government departments, policymakers, decision-makers, parliamentarians, the academia, IPR holders, potential creators and innovators, R&D centres, agencies responsible for building respect for IP, SMEs, consumers and civil society. The WAPBD explained the mandate of WIPO in the following manner:[250]

> A good way is to use a metaphor to describe the role of WIPO. We are the architects. As an architect, we talk to the clients, who are the countries, to see what the client wants to build. So, the client may say, 'I want to build a house with a living a room and a small kitchen' and so on. And we start designing the house knowing the technical needs–whether it is plumbing needs or structural needs—and then, we turn around to our substantive IP sectors and ask them to choose what entity and vendor they need including external experts as well.

---

[248] Interviewee # 20.

[249] Interviewee # 18.

[250] Ibid.

With the ratification of the *TRIPS Agreement*, the WIPO Technical Assistance program changed its focus to consider the challenges resulting from WTO membership, which implied the acceptance of specific norms contained in the *TRIPS Agreement*. Hence, this program became a priority to help developing countries and least developed countries understand their international obligations and make informed policy choices as regards *TRIPS* implementation.[251] To achieve this objective, WIPO and the WTO signed a cooperation agreement in 1995 to provide coordinated legal and legislative support to developing countries. Because the WTO is a rule-based organisation as well as a superstructural node, it influences member states to implement the *TRIPS* minimum standard and most developing and least developed nations that lack resources depend on the WIPO Technical Assistance programs to fulfil their *TRIPS* obligations. The WTO has joined with WIPO to host workshops in Geneva, which Sri Lankans have attended.

3.9 Procedure for Granting Technical Assistance

As regards access to the WIPO Technical Assistance program, the old procedure at the WIPO General Assembly was that WIPO members would have many types of meetings with countries, and ultimately, WIPO would receive a list of requirements from these countries.[252] In 2015, WIPO changed this procedure because the wish list excluded long-term needs, and 'it's not impact oriented and it consists of seminars in most of the cases'.[253] As the WAPBD stated, 'These seminars are easy, nice and good to do, but holding seminars alone is insufficient.'[254] He further emphasised that the changes that a country wants to experience depend on the existing IP structure and the type of change they desire, that is, whether a weaker, stronger, pro-invention or pro-creativity system. Such changes cannot be achieved solely by conducting innumerable seminars.[255]

As a result, WIPO had a series of discussions prior to the General Assembly, and WIPO met the country representatives in Geneva early in the year rather than later in the year. In addition, WIPO held three annual video conferences with member country representatives, including those from Sri Lanka. Hence, WIPO met more often with the country representatives. The WAPBD emphasised: 'In that way, the conversations become deeper and continuing and allow us to have a discussion with countries tailored to their specific needs. For example: What type of seminar is needed or whether there should be on-the-job training or a study visit, rather than a seminar.'[256]

---

[251] WIPO (2013).

[252] Interviewee # 18.

[253] Ibid.

[254] Ibid.

[255] Ibid.

[256] Ibid.

According to the earlier procedure, a wish list consisted of 40–50 activities, and it was necessary to prioritise. In most of the cases, what was in fact necessary was to conduct three or four activities within 5–10 years in order to obtain the needed results. Hence, the present system is more development oriented, demand driven, transparent and country specific for it considers the particular needs, priorities and development level of member states.

It is apparent from this discussion that WIPO is a global actor in promoting the protection of IP globally through cooperation and collaboration among its members and other stakeholders. To achieve this mandate, WIPO specified in its art 4(v) that 'the Organization shall offer its cooperation among states requesting legal-technical assistance in the field of technical assistance'.[257] Hence, this is a demand-driven program. Countries should request WIPO for assistance, and when certain criteria are met, WIPO will provide technical assistance according to their needs. In this sense, while WIPO is a global node for IP, unlike the WTO it cannot influence countries to accept its recommendations. It provides technical assistance through dialogue with member states and provides recommendations to governments, but it is for the governments to accept or reject these recommendations.

3.10 Areas of Technical Assistance

Sri Lanka needs to identify areas in which it requires technical assistance, and then, WIPO works directly with IP office on the basis of the country's request. In accordance with the terms of Sri Lanka's registration system and in terms of its competencies, 'we work with stakeholders directly such as science, technology and research sectors'.[258]

According to the WIPO Technical Assistance Database, from 2009 February to 2017 October, WIPO conducted 55 Technical Assistance programs in Sri Lanka.[259] These include workshops and seminars on; TT and IP management, patent drafting, patent database searches, patent examiner training, IP for judges, integrating IP into innovation policy formulation, IP office diagnostics and upgrading the IP office of Sri Lanka. In addition, university and stakeholder visits were arranged focussing on the context of creating an IP environment to bridge the gap between academic institutions and industry in Sri Lanka through regional seminars on TT and collective management.[260]

In this context, Sri Lanka has made specific requests for assistance in three main areas. The first area is to upgrade the NIPO, the second is to assist IP stakeholders directly and through the IP office and the third is to develop an IP framework.[261] It

[257] WIPO (2014).

[258] Ibid.

[259] WIPO (2021).

[260] Ibid.

[261] Interviewee # 18.

is important to build these three pillars and identify the current silos in Sri Lanka. This process will enable all interested parties to collaborate in IP areas. In Sri Lanka, WIPO coordinates with COSTI and other public sector entities to develop policy and frameworks.[262]

A starting point would be the national IP strategy discussion, and WIPO is also discussing a technical assistance implementation plan to inform interested parties about relevant activities. The WAPBD emphasised: 'I have met the new Sri Lankan Ambassador to the UN to present the comprehensive framework for Sri Lanka. It is a study for a country's technical assistance implementation plan to capture all assistance to Sri Lanka. WIPO has captured the output and all the outcomes of technical assistance.'[263]

This policy document titled 'A Comprehensive Country Technical Assistance Implementation Plan to Manage the Various Cooperation Activities Relating to Industrial Property in Countries in the Asia and Pacific Region' is an IP development road map for the country. WIPO had requested the Government of Sri Lanka for such a road map to facilitate the use of IP for development through a coherent IP policy and strategy, appropriate legislative and regulatory frameworks, enhanced technical infrastructure and capacity of national IP institutions to administer and manage IPR and enhanced access to global IP systems and knowledge base.[264] Since 2015, WIPO has been discussing the adoption of the 10 PAP in this framework for Sri Lanka. In fact, it is a more elaborate plan than the 10 PAP because Sri Lanka needs a more coherent plan for technical assistance that focuses on SME involvement.[265]

WIPO workshops and seminars have been open to Sri Lanka under the Technical Assistance program, and representatives have been attending these seminars for the past 10 years. However, an effective system to choose the right individuals for these seminars was lacking, and often, certain seminar participants were free riders. In 2016, the UN representative adopted a firm attitude and informed WIPO that it is important to have the right people attend future workshops. As a result, after many years qualified resource persons attended the WIPO workshops in 2016.

The UN representative made the following observation regarding the selection process:[266]

> Not always right people come. But out of six, if you have four right people, I suppose it's a kind of win because earlier there have been fights to come, which Ministers have had to reconcile. Sometimes, I had to be somewhat arbitrary about this in a good way, and I have recanvased some of the nominations saying it was not the right person. We were trying to do something, and it was worthless when jokers come and sit through meetings without making any contribution.

WIPO's technical assistance is important to a resource-poor, financially handicapped country such as Sri Lanka for developing its IP system. Sri Lanka is now within the

---

262 Ibid.

263 Ibid.

264 WIPO (2018).

265 Interviewee # 18.

266 Ibid.

middle-income category, and all the countries who have moved from the middle-income category to a higher category have done so through IP.[267] The difficulty is that WIPO can only negotiate with government institutions, and hence, NIPO or any other government ministry should treat WIPO recommendations as a discursive strategy to shift the discourse towards law reforms. As discussed in Sect. 3.8.6, many negotiations are deadlocked because the NIPO official has been unwilling to coordinate with other local bodies in progressing interconnected communities or discursive conversations for developing IP.

3.10.1 WIPO Enabling the Intellectual Property Environment Project

The Enabling the Intellectual Property Environment ('EIE') Project is a global initiative by WIPO that aims to develop the appropriate innovation system, institutional organisation and efficient processes and to increase the number of people with adequate skills to facilitate the process of knowledge creation and transfer and to transform the knowledge into products and services to society.[268] The target beneficiaries of this initiative are WIPO member states, such as Sri Lanka, universities, R&D institutions, IP and technology managers, innovation-supporting institutions and industry.[269] The focus areas of the EIE Project are TT and innovation systems, technology development, IP protection, capacity building, technology management and commercialisation and engaging all stakeholders.[270] Already, the EIE Project has proved to be a success in Malaysia through an interconnected network of actors, such as government institutions, IP practitioners, science parks, incubators and industries including the automobile, agriculture, and information and communications technology ('ICT') industries, which communicate with each other to develop, manage and commercialise IP.[271] The long-term plan of the EIE Project is to foster strong linkages, networks and collaborations with other stakeholders and actors in the innovation ecosystem. This aspect will be discussed in Chap. 5.

In Sri Lanka, the EIE Project was launched in 2017 for increasing the country's human capacity for technology development, management and commercialisation.[272] WIPO has been providing technical assistance for the project, and the NIPO has been implementing it for NIPO is the focal point to regulate IP. The project involves implementing a networked community using a hub-and-spoke structure to sustain results in capacity building and other technical assistance endeavours.[273]

[267] Interviewee # 20.

[268] WIPO (2017a, b).

[269] Ibid.

[270] Ibid.

[271] Ibid.

[272] COSTI (2020).

[273] Ibid.

COSTI acts as the hub that is an administrative and infrastructural centre and the remaining institutions, such as government agencies, universities, research institutes and public–private partnerships, function as the spokes that support the establishment of a community of technology-generating institutions.[274] In each country, WIPO and each hub work to build the capacity of technology generators, individuals and other actors to use IP to engage actively in the process of transforming inventions and technologies into products, services and enterprises using IP tools and methods.[275]

TISCs come under the EIE Project. Establishing a TISC is one of the plans under the 10 PAP discussed earlier in this chapter. Its objectives include improving the intensity and quality of (technical) innovation in the country by raising awareness of patents and scientific and technical databases among inventors in Sri Lanka and providing state-of-the-art search services. TISCs are expected to be hosted in universities, research institutes, government departments and other locations throughout the country.[276] Currently, five universities[277] and five research institutes[278] function as spokes and COSTI acts as the hub that has the overall responsibility to ensure the objectives of the EIE Project are achieved. The vision of the hub-and-spoke approach is 'not a hierarchy structure but performing like an "organism"'.[279]

The WIPO official explained TISCs' mandate as follows:[280]

> A TISC is a kind of a holy grail for IP. We have a big IP world. Those who want to use IP for their purposes can use this. All developed countries that are able to harness IP for their purposes are in the first group. This is the area of technology, area of utilisation of technology and area of commercialisation of IP. This is not happening on a wide scale in developing countries. So, we are experimenting on the hub-and-spoke concept. So, instead of going to a country and training 1,000 people on a few things, which means nobody is going to be an expert, we try to train a limited number of people on everything. So, research institutions, universities and SLINTEC are going to be the country's foremost experts in that area, in the area of technology commercialisation. These are the spokes, and the hub will be COSTI.

This statement indicates the basic purpose of a TISC is to develop a system for achieving a quality patent because the NIPO mandate is not to teach and how to draft a patent application but to provide information and procedures regarding granting patents.[281] TISCs were developed to support the community by increasing the efficiency of the innovation process by helping innovators (researchers in government agencies and universities) and investors avoid allocating resources to 'reinventing the

[274] WIPO (2017a, b).

[275] Ibid.

[276] Mendes (2015) (n 57).

[277] University of Moratuwa, University of Peradeniya, University of Ruhuna, University of Colombo and University of Kelaniya.

[278] Industrial Technology Institute, Sri Lanka Institute of Nanotechnology, Tea Research Institute, National Engineering R&D Centre, National Institute of Fundamental Studies.

[279] WIPO, EIE Project (n 274).

[280] Interviewee # 18.

[281] Interviewee # 16.

wheel'.[282] TISCs could act as intermediaries to help clear the backlog of patent applications in future, for the patent drafting guidance provided by TISCs will increase the patent drafting process for prospective innovators.[283]

Hence, the EIE Project and TISCs have introduced a new discourse for IP. Both initiatives comprise an influential node for IP because it provides access to online patent resources, scientific and technical literature and other IP-related publications; assists users to undertake patent searches and retrieve other technology-related information; and provides training in the use of these resources and information on IP laws, management, strategy, commercialisation and marketing.[284] It is too early to determine the impact of TISCs and their influence on the IP system, but this is a forward-looking initiative to push IP for economic development and will be discussed further in Chap. 5.

3.11 Integrating Intellectual Property into Innovation Policy in Sri Lanka

When the 10 PAP was proposed in late 2013 to enhance the IP system in Sri Lanka, there was a sudden drive to assess the country's IP ecosystem. WIPO took the initiative to conduct a comprehensive study on *Integrating Intellectual Property into Innovation Policy Formulation in Sri Lanka* in 2014 with the financial support of the Government of Japan.[285] The objective was to understand the innovation ecosystem; to examine the extent to which IP considerations have served or could serve to strengthen innovation; and to make recommendations to the government. This became vital to Sri Lanka, given the dire need to accelerate its economic development after emerging from a civil war that hampered its development for 30 years.

The WIPO study identified the main actors, institutions and policy initiatives in Sri Lanka through face-to-face interviews held in June 2014.[286] Its findings were based on policies and status of ST, IP management, skills and good practices. Recommendations were provided regarding creating and implementing policies and a legal framework, improving research capability, managing research output, conducting patent database search, building linkages between research and industry and developing skills and biodiversity. Some of the recommendations were considered by the Government of Sri Lanka in integrating IP considerations into its innovation policy.[287] The findings of the report will be further discussed in Chap. 5. The WIPO Report was submitted to Mr Rishad Bathiudeen, former Minister for Industry and

[282] Interviewee # 18.

[283] Ibid.

[284] Mendes (2015) (n 276).

[285] Ibid.

[286] Ibid.

[287] More information on the innovation policy will be discussed in Chap. 5.

Commerce through a letter dated 16 January 2015.[288] It is assumed that the report is still with the Minister for Industry and Commerce.

Notably, similar comprehensive studies on upgrading the innovation support structure in Sri Lanka were conducted in 2000 and 2002,[289] and these studies have been proven to be unproductive owing to the NIPO's lack of commitment to implement the stated recommendations. This is one of the reasons that the WAPBD said that WIPO assistance to upgrade the IP system is being wasted because Sri Lanka's IP office does not have the minimum standard for capacity building. A similar view was stated by the former WAPBD.

> In 2000, I was able to carry out a study for Sri Lanka regarding its innovation support structure. Some statistics may be outdated, but certain facts and recommendations are valid to date. At that time, I was the desk officer for Sri Lanka at WIPO, so I thought I should help my country to develop the capacity to invent as part of our regular Technical Assistance program. After this visit, I arranged another follow-up visit to upgrade the innovation support structure. Then, I followed up with another study in Sri Lanka in 2002 for enhancing Sri Lanka Inventors Commission within the framework of upgrading the main project. We did the basic study, and in the context of the basic study, we recognised how this Commission can be strengthened. All these were done with a view to giving the opportunity to use IP for development. From time to time, studies come up, but recommendations are not taken seriously.

The MIC should settle this situation as a responsible node by appointing a senior level officer who could exclusively deal with WIPO and other international collaborations. If not, as discussed previously, most of the WIPO Technical Assistance programs offered to Sri Lanka will be wasted.

The previous sections have highlighted how the nodes are structured within the IP ecosystem in Sri Lanka and how they act within the local and global legal processes communicating with others influencing their power. With regard to local legal processes, the book should also note there will be various actors, striving discursively and otherwise, for influence over lawmaking. Thus, in this case study of patent grant administration, it has been found that the DG of NIPO does not operate as a governing node is supposed to. The functions of communicating and influencing the associated offices and relevant stakeholders for the smooth functioning of matters relating to patents and PVR are not occurring. This weak or recalcitrant administration of NIPO was a reason repeated by several interviewees[290] for the IP inertia on the local legal process. As discussed previously, these interviewees expressed concerns about the refusal of the DG of NIPO to interact with other local agencies to streamline IP issues[291]; the shifting of IP policy formulation from NIPO to the MIC, given NIPO's lack of progress[292]; and personal conflicts between NIPO staff and

[288] Email from Nanayakkara Tamara (tamara.nanayakkara@wipo.int) to Asanka Perera, 3 November 2021.

[289] Chin (2000, 2002). Both these studies were obtained by the former WIPO official in 2018 while conducting interviews in Geneva.

[290] Interviews conducted in 2017 and 2018 in Sri Lanka.

[291] Iinterviewee # 21.

[292] Interviewee # 11.

the DG, which have resulted in the backlog of trademark and patent applications[293] and delays in finalising the PVR law. This implies a lack of discourse from the DG of NIPO and the DoA', which are important nodes under nodal governance in the drafting and passage of PVR legislation.

3.12 Conclusion

It is apparent from the discussion in this chapter that patent administration in Sri Lanka has been subject to a series of discourses over the past few years. Most such discourses relate to reforms of the existing patent administration system in areas such as the patent examination and the patent granting processes. The present system is underdeveloped compared with those of other countries in the Southeast Asian region.

Local policymakers play a key role in patent administration in Sri Lanka. As discussed in this research, some local actors have deployed strategic discourses to change the IP discourse, while other actors, such as the NIPO as a prominent node, have been reluctant to communicate with other agencies to coordinate IP-related matters, which has become a bottleneck in the patent administration system.[294] Meanwhile, global actors, such as WIPO, have been pushing for the modernisation of the system but mainly with patient offers of assistance and involvement rather than the threat of coercive measures.

As discussed above, the discourse on IP has been changing since 2010. This change is driven by the progressive thinking of some in the government sector as well as the private sector and professional groups that have come to the view that Sri Lanka will never prosper unless people generate new leading-edge high-technology research that can be converted into industries and money to add value to such innovation. This view supports the neo-liberal thinking that the presence of strong IP will promote local innovation and foreign investment.[295] This aspect will be discussed in Chap. 6 of this book.

In this context, the local discourse suggests a developing country such as Sri Lanka need to establish an IPR system that encourages learning and follow-on innovation. For example, a utility model system should be introduced for independent local inventors in order to ensure high-technology applications are properly screened. Such reforms would strengthen the provision and administration of IP protection, shift the discourse from a weak IP system, encourage local innovation and attract FDI inflows that would generate local employment and TT to boost the economy, at least with the mobilisation of other government incentives and conditions to harness that IP.[296] Therefore, Sri Lanka, while retaining its sovereignty over patent administration,

[293] Ibid.

[294] Interviews conducted in 2017 and 2018 in Sri Lanka.

[295] Arup (2012) (n 225), p. 136. See also Chap. 5 of this book.

[296] Ibid 136.

needs to design a system that adjusts global patent principles to suit its local economic and social contexts.[297]

As the first case study, the theoretical framework of this book has assisted me to understand the actors, processors and discourses in the administration of the patent system in Sri Lanka. As stated at the beginning of this chapter, the main legal policy discourse on patent administration was local rather than global, mainly because patent lawmaking is territorial in nature and predominantly subject to national laws of any country. For example, NIPO and the local actors such as the ministries, ministers and other officers within NIPO act as influencers in the patent administration of Sri Lanka. This has been discussed in Chap. 2 of this book. This does not mean that global lawmaking is absent in the patent administration discourse in Sri Lanka. For example, WIPO has been a prominent global node in providing technical assistance to upgrade the patent administration in Sri Lanka, but their recommendations are demand driven, rather than mandatory, and as discussed in this chapter Sri Lanka has disregarded many recommendations by WIPO in the global lawmaking process. As a result of this lack of discourse by the local actors, patent administration system still remains outdated in Sri Lanka as discussed in this chapter. Patent examination is based on formality, rather than substantive or modified examinations and this method has restricted patent examiner to undertake only inventions based on low-technology protection due to lack of resources. Moreover, as stated by a patent examiner, they are not properly trained to undertake, high-technology inventions and as a result majority of patents are grated for engineering developments, which are based on low-technology protection.

Undoubtedly, the patent discourse has been influenced by superstructural nodes, including the TRIPS, WTO, and through WIPO by providing technical assistance to upgrade IP administration, but the theories have also revealed that local actors like the NIPO, ministries and ministers have become more influential in the IP administration discourse. For example, it was acknowledged globally that patent administration in Sri Lanka is not up to the standard, unlike that of other developing countries, but no reforms have been introduced to change the system. Moreover, WIPO's Technical Assistance programs were not used prudently to upgrade the system. This demonstrates that local power dynamics have played a crucial role in the IP policy making in Sri Lanka. However, the interviews identify in this power dynamic there has been no coercion globally to focus or streamline patent discourse in Sri Lanka, through global processes established by TRIPS or trade retaliations.

Discourse was an appropriate medium or mode to study and?, to identify the participants interacting with each other about lawmaking and patent reforms, given the contrasting views and the lack of resolution of the system in Sri Lanka. It was interesting to note that dialogue, interaction and communication between nodes have become influential tools in the patent administration discourse to elucidate the dynamics in the Sri Lankan IP policy developments. Certainly, treaties are made and legislation is passed, but this aspect is indeed discursive, even globally. The fact that patent administration has not undergone any reforms implies that local power

297 Drahos (2010) (n 239), p. 331.

dynamics mean that regardless of the global rules, the future of Sri Lanka's patent administration is ultimately left to the Sri Lankan Government. Exposure to lower-level influence from outside, such as from contact with foreign patent offices to assist in examinations and training identifies avenues of discourse. All the findings in this chapter are reached based on the contributions of the interviews conducted on patent administration of Sri Lanka. The next chapter will present the second case study on discourses on protection of plant varieties in Sri Lanka.

Competing Interests The author has no conflicts of interest to declare that are relevant to the content of this chapter.

References

Alikhan S (2000) Socio-economic benefits of intellectual property protection for developing countries WIPO

Arup C (2012) The transfer of pharmaceutical patent laws: the case of India's paragraph 3(d). In: Gillespie J, Nicholson N (eds) Law and development and the global discourses of legal transfers. Cambridge University Press, Cambridge

Australian Patent Office (2020) Manual for practice and procedures. http://www.ipaustralia.gov.au/pdfs/patentsmanual/WebHelp/Patent_Examiners_Manual.htm

Bailas A (2007) European patent office, examiner training at the EPO. http://www.tokugikon.jp/gikonshi/247tokusyu6.pdf

Bhatangar P (2021) Patent pre-grant and post-grant opposition procedure in India versus re-examination in the US. Pleaders Intelligent Legal Solutions. https://blog.ipleaders.in/patent-pre-grant-post-grant-opposition-procedure-india-vs-re-examination-us/

Bodenhausen GHC (1969) Guide to the application of the Paris convention for the protection of industrial property. United International Bureaux for the Protection of Intellectual Property

Chattejee P (2017) Is India's expedited examination of patents a big deal? Intellectual Property Watch. http://www.ip-watch.org/2017/09/04/indias-expedited-examination-patents-big-deal/

Chin LY (2000) Report of the WIPO mission on the assessment of needs for establishing/upgrading the innovation support structure and services in Sri Lanka

Chin LY (2002) Mission report on enhancement of the Sri Lanka inventors commission (SLIC) within the framework of the project for upgrading the innovation support structure and services in Sri Lanka

COSTI (2020) EIE project: Sri Lanka. http://costi.gov.lk/index.php/en/com-dpcalendar-submenu-locations/eie-project-sri-lanka-tmp

Daily Mirror (2012) Supreme court issues landmark order on intellectual property law. http://www.dailymirror.lk/business/other/22452-supreme-courtissues-landmark-order-on-intellectual-property-law-.html

Drahos P (2010) The global governance of knowledge: patent offices and their clients. Cambridge University Press, Cambridge

Evenson RE, Westphal LE (1994) Technological change and technology strategy. Discussion Paper Yale University 709. http//hdl.handle.net/10419/160630

Federal News Network (2018) USPTO director looks to decrease patent backlog by improving workforce efficiency. Podcast. USPTO director looks to decrease patent backlog by improving workforce efficiency | Federal News Network

Foreign Ministry Sri Lanka (2018) Unveiling of painting of Lakshman Kadirgamar at WIPO. Unveiling of painting in honour of the late Lakshman Kadirgamar at WIPO—Foreign Ministry—Sri Lanka (mfa.gov.lk)

Gee LH et al (2009) Reforms towards intellectual property-based economic development in Malaysia. J World Intell Prop 12:4

Geeganage A (2013) Sri Lanka's role in the world trade organization. Int J Bus Soc Sci 4:1

Gillespie J (2008) Towards a discursive analysis of legal transfers into developing East Asia. N Y Univ J Int Law Polit 40:1154

Gujarat National Law University (2021) The need to protect utility model in India. Discussion Paper

Hewage NS (2015) Promoting a second-tier protection regime for innovation of small and medium-sized enterprises in South Asia: a case of Sri Lanka. Nomas

Ho C (2011) Access to medicine in the global economy: international agreement on patents and related rights. Oxford University Press, Oxford

Hoekman BM, Maskus KE, Saggi K (2005) Transfer of technology to developing countries: unilateral and multilateral policy options. World Develop 33:10

Indian Patents Act 1970

IP Australia (2020a) Expedited examination for standard patents. https://www.ipaustralia.gov.au/patents/applying-patent/standard-patent-application-process/examination-standard-patent/expedited-examination-standard-patents

IP Australia (2020b) Global patent prosecution highway pilot program: requirements and procedures. https://www.ipaustralia.gov.au/patents/applying-patent/standard-patent-application-process/examination-standard-patent/expedited-examination-standard-patents

Iran Patent Centre (2020) Local working requirements of patents. https://en.patentoffice.ir/paper/5296/Local-Working-Requirements-of-Patents

Japan Patent Office (2021) Procedures for obtaining a patent right. http://www.jpo.go.jp/tetzuki_t_gaiyo_e/pa_right.htm

Julius and Creasy (2012) Patent Law in Sri Lanka

Kadirgamar S (2013) Lakshman and the intellectual property laws. Colombo Telegraph. Lakshman and the Intellectual Property Laws-Colombo Telegraph

Kannangara P, Kern D (2018) Understanding the world trade organization. Lakshman Kadirgamar Institute. https://www.lki.lk/publication/understanding-the-world-trade-organization

Karunaratna DM (2010) Elements of the law of intellectual property in Sri Lanka. Sarasavi Publishers

Kerry VB (2007) TRIPS the Doha declaration and paragraph 6 decision: what are the remaining steps for protecting access to medicines? Global Health 3(3):1124

Kim YK, Lee K, Park WG (2012) Appropriate intellectual property protection growth in countries at different levels of development. Res Policy 41:2

Kuanpoth J (2008) Appropriate patent rules in developing countries—some deliberations based on Thai Legislation. J Intell Prop Rights 13:5

Legal Aid Commission of Sri Lanka. http://www.legalaid.gov.lk/index.php/2016-01-13-09-16-07/about-us

Lumley MA (2001) Rational ignorance at the patents office. North Western University Law Review, p 95

Madrid Agreement (1979) Concerning the international registration of marks. as amended. Accessed 28 Sept 1979

Marsoof A (2012) TRIPS compatibility of Sri Lankan trademark law. J World Intell Property 15:1

Marsoof A (2018) Exclusive patent rights and local working requirements: a developing country's perspective. In: Bharadwaj A, Devaiah VH, Gupta I (eds) Multi-dimensional approaches towards new technology. Springer, New York, p 315

Maskus KE (2000) Intellectual property rights and economic development. West Res J Int Law 32:11548

Mathews D (2005) TRIPs flexibilities and access to medicines in developing countries: the problem with technical assistance and free trade agreements. Eur Intell Property Rev 11:364

Mendes P (2015) Integrating intellectual property into innovation policy formulation in Sri Lanka. WIPO. https://www.wipo.int/edocs/pubdocs/en/wipo_report_inn_lk.pdf

Merges RP (1999) As many as six impossible patents breakfast: property rights for business concepts and patent system reform. Berkeley Technol Law J 14:64–98

Merrill SA, Levin RC, Myres MB (eds) (2004) A patent system for the 21st century. The National Academies Press

Ministry of Industry and Commerce (2018) Terms of reference. National Intellectual Property Policy for Sri Lanka

Mitchell A, Voon T (2009) Patents and public health in the WTO, FTAs and beyond: tension and conflict in international law). J World Trade 43:3

Moir HVJ (2013) Inventive step for a patent system. Eur Intell Property Rev 3

National Intellectual Property Office. https://www.nipo.gov.lk/

NIPO (2022) Statistics. https://www.nipo.gov.lk/web/index.php?option=com_content&view=article&id=8&Itemid=130&lang=en

Pathiraja K (2013) Kadirgama memorial oration. Daily FT. https://www.ft.lk/News/kadirgamar-memorial-oration-2013/56-211372

Perera A (2014) The administration of patent system in Sri Lanka: a critical appraisal. 43 Common Law World Rev 43: 154

Perera C, Dasanayaka S (2004) Technology development: key issues in productivity. In: Kelegama S (ed) Economic policy in Sri Lanka: issues and debates. Sage Publications, New York

Permanent Mission of Sri Lanka to the UN (2018) WIPO and Sri Lanka to initiate 10 point action plan for Sri Lanka. http://www.lankamission.org/intellectual-property/1678-wipo-and-sri-lanka-to-initiate-a-10-point-action-plan-on-intellectual-property.html

Pitts S, Kim J (2009) The patent prosecution highway: is life in the fast lane worth the cost. Hast Sci Technol Law J 1:2

Reichman JH (2009) Compulsory licensing of patented pharmaceutical inventions: evaluating the options. J Law Med Ethics 37:2

Restrepo CP (2016) Patent cooperation mechanisms in the Pacific alliance: an initial assessment of the effectiveness of the patent prosecution highway for intra-regional trade negotiation. World Trade Instit 16:2016

Shikha N (2009) Comparative study on pre-grant and post-grant patent opposition in India. http://www.ssrn.com/abstract=1503188

Sirimanna B (2019) Intellectual property office expedites the issuance of patent and trade marks. Sunday Times. https://www.sundaytimes.lk/190616/business-times/intellectual-property-office-expedites-the-issuance-of-patent-and-trade-marks-353158.html

Sri Lanka Commercial High Court (2017) Sri Lanka's commercial high court has over 5000 pending cases. https://www.lankabusinessonline.com/sri-lankas-commercial-high-court-has-over-5000-pending-cases/

Sri Lanka Inventors Commission Home (2022). http://slic.gov.lk/

Sri Lanka Parliament (1979) Parliamentary debates

Sri Lanka Parliament (2003) Parliamentary debates

Supreme Court Special Determination Nos. 14, 15, 16/2003 Hoen EFM (2002) TRIPS, pharmaceutical patents and access to essential medicines: Seattle, Doha and beyond. Chicago J Int Law 3:1

Suthersanen U (2006) Utility models and innovation in developing countries. Issue Paper 13. UNCTAD-ICTSD projects on IPRs and sustainable development. http://www.iprsonline.org/unctadictsd/description.htm

Taylor J (2017) Compulsory licensing: a misused and abused international trade law. Phrma. https://catalyst.phrma.org/compulsory-licensing-a-misused-and-abused-international-trade-law

The Office of Controller General of Patents (2011) Designs and trade mark India. Manual of patent office practice and procedures. http://www.ipindia.nic.in/writereaddata/Portal/IPOGuidelinesManuals/1_28_1_manual-of-patent-office-practice_and-procedure.pdf

Weatherall K, Rotstein F, Dent C (2011) Patent opposition in Australia: The facts. Univ New South Wales Law J 34
Wickramasinghe CN, Ahamed N (2012) Influence of demographic and technical profile on success of independent investors in Sri Lanka. J World Intell Property 15:789
Wilson J (2007) Sri Lanka report on patent harmonization. http:www.apaaonline.org/.../2007Sri%20LankaGroupFinaladd-071210.doc
WIPO (1979) WIPO model law for developing countries on inventions PATENT LAW IN SRI LANKA (juliusandcreasy.com)
WIPO (1991) The PCT now has 156 contracting states. http://www.wipo.int/pct/en/pct_contracting_states.html
WIPO (2013) Delivery of WIPO technical assistance manual. https://www.wipo.int/export/sites/www/cooperation/en/docs/ta_manual.pdf
WIPO (2014a) Alternatives in patent search and examinations policy guide. http://www.wipo.int/edocs/pubdocs/en/wipo_pub_guide_patentsearch.pdf
WIPO (2014b) Protecting your inventions abroad: frequently asked questions about the PCT. https://www.wipo.int/pct/en/faqs/faqs.html
WIPO (2017a) Enabling the intellectual property (IP) environment (EIE) project implementation. ETInternational. https://www.wipo.int/edocs/mdocs/aspac/en/wipo_ttos_kul_18/wipo_ttos_kul_18_p1.pdf
WIPO (2017b) The enabling innovation environment (EIE) project for intellectual property and technology. https://www.wipo.int/export/sites/www/cooperation/en/funds_in_trust/docs/eie_summary.pdf
WIPO (2018) Project summary: a comprehensive country technical assistance implementation plan (CTAIP) to manage the various cooperation activities relating to industrial property in countries in the Asia and Pacific Region
WIPO (2021) Technical assistance database: search results, Sri Lanka. http://www.wipo.int/tad/en/activitysearchresult.jsp?vcntry=LK
WIPO (2022a) PCT applicant's guide: international phase annex 3. https://www.wipo.int/export/sites/www/pct/guide/en/gdvol1/annexes/annexc/ax_c_ib.pdf
WIPO (2022b) Receiving officers international bureau of the world intellectual property organisation. PCT Applicant's Guide—International Phase—Annex. https://www.wipo.int/export/sites/www/pct/guide/en/gdvol1/annexes/annexc/ax_c_ib.pdf
WIPO Manual (2014) Delivery of WIPO technical assistance. Delivery of WIPO Technical Assistance, p 4
WIPO Project Summary (2020) A Comprehensive Country Technical Assistance Implementation Plan (CTAIP) to Manage the Various Cooperation Activities Relating to Industrial Property in Countries in the Asia and Pacific Region
WIPO Project Summary (2021) A Comprehensive Country Technical Assistance Implementation Plan (CTAIP) to Manage the Various Cooperation Activities Relating to Industrial Property in Countries in the Asia and Pacific Region
WIPO Unveils Kirinde Masterpiece to Honour Lakshman Kadirgamar (2018) The sunday times online. https://www.sundaytimes.lk/180624/news/wipo-unveils-kirinde-masterpiece-to-honour-lakshman-kadirgamar-299601.html
WTO (2016) Trade policy review: Sri Lanka. http//:WTO|Trade policy review-Sri Lanka2016
WTO (2022) Sri Lanka and the WTO. https://www.wto.org/english/thewto_e/countries_e/sri_lanka_e.htm
Yang D (2011) Compulsory licensing: for better or for worse, the done deal lies in the balance. J Intell Property Rights 17:2145

Chapter 4
Discourses on Legal Framework for Protection of Plant Varieties in Sri Lanka

Abstract This chapter focuses on Sri Lanka as a relatively unexplored PVR case study in the general comparative literature in the South Asian region based on ownership and stewardship approaches. Comparing ownership with stewardship approaches, the researcher finds that the ownership discourse is inadequate, and stewardship is more suited to Sri Lanka, considering its subsistence agricultural economy. A stewardship approach is attractive if it will uphold the legal space of farmers for maintaining genetic resources through a recognition and reward system rather than just trying to balance FR with breeders' rights merely within an IP ownership approach. The researcher argues that (Sri Lankan) FR realisation can be achieved, not only through implementation of a *TRIPS*-consistent sui generis system of IP protection, and uptake of the *CBD* and *FAO Treaty* measures for sharing benefits, although these may be required, but also through integrating government policy and collaborating with all stakeholders relevant to agriculture in favour of farming communities. This assessment is borne out by the reluctance so far to enact and apply the draft PVR/PBR legislation and the deployment of alternative means to recognise and reward the local farmers' cultivation of plant varieties. These competing global and local legal discourses will now be analysed.

4.1 Introduction

Until the twentieth century, discourse on IP protection for plants was scarce, almost to the point of being non-existent. Thus, farmers worldwide could freely use biological resources to conserve and cultivate PGR, which includes seeds, plant varieties, genetic codes, sequences, DNA and germplasm for food and agriculture, as stewards or custodians of agrobiodiversity. Virtually the entire history of agricultural production, up until the second half of the twentieth century, placed seed collection and distribution in the hands of farmers and the public domain because crops were brought from the new world to the old world.[1] As a local practice, farmers collected seeds after the harvest and used them for the next crop, exchanging any

[1] Borowiak (2004), p. 511.

A. Perera, *Dilemmas of Intellectual Property Discourse in Sri Lanka*,
https://doi.org/10.1007/978-981-97-6117-3_4

excess with neighbours and adapting them to changes in the environment. These practices are commonly known as farmers' rights ('FR'). Through this process, farmers contributed to the sustainable development of plant varieties.[2]

However, during the late twentieth century, these traditional farming practices were increasingly subjugated to IPR in plants by virtue of their countries' adherence to the UPOV[3] and later the World Trade Organization's *TRIPS Agreement*. Article 27.3(b) of the *TRIPS Agreement* mandates member states to protect their plant varieties 'either by patents or by any sui generis law or any combination thereof'. Hence, for most developing countries, including Sri Lanka, given that UPOV membership was optional, the need for the protection of plant varieties surfaced after the ratification of the *TRIPS* script,[4] which comes under the global lawmaking process as discussed in Chap. 2.[5]

The increase in the recognition of IPR providing ownership of economic rights to developed plant varieties can be predominantly observed in countries such as the US and Australia, which rely highly on industrial and commercial/export farming. However, this situation has created conflicts with rights of farmers in developing and least developed countries.[6] This is because with the recognition of IPR on plants, traditional farming practices used by farmers for generations, such as seed sharing with other farmers and keeping the excess seed for the next harvest, were restricted under a PVR regime that gave property rights to one person, such as the 'breeder'. These practices come under the purview of FR, and in recent decades, FR has become a continuing discourse now in tension with the discourse on the new breeders' property rights (designated PBR) strengthening progressively under the iterations of the conventional PVR under the *UPOV Convention*, adopted in 1961 and revised in 1972, 1978 and 1991 and the *TRIPS Agreement* of 1995, particularly in developing and least developed countries. This aspect will be discussed later in this chapter.

4.1.1 Competing Discourses on PVR

Hence, following the recognition of PVR, competing discourses have emerged between the breeders of new varieties and farmers' traditional rights. Breeders' varieties are protected under the NDUS criteria, which are considered a high-technology protection under a PVR regime.[7] A breeder must fulfil these criteria if a new variety is to be protected and registered under the PVR law. In contrast, farmers who have been breeding varieties in an informal incremental manner for generations are unable

---

[2] Perera (2017).

[3] The UPOV was established by the *International Convention for the Protection of New Varieties of Plants*, which was adopted in Paris in 1961 and revised in 1972, 1978 and 1991 (*UPOV Convention*).

[4] Gervais (2013). See also Gervais (2010).

[5] See *TRIPS Agreement*.

[6] De Wit (2017).

[7] *UPOV Convention*.

to protect these under a PVR regime for their varieties could not satisfy the NDUS criteria. Therefore, such farmer-bred varieties will not be recognised as new varieties under the PVR law although their conservation and adaptation stewardship take skill and experience. Indeed, their improvements could be appropriated by others (sometimes regarded as biopiracy). Instead, they need to look for space within breeders' property rights to continue freely with their traditional seed practices.

Moreover, this competing discourse has real-life consequences on farmers' livelihood because, within the Sri Lankan context, subsistence farmers fall below the poverty line and rely highly on agricultural biodiversity for food security purposes. Restrictions imposed by a PVR regime will adversely affect their livelihood and social needs. Hence, a discourse was created between sectors of these two competing production models, which is characterised in this case study as a contrast between private property (ownership) and environmental stewardship, which may be contrasted, again, as high- and low-technology protection. Therefore, it is important to consider resolving or possibly balancing the competing discourses of breeders and farmers under a PVR regime.

Andersen described the competing discourses as one of ownership versus stewardship.[8] This conflict is particularly relevant in developing countries for national implementations of IPR have produced various hybrid sui generis systems endeavouring to incorporate FR within the PVR/PBR IPR framework required by UPOV and WTO membership. The livelihoods of many small farmers are at stake. Moreover, the contribution they make to agricultural biodiversity and environmental sustainability is important to all humans. However, in recent decades, traditional crop varieties historically conserved and cultivated by many small farmers have been neglected owing to the breeding of new varieties, where IPR are paramount.

One method of balancing these competing discourses is to recognise and realise FR and include a section of FR in the PVR legislations of many developing countries. This was possible under a sui generis system, considering that *TRIPS* allow countries to interpret art 27.3[9] and opt for the *UPOV Convention* revised in 1978 rather than in 1991 or indeed not sign the *UPOV Convention* because FR retention was considered essential to sustainable agricultural development in developing countries.

4.1.2 Levels of Lawmaking in PVR

This chapter pursues its enquiry by means of a case study of Sri Lanka's lawmaking for its vital agricultural sector.[10] For this case study, lawmaking can be considered under three levels; domestic, national and international. The first level is vital for this chapter since the discourse on PVR has particularly affected grassroot farmers and stakeholder alliances. Discourse on grassroot farmers is a major reason that the PVR

[8] Andersen (2017), p. 449. See also Andersen (2006), p. 5.

[9] Gervais (2005), p. 137.

[10] Perera (2021).

law is not yet enacted in Sri Lanka. This group has rejected IPR on plants and thus has become a governing node in the PVR discourse. Most farmers in Sri Lanka play an important role in in situ conservation and the sustainable use of agrobiodiversity, thus fostering innovation in agriculture as well as conservation.[11] Grassroot farming activities are under the domestic level. Farmers' traditional seed practices can be regarded as an informal customary law system, just as other practices have been regarded, such as the sharing of water courses.[12]

As for the second level, all legislation relevant to agricultural development, including biodiversity-related matters, are under the national level. National lawmaking processes were first identified in Chap. 2 of this book. However, politically and economically, national lawmaking cannot overlook the concerns of significant domestic-level actors, such as farmers in this case, as well as any global actors with interests, such as produce importers and foreign-owned plantations.

The third is the international level. This level is contested too, although *TRIPS* does put a hard-law requirement, possibly high-technology protection, into play. Intriguingly, most other countries, and not withstanding its international obligations under *TRIPS* as a member of the WTO, Sri Lanka, have not yet implemented a PVR law. However, Sri Lanka has a PVR Bill ('2001 Bill'),[13] first drafted in 2001 and redrafted in 2011; a third 2019 version of the Bill is currently with the Ministry of Agriculture, but the researcher does not have access to it.

Sri Lanka has not signed any of the versions of the *UPOV Convention*. Sri Lanka is also a member of both the *CBD*[14] and the *FAO Treaty*.[15] As yet, Sri Lanka does not have a formal legal framework that recognises PVR or FR.[16] The impact of the *TRIPS Agreement* as a superstructural role was discussed in Chap. 2 and its influence on agriculture in developing countries, such as Sri Lanka, will be further discussed under the section on *TRIPS Agreement* in this chapter.

---

[11] Perera (2011). See also Perera (2017) (n 2).

[12] McGuire and Sperling (2016).

[13] Protection of Plant Varieties Bill 2001 ('2001 Bill').

[14] The *CBD*, which entered into force 29 December 1993, is an international legal instrument for 'the conservation of biological diversity, the sustainable use of its components and the fair and equitable sharing of the benefits arising out of the utilization of genetic resources' that has been ratified by 196 nations.

[15] The *International Treaty on Plant Genetic Resources for Food and Agriculture* ('*FAO Treaty*'), 29 June 2004 is a global response to promote the conservation of PGR and to protect farmers' rights to access and have fair and equitable sharing of benefits arising out of their use. Sustainable use of PGR is fundamental for achieving food and nutrition security and for a progressive realisation of the right to food.

[16] The proposed 2001 Bill has been floating in Sri Lanka for the past 20 years in several different versions without implementation and consists of a section on FR.

4.1.3 PVR as Low-Technology Protection Regime

This chapter examines reasons as to why PVR case study favours low-technology protection. It is because PVR regime has real-life consequences on farmers' livelihood, within the Sri Lankan context and these farmers are not aware or educated regarding the NDUS criteria used by the PBR regime which is based on high technology. Moreover, majority of farmers in Sri Lanka are subsistence farmers who fall below the poverty line and rely highly on agricultural biodiversity for food security purposes. Restrictions imposed by a PVR regime will adversely affect their livelihood and social needs. Hence, a discourse was created between sectors of these two competing production models, which is characterised in this case study as a contrast between private property (ownership) and environmental stewardship, which may be contrasted, again, as high- and low-technology protection. Therefore, it is important to consider resolving or possibly balancing the competing discourses of breeders and farmers under a PVR regime.

To examine how global and local governance actors or nodes play power dynamics in developing an PVR/PBR regime in Sri Lanka, it is crucial to discuss the role of nodes in this case study. Nodes that exist in PVR include the TRIPS Agreement and WTO as a superstructural node, through its ability to require compliance by every member country to the implement the TRIPS requirements into local legal frameworks. In the arena of PVR, TRIPS has the mentalities, technologies, resources and institutional force to mobilise, assist and influence developing countries towards implementing a PVR/PBR system. However, in spite of this global requirement Sri Lanka still does not have a PVR law, suggesting there is no coercion or influence by the WTO to change the PVR. Nevertheless, divergences identified from the interviews for this book revealed local discourses challenges the global pressure and conflict in introducing PVR laws. The protests by farming communities and environmental groups in Sri Lanka is a key factor in Sri Lanka, which will be discussed later in this chapter. To elucidate the power dynamics in the PVR regime in Sri Lanka, this case study will also examine how variety of actors within the PVR regime have exerted influence with the other nodes through interaction and communications creating a social discourse thus, introducing and promoting recommendations to PVR in Sri Lanka.

Based on the above background, this case study provides a unique opportunity to develop a sui generis structure, where no formal framework currently exists in Sri Lanka. Hence, developing a sui generis framework for PVR conducive to Sri Lankan FR requires the investigation of several essential questions, expressed as follows:

What legal regime and government program might be implemented:

1. to safeguard farmers' ability to access both existing agrobiodiversity and new breed innovations in plant varieties, especially their freedom to save and share seeds; and
2. to reward farmers for their conservation and cultivation of traditional and local varieties, both defensively to protect them against misappropriation by

others and proactively to encourage their collective economic and environmental contributions.

Resolving these questions is vital if local farmers are to compete and coexist with the IPR proposed within the PVR regime. However, before identifying findings, it is necessary to map the terrain of conflict between FR and PVR, employing Andersen's stewardship–ownership contrast.[17] The tussle between the two is crucial to the realisation of PVR and FR in Sri Lanka and indeed other countries. By using *TRIPS* flexibility in conjunction with other international treaties and striving to achieve a legal cohabitation between them,[18] Sri Lanka could realise FR by balancing the needs of small subsistence farmers and modern plant breeders.

4.2 Stewardship versu Ownership Framework

This chapter's analysis of the PVR versus FR lawmaking discourse in Sri Lanka is guided by Andersen's contrast between stewardship and ownership approaches, which are individual rights. The ownership approach aims to establish individual or collective ownership of genetic resources, in order to provide incentives to promote innovative breeding as well as the conservation and sustainable use of agrobiodiversity.[19] Ownership, while also granting PVR to corporate science, offers knowledge protection to farmers from misappropriation by enabling its holders to have rights to make decisions with other stakeholders on mutually agreed terms.[20] Underlying this approach is the concept that farmers, similarly to commercial breeders, should be granted property rights to control their knowledge, together with participation in access and benefit-sharing ('ABS') schemes, as measures of creating an incentive structure for farmers.[21] The aim of adding ABS legislation is to reduce the inequity that farmers investing and bargaining in an ownership system are likely to face.

The ownership approach is preferred by countries with industrialised agriculture, such as Australia, which is oriented towards export markets, preferring patent protection and a strong sui generis system for the protection of plant varieties.[22] Such a system facilitates imports of propagating material, such as terminator seeds, for breeders may be reluctant to transfer or sell any material to countries that do not provide such protection.[23] A strong IPR system developed using the ownership approach is considered a crucial mechanism to protect and encourage investment in R&D in these countries, to facilitate commercialisation alliances with companies in other countries and also to facilitate trade in biotechnology products. Therefore,

[17] Andersen (2016) (n 8).

[18] Ibid.

[19] Ibid 456.

[20] Andersen (2016).

[21] Ibid.

[22] Perera (2017) (n 11).

[23] International Plant Genetic Resources Institute (1999).

countries with a strong capacity in biotechnology are likely to gain many benefits from a strong IPR system.[24] Sri Lanka may aspire but will not qualify currently. This issue will be further discussed in Chap. 5.

In contrast, a stewardship approach is a more comprehensive system whereby farmers continue to act as stewards of biodiversity on their own terms. In terms of FR, a stewardship approach requires that farmers must be granted rights collectively, to enable them to continue as stewards and innovators of agrobiodiversity and to reward them for their contribution.[25]

A principal difference between the ownership and stewardship approaches is that while the former emphasises IPR for farmers, the stewardship approach is a non-IPR mechanism for the protection and cultivation of farmers' varieties. The latter approach first seeks to exempt farmers' varieties from breeders' rights system. It has a defensive dimension. In other words, proponents of stewardship promote 'farmers privilege', such as saving, sharing and exchanging seeds for the next harvest.[26] The idea is to provide the 'legal space' required for farmers to continue and uphold their roles in the maintenance and conservation of agrobiodiversity.

If the ownership approach were introduced to realise PVR or FR in Sri Lanka, it would pose the following obstacles in the implementation process. First, as farming communities generally have collective responsibility over the innovation process,[27] it is extremely difficult to identify a single farming community as a potential right holder.[28] Second, depending on the farmers' privilege, other traditional farming communities need to pay royalties to use another community's traditional varieties, which would negate the underlying rationale of FR because revenue is transferred from one group of resource-poor farmers to a similar group. Hence, stewardship is a non-IP approach to recognise farmers' role for the benefit of all humankind. Furthermore, it suggests that proactively, government should positively reward and support farmers for their contributions in this context.

Stewardship is not just a localised discourse; it has international support through the UN's *CBD* and *FAO Treaty*. These instruments also view farmers as the stewards or custodians of agricultural diversity, charged to preserve such diversity for the greater good, rather than to protect their own rights as ownership rights.[29] Hence, the conservation and cultivation rationale of FR promotes stewardship conceived as collective community rights to farmers' contributions to biodiversity on their own terms in accordance with their local ecosystem, climatic conditions, economic resources, community values and topographic conditions. Sri Lanka acceded to the *FAO Treaty* on 17 September 2013 and is also a member of the *CBD*; it is hence

[24] Ibid.

[25] Andersen (2006) (n 17).

[26] Andersen (2005).

[27] However, there could be individual farmers who engage in the innovation process similarly to the Khobgradge case cited in FN 169.

[28] Correa (2000).

[29] Guneratne (2008), p. 144.

bound, insofar as these treaties are hard law, or encouraged, so far as they are soft law, to protect FR through the implementation of national legislation.

4.2.1 The Indian Experience on FR

The Indian system has been considered a benchmark for it is viewed to protect and incentivise FR while adopting a plant variety protection statute. The chapter on FR introduced by the Indian policymakers as the *Protection of Plant Varieties and Farmer's Rights Act, 2001* (*'Indian Plant Act'*)[30] in conjunction with PVR required by *TRIPS* and allied treaties, such as the *UPOV Convention*, came into reality with strong stakeholder motivation. In the Indian context, NGOs and local stakeholder alliances influenced policymakers to change the law, and hence, they can be regarded as governing nodes because they participate in discourse or communicative acts using their own criteria to assess and prioritise the relevance and value of the needs of Indian farmers and Indian policymakers.[31] The Indian experience provides guidance on how Indian NGOs and stakeholder alliances and activists mobilised public opinion through simultaneously deploying multiple nodes to communicate, such as unprecedented public demonstrations, which resulted in India introducing of a sui generis law. These nodes 'spoke back' to global nodes, such as Monsanto and other MNCs that have monopolised the production of GM seeds[32] under PVR laws. However, ultimately, amid local nodes speaking back, the global nodes win.[33]

The *Indian Plant Act* was seen to fulfil both India's international obligations under the *TRIPS Agreement* and its commitment to local farmers' welfare. The Indian system has features to implement FR, which include protection, access and reward. It shows how local interests can shape change and inclusion. Hence, Indian PVR legislation is often referred to as the most progressive, inclusive or advanced worldwide.[34] However, the *Indian Plant Act* is a benchmark for implementing the 'ownership' approach to offer IPR for farmers because the this Act treats farmers as breeders and farmers who want to register their varieties must fulfil the criteria stipulated in the Act, similarly to commercial breeders.[35] However, as will be analysed in the next section, without stewardship provisions, India's ownership approach that allows IPR for farmers has been unsuccessful in realising FR within a conventional IPR framework.

---

[30] *Protection of Plant Varieties and Farmer's Rights Act, 2001* Act No. 53 of 2001.

[31] Peschard (2016).

[32] Thomas and De Tavernier (2017).

[33] Bhardwaj and Jadhav (2019).

[34] Santilli (2012). See also Prajeesh (2015).

[35] This aspect is discussed in detail under ownership protection for farmers' varieties in Sect. 4.7 and registration of farmers' varieties in Sect. 4.7.3 of this chapter. Also see, Rangnekar (2016), p. 285.

4.3 Farmers Rights: Origins and Approaches

4.3.1 International Treaty Context

4.3.1.1 FAO Treaty

The presence of these treaties alongside the WTO's *TRIPS* shows that the global discourse is not uniform and unidirectional. FR have emerged through a range of international instruments. In the early 1990s, the demand to recognise FR garnered attention in international agricultural circles following a series of debates in FAO. This groundswell led to the adoption of three FAO Conference resolutions[36] that simultaneously recognised the rights of plant breeders as well as farmers. The FR concept was then included in the FAO Undertaking on Plant Genetic Resources,[37] and later, in the *FAO Treaty*, which came into force in 2004. Sri Lanka is a member of the *FAO Treaty*.[38]

The *FAO Treaty* recognises the right of farmers and emphasises the need for promoting and protecting FR at both national and international levels. Article 9 of the Treaty recognises the enormous contribution of farmers and local communities to the conservation and development of PGR for food and agriculture and identifies measures to protect and promote FR.[39] It recommends national governments implement national measures to realise FR.

4.3.1.2 CBD

Similarly, the *Nagoya Protocol on Access to Genetic Resources and the Fair and Equitable Sharing of Benefits Arising from their Utilization* under the *CBD* supports and protects FR by seeking the prior informed consent of related communities for access to genetic resources and traditional knowledge.[40] It makes provisions for the equitable sharing of benefits accruing from the use of genetic resources and associated traditional knowledge.[41] Article 6 of the *CBD* requires Contracting Parties to develop a National Biodiversity Strategy and Action Plan, or an equivalent instrument. Sri Lanka ratified the *CBD* in 1994. Hence, both *CBD* and the *FAO Treaty* view farmers

---

[36] Food and Agricultural Organisation, Resolutions 4/89 (Agreed interpretation of the International Undertaking agreed interpretation), 5/89 (Farmers' Rights) and 3/91 (concerning public land).

[37] FAO Undertaking on Plant Genetic Resources, Res 4/89 (Agreed interpretation of the International Undertaking agreed interpretation) and 7/93 (Revision of the International Undertaking agreed interpretation).

[38] *FAO Treaty*.

[39] Ibid.

[40] Peschard (2016) (n 31). See also Flach et al. (2009); Sherman (2003); Blakeney (2011).

[41] *CBD* art 8(j).

as stewards or custodians of agricultural diversity, who preserve such diversity for the greater good instead of personal gains or property rights.[42]

4.3.1.3 Declaration on the Rights of Peasants and Other People Working in Rural Areas

The UN *Declaration on the Rights of Peasants and Other People Working in Rural Areas*, which was ratified in December 2018, grants individual and collective rights to land, seeds and natural resources. These rights are granted not only to farmers—indigenous peoples, minorities and local communities are also recognised as legitimate rights holders.[43] It includes the right to life through agricultural production (art 18), right to seeds (art 19) and right to traditional knowledge and protection of biological diversity (art 20). Article 19 specifically reproduces the FR provisions of the *FAO Treaty*, including 'the right to save, use, exchange and sell their farm-saved seeds or propagating material'.[44] These rights are recognised in the literature as the main components of FR.[45] The right to seed is the central construct of FR and the conflict that arises between stewardship and ownership approaches.

The right to seed thus has conceptually expanded from its main components, to become a powerful expression described as 'seed activism' that encompass semantic innovations, such as seed commons, peasant seeds and seed sovereignty.[46] Seed-saving practices have been described as a form of 'quiet activism' that cuts across the rural–urban and global South–North divides.[47] This aspect will be discussed later in this chapter.

4.3.1.4 TRIPS Agreement

The implications of complying with art 27.3(b) of the *TRIPS Agreement* for small farmers and rural communities in developing countries, such as Sri Lanka, are likely to be considerable. Article 27.3(b) of the *TRIPS Agreement* deals with the protection of plant varieties as follows:

> Members may also exclude from patentability plants and animals other than micro-organisms, and essentially biological processes for the production of plants or animals other than non-biological and microbiological processes. However, members shall provide for the plant variety protection either by patents or by an effective sui generis system or by any combination thereof.

---

[42] Andersen (2005) (n 26).

[43] Peschard and Randeria (2021). See also Elderman and James (2011).

[44] UN *Declaration on the Rights of Peasants and Other People Working in Rural Areas*, GA Res. 73/165 on 17 December 2018, 14/17.

[45] Peschard and Randeria (2021) (n 43).

[46] Ibid.

[47] Ibid 8.

The term sui generis means unique or of its own kind. Plant variety protection is a special system adapted specifically to address the issues of plant varieties and their protection. The *TRIPS Agreement* is silent about the components that constitute an 'effective sui generis system'. It is entirely left to national governments to design such a system suitable to the national needs, provided it is effective in providing plant variety protection.[48]

Hence, the inclusion of art 27.3(b) is an example of a global discourse initiated by the WTO, and within the process, developed countries can be classified as governing nodes because they have the thinking that could shape and influence the developing countries' response to the inclusion of art 27.3(b). Moreover, they have all the support and resources to fuel its influence and a system to enforce on all nations that are unwilling to corporate with the inclusion. Moreover, the WTO and developed countries are a superstructural node because they can channel resources to exert simultaneous influence at the national and global level. However, developed countries, such as the US, the UK, the EU and the Andean Community wanted to drop art 27.3(b) since most of these countries already had plant variety protection laws based on the *UPOV Convention*, as revised in 1978 or 1991 on the basis of the ownership approach, which is considered *TRIPS* compliant as a sui generis system.

Because art 27.3(b) was controversial from inception, it was agreed that the article be reviewed after four years of its operation, but the review has never been completed. The review is for the primary purpose of gathering information on the ways that the plant and animal invention provisions are implemented under domestic laws.[49] However, some members, mainly the developed countries, prefer dropping the exception, in order to provide patent protection for plants and animals because the patent protection discourse is regarded as stronger than PVR.[50]

In 1999, at the Seattle Meeting of Ministers, the summit was closed because of public protests and developing country withdrawals because countries were unable to bridge the differing viewpoints on issues in the areas of agriculture, labour, anti-dumping, investment and implementation and on other issues, including biotechnology.[51] The mere fact that the Meeting was closed because of protests implies the influence of those indirect actors over decision-making.

The next review was held in 2001 at Doha. Paragraph 19 of the *Doha Declaration* broadened the discussion about protecting plant varieties. It states that the TRIPS Agreement Council should also examine the relationship between the *TRIPS Agreement* and the *CBD*. The trend in the discourse was for any patent protection to be linked with recognition and reward for traditional knowledge and folklore.[52] The fifth ministerial summit of the WTO was held in Cancun, Mexico, in September 2003.[53] At this point, many developing countries expressed the desire to review art 27.3(b),

[48] Perera (2010).

[49] Ibid.

[50] Perera (2010) (n 48).

[51] Ibid.

[52] WTO (2011).

[53] Gunawardena (2003).

ranging from the total exclusion of patents on life to restricting to, and narrowing down, protection further. Sri Lanka's position, both in 1999 and in 2003, was that there should be no life-patenting provisions in the *TRIPS Agreement*.[54] It favours the current position.

However, at Cancun, the talks broke down when Kenya, the leader of the African Group, walked out of the ministerial-level discussion.[55] The main reason for this breakdown was the inflexibility of the US about granting any trade concessions in agriculture negotiations, especially about cutting back the heavy cotton subsidies, which resulted in hurting cotton farmers in Africa.[56] Hence, the revision of art 27.3(b) has not advanced.

The breakthrough during the Doha round was the agreement to include the *TRIPS* disclosure requirement within the draft modalities for *TRIPS*-related issues. In 2006, submissions in response to the communication from Switzerland listed many issues that are relevant to the implementation of the disclosure requirement.[57] On 27 May 2006, at the request of the Indian delegation, the following communication was circulated:[58]

> Members agree to the inclusion in the TRIPS Agreement of a mandatory requirement for the disclosure of origin of biological resources and/or associated traditional knowledge in patent applications. Text based negotiations shall be undertaken in Special Sessions of the TRIPS Council, and as an integral part of the single undertaking, on an amendment to the TRIPS Agreement establishing an obligation for Members to require patent applicants to disclose the origin of biological resources and/or associated traditional knowledge, including Prior Informed Consent and Access and Benefit Sharing.

In July 2008, many developing countries, including Sri Lanka, submitted the following draft modalities for consideration by Ministers for *TRIPS*-related issues.[59]

- Members agree to amend the *TRIPS Agreement* to include a mandatory requirement for the disclosure of the country providing/source of genetic resources, and/or associated traditional knowledge for which a definition will be agreed, in patent applications. Patent applications will not be processed without completion of the disclosure requirement.
- Members agree to define the nature and extent of a reference to Prior Informed Consent and Access and Benefit Sharing.
- Text-based negotiations shall be undertaken, in Special Sessions of the TRIPS Council, and as an integral part of the Single Undertaking, to implement the above. Additional elements contained in members' proposals, such as prior informed

[54] Ibid.

[55] Sahai (2002).

[56] Gunawardena (2003) (n 53).

[57] *Communication from Bolivia, Cuba, Ecuador, India, Sri Lanka and Thailand, Submission in Response to the Communication from Switzerland*, WTO Doc IP/C/W/470 (21 March 2006).

[58] WTO Secretariat (2006).

[59] WTO (2022).

consent and ABS as an integral part of the disclosure requirement and post-grant sanctions, may also be raised and shall be considered in these negotiations.[60]

In 2011, the proposals dealing with the relationship between the WTO's IP (*TRIPS*) agreement and the UN *CBD*, including an element sometimes called biopiracy, were discussed. On this issue, delegations differed in interpreting the 2001 *Doha Declaration* mandate, and hence, the issue is unresolved to date.[61]

4.3.1.5 UPOV Convention

Although several different sui generis systems are under contemplation, the term sui generis has most often been used with respect to the *UPOV Convention* although it is not mentioned in *TRIPS*. This move emptied the sui generis system of its quintessence and put at risk smallholder farmers, whose practice of saving, sharing and replanting seeds is embedded in a long, generational tradition.[62] Distinctions can be made between the *UPOV Convention* revisions of 1978 and 1991 between which signatories may choose. For example, the 1991 *UPOV Convention* narrows farmers' exceptions, which were recognised under the 1978 *UPOV Convention.*[63] This distinction is crucial to FR realisation.[64]

The modification introduced by the 1991 *UPOV Act* implies nodal influence by the US. In fact, the US enacted its own *Plant Variety Protection Act* ('*PVPA*') in 1970, and this has extended IP protection to sexually reproduced or tuber-propagated plant varieties (other than fungi and bacteria).[65] Unlike the US *Plant Patent Act,*[66] this Act of 1970 granted a 'brown-bag'[67] exemption to farmers to save, replant or sell the protected variety they have purchased from the owners: the private biotechnology companies. This exemption, which is similar to farmers' privilege, was detrimental to industrial agriculture owing to the pressure of the seed companies who are also governing nodes in the PVR regime.[68] By fostering the idea of protecting US PVR

---

[60] Ibid.

[61] WTO (2008).

[62] Dogbevi (2017). See also Verma (2007).

[63] Arup (2008).

[64] Correa has proposed an alternative to a UPOV-type regime of PBR, one that is suitable for the seed supply and agricultural systems prevailing in developing countries, on the basis of three categories of plant varieties: 'new uniform plant varieties', 'new farmer and other heterogeneous varieties' and 'traditional farmers' varieties'. See Correa (2015).

[65] 7 USCS § 2402—Right to plant variety protection; plant varieties protectable.

[66] The US *Plant Patent Act* was enacted by the Congress in 1930 and has conferred patent protection to asexually reproduced plants (see 35 USCS § 161 et seq 4).

[67] 7 USCS § 2543—Right to save seed; crop exemption ('it shall not infringe any right hereunder for a person to save seed produced by the person from seed obtained, or descended from seed obtained, by authority of the owner of the variety for seeding purposes and use such saved seed in the production of a crop for use on the farm of the person, or sale as provided in this section.').

[68] Dogbevi (2017) (n 62).

beyond national borders, the US became a signatory to the 1991 *UPOV Convention*.[69] At the national level, and in conformity to the 1991 *UPOV Convention*, the US Congress repealed the 'brown-bag' exemption in 1994. Thus, overall, UPOV advances the interests of commercial plant breeders and MNCs.

Notably, Sri Lanka has not yet joined UPOV has not been pressed to do so by countries such as the US. However, Sri Lanka entered into the first *Trade and Investment Framework Agreement* with the US in 2002 to reaffirm its support to the WTO and to the Doha Development Agenda.[70] By 2016, Sri Lanka has entered into 12 such agreements to boost bilateral trade and investment.[71] However, no available information suggests that such agreements include trade in agriculture.

This analysis has identified certain key global discourses on PVR. The *TRIPS* discourse is a clear global influence by the WTO, developed countries and MNCs on developing and least developed countries over the interpretation of art 27.3(b). Although developing countries obtained some concessions in the ministerial meetings, most meetings were discontinued because developing countries were not satisfied with the solutions provided by the WTO, developed countries and MNCs for the issues raised by the developing countries. All the other global discourses were not mandatory for the countries to follow, unlike the *TRIPS*.

4.4 Farmers' Rights as a Collective Right

FR, as a collective right, can be observed in the agricultural sectors of many developing countries, including Sri Lanka, which could be classified under the stewardship approach. This approach is tailored to provide incentives and support to farmers.[72] Local farmers represent the primary workforce population in developing countries as a collective group, and they imbibe their practices of selecting, saving, sharing and replanting seeds from socio-cultural and religious values transmitted from ancestors

---

[69] See *Plant Variety Protection Act Amendments of 1993*, 140 Cong Rec H 8026, August 12, 1994. In order to provide our plant breeders protection in other countries as well, the United States became a member of the *UPOV Convention* in 1981. UPOV, *Members*. https://www.upov.int/members/en/. The UPOV currently has 25-member countries and provides for uniform practices in the construction and administration of plant variety protection laws in the various member states. After several years of negotiations, the *UPOV Convention* was significantly revised in 1991 to provide improved protection for innovative plant varieties. The United States is a signatory to the 1991 agreement. The Bill before the House today would conform the current *Plant Variety Protection Act* to the 1991 *UPOV Convention*.

[70] Office of the United States Trade Representative (2022).

[71] Ministry of Foreign Affairs Sri Lanka (2016).

[72] Department of Agriculture, Fisheries and Forestry, Australia (2022).

to new generations, which have been engraved in their customs, traditions and identity for centuries.[73] These practices belong to the customary traditional order and the patrimony of these communities.[74]

Moreover, the collective right concept now has its roots within FAO and the *CBD*, but it is not well recognised in national legislation.[75] It is difficult to find legal means to realise the stewardship approach or farmers' collective rights in biodiversity on their own terms within their local ecosystems, climatic conditions, economic resources and topographic conditions. Farmers within a community collectively take part in sharing seeds, breeding plants and adapting varieties to climate, water and topographic conditions by applying their indigenous knowledge and skills and customary practices.[76] Some scholars have argued for the recognition of the socio-political and agro-ecological contexts in which the practices of seed repossession appear and the value of these customary practices for the commonisation of seeds.[77] Within these contexts, Gibson argued:

> it is imprecise to say there is no proprietary system or entitlement within indigenous and traditional communities. By doing so we deny indigenous and traditional practices and relationships of stewardship. We also deny the community's right to respect through its knowledge if that community is unable to access and practice traditional system and customs of stewardship and guardianship of the land, resources.[78]

For this reason, any infringement of the age-old ordinary practices and customs of indigenous people ought to be considered a violation of the essence, the intrinsic value and the identity of these communities as a collective right.

There are several instances in which such a community-based system has been used in practice in Sri Lanka, to give farmers legal space and form to engage in their agricultural activities collectively. The first example relates to rice paddy cultivation, paddy management, soil conservation, plant protection, fertilisation and pesticide control techniques that farmers undertake as a collective group.[79] The second example relates to the collective agricultural wisdom of farmers in the areas of water collection and conservation and irrigation practices.[80]

These collective rights have permitted and empowered farmers to use traditional cultivation-related practices for generations. These are examples of the stewardship approach, which provides an existing foundation for the conceptual framework for FR realisation in Sri Lanka. Sri Lankan policymakers need to be mindful about these issues because farmers belong to an interpretive or epistemic community that shares similar epistemological assumptions, beliefs and preferences on FR. They communicate with each other and build their shared assumptions and understandings on issues

[73] Dogbevi (2017) (n 68).

[74] Ibid.

[75] European Agroecology Knowledge Exchange Network (2017). See also GRAIN (2005).

[76] Phillips (2016).

[77] Patnaik et al. (2017).

[78] Gibson (2005).

[79] Abeywardana et al. (2019).

[80] News First (2019).

that affect farmers, and therefore, any solutions should be proposed after consulting them. These traditional resource rights could lead to conflicts if the governments fail to engage in consultations with farmers prior to implementing laws that affect them.[81] In other words, government failure to engage farmers suggest that the government has failed as a governing node to listen to farmers needs and wants. This failure will lead to further unprecedented conflicts.

4.5 Sri Lanka: Case Study

4.5.1 High-Technology Breeders' Intellectual Property Rights

At present, nationally and internationally, different forms of legal protection are available to breeders of new plant varieties. In the international arena, the *UPOV Convention* is the first multilateral effort to provide them with sui generis protection. Hence, UPOV created a new type of IP protection for new plant varieties and this new right was called plant breeders' rights ('PBR').[82]

The main aim of the *UPOV Acts* is to promote the protection of the breeder of new plant varieties. It provides protection not only for new plant varieties, but also contains explicit and detailed rules on the conditions and arrangements for granting protection.[83] For example, the Acts contains rules relating to the scope of protection of breeders' rights, the duration of protection, the possible restrictions and exceptions, and the forfeiture of protection.

Countries such as the US and Australia are members of the *UPOV Convention* of 1991. The US has had its *Plant Patent Act* since 1930 and its *Plant Variety Protection Act* since 1970. Australia enacted the *Plant Breeders' Rights Act 1994* (Cth) principally to be in conformity with the 1991 revision of the *UPOV Act*. Importantly, under the PVR legislation, plant varieties themselves are registrable, and although these varieties must have a breeder, it is the variety itself that rights are granted for, and not a process or a technique, as in the case of patent protection.[84] The breeder has exclusive control over the propagating material (e.g. seeds, cuttings, divisions and tissue culture) and harvested material (cut flowers, fruits and foliage) of a new plant variety.[85]

Most of these developed countries have a patent system to protect plant varieties, which restricts anyone from using a protected variety unless authorised by the patent owner. For example, both the US and Australia, which have industrialised agriculture,

[81] Rodríguez-Garavito (2011).

[82] Perera (2010) (n 50).

[83] Ibid.

[84] IP Australia (2019).

[85] Ibid.

are oriented towards export markets and prefer patent protection and a strong sui generis system for protecting plant varieties. Such a system facilitates imports of propagating material, for breeders may be reluctant to sell any material to countries that do not provide protection. A strong IPR system is considered a crucial mechanism to protect investment in R&D, to facilitate alliances with companies in other countries and also to facilitate trade in biotechnology products. Therefore, countries with a strong capacity in biotechnology are likely to gain many benefits from a strong PVR system based on the *UPOV Act*. Hence, PVR and patent protection for plant varieties was a double-barrelled gun for developed countries, who could anyway enjoy a high level of protection for their plant varieties under this dual system.[86] Such a system is considered a high-technology protection for plant varieties since both patent and PVR requires specialised competences and breeders are required to fulfil number of the criteria under the Act, for their varieties to be protected under the Act.

After ratifying the *TRIPS Agreement*, some developing countries ratified the *UPOV 1991 Act* as a possible sui generis system under art 27.3(b) of the *TRIPS Agreement*, but others chose the 1978 version. Countries such as India and Thailand enacted PVR Acts to comply with the *TRIPS Agreement*, but these countries deviated from the UPOV-style protection. For example, India enacted the *Protection of Plant Varieties and Farmers' Rights Act (2001)* and Thailand the *Plant Varieties Protection Act (1999)*. Both India and Thailand used the word Plant Variety Protection as the title for their respective Acts, rather than PBR. Technically both these terms refer to IPR on plants but have a subtle difference. While PBR is the more high-technology ownership version, which allows breeders of new plant varieties to fulfil many criteria, PVR are the broader, more neutral category, possibly allowing protection of the traditional varieties, although still through an ownership approach. For example, the Acts of both India and Thailand while protecting breeders of new plant varieties also protect traditional varieties bred by farmers. Under PBR, only breeders are protected and as discussed earlier, the criteria for protection are more technical.

Accordingly, the Sri Lankan Government titled its Bill as 'Protection of Plant Varieties', which implies that Sri Lankan policymakers have acknowledged subsistence farming as the country's norm. Its farmers rely heavily on traditional varieties for their survival, and high-technology PBR that does not recognise farmers' exceptions will adversely affect their livelihood. Hence, it is important to identify the competing discourses for breeders and farmers when drafting PVR legislation in Sri Lanka, similar to India and Thailand.[87]

---

[86] Antons (2016).

[87] Perera (2017) (n 22). See also Perera (2010) (n 82).

4.5.2 Intellectual Property Law for Plant Varieties in Sri Lanka

The *IP Act No. 36 of 2003* of Sri Lanka does not provide patent protection for plant varieties. Section 62(1) defines an invention and s 62(3) states that the following are not patentable:[88]

> plants, animals and other microorganisms other than transgenic microorganisms and an essentially biological processes for the production of plants or animals, other than non-biological and micro-biological processes.

Instead, the NIPO of Sri Lanka proposed a separate, sui generis system of IP for plant varieties, focusing on the new varieties that professional breeders develop, through a *TRIPS*-compliant framework. That took form in the 2001 Bill. The 2001 Bill, which a former official of NIPO drafted, was a verbatim copy of *UPOV 1991*. According to the official, this was a working document[89] and it was not sent to the Parliament. The primary purpose of the Bill is to provide for the registration of new plant varieties, but it also seeks to encourage the development of new varieties of plants; to protect the rights of farmers, breeders and researchers who develop these new varieties; and to provide for matters connected therewith or incidental thereto.[90] However, the Bill lacks a fully integrated FR provision.

Yet, notably, the *Seed Act No. 22 of 2003* (‘*Seed Act*’) was enacted and a new Seed Bill was proposed to amend this Act, which Parliament has not yet passed because of stakeholders’ opposition. Therefore, the current and future position of PVR is uncertain in Sri Lanka. Nor is FR consolidated. The main features of the *Seed Act* and the new Seed Bill will be examined in this section, but, in summary, it does not comprehensively establish a system consonant with either of Andersen’s approaches to FR. However, the policymakers interviewed in this research and the FR literature have appreciated the significance of this lawmaking and the need to demonstrate and mobilise to protect existing practices and rights recognised by custom and in agricultural ordinances.[91] In line with the stewardship approach, most Sri Lankan farmer activists, NGOs and stakeholders also oppose the introduction of any type of property rights on traditional varieties as well as any type of centralised registries of information on these varieties under the PVR Bill.

The local discourse on the PVR Bill was the result of a collaboration between the NIPO and the Sri Lankan DoA. In July 2001, both invited stakeholder alliances consisting of representatives of civil society organisations, grassroot-level farmers, NGOs, law firms, biotechnology industry agents, universities and research institutes through a national seminar, to create a national consensus about the contents of a

---

[88] *IP Act No. 36 of 200*, s 63(2) 49.

[89] Interviewee # 23.

[90] See the long title of the 2011 Bill.

[91] These interviews were conducted in 2002. However, the context is still valid since the PVR Bill is still not enacted in Sri Lanka. Interviewee # 27; Interviewee # 28; Interviewee # 29; See also Gunawardena (2000a, b).

proposed IP system for plant varieties.[92] Within the PVR discourse, these entities can be regarded as interpretive communities. These members communicate with each other, develop their shared epistemological assumptions and implicit understandings on PVR and attempt to find appropriate solutions. Some of these members are often embedded in more than one interpretive community and their communicative acts motivate the government to change its regularity preferences.

Given that the PVR Bill was designed to grant IP protection for breeders of new varieties, which is similar then to *UPOV 1991*, critics argued that the law would not address the needs of Sri Lankan farmers. A specific concern was that PVR Bill did not contain parallel protections for the conservation, use and exchange of traditional plant varieties.[93] Therefore, NGOs made the following suggestions for amending the draft:[94]

- It should not only cover 'breeders' but should be expanded to cover community rights and traditional crop varieties bred by farmers.
- It should not only cover 'new varieties' but also traditional varieties, those bred by the DoA and varieties bred by other bodies.
- It should not extend rights to all varieties of plants. Crops essential for the nation's food security needs, such as rice, cereals and some legumes, should be excluded.
- It need not grant long-term monopoly rights for new varieties. The NGOs consider it is important to reduce the period of protection for food crops and for commercial crops, such as tea and rubber.
- A new variety should be distinct by not one characteristic, but by a wider margin in order to prevent a series of genetically homogenous or closely related lines being protected. Narrow genetic diversity in a crop is detrimental to the country for it increases vulnerability to adverse events.
- The breeder's application should mention the parental lines and the country of origin. If one or more lines have been taken from Sri Lanka, a royalty should be paid to the farmers, communities or research institutes who have developed these varieties. In cases where it is not possible to determine the above or when the beneficiaries do not seek any royalty, the evaluated amount should be added to a fund established under the Act.
- Varieties bred or developed by a public body, an interest venture or an individual who does not seek profits shall be awarded a certificate, with costs being borne by the fund referred to above.
- If a variety registered for public interest is to be used to breed other varieties for commercial use, the user should secure explicit approval from the rights holder, abide by the terms and conditions and pay a royalty to the fund.
- The principle of essentially derived varieties should be excluded from the Draft, and a section should be incorporated to grant rights and privileges to farmers.

---

[92] Ibid.

[93] Ibid.

[94] Perera (2010) (n 87).

- Privileges should be granted to research institutes or the public to use protected varieties for developing varieties for non-profitable, public interest uses.
- It should include a CL provision.

These observations and suggestions were sent by the NGOs to the Seed Certification Office for perusal, and this Office submitted its views to the NIPO. Unfortunately, Sri Lankan legislators overlooked above recommendations and the existing economic and social conditions and drafted the proposed Bill in 2001 based on the 1991 UPOV Convention that does not address the needs of local farming communities. The effects of transplanted law to the recipient state has been discussed in Chap. 2 of this book.

In late 2001, a group of NGOs, including the Law and Society Trust and the Institute of Policy Studies, submitted recommendations to the NIPO to not follow the UPOV model but, instead, revise the scope of the Bill to recognise the rights of local farmers over their varieties. Furthermore, the recommendations argued that the Sri Lankan system of plant variety protection should promote the conservation, use and improvement of traditional varieties, including those bred by public entities, such as the DoA.[95] Significantly, during the initial period of the PVR discourse the NGOs were regarded as a governing node. They had the necessary thinking power, processes, resources and support to mobilise the public against enacting the 2001 Bill. Mainly, the NGOs lobbied against the 2001 Bill rather than through public campaigns as in India. This suggests that the interpretive community in Sri Lanka was not aware or not fully informed about the 2001 Bill. These NGOs became powerful communicative actors because they were not only learning from each other but also simultaneously deploying multiple modes to communicate and disseminate about the PVR discourse.

For more than a decade later, there was little discourse on the PVR Bill among the local actors. The local reasons could be that during 2001–2009, Sri Lanka experienced a civil war, which put it into a vulnerable economic position locally and globally, and hence, it did not consider the implementation of national legislations, such as PVR, a priority. More importantly, the IP subsystem lacked a champion to push the PVR Bill. Another reason could be that farmers and environmentalists were against a PVR that lacked amendments to address their specific local needs.

Interestingly, there was no global pressure to implement the 2001 PVR Bill from the WTO or any other developed or developing county. A likely reason is that since agriculture is not modernised in Sri Lanka, productivity remains low, market and value addition activities are underdeveloped and the potential for niche commodities remains significant for the domestic and export markets.[96] Given the lack of robust investment and innovation in agribusinesses, there is no threat of the international community pushing Sri Lanka for PVR implementation.[97]

---

[95] Ibid.

[96] Ministry of Agriculture Sri Lanka (2018).

[97] Perera (2010) (n 94), p. 302.

During the 2001–2010 period, the NIPO and the DoA did convene several consultations with stakeholder groups, such as farming organisations, NGOs and environmental organisations, and eventually released a revised version of the PVR (2011 Bill). Compared with the PVR 2001 Bill, which adopts an ownership approach, this version of the Bill recognises certain privileges and safeguards for farmers, which supports a stewardship approach. For example, the 2011 Bill would permit farmers to 'save, use, sow, re-sow, exchange, share or sell [their] farm produce including [the seed of a protected variety]'.[98] Moreover, the 2011 Bill also would exempt farmers from penalties for the infringement of plant breeders' IPR under *certain* situations. For instance, farmers would not be considered to have infringed if they were not aware that a particular variety was protected as IP at the time of infringement.[99] Another key feature of the 2011 Bill is that it recognises the role of farmers in crop genetic diversity, namely, that of a farmer 'who conserves and preserves, severally or jointly, with any person any wild species or traditional varieties or adds value to such wild species or traditional varieties through selection and identification of their useful properties'.

The 2011 Bill defines 'farmer' as any individual who (1) grows crops by cultivating the land himself/herself; (2) oversees the cultivation of crops by another person; (3) is a 'tenant cultivator'; or (4) conserves and preserves—whether individually or collectively—any wild species or traditional variety, or adds value to these plants through the selection and identification of useful properties.[100] Furthermore, the revised Bill provides a definition of 'farmers' variety', which is conceptualised as a variety that has been 'traditionally cultivated and evolved by ... farmers in their fields' or that is a 'wild relative or landrace of a variety about which ... farmers possess the common knowledge'.[101]

Although these changes may be understood as improvements over the initial, 2001 Draft, notably, the proposed framework has been stalled since 2011. Part of the reason for this 'inertia' within government is that stakeholder groups, such as farmers' groups and NGOs, have continued to express concerns over the contents of the 2011 Bill. For instance, notwithstanding its expressed recognition of farmers and their varieties, the 2011 Bill fails to create an enabling environment to obtain legal rights over traditional varieties that come under FR.[102]

When the 2011 Bill was sent to the Parliament subcommittee for consideration, the subcommittee recommended that the DoA be the authority to deal with this Bill since its content is scientific and technical and the DoA has the relevant expertise to handle the drafting.[103] From this point onwards, the discourse on the PVR changed, and thus, the DoA became a governing node in the drafting process. The revised

---

[98] Bill on the Protection of Plant Varieties (Breeder's Rights) of Sri Lanka s 34(ii).

[99] Ibid ss 35(i)–(ii).

[100] Ibid s 4.

[101] Ibid.

[102] Perera and Adhikari (2019), p. 161.

[103] Interviewee # 30. The researcher does not possess a copy of the 2019 revised Bill for any further comment. The interviewee did not hint at any changes to the Bill.

PVR Bill has been submitted to the Ministry of Agriculture in 2019 for comments. If this Ministry is satisfied with the 2019 revision, the Bill will be submitted to the Parliament subcommittee for their recommendations and finally to the Legal Draftsman department to formally draft the Bill. However, there has been no public exposure on the 2019 revised Bill and under the conditions of the present global crisis, and Sri Lanka's own economic problems, it is doubtful that any necessary action will take place in the near future.[104]

Yet, remarkably, there has been no pragmatic pressure on the Government from the WTO, other countries, plant breeders or corporate farmers to implement the PVR Bill. A likely reason for this indulgence is that agricultural production in Sri Lanka is a considerably low-technology activity, and as a result, Sri Lanka is not considered a lucrative market by multinational seed corporations nor a threat to high-technology imports.[105] It might also be because of its civil war and other political difficulties; Sri Lanka has been afforded extra time to address its international obligations.

Hence, the practical position is that most Sri Lankan farmers, farmer organisations and FR activists support a stewardship approach because farmers are the backbone of Sri Lanka, who are the major seed providers for agriculture. They have rejected the ownership approach for Sri Lanka for this approach is focused on awarding IPR for farmers (and others, notably breeders).

4.6 Strategies to Realise Farmers' Rights

As discussed, neither the 2001 nor the 2011 PVR Bill of Sri Lanka adequately supported FR and agrobiodiversity conservation. In this chapter, three strategies are investigated:

1. What measures could be used to protect farmers' ability to access and use existing agrobiodiversity and innovations?
2. What incentives can be introduced to encourage farmers to sustain on-farm conservation and access to seed banks?
3. What type of reward system can be implemented to protect and register farmers' varieties without ownership?

4.7 Ownership Protection for Farmers' Varieties

Although farmers' varieties are not protected under the conventional PVR system, countries could create a sui generis plant variety protection system that would comply with the *TRIPS Agreement* and provide protection for these varieties. As stated above,

---

[104] Ibid.

[105] However, the local seed propagators from the private sector can obtain incentives by importation of foreign varieties.

countries such as India have used *TRIPS* flexibilities to provide such a system.[106] For example, by using an ownership approach, India allows its farmers to protect their traditional varieties under the PVR law provided they satisfy the NDUS criteria, meaning breeders and farmers are both equally eligible for IPR.

In contrast to the Sri Lankan PVR Bill, the *Indian Plant Act*[107] offers protection to three categories of varieties, namely, extant varieties,[108] farmers' varieties[109] and essentially derived varieties.[110] Clause 39 (1) (i) states that 'a farmer who has bred or developed a new variety shall be entitled to registration and other protection in like manner as a breeder of a variety under this Act'.[111] This implies that farmers are recognised as breeders and generally have the same rights as those guaranteed to public and private breeders. However, under the Sri Lankan Bill, farmers are not considered breeders, nor are rights given to traditional varieties.

Although the *Indian Plant Act* purports to protect farmers' varieties, s 15(2) says that the registration criteria are the same as for new plant varieties, such as the NDUS criteria of *UPOV 1991*. Farmers face difficulties to fulfil the NDUS criteria because their varieties lack a high level of genetic uniformity and stability. For the registration of farmers' varieties, the Indian criteria have been modified to require farmers to submit half the quantity of seed material required for a commercial variety, and the number of 'off types' cannot exceed double the number of off types specified for the new variety.[112] This modification does not resolve the underlying problem of the inadequacy of NDUS criteria for FR.

Similarly, the 2011 Bill of Sri Lanka does not create a separate category of protection for farmers' plant varieties. Ownership rights are linked only to the development of a new variety. Although it could be argued that farmers might apply for protection when they act as breeders of new varieties, for several reasons, this possibility is an insufficient means to advance their interests. First, the NDUS requirements are typically difficult for farmers to meet, thus rendering it difficult for them to obtain rights as breeders over traditionally cultivated or farmer-bred varieties. Specifically, it is unlikely that they could claim that their traditional varieties are novel, for these varieties typically have been sold 'or otherwise disposed of' for periods greater than one year prior to the date of application.[113]

---

[106] Rangnekar (2016) (n 35).

[107] *Protection of Plant Varieties and Farmer's Rights Act No 53 of 2001* ('*Indian Plant Act*').

[108] Ibid cl 2(j). Extant varieties refer to a variety available in India under the *Seed Act No 22 of 2003* ('*Seed Act*'), or farmers' variety or variety of common knowledge or any other variety that is in the public domain.

[109] Ibid cl 2(l). Farmers' variety refers to a variety that has been traditionally cultivated and evolved by the farmers in their fields, or is a wild relative or a land race of a variety about which the farmers possess common knowledge.

[110] Ibid cl 2(h)–(i). Essentially, derived variety includes a variety predominantly derived from a variety protected under the law.

[111] See ibid, cl 39.

[112] Government of India, *The Gazette of India: Extraordinary* (Part 11, Sect. 4.3, Sub Section (i) GSR 452 (E) June 30, 2009).

[113] Bill on the Protection of Plant Varieties (Breeder's Rights) of Sri Lanka s 10.

Furthermore, it would likely be challenging for Sri Lankan farmers to meet the criteria of uniformity and stability, because traditional varieties are often characterised by genetic heterogeneity. It is unlikely that these varieties could be understood as 'sufficiently uniform'[114] and that the essential characteristics of these varieties would 'remain unchanged after repeated propagation', one of their virtues being the continuing adaptation to local ecological variations·[115] Hence, within the Sri Lankan context, the criteria for the protection of farmers' varieties under the 2011 Bill become meaningless.

4.7.1 Protection from Biopiracy

The ownership approach could lead to unjust outcomes when farmers' varieties are used for plant breeding and development. For example, under the 2011 Bill, plant breeders may use farmers' varieties as source of germplasm, without any obligation to obtain prior informed consent from farmers. Likewise, the Bill does not require breeders to share any benefits that may result from the use of farmers' varieties with the providers of this source germplasm.

The 2011 Bill would require applicants for plant variety protection to declare that 'the genetic material or parent material was lawfully acquired for [the] breeding [of the new variety]'.[116] However, it does not explicitly state whether this provision would require applicants to seek prior informed consent or to conclude ABS agreements with the providers of the genetic or parent material used to develop the new variety. Given that the 2011 Bill does not contain any ABS language, and that there is no other legal regime in Sri Lanka to govern this subject matter, 'lawfully acquired' in this context will likely only be interpreted to mean not in violation of any private contract or criminal law. Thus, breeders of new plant varieties could exploit this ambiguity to appropriate farmers' varieties for use as parent material, without the need to fulfil any ABS obligations. It could be argued that the non-inclusion of a benefit-sharing provision was a negligent act by the drafters since this was one of the critical issues raised by the stakeholders against the 2001 Bill. Moreover, when the 2011 Bill requires applicants to make a declaration regarding how they acquired the material for breeding purposes, having a provision on prior informed consent is essential to implement this declaration. Hence, this could be regarded as a deliberate omission rather than a lack of knowledge or expertise of the drafters.

Hence, Sri Lankan lawmakers should be concerned about the potential appropriation of farmers' varieties. Evidence indicates that Sri Lanka is extremely vulnerable to biopiracy,[117] a concept that may be understood as the misappropriation or

[114] Ibid s 12.

[115] Ibid s 13.

[116] Ibid s 17.2(x).

[117] Amarasinghe (2018).

unauthorised exploitation of a country's national biodiversity.[118] One example is *Kotala-himbutu* (*Salacia reticulata*), which is a plant that is traditionally used in Sri Lanka for different health benefits, including to help control hyperglycaemia (high blood sugar).[119] As of 2020, numerous parties have already exploited this plant and, by 2006, this exploitation had resulted in 30 patents claiming different properties of *Kotala-himbutu* for different commercial purposes, without obtaining any prior informed consent from the providers of this plant and without executing any benefit-sharing agreement.[120] To minimise biopiracy, in 2006 the Sri Lankan Government banned the export of all *Kotala-himbutu* plant material and other related species, but this export ban did not go far enough.[121]

Instead, to mitigate the risk of biopiracy and the misappropriation of traditional plant varieties, Sri Lanka must incorporate ABS provisions into its 2011 Bill. In doing so, the country should follow the principles articulated in the 1992 *CBD* and the ensuing 2010 *Nagoya Protocol on Access to Genetic Resources and the Fair and Equitable Sharing of Benefits Arising from their Utilization.*[122] Sri Lanka is a Contracting Party to both of these treaties, and the Sri Lankan Government has expressed its commitment to implementing national rules to regulate the access and utilisation of genetic resources and associated traditional knowledge.

A Draft Legal Framework on the *Access to Biological Resources Law 2000* ('*Access Law*') was developed by Ministry of Forestry and Environment to develop a legal and institutional framework for regulating access to genetic resources for fair and equitable sharing of benefits.[123] Under the *Access Law*, access was proposed to be regulated by an 'inter-agency committee' that among other things is required to monitor any informed consent requirements from individual resource owners other than the state.[124] This was the first and the last effort to draft an access law, and as of 2020, this Draft was also part of the Sri Lankan legal lacunae in local lawmaking; the country has not yet created a system of fair and equitable benefit sharing.[125] However, access can be regulated in terms of the standard provisions in the *Fauna and Flora Protection Ordinance, No 2 of 1937* and the *Forest Ordinance, No 16 of 1907* but there are no provisions whereby benefits could accrue to resource owners other than the State, be they individuals or communities.[126]

---

[118] Robinson (2010).

[119] Li et al. (2008).

[120] Gunawardena (2006).

[121] Rodrigo (2013).

[122] Hirimuthugodage and Samaratunga (2016).

[123] Nanayakkara and The World Conservation Union (2000) (Consultant's Report No. 75243 L1, Biodiversity Secretariat of the Ministry of Forestry and Environment, Sri Lanka, July 2000). The text is not available at present but the *Access Law* has been cited in Law and Society Trust, *Our Common Heritage: Farmers Rights to Plant Genetic Resources in Sri Lanka* (Law and Society Trust Sri Lanka, 2007) 17 (*Our Common Heritage*).

[124] Law and Society Trust (2007), p. 30.

[125] See Perera and Adhikari (2019) (n 102).

[126] Law and Society Trust (2007) (n 124).

4.7.2 Enabling Farmers to Access and Use Existing Agrobiodiversity and Innovations

With the PVR law looming, the major concern has been the potential restrictions on farmers' ability to access and use innovations from farm-saved seeds of a protected variety. The right to save, use, exchange and even sell these seeds and propagating material continues to be on the basis of ownership and has been exercised by farming communities for generations. The introduction of PVR in Sri Lanka has now become a controversial issue within the debate. This right is generally known as 'farmers' privilege'. It operates within the framework of FR irrespective of the rights of others, which conflicts directly with the ownership objective of PVR.[127]

The concept of saving seeds is a customary and cultural practice, which is an important method by which farmers have traditionally selected and improved their own plant varieties.[128] The farmers not only kept seeds but also exchanged and shared crops freely with neighbours.[129] If the farmers are denied the right to share or perhaps to sell seeds, it would not only result in a substantial loss of income for them, but more importantly, it would displace them as one of the seed providers of the country. Most developing countries have incorporated provisions on the right to save seeds to continue this practice within a PVR *TRIPS*-compliant framework.[130] This incorporation will generally allow farmers to share seeds while restricting them from selling seeds commercially, for example, by running a business or selling seeds to a third party.

Seed-saving practices in recent times have given rise to seed activism, which encompasses all actions that oppose the enclosure of seeds and defend the individual and collective rights to seeds.[131] Seed activism appeals to broad constituencies because, as the basis of our food supply, the seed carries symbolic power, even for urban dwellers. However, the biggest challenge to seeds is that they lack commodification[132] because seeds defy the necessary criteria of property: excludability and divisibility.[133] Seeds are not a form of classic commodity with fixed embodiments because the neighbour is not excluded from enjoying the same benefits as the first owner.[134] In other words, the exclusionary premises for the extension of 'full liberal ownership' to seeds are weak.[135] However, seed commodification can be pursued

[127] Guneratne (2008) (n 29), p. 200.

[128] Sampath (2001). Varieties selected and improved by farmers are preserved by seed banks in Sri Lanka. See also Moonka and Mukherjee (2018).

[129] Phillips (2016). See also Montúfar and Ayala (2019).

[130] Correa (2000) (n 28), pp. 32–33.

[131] Peschard and Randeria (2021) (n 45).

[132] Chandra (2015).

[133] Kaushik (2006), p. 284.

[134] Chandra (2015) (n 132).

[135] Honore (1961), p. 107. Liberal ownership is the right to possess, the right to use, the right to manage, the right to income, the right to capital, the right to security, etc.

through two routes: the technological and the institutional or social routes.[136] Hence, within the context of agriculture, seed ownership has received a significant amount of attention in the PVR discourse.

Pottinger defined seed-saving practices as 'quiet activism' that encompass 'small, every day, embodied acts, often making and creating, that can be either implicitly or explicitly political in nature.'[137] These practices include, 'modest, quotidian acts of kindness, connection and creativity' that nonetheless 'critique, subvert and rework' dominant modes of production and consumption.[138] To indigenous farmers, seed saving represents a form of resistance mobilised through narratives of tradition, sovereignty, freedom and environmental protection.[139] Seed saving can also constitute an overtly political or militant form of activism in situations where the practice is criminalised.[140] In addition to quiet activism, numerous types of mobilisation have emerged, for example, the Global March against Monsanto, seed swaps and guerrilla gardeners.[141] These 'quiet activism' modes or militant acts are examples of how interpretive communities communicate with each other and build their shared epistemological assumptions on seed-saving practices. Moreover, since these communities use multiple discourse modes to communicate, it is important to understand which mode is dominant for seed saving.

The 2011 Sri Lankan PVR Bill has FR provisions. Some are ownership oriented—indeed, PBR-based rather than PVR-based ones.[142] Section 34(1) states that 'a farmer who has bred or discovered and developed new varieties shall be entitled to the registration and other protection in like manner as a breeder of a variety under this Act'. A farmer will be able to benefit from this section only if they breed a new variety. Unlike the *Indian Plant Act*, this section does not give any concessions for the registration of traditional varieties, which are the type of varieties that most farmers conserve and develop.

Other provisions are access oriented. Section 34(2) of the 2011 Bill states that 'a farmer shall be deemed to be entitled to save, use, sow, re-sow, exchange or share, sell his farm product, including a seed of a variety protected under this Act, in the same manner as he was entitled to before the coming into force of this Act'. Section 34(2) gives rights, to sell 'in the same manner as they were entitled before the Act', but since no rights to sell protected varieties exist before the Bill is enacted, it is in effect only giving rights to sell non-PVR seeds or traditional varieties. However, similarly to the *Indian Plant Act*, under s 34(2) of the 2011 Bill, farmers are prohibited from selling

[136] Chandra (2015) (n 134).

[137] Pottinger (2017), p. 215.

[138] Ibid.

[139] Garz'on and Escobar (2019).

[140] Ibid.

[141] Ibid. See also Peschard and Randeria (2020).

[142] PBR, which is the more high-technology ownership version, contrasts with PVR, which is the broader, more neutral category, possibly allowing protection of the traditional varieties, although still an ownership approach similar to those of India and Thailand. See Sect. 4.7 of this book on 'Ownership Protection for Farmer's Varieties'.

branded seeds[143] of a protected variety, although under s 35(1) they are immune from infringement action if at the time of the infringement they were not aware of the existence of the right so infringed. Furthermore, s 25(a) states that the breeder's rights shall not extend to 'acts done privately and for non-commercial use', thus providing additional limitations to breeders' rights.[144] Yet, still, a main reason for the stakeholders' criticism of the FR provision in the 2011 Bill is its ownership-oriented structure.

4.7.3 Registration of Farmers' Varieties

The registration of farmers' varieties generally follows the ownership approach, when it could be crafted to support the stewardship approach. The following section examines the different approaches to seed registration in developing countries[145] and compares these with Sri Lanka's approach.

The original objective of variety registration was ensuring transparency in the market, enforcing quality control, providing information to farmers and increasing agricultural production.[146] Countries have the flexibility to use either the mandatory or voluntary variety registration but need to balance the different policy objectives under the overall goal of promoting agricultural growth. Mandatory registration implies that a plant variety cannot be sold unless it has been registered in a national register of varieties. It will allow farmers to view the seed tag and know it is a quality-controlled seed.

Documenting the existence of these varieties shows that such varieties are not new, thereby preventing third parties from claiming these varieties in applications for patents or PVR. Moreover, information contained in plant variety registers provides the interested parties details about those with whom they must share benefits if they generate income through the use of the registered variety.[147]

In contrast, in voluntary registration there is an obligation to print the quality parameters in the label, but this requirement is not compulsory. Hence, this system provides reduced transparency in naming the varieties.[148] However, the advantage of voluntary registration is that a large array of varieties may be allowed in the seed market, which provides an enormous opportunity to develop commercial markets for both farmers' varieties and imported seeds.[149] Different countries have varied farming and seed systems and obviously will adopt different solutions. Regardless,

---

143 Branded seed means any seed put in a package or any other container and labelled in a manner indicating that such seed is of a variety protected under the PVR law.

144 Anver (2016).

145 Louwaars and Burgaud (2016), p. 184.

146 Ibid.

147 Noriega (2016), p. 213.

148 Louwaars and Burgaud (2016) (n 145).

149 Ibid.

according to the system the countries have ratified in the *CBD* and FAO Treaty, they have a responsibility to promote the treaty obligations.[150]

Seed regulations negatively affect the registration of farmers' varieties by imposing NDUS criteria for plant breeding and industrial agriculture commercial 'value for cultivation and use' criteria, for two reasons.[151] First, since farmers' varieties are not normally genetically homogeneous enough to meet the NDUS requirements for approval and certification for commercial sale, they are excluded from the market and gradually disappear from active commercial use.[152] Second, farmers' varieties must fulfil the value for cultivation and use criteria based on the use of chemical fertilisers, herbicides and pesticides. These varieties do not fulfil either of these criteria because they are genetically unstable.[153] Therefore, such varieties are no longer considered to be seeds, but instead are conceptualised as grains. Many seed laws prohibit all other exchange and sale of grains, since grains are unregistered seeds.[154] As a result, farmers' movements and organisations have struggled for many years to amend laws that discriminate against traditional seeds. For example, small farmers and their allies in Brazil have fought and obtained a provision that recognises local, traditional varieties.[155]

In 2003, the Sri Lankan Government, with the recommendation of the Ministry of Agriculture, enacted the *Seed Act* to regulate the quality of seed and planting material and to safeguard farmers as well as seed handlers, distributors and users from malpractices that would harm the country's seed industry.[156] Although the Act was passed in in 2003, it came into practice only in 2008, another legal lacuna.

The *Seed Act* has features to regulate the quality of seed and planting materials supplied to farmers and distributed by seed handlers[157] under the Act.[158] It has established a National Seed Council with wide powers to regulate policies regarding seed distribution, quality, supply and import; the registration of seed handlers; and the Establishment of a Seed Certification Service to monitor the certification standards of seeds.[159] To date, about 1,926 seed handlers have been registered under this Act.[160] The National Council is also meant to take appropriate action to protect new plant varieties under s 6(h) of the *Seed Act* but this Act does not contain provisions on mandatory variety registration. The above discussion on seed regulation demonstrates how the lawmaking process is dominated by the local political process in Sri Lanka.

---

150 Ibid.

151 See Peschard and Randeria (2020) (n 141), p. 11.

152 Ibid.

153 Ibid.

154 Ibid.

155 Ibid.

156 Hirimuthugoda (2014).

157 *Seed Act* s 22. Seed handler means any person who is a producer, importer, distributor or co-ordinator.

158 Ibid s 5.

159 Ibid.

160 Hirimuthugoda (2014) (n 156).

The 2011 Bill did provide an adequate system of variety registration.[161] Part 3 of the Bill mandates the DG of NIPO to establish and maintain a register, known as the Register of New Plant Varieties, in which all the qualified new plant varieties should be recorded. Such records should include, inter alia, the name of each registered new plant variety; the name and address of the rights holder; the name and address of the agents of the rights holder, if any; dates of application and registration; and the date of priority, if applicable.[162] The draft also provides for the creation of a registry called the National Registry of New Plant Varieties. This is to be located at the Plant Genetic Resources Centre. This Registry will be under the administration and supervision of the DG, Agriculture, and will exist for the collection and maintenance of information on extant varieties and the reception and maintenance of technical data and samples of new plant varieties. The head of the Plant Genetic Resource Centre shall act as the Registrar of the Registry of New Plant Varieties as directed and supervised by the DG, Agriculture.[163] The National Registry of New Plant Varieties is also to have a panel of experts chaired by the DG, Agriculture, to facilitate the implementation of the provisions of this Act. Apart from the DG, Agriculture, and NIPO, the panel includes the directors of research institutes operating in Sri Lanka.[164]

Mandatory variety registration is rejected in a growing number of countries. For example, in India, activists organised a campaign to stop a 2004 Seed Bill being enacted that required such registration.[165] As a result, the *Indian Plant Act* does not have mandatory seed registration. It contains a section on registration but the purpose of registration in this Act is to prevent farmers' varieties from being privately appropriated without compensation. However, in practice, it is a difficult to ascertain whether such varieties have been used in the development of a commercial variety because identifying landraces from which these varieties are derived is a cumbersome procedure.[166]

As a result, the registration of farmers' varieties has not resulted in a single benefit-sharing mechanism because no breeder or a company has disclosed the use of a farmer variety under the Act. Moreover, due to the wording of the Act, it provides few other opportunities for benefit sharing. For example, the Act says that farmers are entitled to benefit from the government-funded Gene Fund if they engage 'in the conservation of PGR of land races and wild relatives of economic plants'.[167] To be eligible, a farmer breeder must disclose that a tribal or rural family involved

[161] According to the Bill, 'variety' means a plant grouping within a single botanical taxon of the lowest known rank, which grouping, irrespective of whether the conditions for the grant of a registration under this Act are fully met, can be (i) defined by the expression of the characteristics resulting from a given genotype or combination of genotypes; (ii) distinguished from any other plant grouping by the expression of at least one of the said characteristics; and (iii) considered a unit with regard to its suitability for being propagated, which remains unchanged after such propagation.

[162] Bill on the Protection of Plant Varieties (Breeder's Rights) (Sri Lanka) s 6.

[163] Ibid s 7.

[164] Ibid s 8. Kamardeen (2013), pp. 50, 53.

[165] Mulleriyawa (2016).

[166] Ibid.

[167] Peschard (2016) (n 40).

in the breeding or development of such a variety has conserved the use of genetic material.[168] In practice, if farmers develop a variety by selecting and breeding a public sector variety, as in the case of Khobragade,[169] they are not entitled to benefit sharing.[170]

The Indian experience on the registration of farmers' varieties amply suggests that a registration system is only a defensive strategy to realise FR. As Peschard argued, 'the fact that farmers' varieties are being registered under the Act is not in itself an indicator or a guarantee of realisation of FR'.[171] According to the number of applications received and registration certificates issued yearly for farmers' varieties, farmers individually have made clear progress annually in India.[172] As regards implementation of the Act, farmers have an unequal status to realise FR, because the *Indian Plant Act* only provides IPR for farmers in the same manner as breeders. This is a common weakness of the ownership approach.

Moreover, in 2013, since the government felt there were discrepancies in the current *Seed Act* 2003, a new Seed Bill was introduced by the DG, Agriculture, in Sri Lanka as the Seed and Planting Material Act No.—of 2013 (hereinafter referred to as the 'Newest Seed Bill'). However, the Newest Seed Bill has not yet been enacted. One purpose of introducing this Bill was to address the interest of consumers because with more commercial involvement in seed production and marketing, there have been reports across Sri Lanka about substandard seeds being distributed to farmers.[173]

The Newest Seed Bill has the following controversial provisions that affect FR:[174]

- the mandatory variety registration of farmers and the certification of seed and planting material in Sri Lanka by Seed Certification Service;
- the maintenance and publishing of a list of producers and suppliers of certified seeds, by the DoA;
- the enforcement provisions that enable officials to raid farms in search of illegal seeds;
- the penalty provisions of imprisonment of not less than one month and not exceeding six months, or a fine not less than 50,000 rupees, or both; and
- the centralising of authority over seed-related activity to the DoA. Activists fear that it could edge out small farmers who have historically protected and improved plant crop varieties.

---

[168] Ibid.

[169] By collecting seeds and replanting them year on year, Dadji Ramji Khobragade developed a new rice variety that became popular throughout the region. Khobragade was happy to share his seeds with farmers from other villages. However, when university researchers took his seeds to conduct experiments, and four years later released an improved variety, they did not credit Khobragade. Furthermore, under a law governing intellectual property and plant varieties, Khobragade was not entitled to any share of the profits from the sale of this new variety.

[170] Bavadam (2011).

[171] Peschard (2016) (n 167).

[172] Agrawal (2017).

[173] Ibid.

[174] Mulleriyawa (2016) (n 165).

Seed certification in the Newest Seed Bill promotes an ownership approach on the basis of concepts from the *Indian Plant Act* because it supports mandatory registration. FR proponents have proposed that the legal requirement for registration should be accommodated within the variety registration system by adopting 'looser' identifiability criteria for the commercial marketing of farmers' varieties to realise FR.[175] Through this system, the unequal status faced by farmers in the registration of farmers' varieties could be minimised. Hence, the modification of the existing variety registration system will be a crucial prerequisite to the realisation of FR in Sri Lanka.[176]

4.8 Reward System for Farmers' Stewardship

In Sri Lanka, farmers can obtain direct and indirect benefits from the use and conservation of PGR. The development of varieties that have high yields; increased resistance to pests, diseases and environmental stresses; and better quality are some direct benefits. Increased average yield and farmer income are major indirect benefits.[177] However, in Sri Lanka at present, 90% of farmers are recipients of poverty alleviation subsides,[178] which are similar to social security cash transfers, but there is no direct benefit-sharing system to reward them for utilising their PGR. Rewarding them supports the stewardship approach, which is recognised under the customary law in Sri Lanka.

4.8.1 Recognition of Customary Law

The agricultural management system in Sri Lanka is a community-based system that has roots in customary law.[179] Rice growing serves as a good example. Water is vital to rice growing. According to ER Leach, the small tank system in Sri Lanka was developed and managed by local communities collectively from the third and fourth century onwards.[180] In the early days of British administration, village-level administration was carried out under the responsibility of a headman[181] and, later, the

[175] Srinivasan (2016), p. 252. This criterion is not based on the NDUS criteria but through the person 'skilled of art'. Farmers could be able to identify varieties in their fields, even such varieties that are unstable.

[176] Ibid.

[177] Department of Agriculture Sri Lanka (2008).

[178] Gunawardene (2010).

[179] Abeywardana et al. (2019) (n 79).

[180] Leach (1959).

[181] Karunanada (2006).

British formalised the position under the village committee system.[182] The headman system helped to conduct irrigation as a collective effort by the whole village. The village obeyed the verbal orders of the headman.[183]

After independence, rapid changes occurred within the agricultural management system. Cultivation Committees were first introduced and later the farmer organisation approach was introduced. *The Agrarian Services Act No. 4 of 1991* legitimised farmer organisations.[184] The rationale behind this community-based system is to give farmers the leadership to take part in agricultural management in a participatory manner, supervised by the officers of the Agrarian Services Department together with the farmer organisation.[185]

In several instances in Sri Lanka, this community-based system has been used in practice to realise FR. The first example relates to rice paddy cultivation, paddy management, soil conservation, plant protection, fertilisation and pesticide control techniques, which farmers undertook as a collective group.[186] Moreover, farmers in Sri Lanka were known to not only share crop varieties, but also help each other collectively, in preparing the land, sowing seeds, maintaining the crop, harvesting and taking measures against pests and diseases when necessary.[187] Furthermore, *chena*-style cultivation (involving slash/burn techniques) was conducted as a collective farming method because the various chena cultivation processes involve cleaning the ground by cutting and burning the debris of existing vegetation in a collective manner.[188]

To return to the topic of water management, in addition to cultivation techniques, a few routines or rituals were identified as part of the irrigation landscape in the Dry Zone and most of these rituals were conducted as collective efforts led by the village elders, astrologers and temple priests.[189] Farmer organisations initiate these rituals. Furthermore, decisions on matters related to irrigation agriculture are taken collectively. Government officials consult and provide recommendations, while decisions are taken by farmers' vote, for which a two-thirds majority of the votes are required.[190] In general, decisions on the irrigation water and the type of seeds to be used, the cultivation period, the fertiliser benefits and the loan schemes for farmers are taken at seasonal meetings by farmers collectively.[191]

The second example relates to the collective agricultural wisdom of farmers in Sri Lanka in the areas of water collection, conservation and irrigation practices. The water management system introduced in ancient Sri Lanka continues to equal the

[182] Ibid.

[183] Abeywardana et al. (2019) (n 179).

[184] Ibid.

[185] Ibid.

[186] Ibid.

[187] Gunawardena (2000a, b).

[188] Abeywardana et al. (2019) (n 183).

[189] Ibid.

[190] Ibid.

[191] Ibid.

achievements of modern science. The system collects rainwater in an elaborate series of tanks and reservoirs known as 'the Cascade system' which is then used to irrigate fields in the Dry Zone.[192] According to FAO, this ancient initiative aims to protect and promote valuable agricultural heritage and preserve biodiversity and traditional knowledge to create resilient ecosystems, which fall within the realm of FR.[193]

A third example relates to realising the adaptation[194] capacity of farming communities in coastal Sri Lanka. This research has indicated that community-based adaptation activities have the capacity to reintroduce traditional rice varieties to restore yields—varieties that were neglected by formal research institutes—following the failure of fertiliser-dependent hybrid varieties.[195] The research also found farming organisations in each village acted as the decision-making forum for issues such as the farming calendar, water distribution and seed selection. This history illustrates the collective nature of farming communities extending their support to other farmer groups in the learning process.[196]

As will be illustrated later in this chapter, the number of campaigns conducted regarding the Sri Lankan PVR Bill and the Newest Seed Bill are examples of the collective rights of farmers attempting to block laws that they consider detrimental to their interests.

Within the Sri Lankan context, these examples illustrate collective community rights, which are a bundle of rights known as 'traditional resource rights'.[197] Scholars have identified these rights as cultural rights based on the collective cultural property of communities.[198] Traditional resource rights permit and empower farmers to carry on traditional cultivation-related practices for generations. They are examples of the stewardship approach, which provides an existing foundation for the conceptual framework for the realisation of FR in Sri Lanka.

For instance, certain aspects of FR are recognised and articulated under the *Irrigation Ordinance Act No 32 of 1946* and the *Land Development Ordinance Act No. 19 of 1935*, a subordinate legislative function that provides for the recognition of custom as a source of law.[199] For example, in irrigation, agriculture and fisheries, custom appears to have been recognised by law to a limited extent, and becomes part of the national legal discourse.[200] However, informal customs and traditions relating to irrigation and cultivation are still widely practised in Sri Lanka but some concepts do not have a parallel in its common law, which is the Roman–Dutch law.[201]

---

192 News First (2019) (n 80).

193 Ibid.

194 Adaptation here refers to the process through which farming communities adjust to the effects of climate change.

195 Ensor and Weragoda (2009).

196 Ibid.

197 Nanayakkara (2007), p. 48.

198 Coombe (2017), p. 373.

199 Nanayakkara (2007) (n 197), p. 25.

200 *Irrigation Ordinance No 32 of 1946* ss 23, 96; *Agrarian Development Act No 46 of 2011*s 87.

201 *Haramanis v Amarasekera*, 16 NLR 207.

Although custom serves as an informal source of law in Sri Lanka, the examination of case law has indicated that there has been no widespread recognition of custom and nor has written law modified customs.[202] These traditional resource rights could lead to conflicts if the governments fail to engage in consultations with farmers prior to implementing national laws that affect them.[203] Sri Lankan policymakers need to be mindful about these issues and the character of the customary discourse.

4.8.2 Positive Rewards

The reward system and benefit sharing go hand in hand. Benefit sharing for food security and environmental sustainability results in compensating and rewarding farmers for their contributions, which is an important element of stewardship. To achieve these goals, the 2011 PVR Bill should be revised, or some other legislation such as the *Fauna and Flora Ordinance* should be added in a way that would create an enabling environment for the Sri Lankan Government's breeding and extension institutions and the domestic private sector to collaborate with local farmers. This could take the form of, for example, varietal development research and participatory breeding and conservation programs that focus on the use and improvement of traditional varieties for commercial cultivation.

Furthermore, the prospective Sri Lankan IPR system for plant varieties should recognise and reward farmers as innovators and the conservators and cultivators of traditionally cultivated plant varieties. This could be achieved through strategies similar to those implemented in India, for instance, by creating a system of awards or grants to recognise individual farmers and communities as 'plant genome saviours'.[204] Evidence from other countries suggests that farmers would be motivated to conserve and develop traditional varieties, including crop wild relatives, if they were able to obtain economic incentives and social or legal recognition for their contributions.[205] However, under the *Indian Plant Act*, the reward is for only those farmer varieties that have some economic value for breeders based on further development by breeders. Hence, some have argued that giving awards to farmers results in the privatisation of PGR and undermines the purpose of FR.[206]

Some countries have introduced schemes designed to reward farmers for improvements in farmland biodiversity.[207] Australia has a program related to environmental management for improving biodiversity and particularly for sequestering carbon.[208]

---

[202] Nanayakkara (2007) (n 199).

[203] Rodríguez-Garavito (2011) (n 81).

[204] This scheme is criticised because such awards are given only for farmers' varieties that have economic value.

[205] Perera and Adhikari (2019) (n 125).

[206] Peschard (2016) (n 171).

[207] Ibid.

[208] Ibid.

These 'innovative farmer-led programs' acknowledge the important role of farmers as stewards of biodiversity and environmental sustainability, styled in economic terms as ecological services.[209] For instance, plant breeders involved in the Participatory Plant Breeding initiative in South West China have a system to enter into contractual agreements with the farmers they are working with to reward them for conserving the landraces and share the benefits they derive with the farmers.[210] The Green Box subsidies of the EU's Common Agricultural Policy are another example of government-funded subsidies for farmers, provided they do not distort production or trade, or at most, cause minimal distortions.[211]

Reward systems properly fit within the stewardship approach to FR. Namely, a reward system generates income for farmers' contributions towards the conservation of local ecosystems, and in contrast, it reduces the likelihood that agricultural businesses will misappropriate local genetic resources without giving fair consideration and compensation.

4.8.3 Providing Incentives for On-Farm Conservation and Access to Seed Banks

As noted above, farmers' contribution to on-farm conservation and the sustainable use of food and agriculture comes within stewardship; it is recognised by FAO and is in harmony with the *CBD*.[212] In Sri Lanka, traditional varieties bred by farmers are important for both increasing agricultural production and maintaining sustainable ecosystems. However, the genetic erosion of cultivated traditional varieties and wild relatives of crop plant species in Sri Lanka has been occurring rapidly in natural habitats over the years. This is the result of neglect, and thus far, it is not the result of competition from high-technology plant breeds, such as genetically modified organisms and other high-yielding varieties within local farming or within food imports. However, that competition may arise.

To provide incentives to farmers and the farming community and to strengthen on-farm management, several 'on-farm conservation' programs have been implemented in Sri Lanka.[213] The national herbarium at the Royal Botanical Gardens in Peradeniya and the herbariums in Hakgala and Gampaha have a large collection of about 132,000 plant specimens. By using the information collected by the Plant Genetic Resource Centre, an atlas of 35 maps identifying the collection sites of 46 traditional crop species has been published, thus developing an inventory and databases for locally adapted varieties.

---

[209] Godden (2009), p. 807.

[210] Song et al. (2016).

[211] Banga (2014).

[212] Perera (2011) (n 97).

[213] Department of Agriculture Sri Lanka (2008) (n 177), p. 45.

On-farm conservation programs and about 1.3 million home gardens in different agro-ecological zones also play important roles in in situ conservation of plant genetic resources for food and agriculture.[214] Moreover, to help farmers develop and improve their varieties, the establishment of on-farm conservation centres for traditional varieties, the promotion of on-farm seed production from seed banks, the establishment of seed exchange mechanisms and the compilation of traditional knowledge, and of information on the cultural and traditional farming system of the country is under way.[215] Hence, on-farm conservation of PGR is a stewardship initiative that provides farmers with incentives to accomplish the maintenance of PGR in a sustainable manner under the FR concept.[216]

On the issue of ex situ conservation as a global initiative, member states of the South Asian Association for Regional Cooperation ('SAARC'), comprising Afghanistan, Bangladesh, Bhutan, India, the Maldives, Nepal, Pakistan and Sri Lanka signed the agreement establishing the SAARC *Seed Bank Agreement* and the *Framework of Material Transfer Agreement* at the 17th SAARC Summit held in November 2011.[217] The objective of this Agreement is to recognise 'the importance of regional and sub-regional collective self-reliance in agriculture with respect to attaining seed security as a means of food security'.[218] In this global discourse, the policy attention of the SAARC governments is to address the competing discourses, that is, the concern about the expansion of the global IP on plants and its effects on the traditional seed system, and limit, among others, FR to save, use, exchange and sell seeds to meet the ends of farmers. Hence, the operationalisation of the Agreement should focus on balancing these competing discourses.

Locally, Sri Lanka has a system in place for ex situ conservation, which provides an incentive for farmers. Ex situ conservation of the PGR of various crop species in Sri Lanka is performed by several organisations, while the Plant Genetic Resource Centre is the focal point of national programs on ex situ conservation. Seed gene banks is an example of the ex situ conservation method. In Sri Lanka, there are about 15–500 accessions recorded in ex situ conservation centres and the Plant Genetic Resource Centre's seed gene bank has about 10,000 accessions. These include rice-related species, grain legumes, vegetables and oil crops. Field gene banks of several organisations also operate as effective ex situ conservation programs.[219] Hence, community seed gene banks can be effective platforms to ensure that landraces are preserved for future usage, especially for seed improvement processes, such as participatory plant breeding.

---

[214] Ibid.

[215] Ibid.

[216] Vernooy et al. (2020).

[217] Adhikari (2012). Also see, *Agreement on SAARC Seed Bank Agreement* and the *Framework of Material Transfer Agreement* (signed on 11 November 2011). https://www.saarc-sec.org/index.php/resources/agreements-conventions/33-agreement-on-establishing-the-saarc-seed-bank/file.

[218] SAARC *Seed Bank Agreement* art 1.

[219] See Vernooy et al. (2020) (n 216).

To alleviate the economic and food security pressures within civil-war-affected communities in Sri Lanka, Responsible Research, and Innovation has developed a community-managed seed bank to implement home garden systems, and under this project, has taught organic cultivation techniques; promoted ecologically appropriate design ideas, such as live fencing; and resorted to traditional water catchment systems.[220]

As discussed earlier, the maintenance of seed banks in Sri Lanka has shown progress;[221] however, currently there is no legislation to regulate the access to, or the utilisation of, resources. FAO says it is important to have an efficient, effective system to regulate the access to genetic resources and to ensure fair and equitable sharing of benefits arising from the use of these resources.[222] Article 8 of the *FAO Treaty* states that Contracting Parties to the Treaty are required to provide technical assistance, especially to those that are developing countries, for facilitating the implementation of the Treaty. This suggests that while the Treaty provides the Framework, it is the Contracting Parties who provide technical assistance to each other.

4.8.4 Non-ownership Commercialisation of Farmers' Varieties

As stated earlier, the conservation and development of traditional varieties adapted to local conditions by farming communities in Sri Lanka maintain the discourse on stewardship. However, these farmers' varieties are seldom part of the mainstream organised commerce in seeds because transactions in the seeds of these varieties are highly localised and restricted to informal exchanges between farmers, which provide few economic benefits for communities that conserve and develop these varieties.[223] If larger markets could be established for these varieties and their seeds handled in commercial quantities, and if these varieties could be commercially marketed, incentives would be provided for continued conservation and adaptation of varieties by farmers. Hence, the rationale for the commercialisation of farmers' varieties would be to provide self-sustaining market-based incentives for farmers' conservation efforts.[224]

The most important obstacle to the commercialisation of farmers' varieties in developing countries, including Sri Lanka, is the seed regulatory system that excludes these varieties from organised seed sector activities, including marketing. This is neglected in the lawmaking process to date.[225] As discussed above, through quality

[220] International Analog Forestry Network (2014).

[221] Sri Lanka has signed a Memorandum of Understanding with India and Pakistan to exchange germplasm.

[222] Department of Agriculture Sri Lanka (2008) (n 213).

[223] Srinivasan (2016) (n 175).

[224] Ibid. See also Sect. 4.8.

[225] See Sect. 4.7.3.

control requirements, the *Seed Act* system not only regulates the physical quality of seeds sold to farmers, but also the varietal identity of the seeds they purchase.[226] For example, s 14 of the *Seed Act 2003* highlights the certification monopoly of the Seed Certification Service, which includes monitoring the production and processing of seeds and reviewing their quality to ascertain their suitability. Most farmers' varieties do not satisfy this quality control system, and hence, such varieties are categorised as unregulated varieties. Thus, these seeds may not be marketed. Given that Sri Lanka still does not have a PVR law, at present, the commercialisation of seeds is regulated under the *Seed Act* 2003. The 2011 PVR Bill does not mention the commercialisation aspect, and hence, it could be argued that the *Seed Act* can be considered a de facto PVR law.

Owing to the quality control requirements of the *Seed Act 2003*, farmers are obliged to compete with the industrial model of production to market the seeds of the local plant varieties. Hence, it is recommended that an alternative certification mark system or fair-trading provision be introduced to enable such local farmers' products to obtain a good price. Certification and accreditation systems are not wholly dependent on government uptake. Civil society groups have come forward to fill the gap with a private standard setting. Sri Lanka has a product certification mark system managed by the Sri Lanka Standards Institution, which is commonly known as SLS Marks.[227] It denotes that the product has been manufactured in conformity with the relevant Sri Lanka Standard Specification. By implementing the SLS Marks scheme for seeds, manufacturers and consumers will both reap benefits. The latter will benefit by being able to identify a quality product from the appearance of this Mark. The former will benefit by being able to convince their customers that they consistently manufacture quality products, since they face competition not only from high-technology varieties but also from substandard and even counterfeit products in the market.

The Oxfam Fair Trade program is another example of an NGO system to support local producers. Oxfam purchases products directly from producers who meet the standards of a fair-trading certificate. It also supports the social and economic development of the entire community by paying the minimum fair-trade price and a premium price for a range of products.[228] Moreover, as in the case of quinoa, when a local product becomes popular, large companies begin producing it and, as a result, local farmers are marginalised.[229] Hence, a product certification mark system could be introduced to commercialise farmers' local varieties in order to find a niche market for their products.

---

226 Ibid.

227 Federation of Chambers of Commerce and Industry of Sri Lanka (2020).

228 OXFAM (2022).

229 The Economist (2021). See also Philpott (2013). See also Berson (2014).

4.9 Impact of Stakeholder Alliances in Sri Lanka

Thus, which discourse is prevailing? The PVR discourse has resulted in the rise of many stakeholder alliances in Sri Lanka. These alliances had competing discourses about the impact of implementing a PVR Act in Sri Lanka. From the first draft onwards, one group of stakeholders, including farmers' groups, environmentalists, grassroot farmers, NGOs, activists, and civil society, has criticised the Bill, claiming possible implications that the PVR Bill could have for smallholder farmers and traditional agriculture systems. They argue that the Bill does not address the local needs of the Sri Lankan agricultural economy, such as not recognising farmers' privilege and the inability to protect the country's traditional varieties.[230]

The other concerns were the impact of PVR on the relative positions of the public centre research capabilities and the private sector research agenda. Before the enactment of PBR, countries such as the US and Australia had concerns over shifting the research priorities of public research institutions.[231] The increased prominence of private companies in the seed sector could cause public institutes to back out of developing and conserving finished varieties and to concentrate on a more facilitating role in breeding, shifting towards basic research.[232] Given the relatively low level of innovation in agriculture in Sri Lanka, this group fears that the creation of PVR would permit new plant varieties to be owned and registered, and literally 'open up a space' that would be invaded by foreign applicants, who would then stifle local competition, which is in any case in its infancy.[233] If this were to happen, one of the objectives of the Act, which is 'to encourage the development of new plant varieties', would be self-defeating.[234]

In contrast, local industry representatives, such as seed exporters and seed regulators, have expressed support for the exclusive exploitation rights that the PVR Bill would grant to plant breeders[235] Their view was PVR may induce a shift towards applied research. PVR could lead to a reallocation of resources in the sense that public breeders, trying to maximise royalty income, may give a higher priority to the breeding of commercial crops than to basic research and the breeding of crops for marginal areas.[236] Hence, it is important to see how the government policy-makers reconcile these competing discourses before finalising the Bill. At present, the Government's position remains uncertain.

Moreover, further stakeholder motivation was seen when the Newest Seed Bill was introduced in 2013. This Bill has also been criticised by interest groups, including environmental activists, scientists, grassroot farmer organisations, the Movement for National Land and Agricultural Reform and concerned citizens. They say this

[230] Perera (2021) (n 10).

[231] Jaffe and Wijk (1995).

[232] Ibid.

[233] Kamardeen (2013) (n 164), p. 51.

[234] Ibid.

[235] Jaffe and Wijk (1995) (n 231).

[236] Ibid.

Bill would benefit the seed industry, controlled by big transnational corporations, at the expense of the country's small-scale farmers who are the mainstay of the rural economy.[237] According to these parties, the present *Seed Act* 2003 provides adequate law to safeguard the farmer community, to prevent illegal imports and exports of seeds and to protect indigenous paddy varieties.[238]

As a mark of protest, more than 700 organisations working for the rights of farmers and agricultural workers, and people supporting food sovereignty[239] and land reforms have held marches in different cities, mass protests and community theatre presentations in order to convey to the public what they are struggling to protect and defend.[240] Moreover, the alliance known as the National Movement to Protect Seed Rights is currently campaigning against the adoption of the Newest Seed Bill 2013 through an online petition, 'Stop Proposed Seed Bill in Sri Lanka'.[241] Vandana Shiva, a prominent Indian environmental activist and seed rights campaigner, commented that the Newest Seed Bill is designed for the transnational seed industry, which by promoting uniformity, destroys indigenous biodiversity, and by promoting its rights, undermines FR.[242]

In contrast, proponents of the Newest Seed Bill, such as seed importers and private sector seed producers and distributors, argue that this Bill has been introduced in the Parliament to narrow the gaps in the present system. It will build a proper system whereby only registered producers can supply seeds, to ensure seed quality and to generate higher productivity and yields. Presently, only 20–25% of seeds and planting material are from registered producers and 75% are from unregistered sources, which, they argue, results in farmers receiving substandard seeds.[243] Most new seeds are imported into Sri Lanka.[244]

However, farmers argue that this is not a main concern for them because, at the village level, they purchase seeds locally and from reliable sources whom they can trust. They also argue the issue of bad quality seeds in the market is a weapon for corporate farmers in Sri Lanka and for seed sellers who want to safeguard not only their seed monopolies but other 'planting material' monopolies, which are substitutes, for instance, for green manure made by farmers, in favour of the companies who produce synthetic inputs. According to these parties, the present *Seed Act* already provides adequate law to safeguard the farmer community, to prevent illegal imports and exports of seeds and to protect indigenous paddy varieties.[245]

---

237 Kannangara (2014).

238 Ibid.

239 The researcher acknowledges that food sovereignty is an issue in FR, but it is not the focus of this research.

240 La Via Campesina (2015). See also La Via Campesina (2014).

241 Environmental Justice Organisation (2016).

242 Kurukulasuriya (2014).

243 Warushamana (2014).

244 Hirimuthugoda (2014) (n 160).

245 Kurukulasuriya (2014) (n 242).

Moreover, the Movement for National Land and Agricultural Reform has stated that to ensure the conservation of PGR, the Technical and Advisory Committee to be established under the new Act has no representatives from the farming community nor any biodiversity experts.[246] It is important to include them because the Bill directly affects them. This demonstrates policymakers have violated the core principle of the *FAO Treaty* by not considering farmer participation and consultation in the lawmaking process regarding FR. This further demonstrates the lack of receptivity by the government to the discourse to realise FR in Sri Lanka. However, the former Minister of Agriculture has said the Newest Seed Bill would not be implemented without the consent of all sections of society and that it is a national duty to amend the existing *Seed Act* to protect farmer communities.[247]

Notably, these groups/organisations acting as governance/governing nodes have used multiple discourse modes to communicate their dislike regarding the Newest Seed Bill and these types of protests, marches and publications show how communities communicate with each other and build their shared epistemological assumptions against the Newest Seed Bill. In contrast, since there are competing high-technology discourses regarding the PVR Bill and the Newest Seed Bill, the government is in a quandary about these concerns.

4.9.1 Way Forward for Sri Lanka

The 2011 PVR Bill was an improvement over the 2001 PVR Bill for it acknowledged FR to some extent. Nevertheless, it is argued that the failure to enact any PVR legislation is better for farmers. National interests prevail. As long as Sri Lanka does not implement PVR, the discourse on FR will not become a political concern, but conflict remains a prospect because policymakers have become a pragmatic obstacle by overlooking the inherent features of the agricultural economy of Sri Lanka when drafting the 2001 and 2011 PVR Bills.[248] In other words, these policymakers as a governing node were unable to influence the government to consider the social needs of Sri Lanka, other than a position of no PVRs at all, which is perhaps not tenable in the longer term.

This was also evident when the Newest Seed Bill was introduced. Farmers and stakeholders mobilised to stop this Bill since it tried to introduce mandatory seed registration and raid farmers in search of illegal seeds. As indicated, these types of communicative acts are overtly political or militant. By using this defensive mode of discourses, farmers seek seed sovereignty and legal space to continue their customary farming practices and commercialise their traditional varieties to improve their livelihood. Policymakers should not overlook these types of communicative acts because, the evidence shows, these acts too have a regulatory function.

[246] Ibid.

[247] Kurukulasuriya (2014) (n 245).

[248] Perera (2017) (n 87).

The introduction of the PVR Bill in Sri Lanka could be seen as a direct global process flowing from Sri Lanka's WTO membership and *TRIPS* obligations. However, the data reveal that there was no nodal influence locally, nationally or globally to enact a PVR Act suitable to Sri Lanka. Intriguingly, there is no evidence of representations from the WTO, developed countries or MNCs, at least publicly, to pressure Sri Lanka to enact the legislation. For example, unlike in the case of India and Latin American countries, there has been no international pressure, it seems, from the WTO or any powerful states, or other entities, to implement PVR, in line with the adherence to *UPOV 1991*. Unlike the international pressure exerted on Colombia, for example,[249] the Sri Lankan Government has not been forced to confiscate seeds handled by farmers. The fact that the PVR Bill has not been implemented as of 2022 suggests that PVR are not a global issue for Sri Lanka. The 2019 revision of the PVR Bill has been submitted to the Ministry of Agriculture with no positive outcome to date. Hence, the researcher is unable to comment on the contents of this revision or its prospects of passage.

From this discussion, it is apparent that a stewardship approach would thus be the appropriate solution. This approach recognises and rewards their conservation and cultivation within farmers 'legal space' without tying them up in ownership issues and losing the commons entirely. It provides the following positive features:[250]

- It would recognise the informal, collective and cumulative systems of innovation of local and indigenous communities and farmers.
- No novelty, inventiveness or secrecy would be required for traditional varieties.
- No one will be singled out as legal owner.
- There would be no arbitrary time limits for protection.
- The conferred rights would be 'non-monopolistic' and would not hinder the non-commercial use and exchange of seeds within and among communities.
- Royalties would not have to be paid, although farmers could be paid for quality control.
- Registration, and therefore administrative machinery, would not be necessary.
- It would not oblige farmers or community members to keep secrets or change their traditional practices.
- Because no monopolies would be recognised, the possession of the same knowledge by different communities would be legitimate.
- The rights against infringement would arise when a variety has been acquired in a manner contrary to certain rules, such as national access legislation or other acceptable practices on the collection of germplasm.[251]

Taking into consideration the low economic status of the country and the importance of small farm holdings and subsistence farming,[252] it is the opinion of this

[249] Garz'on and Escobar (2019) (n 139).

[250] Correa (2000) (n 130), pp. 32–33.

[251] Ibid.

[252] Farming is a livelihood for Sri Lankan farmers and if there is excess, they will sell or share their produce with their neighbours for other goods.

researcher that Sri Lanka should continue to apply the local discourse for devising a mechanism to realise FR for their contribution based the stewardship approach, which is a non-IP regime. Under this system, farmers can be regarded as stewards or custodians of PGR. Sri Lankan farmers depend on farming for subsistence purposes. How Sri Lanka reconciles this approach with the impending global discourse on PVR remains to be seen.

Nonetheless, the Sri Lanka government could do more than keep a legal space for farmers to realise FR. Finding solutions to the strategies identified at the beginning in this chapter could be a starting point to provide recommendations. Regarding farmers' ability to access and use existing agrobiodiversity and further innovations, a novel legislation needs to be introduced that gives concessions for the registration of traditional varieties, which are the type of varieties that most farmers conserve and develop. The law must also provide positive reward systems for conservation and cultivation and a mechanism to commercialise farmers' varieties as discussed in the previous sections. As a means of providing farmers with incentives to encourage on-farm conservation and access to seed banks, legislation needs to be introduced to regulate the access to, or the utilisation of, resources. The new law should also have a mechanism on how government and private funding could be extended to allow farmers to protect traditional practices along with local knowledge, to adapt varieties to changing local conditions.[253] Hence, the government needs to balance the new commercial incentives with biodiversity considerations, so that the system can be made sufficiently attractive, both for knowledge holders and potential knowledge users.[254]

4.10 Conclusion

As discussed in the previous sections, the main discourse on PVR from the introduction of the first Bill is the difficulty in reaching a consensus regarding the FR provision in the Sri Lankan PVR Bill. This is the main reason that the PVR Bill has not yet been adopted in Sri Lanka. Yet, this must attract the criticism of delay in implementing the law. After all, *TRIPS* requires an effective system of protection. About the substance, the Sri Lankan 2011 PVR Bill has recognised FR to some extent, but essentially takes the ownership approach—presumably the 2019 version as well. This was not accepted by all the stakeholders for this affects the majority of the farming community in Sri Lanka. While Sri Lanka is also a member of both the *CBD* and the *FAO Treaty*, legal policy and institutional support are required for conserving its biodiversity resources.

Moreover, to realise FR in Sri Lanka, as stated above, it is important to find solutions via the strategies addressed in this chapter. In finding solutions, it is crucial to examine the measures taken by other countries as a benchmark, while adopting a

[253] Gunawardene (2010) (n 56).

[254] Antons (2010).

less legalistic and more consultative approach to give Sri Lankan subsistence farmers a 'legal space' for their practices as stewards, which has been supported by farmer groups and activists as the means for the realisation of FR. The stewardship approach aims to prevent the misappropriation of farmers' varieties and avert the establishment of any form of monopolisation that denies farmers' practices and values. The lobbying and mobilising by local farmers' groups and organisations against the seed-saving practice under the Newest Seed Bill show that there is a rising discourse among stakeholders while simultaneously policymakers are not listening to their concerns. These discourses are not merely political, but economic and environmental as well.

As discussed at the beginning of this chapter, PVR protection for Sri Lanka is an international treaty obligation, from which it will not be able to withdraw. Both India and Thailand faced similar concerns, controversies and challenges when introducing the PVR in their countries but were able to negotiate these differences and finally a PVR was agreed upon that recognises the interest of breeders as well as farmers. In contrast, Sri Lanka's 2011 PVR Bill puts both farmers and breeders under the same criteria of protection.

Therefore, common challenges for Sri Lanka are to implement the PVR Bill without further delay and to identify ways to make a non-IP regime work for sustainable and inclusive agricultural development for farmers. In other words, the government should consider the competing interests of breeders as well as farmers. Both these groups are crucial for the economic development of Sri Lanka. As discussed in this chapter, while recognising the rights of commercial breeders, it is important to support the rights of local and traditional farmers who rely on conservation, sustainable use, cultivation, development and sale of traditional plant varieties and customary forms of seed use, exchange and circulation for food security and livelihood enhancement. This is an inherent feature of Sri Lankan agriculture that cannot be forgotten by the country's policymakers.

Sri Lanka's local and global legal processes have not, intriguingly, made any progress either in the implementation of PVR or realisation of FR. This could not materialise merely through acceding to international treaties. The international treaties in this field are not uniform, and their expectations need to be reconciled at the level of national implementation. Furthermore, international treaty requirements should be accompanied by the leadership of a champion or a governing node who could influence the policymakers or the government for reforms.

The responsibility of implementing the PVR Bill is currently with the DoA in Sri Lanka, but data indicate that it has not acted as a governing node to influence the government to fast track the Bill by emphasising the benefits it could bring to the Sri Lankan economy. In other words, the DoA has neglected its regulatory function as a governing node, or it has been neglected by others. That the 2019 revision is still in the Ministry without any further action is a good example of this neglect. The lack of a bridge and a resolution in the discourse can be attributed to a range of factors; it cannot be explained by just one factor. Those factors, it would seem, include the absence of national political will, domestic civil unrest, missing global pressures, unplanned agricultural policies and regulations and weak technical and legal infrastructure. Unfortunately, as discussed to date at least, these features hold back the Sri Lankan IP ecosystem. Hence, the greatest bottleneck for PVR in Sri Lanka thus far has been the state of inertia in this regard.

In this second case study, the data analysis has highlighted that local discourses matter more than global discourses because in the Sri Lankan context, PVR law discussions and negotiations were initiated in the domestic and the national levels and still PVR has not been implemented in Sri Lanka.

The nodal governance and systems theory have helped to understand that there are different actors, local and global, in the PVR power dynamics in Sri Lanka. This framework also enabled me to identify the actors who influence PVR discourse through the *TRIPS Agreement*, which has made it mandatory to have PVR legislation, but so far there is no evidence of pressure or coercion by global actors to implement such an Act in Sri Lanka. However, as discussed previously in this chapter, within the local level protests by farming communities, organisations, action groups and environmental groups in Sri Lanka have expressed resistance regarding introducing a new Seed Act since it undermine the rights of farmers. This demonstrates power dynamics of the stakeholder communities against introducing the PVR laws.

Moreover, discourse was an appropriate mode of study for this chapter on PVR lawmaking. In the absence of soft law, evidence suggests that there was not only influence by nodes such as the stakeholder alliances, that comprised with farmers, environmentalists, academics and NGOs, various policymakers inside and outside the government, ministries, offices, but also inertia in dialogue and interaction, which has delayed the implementation of the PVR law to date. Discourse identified through dialogue, interaction and communication between nodes is an influential tool in the PVR regime to elucidate the dynamics in the developments of PVR regime. Although the *TRIPS*-mandated PVR should be implemented, the analysis in this chapter showed that in the absence of global pressure, the ultimate decision on whether to have a PVR law depends on the decision-making of Sri Lankan policymakers.

The next chapter will discuss whether the STI discourse has influence the innovation eco- system in Sri Lanka.

Competing Interests The author has no conflicts of interest to declare that are relevant to the content of this chapter.

References

Abeywardana N et al (2019) Indigenous agricultural systems in dry zone of Sri Lanka: management transformation assessment and sustainability. Sustain J 11:3

Adhikari K (2012) Seed banking in South Asia. In: South Asia watch on trade, economics and environment

Agrawal RC (2017) Opportunities and challenges created by plant variety protection and farmers' rights act in India. In: Reimagining the governance of genetic resources and intellectual property for agriculture and food security in Asia Kathmandu

Amarasinghe KK (2018) Bio-piracy and its impact on biodiversity: a special review on Sri Lankan context. J Environ Protect 3:164
Andersen R (2005) The history of farmers' rights: a guide to central documents and literature. The Farmers Rights Project
Andersen R (2006) Realising farmers' rights under ITPGRFA: summary findings from the farmers rights project.' FNI Report No 11
Andersen R (2016) The evolution of farmers' rights'. In: Halewood M (ed) Farmers' crop varieties and farmers' rights: challenges in taxonomy and law. Routledge, New York
Andersen A (2017) "Stewardship" or "ownership": how to realise farmers' rights. In: Hunter D et al (eds) Routledge handbook of agricultural biodiversity. Routledge, New York
Antons C (2010) Sui generis protection for plant varieties and traditional knowledge in biodiversity and agriculture: the international framework and national approaches in the Philippines and India. Indian J Law Technol 6:121
Antons C (2016) Article 27(3)(b) TRIPS and plant variety protection in developing countries. In: Ullrich H et al (eds) TRIPS plus 20: from trade rules to market principles. Springer, New York
Anver G (2016) Breeders' rights detrimental to Sri Lankan farmers'. The Sunday Leader (Sri Lanka)
Arup C (2008) The world trade organization knowledge agreements. Cambridge University Press, Cambridge
Banga R (2014) Impact of green box subsidies on agricultural productivity, production and trade. Centre for WTO Studies
Bavadam L (2011) Bitter Harvest. Frontline India
Berson J (2014) The quinoa hack. New left review. 85. https://newleftreview.org/issues/II85/articles/joshua-berson-the-quinoa-hack
Bhardwaj M, Jadhav R (2019) Monsanto patent victory seen as a boost to biotech investment in India. US Legal News. https://www.reuters.com/article/uk-india-monsanto-idUSKCN1P2092
Blakeney M (2011) Trends in intellectual property rights relating to genetic resources for food and agriculture. FAO Commission
Borowiak C (2004) Farmers' rights: intellectual property regimes and the struggle over seeds. Polit Soc 32:4
Chandra R (2015) The inscription of law in life. Centre for Policy Research
Coombe RJ (2017) Frontiers of cultural property in the global South. In: Anderson J, Geismar H (eds) Routledge companion to cultural property. Routledge, New York
Correa CM (2000) Options for the implementation of farmers rights at the national level. South Centre
Correa CM (2015) Plant variety protection in developing countries: a tool for designing sui generis plant variety protection system: an alternative to UPOV 1991. Association for Plant Breeding for the Benefit of Society. https://www.apbrebes.org/news/new-publication-plant-variety-protection-developing-countries-tool-designing-sui-generis-plant?pk_campaign=tool
De Wit MM (2017) Stealing into the world: conservation science, plant breeding and the makings of new seed enclosures. J Peasant Stud 44:1
Department of Agriculture Fisheries and Forestry Australia (2022) Agriculture stewardship packages. https://www.agriculture.gov.au/ag-farm-food/natural-resources/landcare/sustaining-future-australian-farming
Department of Agriculture Sri Lanka (2008) State of plant genetic resources for food and agriculture in Sri Lanka. FAO/Government Cooperative Programme
Dogbevi K (2017) The sui generis system of plant variety protection under the TRIPS agreement: an empty promise for developing countries. SSRN
Elderman M, James C (2011) Peasants' rights and the UN system: quixotic struggle? Or emancipatory idea whose time has come? J Peasants Stud 38:1
Ensor J, Weragoda R (2009) Realising the adaptive capacity of farming communities in coastal Sri Lanka. Waterlines 28:3

Environmental Justice Organisation (2016) Farmers defend their rights against a new seed law, Sri Lanka. https://ejatlas.org/conflict/sri-lankan-farmers-defend-their-rights-against-a-new-seed-law

European Agroecology Knowledge Exchange Network (2017) Secure farmers' collective rights to their own seeds European coordination via compesina. https://www.eurovia.org/secure-farmers-collective-rights-to-their-own-seeds/

Federation of Chambers of Commerce and Industry of Sri Lanka (2020) Sri Lanka standard institution (SLS) product certification mark. http://www.fccisl.lk/featured-topic/sri-lanka-standards-institution-sls-product-certification-mark/

Flach J et al (2009) The Nagoya protocol on access to genetic resources and benefit sharing: best practices for uses of lactic acid bacteria. Pharma Nutr 9

Garz'on DS, Escobar LG (2019)Revolturas: resisting multinational seed corporations and legal seed regimes through seed saving practices and activism in Colombia. J Peasant Stud 47:4

Gervais DJ (2005) Traditional knowledge and intellectual property: a TRIPS-compatible approach. Michigan State Law Review

Gervais DJ (2010) TRIPS agreement: drafting history and analysis

Gervais DJ (2013) TRIPS and development. Vanderbilt Public Research Paper No. 13/46

Gibson J (2005) Community resources: intellectual property, international trade and the protection of traditional knowledge. Routledge, New York

Godden L (2009) Book review: the principle of sustainability: transforming law and governance. Osgood Hall Law J 47:4

GRAIN (2005) Collective rights over farmers' seeds in Italy. Extracts from an interview with Antonio Onorati. https://www.grain.org/en/article/538-collective-rights-over-farmers-seeds-in-italy

Gunawardena J (2000a) Traditional crop varieties and plant variety protection-Sri Lanka must tread cautiously. The Island (Sri Lanka)

Gunawardena J (2000b) Traditional crop varieties and plant variety protection: Sri Lanka must tread cautiously

Gunawardena J (2003) Throwing Lankan farmer to corporate dragon. The Island (Sri Lanka)

Gunawardena J (2006) Kothala-Himbutu: decisive victory over bio-piracy. The Island (Sri Lanka).http://www.island.lk/2006/07/12/midweek4.html

Gunawardene N (2010) Who speaks for small farmers, earthworms and cow dung. Groundviews. https://groundviews.org/2010/08/19/feature-article-who-speaks-for-small-farmers-earthworms-and-cow-dung/

Guneratne C (2008) Genetic resources and international law. PhD Thesis, University of Waikato

Hirimuthugoda D (2014) Does Sri Lanka need a new seed act? The Island (Sri Lanka). http://www.island.lk/index.php?page_cat=article-details&page=article-details&code_t...

Hirimuthugodage D, Samaratunga PA (2016) Intellectual property rights in protecting new plant varieties and farmers' traditional knowledge. Institute of Policy Studies

Honore AM (1961) Ownership. In: Guest AG (ed) Oxford essays in jurisprudence. Oxford University Press, Oxford

International Analog Forestry Network (2014) RRI inaugurates community seed bank: hope in the wake of war. IAFN-RIFA. https://www.analogforestry.org/rri-inaugurates-community-seed-bank/

International Plant Genetic Resources Institute (1999) Key questions for decision-makers, protection of plant varieties under the WTO agreement on trade-related aspects of intellectual property rights' decision tools. IPGRI Working Paper

IP Australia (2019) PBR Basics. https://www.ipaustralia.gov.au/plant-breeders-rights/understanding-pbr/pbr-basics

Jaffe W, Wijk JV (1995) The impact of plant breeders' rights in developing countries: debate and experience in Argentina, Chile, Colombia, Mexico and Uruguay. Inter-American Institute for Cooperation on Agriculture, University of Amsterdam

Kamardeen N (2013) The significance of plant variety legislation in promoting economic growth: an analysis of the proposed law in Sri Lanka. South East Asia J Contemp Bus Econ Law 2:3
Kannangara N (2014) Sowing devastations proposed seed act. The Sunday Leader (Sri Lanka)
Karunanada UB (2006) Nuwarakalawiya and the North Central province under British Administration 1833–1900: an area study of British administration in Sri Lanka. Research Centre for Social Sciences University of Kelaniya Sri Lanka
Kaushik RS (2006) Biocapital: the constitution of postgenomic life. Duke University Press Books
Kurukulasuriya L (2014) Sri Lankan farmers resist new seed law. New Internationalist. https://newint.org/blog/majority/2014/01/28/sri-lanka-seed-law
La Via Campesina (2014) The people's caravan for seed and food security: MONLAR, Sri Lanka. GRAIN. https://viacampesina.org/en/the-people-s-caravan-for-seed-and-food-sovereignty-monlar-sri-lanka/
La Via Campesina (2015) Seed laws that criminalise farmers: additional country experiences. GRAIN. http://www.grain.org/article/entries/5147-seed-laws-that-criminalise-farmers-additional
Law and Society Trust (2007) Our common heritage: farmers rights to plant genetic resources in Sri Lanka. Law and Society Trust Sri Lanka
Leach ER (1959) Hydraulic society in Ceylon. Past Present 15:1
Li Y, Huang TH, Yamahara J (2008) Salacia root, a unique ayurvedic medicine, meets multiple targets in diabetes and obesity. Life Sci 82:22
Louwaars N, Burgaud F (2016) Variety registration: the evolution of registration system with a special emphasis on agrobiodiversity. In: Halewood M (ed) Farmers' crop varieties and farmers' rights: challenges in taxonomy and law. Routledge
McGuire S, Sperling L (2016) Seed system and small holder farmers use. Food Sec 8:1546
Ministry of Agriculture Sri Lanka (2018) Agriculture sector modernization project. http://www.agrimin.gov.lk/web/index.php/en/project/12-project/841-agriculture-sector
Ministry of Foreign Affairs Sri Lanka (2016) US-Sri Lanka trade and investment framework council adopts action plan to boost bilateral trade
Montúfar R, Ayala M (2019) Perceptions of agrodiversity and seed-saving practices in the Northern Andes of Ecuador. J Ethnobiol Ethnomed 15:21
Moonka R, Mukherjee S (2018) TRIPS flexibilities and India's plant variety protection regime: the way forward. BRICS Law J 5:11
Mulleriyawa R (2016) Farmer weeded out in seed act. The Sunday Times (Sri Lanka)
Nanayakkara A (2007) Protecting farmers' rights: historical, contemporary and international perspectives. In: Law and Society Trust (ed) Our common heritage? Farmers' rights to plant genetic resources in Sri Lanka. Law and Society Trust
Nanayakkara A, The World Conservation Union (2000) Recommendations for the regulation of access to genetic resources and the fair and equitable sharing of benefits. Biodiversity Secretariat of the Ministry of Forestry and Environment Sri Lanka
News First (2019) Sri Lanka's ancient "Wewa" water system recognised as global heritage system. https://www.newsfirst.lk/2018/04/19/sri-lankas-ancient-wewa-water-system-recognised-as-global-heritage-system-by-un/
Noriega IL (2016) Defensive protection of farmers' varieties. In: Halewood M (ed) Farmers' crop varieties and farmers' rights: challenges in taxonomy and law. Routledge, New York
Office of the United States Trade Representative (2022) Trade and investment framework agreements. https://ustr.gov/trade-agreements/trade-investment-framework-agreements
OXFAM (2022) About fair trade. https://www.oxfamfairtrade.be/en/why-oxfam-matters/about-fair-trade/
Patnaik A, Jongerden J, Ruivenkamp G (2017) Repossession through sharing of an access to seeds: different cases and practices. Int Rev Sociol 27:1
Perera A (2010) Protection of plant varieties in Sri Lanka. Law and Society Trust Publication
Perera A (2011) Plant variety protection in Sri Lanka and its impact on Sri Lanka's agricultural economy: a critical analysis. J World Intell Prop 14(4):3

Perera A (2017) Legal framework for plant breeders' rights in Sri Lanka: a review. Eur Intell Prop Rev 39:5
Perera A (2021) Searching for a balance: realisation of farmers' rights in Sri Lanka: a case study on ownership and stewardship. Eur Intell Prop Rev 43:10
Perera A, Adhikari K (2019) From neglect to protection: recognising the importance of farmers' varieties in Sri Lanka. In: Adhikari K, Jefferson DJ (eds) Intellectual property law and plant protection: challenges and developments in Asia. Routledge, New York
Peschard K (2016) Seed wars and farmers' rights: comparative perspectives from Brazil and India. J Peasant Stud 44:1
Peschard K, Randeria S (2020) Taking monsanto to court: legal activism around intellectual property in Brazil and India. J Peasant Stud 47:4
Peschard K, Randeria S (2021) Keeping seeds in our hands: the rise of seed activism. J Peasant Stud 47:4
Phillips C (2016) Saving more than seeds: practices and politics of seed saving. Routledge, New York
Phillips C (2019) Saving more than seeds: practices and politics of seed saving. Agricult Hum Values 34:1245
Philpott T (2013) Quinoa: good, evil or just really complicated? The Guardian. https://www.theguardian.com/environment/2013/jan/25/quinoa-good-evil-complicated
Pottinger L (2017) Planting the seeds of a quiet activism. Royal Geogr Soc 49:2
Prajeesh P (2015) Farmers' rights to seeds: issues in Indian law. Econ Polit Week 1:12
Rangnekar D (2016) Commentary on the Indian protection of plant varieties and farmers' rights act 2001. In: Halewood M (ed) Farmers' crop varieties and farmers' rights: challenges in taxonomy and law
Robinson DF (2010) Confronting biopiracy: challenges, cases and international debates. Earthscan
Rodrigo M (2013) Biopiracy on rise. The Sunday times (Sri Lanka). http://www.sundaytimes.lk/130224/news/biopiracy-on-the-rise-34295.html
Rodríguez-Garavito C (2011) Ethnicity gov: global governance, indigenous peoples, and the right to prior consultation in social minefields. Indiana J Glob Legal Stud 18:1
Sahai S (2002) Protection of plant varieties and farmers' rights law making and cultivation of varietal control. Econ Polit Weekly 37
Sampath P (2001) Protection of plant varieties and framers' rights bill. Indian J Environ Law 2:1
Santilli J (2012) Agrobiodiversity and the law. Regulating genetic resources, food security and cultural diversity. Earthscan
Sherman B (2003) Regulating access and use of genetic resources: intellectual property law and biodiversity. Eur Intell Property Rev 25:7
Song Y et al (2016) Access and benefit sharing in participatory plant breeding in Southwest China. Farming Matters
Srinivasan CS (2016) Institutional capacity and implementation issues in farmers' rights. In: Halewood M (ed) Farmers' crop varieties and farmers' rights: challenges in taxonomy and law. Routledge, New York
The Economist (2021) Quinoa: against the grain. The fad for the Andean staple has not hurt the poor—yet. https://www.economist.com/finance-and-economics/2016/05/21/against-the-grain
Thomas G, De Tavernier J (2017) Farmer-suicide in India: debating the role of biotechnology. Life Sci Soc Policy 13:8
Verma SK (2007) Protecting traditional knowledge: is a Sui generis system an answer? J World Intell Property 7
Vernooy R et al (2020) The role of community seed banks in achieving farmers' rights. Develop Pract 30:5
Warushamana G (2014) Proposed act will ensure seed quality. The Sunday Observer (Sri Lanka)
WTO (2008) TRIPS: reviews. Article 27(3)b and related issues: background and the current situation. https://www.wto.org/english/tratop_e/trips_e/art27_3b_background_e.htm

WTO (2011) The Doha declaration on TRIPS and public health ten years later: the state implementation. South Centre. https://www.southcentre.int/wp-content/uploads/2013/06/PB7_-Doha-Declaration-on-TRIPS-and-Health_-EN.pdf
WTO (2022) Draft modalities for TRIPS related issues, trade negotiations committee. https://www.wto.org/english/tratop_e/trips_e/art27_3b_e.htm
WTO Secretariat (2006) The protection of traditional knowledge and folklore summary of issues raised, and points made. https://www.wto.org/english/tratop_e/trips_e/art27_3b_e.htm

Chapter 5
The Science, Technology and Innovation Discourse in Sri Lanka

Abstract This chapter will examine the role the development of IP policy has played in science, technology and innovation (STI) in Sri Lanka. Aligning with Chaps. 3 and 4 STI discourse too favours a low-technology protection because, STI indicators remain relatively low compared to develop countries. As a result, most public sector ST innovations which are patented at all in Sri Lanka are developed using basic research which is considered low-technology, rather than on applied or demand driven research, which aims for the commercialisation of high technology commonly by licencing or patenting with industry. Furthermore, it seems Sri Lanka's IP policy fails to attract foreign investment and the local access to high technology it should bring with it if it is appropriately embraced and regulated. This chapter consists of two parts; the first part presents discourses on the role of IP in stimulating local innovation and the second discusses its role in stimulating FDI innovation and technology transfer.

5.1 Introduction

Patent law and regulation do not exist in a vacuum; they exist to translate ideas into IPR that can then be commercialised and disseminated, and for this reason, the settings of a patent system and legal structure are intertwined with the development discourse relating to ST in Sri Lanka.

Dasanayaka has documented that long-term development strategies to eradicate poverty involve programs that incorporate R&D in ST for development in Sri Lanka.[1] A recent study on reframing IP in Sri Lanka has further reiterated that Sri Lanka needs to shift its focus towards promoting a culture of innovation through R&D as a matter of policy.[2] Countries such as Singapore and Malaysia would not have achieved their economic growth and industry competitiveness without strong technology and innovation policies and R&D base.[3] The R&D base can be curiosity driven, demand

[1] Dasanayaka (2003).

[2] Marsoof et al. (2022).

[3] Perera and Dasanayaka (2004), pp. 244–245.

A. Perera, *Dilemmas of Intellectual Property Discourse in Sri Lanka*,
https://doi.org/10.1007/978-981-97-6117-3_5

driven, learning based, fundamental (basic) or applied to foster science and innovation, and hence, it comprises a broad spectrum.[4] No single category of research is more important than any other category, but R&D in ST, in the forms of basic and applied research have been considered methods for economic development, although R&D may be largely concerned with the adaptation of global ST to local needs rather than the making of original local breakthrough inventions.

Innovation is defined by the Organisation for Economic Co-operation and Development's *Oslo Manual 2018* as a new or improved product or process (or combination thereof) that differs significantly from the unit's previous products or processes and that has been made available to potential users (product) or brought into use by the unit (process).[5] This conceptually mirrors the focus in patents of advances as an inventive step and novelty, which supports the linkage of patenting to ST, but it also identifies the requirement that innovation must be commercialised. In other words, innovation involves bringing this new idea to the market, though commercialisation. Without commercialisation, there is no value added to the patent or the discovery to be an innovation. Yet, innovation is wider than just the implementation or commercialisation of patents and IP. Innovation is not just linear; it often assumes a loop: It involves the users' learning, application and improvement of the original ST. Thus, the STI-related IP policy is concerned with stimulating both knowledge creation and knowledge uptake. Innovation-related IP is not just codified IP, such as patents, but links to the know-how embodied in people and partnerships.

Hence, to have to access knowledge creation, technology output factors, such as patent applications and registrations, are indicators of the status of the existing industrial base of Sri Lanka. Developments in industry indicate the knowledge impact of IP, whereas knowledge diffusion is observed in the shifting IP discourse through collaborations such as industry–university partnerships, the overseas training of local staff, workshops conducted by foreign IP offices, such as those of Korea and Japan and USPTO and WIPO, to enhance ST knowledge. This aspect will be discussed in this chapter.

Before the case can be examined through explaining the STI development in Sri Lanka, it is necessary to identify the common discourse (which Sri Lanka might adopt) regarding the status of commercialisation of innovation through IP and whether innovation is supported through industry or government, or ideally both. Such developments are achieved when there is an entrepreneurial ecosystem or culture that supports and fosters the commercialisation of scientific research. This is not to say that every invention will be commercialised, but rather the existence of discourse that fosters and enables commercialisation of IP is being described as the basis for ensuring economic prosperity in a knowledge-based economy.[6] It has been

---

[4] Mendes (2015).

[5] OECD/Eurostat (2018).

[6] Dructer (1992). Drucker attributed to economist Fritz Machlup, originating the term' knowledge economy.' The phrase 'knowledge-based economy' describes the new economic environment in which the generation and management of knowledge play a predominant part in wealth creation, as compared with traditional factors of production, namely, land, labour and capital.

recognised in the discourse internationally that, appropriately set, IP is a powerful tool for the development of national innovation policies in many countries when connected with other essential factors.[7]

In the Sri Lankan context, the development debate, from the resource and agricultural to a knowledge-based economy, involves the competing discourses about IP. Does IP aim to protect foreign investors through high-technology protection or does IP aim to protect local businesses, through low-technology protection and licensing or domestic TT? As will be discussed later in this chapter, Sri Lanka's STI sectors aim to foster innovation through localised R&D, technological and commercial innovation and TT with local performance requirements as a condition. This implies that STI and IP discourse is a local or national story based on low-technology protection, rather than a global or international discourse, that focus on high- technology protection. Local policies focus on fostering local innovations rather than on emphasising demand-side innovation policies that attract global competition, which would simply make Sri Lanka a passive site for global high-technology imports and exports. In contrast, the international discourse argues that investment will occur when high-technology IP protection is given to IP developers. These are the two competing discourses that will be discussed in this chapter.

The discourse on commercialisation and innovation identifies that the government is the important local node in developing an environment to support STI, through the utilisation of a tool box of mechanisms, such as establishing innovation clusters, free trade zones, FDI,[8] TT and international production networks, and the utilisation of international aid that the government can access to promote development directly or to operate as a conduit for individuals to connect with appropriate parties. IP is to play a role in this strategy. Further, the NIPO, among others, would in principle be a relevant local node for assistance in the development of STI and the implementation of programs through the policy, but as discussed in Chap. 3, NIPO has initiated discussions with other actors to implement programs and later withdrew from such discussions owing to its inability to interact with them. In the Sri Lankan context, the discourse identifies problems, and solutions developed locally in the discourse on development through R&D and the Science Technology Policy ('STP').

Thus, with this background, the third case study will examine the role of IP on science, technology and innovation (STI) in Sri Lanka based on the theoretical framework outlined in Chap. 2, in this book. Aligning with the first research inquiries. STI discourse favours a low-technology protection because, STI indicators are relatively low compared to the middle-income countries. As a result, most ST innovations which are patented in Sri Lanka are developed using basic research which is considered low-technology, rather than on applied or demand driven research, which involves high technology.

The reasons behind Sri Lanka favouring low-technology protection is that the majority of SMEs in Sri Lanka develop innovations to the local market through a low-technology protection due to the lack of expertise, resources and high cost

[7] WIPO (2017).

[8] Gibbons (2011).

involved in the process. It is only the limited number of multinational companies emphasise the importance of high-technology IP protection as a pre-requisite to attract TT and FDI to increase the innovation activities in Sri Lanka.

To examine how actors or nodes play power dynamics in the STI sector it is crucial to discuss the role of nodes in this case study. STI discourse is predominantly local, where number local nodes, such as the Ministry of Science, Technology and Research, COSTI, SLINTEC and NSF has the mentalities, technologies, resources and institutional force to mobilise, assist and influence develop a stable STI ecosystem in Sri Lanka. This aspect will be discussed in this chapter. To elucidate the power dynamics in the STI in Sri Lanka, this case study will also examine how various actors within the STI eco-system exert influence with the other nodes through interaction and communications creating a social discourse introducing STI policies aimed at fostering an innovation economy in Sri Lanka.

This chapter consists of two parts; the first part presents discourses on the role of IP in stimulating local innovation and the second discusses the role of FDI in stimulating innovation and IP. The first part considers the discourse relating to how IP supports exclusive rights commonly through licensing and collaboration, which are necessary to commercialise inventions. It will examine the STI IP policy for stimulation of local inventions with special emphasis on IP's role in university-industry partnerships. The second part will discuss the role of FDI in attracting TT, joint ventures and upskilling the local economy via IP.

5.2 IP Stimulating Local Innovations

5.2.1 Government Initiatives to Stimulate IP: Primary Discourses

5.2.1.1 The Pre-independence Period

The pre-independence period of Sri Lanka is characterised by the control and influence of three colonial powers. The first was the Portuguese, who ruled the country during 1505–1658, followed by the Dutch, who ruled during 1658–1796, and the British, who ruled from 1796 until Sri Lanka became an independent nation in 1948.

During the colonial period, Western technology was introduced without consideration of existing local operations, but not until British colonisation did modern technology begin to be transplanted into Sri Lanka.[9] The British concept for Sri Lanka was that it would be an agricultural base for them and a market for their industrial products. As Drahos commented in another context, policies were designed to suit the colonisers, not the colonies.[10] To this end, the British structured the Sri Lanka

[9] Ibid.

[10] Drahos (2010).

economy to maximise their profits without consultation or dialogue with local leaders. Consequently, most local industries were ruined and supplanted by tea, rubber and coconut as the main exports from Sri Lanka.

Nevertheless, there were some local benefits. The British period led to engineering advances in the development of infrastructure such as major rail and road networks, ports and education in the form of technical colleges and a Faculty of Engineering in the University of Ceylon. In order to improve the health condition of the settlers, the British established the Medical Research Institute, Ceylon Medical College and the Nurses Training School, which led to substantial advances in the field of health.[11] In the field of agriculture, the DoA, and tea, rubber and coconut research institutes were established, but little attention was paid to the R&D of rice, subsidiary crops and spices. However, in the industrial sector, the British pioneered the establishment of several factories, such as those for coir, steel rolling, plywood, leather, acetic acid, paper, glass and ceramics, owing to the war situation. During this period, the Industrial Research Laboratory was established in the Department of Commerce and Industries to serve local industry. Some technological achievements were also made in the hydropower electricity generation, transport and telecommunications and broadcasting fields during the British occupation of Sri Lanka.[12]

Yet, colonisation reflects a lack of engagement with local leaders on how to preserve the local know-how, because local pressure related to restoring major ancient irrigation works was brought against the colonial administration, mainly owing to pressure from Sri Lankan representatives in the legislature.[13] Thus, during the British colonial period, what really mattered were the legal meanings given to legal transfers via human agents' interpretation. The superstructural nodes of colonial powers meant that the agents of legal transfers interpreted such transfers in strategic ways in order to achieve their own goals, that is, largely the wellbeing of Britain and British firms, through its colonies.

5.2.1.2 Post-independence: From 1948 to Present

The post-independence period demonstrates the discourse among local associations on influencing and developing conversations about the development of ST, and it also illuminates the structural difficulties in the government in implementing policy. During this period, many policies have been promulgated but implementation has been slow for several reasons. The responsibility for research and ST is spread among many ministries and government agencies, which creates inefficiencies, unnecessary duplication and a lack of coordination. Inefficiencies arise owing to the lack of engagement between actors since there was no central authority responsible for coordinating ST until the establishment of COSTI as the governing node. There were many overlaps between ministries and agencies, shifting structures in government

[11] Perera and Dasanayaka (2004).

[12] Ibid.

[13] News First (2019).

and personnel, a lack of genuine interest among policymakers in implementing policies, a lack of local lobbyists to push for policy implementation and a lack of political will owing to numerous changes in the government. Moreover, after the escalation of the ethnic conflict in 1983, government expenditure was diverted to war rather than to industrial development, and thus, little ST development occurred until the civil war officially ended in 2009.

The post-independence discourse was begun by an association of scientists with the mentality that science would assist in development, and not the government. The Ceylon Association for the Advancement of Science (the predecessor to the Sri Lanka Association for the Advancement of Science ['SLAAS']) was founded in 1944 as a voluntary association of scientists committed to the advancement of science. It was a governing node in the discourse at that time because it organised conferences and pressured the government to advance science. For example, it presented proposals for the establishment of a National Council for Science in 1948 to the government by using a model developed by the Indian Council of Industrial Research.[14]

SLAAS was prominent in discourse for the advancement of science in Sri Lanka for it attempted to fill voids that were not being filled by the government, in particular, to the limited extent it was able to establish within its own organisation of activities for promoting ST. A General Research Committee was established to provide some direction on planning and direction to scientists in Sri Lanka.

An example of the activism of the SLAAS is documented in the following statement of the Prime Minister Mrs Sirimavo Bandaranaike at the Ninetieth Annual Session of the SLAAS in 1963:

> I assume that your invitation to me, as Prime Minister, to come to open this Conference is your method of expressing your view that Science and Scientific Research is of primary significance to our country. My acceptance of your invitation will, in itself, indicate to you the fact that I rate your work as the greatest importance.

On this same occasion, the Prime Minister in conclusion said:

> For its part, the government has accepted the need for the formulation of a National Body with the necessary authority to guide scientific activity ... I am glad to announce on this occasion that the Government holds the view that a body such as the National Research Council, which has been proposed for Ceylon by your Association, is most essential, and the necessary steps will be taken to constitute such a body as early as possible.[15]

As result of the push by the Prime Minister, the *National Science Council of Ceylon Act*[16] of 1968 established the National Science Council. The council comprised 21 members appointed by the Minister from 'people closely associated with the pursuit, promotion or application of science', and the selection was based on the representation of six research areas: physical, biological, agricultural, industrial, medical and social sciences. The SLAAS had agitated for the council to be under the direct purview of the Prime Minister, but instead, the government created a new

---

[14] Jaysuriya and De Silva (1972).

[15] Ibid.

[16] *National Science Council of Ceylon Act* No 9 of 1968.

Ministry of Scientific Research and Housing. This decision is interesting for one of the discourses that will be documented later in this chapter identifies that the continual switching of ministries has been a deterrent to developing an IP-related policy.

Later, other local bodies were established, such as the Industrial Development Board in 1966 and the National Engineering Research and Development Centre in 1974, to boost ST. The former was to provide various technical services to SMEs and to inform other R&D organisations about the technology needs and capabilities of other industries, but this did not happen owing to the lack of discourse between other sectors. This Centre was established to conduct and promote research, innovation and commercialisation. This organisation accomplished some research and innovation activities, as will be discussed later, but their commercialisation was not very satisfactory.[17] This also suggest that there was no governing node to push ST in Sri Lanka during this period.

In 1976, an UNCTAD mission, a global discourse, reported that Sri Lanka had the machinery for using imported technology but lacked an R&D sector to foster development.[18] This Report recommended that the Centre for Transfer and Development of Technology be established as a focal point to link R&D institutions with the national economic planning apparatus but no action was taken for such implementation.[19] This is a pragmatic obstacle faced by the then government because the UNCTAD recommendations are not mandatory and political will is required for their implementation.

These governmental initiatives were influenced either by international actors engaged as consultants or advisors, or by local scientific associations that engaged with the private sector and pushed the government to develop ST. During this period, private sector R&D was confined to local subsidiaries of multinationals and associated companies but the most R&D was performed by government-owned corporations in specialist fields, such as ceramics, tyres and mineral sand.

In the 1960–1977 period, little R&D occurred in the private sector owing to the heavy state involvement in the economy.[20] Interestingly, during this period the state was the prominent actor in the ST discourse. As a result, the private sector did not have the opportunity to flourish. However, the discourse changed in the 1977 policy reforms when the centre-right government led by JR Jayawardene came into power in mid-1977 and adopted neoliberalism. In 1979, Sri Lanka became the first country in South Asia to open its economy; it adopted an alternative remedy, with the liberalisation of trade, and accepted export-led growth as its development strategy and the private sector as its growth engine. Consequently, the country's growth rate almost doubled to 8.2% and exports increased to 30.9% of GDP in 1978 from 18.7% in 1977.[21]

---

[17] See Perera and Dasanayaka (2004).

[18] Ibid.

[19] Ibid.

[20] Ibid.

[21] Indraratna (2012).

JR Jayawardene, who later became the President, pioneered the understanding of the importance of ST and R&D for Sri Lanka's economic growth. To achieve this goal, in 1982, he took the National Science Council directly under his purview, and the main role of this body was to advise the President on ST issues.[22] Taking the ST ministry under the auspices of the President is a demonstration of exerting influence within Sri Lanka to push STI. This shows the nodal influence of the President or the ministry, about science-related issues. It also demonstrates the need in Sri Lanka for nodal ability to implement laws. SLAAS requested that a National Science Council be established, and this occurred in 1968. Later, the formulation of a National Science Policy Plan and Implementation document for economic sectors was completed under Jayawardene's guidance.[23]

From 1984 onwards, successive governments in Sri Lanka have implemented initiatives to influence its ST development. Numerous ST agreements were signed with various governments, and various local bodies, such as the Arthur C Clarke Centre, were established, giving recognition to IP in their respective policies. SLIC,[24] NASTEC,[25] NSF,[26] National Science and Technology Policy,[27] National Biotechnology Policy,[28] Science, Technology and Innovation Strategy 2011–2015,[29] COSTI,[30] National Research and Development Framework[31] and National Innovation Agency[32] were established to stimulate STI.

The rationale behind establishing these policies and institutions was to coordinate and develop policies and plans for the advancement of ST for national development and to recognise the value of IP and commercialisation, the need to promote linkages between universities and research institutes and the importance of formulating an IP policy to protect IP in the country.

---

[22] Perera and Dasanayaka (2004).

[23] Ibid.

[24] Sri Lanka Investors Commission, https://slic.gov.lk/.

[25] The *Science and Technology Development Act No 11 of 1994* provided for the establishment of a National Science and Technology Commission (NASTEC).

[26] The NSF was established in 1998 by the *Science and Technology Development Act No 11 of 1994*. The NSF is mandated to serve and strengthen the ST sectors of Sri Lanka.

[27] The National Science and Technology Policy recommended 10 objectives. Objective 8 emphasised developing a culture of innovation and IP, and ensuring the protection of IPR.

[28] Ministry of Science and Technology of Sri Lanka, *National Biotechnology Policy*, http://www.nsf.ac.lk/images/stories/STPRD/biotechnology_policy.pdf. See also Chandrasekera (2017).

[29] Ministry of Technology and Research (2022).

[30] COSTI was mandated to coordinate STI in Sri Lanka.

[31] Ministry of Education Sri Lanka (2022). The purpose of the National Research and Development Framework was to align the activities of ST institutions towards national development and a knowledge economy driven by STI.

[32] Mudalige (2019).

5.2.2 Secondary Discourses

This section will examine government policy initiatives to introduce high-technology protection after the civil war for promoting STI in Sri Lanka and reasons that the high-technology protection concept has not been effective.

The civil war ended more than 13 years ago, but at present, Sri Lanka not only lags in the high-technology area owing to a lack of political will but also faces a grave economic crisis, given its lack of foreign reserves due to mismanagement and corruption. Further, after the end of the civil war, STI became a consistent political mantra without substantive support for implementation or considerations of how these policies should be implemented. For example, *Sri Lanka the Emerging World of Asia 'Mahinda Chinthana'—Vision for the Future, 2010* (Mahinda Vision), the manifesto of the 2010 presidential election, emphasised creating Sri Lanka into a modern economy through STI.[33] Mahinda Vision proposed 10 objectives[34] including to develop and protect a culture of innovation and IP, thus acknowledging IP as a mechanism to foster innovation.[35]

In 2013, the Ministry of Finance and Planning released the *Unstoppable Sri Lanka 2020*[36] policy document, in which Chap. 6 is devoted to 'Building a Culture of Innovation and Research' through research infrastructure at regional universities and many research institutes, by selecting priority areas of development, enhancing the technological and scientific resource base and TT to the grassroots level (i.e. village and to micro enterprises and SMEs). One of the stated aims was to increase high-technology exports from 1.5 to 10% by 2016.[37]

In September 2017, the newly elected Sri Lankan Government launched an ambitious development plan, Vision 2025.[38] The eight-year strategy aims to develop the country into an upper middle-income economy 'by transforming Sri Lanka into the hub of the Indian Ocean, with a knowledge-based, highly competitive, social market economy'. This goal was to be achieved by improving technology acquisition and digitisation. The Technology and Digitisation section of Vision 2025 is crucial for this chapter since it acknowledges that for Sri Lanka to become globally competitive

---

33 Ministry of Finance and Planning (2010).

34 Foster a science, technology and innovation (STI) culture; enhance ST capability for national development and strengthen governance and policy implementation mechanisms; expand and improve the resource base of scientists and technologists; promote basic, applied and developmental research of national importance; develop, or acquire and adapt, scientific knowledge and technology transfer; ensure sustainable use of natural resources for development; promote indigenous knowledge–based technologies; develop and protect a culture of innovation and intellectual property;. ensure the protection of intellectual property rights and promote innovation by introducing IPRs to local entrepreneurs; promote standards of science and technology institutions locally and globally; and promote the application of science and technology for all aspects of human welfare.

35 Abeyratne (2010).

36 Ministry of Finance and Planning (2020).

37 Ibid.

38 World Bank (2017).

and to drive towards a digitally empowered economy, it must develop strategies that encourage the use of digital and other emergent technologies.[39]

Vision 2025 recognises that in the ST field, the country has lagged behind other countries owing to a lack of policies and strategies to develop technology for the manufacturing sector. It further stated that there was minimum focus on promoting innovation technologies, such as artificial intelligence, data mining and other high-quality technological services.[40] This suggests that the economy requires a shift towards innovative, knowledge-based business ventures to foster innovation. Vision 2025 identified reforms to boost STI in the areas of foreign technologies and investment in digital technology and the ICT industry[41] by providing loans to encourage young, educated entrepreneurs to start SMEs.[42] However, Vision 2025 did not emphasise IP as a mechanism to boost ST. This policy was not implemented because of the change in government in 2019.

5.2.3 Governmental Failures in Promoting ST

The following section will examine some of the hindrances related to why Sri Lanka was not ready to embrace high-technology protection to push innovation during the post-independence era.

The post-independent period could be categorised as a system that is fragmented into different communicative social subsystems operating on social discourses. Each subsystem deploys its own program so that its members can communicate with each other and perceive social reality from their own perspectives and in their own way. This was amply visible through the introduction of new STPs, action plans, government policies and various R&D institutions and the intense lobbying to promote and develop the ST sector through communicating and interpreting ideas as government initiatives. During this period, the beliefs and preferences of the interpretive communities who shared similar epistemological assumptions were influenced largely to develop ST discourse and promote IP in Sri Lanka.

Although the discourse was moving towards positive development to boost the domestic market and local innovation implementation through these aspirational policies and strategies, some sectors were wholly neglected and other areas experienced limited implementation.[43] The aspirations listed in the policies were well intentioned, but there was no structured implementation plan, with realistic goals capable of being achieved, and resources to bring these goals to fruition.[44] For example, unlike in Singapore, none of these policies specified a strategy to build

---

[39] Ibid ch 9.

[40] Ibid.

[41] Ibid.

[42] Wickremesinghe (2018).

[43] Mendes, *Integrating Intellectual Property* (n 4).

[44] Ibid.

an ecosystem where Sri Lanka could move from low-cost competition in traditional agriculture, manufacturing and services to developing new high-technology clusters and activities.[45]

Ultimately, with each change of government the rhetoric was there but there was no commitment to R&D or provision of public funding, to develop a rich and diverse research ecosystem by introducing strategies such as open innovation, or attracting world-class researchers to the country.[46] In other words, there was a lack of discourse among policymakers about how to implement the competing needs of the STI ecosystem, such as financial support, resources and the investment climate, rather than just stating policy initiatives. Thus, the IP policy was never refined because there was no prominent node to influence the STI ecosystem in Sri Lanka.

The open economic policy failed to attract high-technology industries, unlike in the case of other South Asian countries that opened their economies later, such as Singapore.[47] Although private R&D and local TT activities showed positive growth in some sectors, such as infrastructure, construction (housing and dams, etc.), garments, communication, ceramics, rubber products and information technology through subcontracting, outsourcing or private R&D work,[48] unlike some of the South East Asian countries, Sri Lanka missed opportunities to coordinate government, industry and finance for attracting high-technology industries to stimulate STI. This implies that although there was a shift in the discourse as a result of change in the economic policy, it did not significantly emphasise the ST and IP landscape in Sri Lanka.

The evidence indicates that amid these ambitious ST policies introduced during 2000 to foster innovation, ST did not make the anticipated progress. The Minister of Finance, in the Budget proposal for 2016, stated:

> Our investment in STI has failed to keep up with the growth in GDP. Its impact is evident in the low percentage of high-technology value addition to our manufactured exports (0.9%), poor contribution of patents and research-based services and industries to our economy. This has to change rapidly if our economy is to be led by innovation. We expect high-technology manufactured exports constitutes at least 10% of our exports by 2020.[49]

In this statement, the Minister duly acknowledged the backwardness of patents and research-based services in the economy, thus emphasising the importance of IP to foster economic development. The Minister further said:

> I propose to set up a National Innovation Centre in the Ministry of Science, Technology and Research, which will manage the Innovation Accelerator Fund set up as a revolving fund. It is proposed to allocate Rs. 100 million as seed capital to this centre while another Rs. 3,000 million will also be provided within a period of 3 years.[50]

---

[45] Poh (2016).

[46] Ibid.

[47] De Silva and Amaradasa (2001).

[48] Ibid.

[49] Sri Lanka Parliament (2016).

[50] Ibid.

However, the allocation of Rs 100 million or the additional Rs. 3000 million was never approved by the Cabinet. This shows the negligence of the policymakers in promoting ST in Sri Lanka. Moreover, the discourse on ST came under multiple ministry jurisdictions depending on the issues involved; for example, research in universities may involve three ministries—the Ministry of Higher Education, Technology and Innovation; the MSTR; and the Ministry of Health, Nutrition and Indigenous Medicine—whereas innovation and ST involve the MIC, and the Ministry of Science, Technology and Innovation. Moreover, as discussed in Chap. 3, in 2019, NIPO was moved from MIC to the Ministry of Science, Technology and Innovation without any valid reason and after a few months was transferred back to the original Ministry. This type of haphazard, trial-and-error decisions have pushed the ST sector in Sri Lanka below the expected level of development.

The above difficulty has been documented by the 2015 WIPO Report, prepared by a WIPO consultant on the request of the Sri Lankan Government, which has identified that 44 research institutes were operating under 17 different ministries.[51] During the period, the ministries have been abolished and Ministers demoted from Cabinet positions, and at present, there are 28 Cabinet Ministers and 38 non-Cabinet Ministers that in various ways determine the acceptance of policy and implementation. This conflicting structure of ministries has been documented in the WIPO Report as an impediment to the implementation of decisions on ST.[52]

Within the Sri Lankan context, it was evident from the data and through the policies that the nodal effort to push the STI ecosystem from aspirational goals was missing owing to the lack of political will of the government and the lack of identification of responsible ministries for implementation. Each governmental change brought new policies without substantive support for implementation or considerations of how these policies should be implemented, which leads to the next discourse related to the development of a National Innovation System ('NIS') as a method to resolve the implementation problems identified in the policy discourse.

5.2.4 Does Sri Lanka Have a National Innovation System for IP Stimulation?

Against the above-discussed discourse on ST, an additional discourse has arisen because of the influence of stakeholders such as industry, academics and scientists on the government regarding the development of a NIS. NIS would enable the nation to profit from its own scientific research through an understanding of the linkages between the actors producing, distributing and applying knowledge. The innovative performance of a country depends on how these actors interact with each other as

[51] Mendes, *Integrating Intellectual Property* (n 43) 27.

[52] Ibid.

elements of a collective system of knowledge creation as well as the technologies they use.[53]

Hence, NIS is a set of institutions that separately and collectively collaborate to the dynamic of government policies in order to stimulate the local innovation process.[54] The development of an NIS reflects the interface between the main actors, such as universities, research centres, think tanks, firms, business associations, bridging institutes and, more generally, producers and users of knowledge in the country, both public and private.[55] Hence, an NIS supports knowledge-interaction and commercialisation among various parties, which is critical for building a knowledge-based economy.[56] The linkages such as joint research, personal exchanges, cross-patenting, purchase of equipment, licensing and TT and a variety of other channels are used by actors in knowledge generation via IP within the innovation ecosystem as critical drivers of economic growth. Sri Lanka, as noted in the policy discourse earlier in this chapter, has recognised innovation as a critical driver for development specifically though patents.

Hence, Sri Lankan policymakers have not adopted a pragmatic approach to its STP for IP generation, which is very much lacking in policies. The policies rarely mention IP and the commercialisation of research through patents.[57] To develop a dynamic IP ecosystem, it is important to recognise the growing importance of collaboration with the private sector and university–industry partnerships in bringing research to the market and the positive role of the government in promoting IP through SMEs.[58] This aspect will be discussed later in this chapter. Hence, as discussed earlier, although Sri Lanka put forward many ambitious policies to promote ST, very few policies used IP as a tool for economic development. However, the interviews revealed there are a few like-minded stakeholders and individuals who are continuing the discourse to push IP through dialogue and communication.

In this regard, a Director of COSTI, stated:

> There is an innovation system in Sri Lanka, but nothing happens with innovation. It is still immature. First, we need to build the culture, and once it is in place, the processes we have developed can be implemented. If the culture does not change, the innovation doesn't occur very quickly. Our mindset needs to change. What Sri Lanka needs are not graduates—it needs a leap forward if we are to catch up with other countries. If not, we will remain a developing country and never become a developed country.[59]

A senior academic of the University of Moratuwa made a similar statement:

> Actually, there is no issue with the innovation system. We have a population of 22 million, and the AL [university entrance] population is only 300,000 every year. Out of these people,

---

[53] Govindaraj (2010).

[54] Ibid.

[55] Ibid.

[56] Wijesinha (2011).

[57] Ministry of Technology and Research, Sri Lanka (2022).

[58] Wijesinha (2011).

[59] Interviewee # 1.

just check how many patents are published per annum by the schools. I'm sure it is higher than that of some other countries. The issue is there is no industry to absorb these inventions.[60]

The statement 'there is no industry to absorb these inventions' is one of the root causes for the lack of innovation in Sri Lanka, because without the financial support of industry, innovations cannot be commercialised through patents, licensing and royalties. Although institutions such as COSTI, whose motto is 'research into rupees', were established to coordinate ST, industry contribution is a core factor to commercialise innovation. This aspect will be discussed later in this chapter.

Further, an official of SLIC explained the current status of the innovation sector in Sri Lanka and the steps the Commission has taken to uplift Sri Lankan innovation by facilitating inventors to convert their inventions to innovations[61]:

Actually, we Sri Lankans are not short of creativity; we have some of the best human resources in this country who are born innovators, but, as a society, we are not yet using these talents towards uplifting the economy. For example, there were only about 260 patent applications from Sri Lanka so far in 2020. So, as a society, we should push our innovators to patent their ideas that come out as new inventions to protect their intellectual property rights.

At the same time, as a country, we are not doing well in converting inventions to innovations. If we are to establish a new culture of commercialisation of innovations, society should be ready to accept locally manufactured products instead of imported items. So, as Sri Lankans, we all have a collective responsibility to popularise products manufactured by local industries while taking steps to discourage importation.

Sri Lanka at present is more a service-based economy and converting it to a production-based economy is no easy task. As of now, we only have about 100,000 local industries, which is a very low number compared with the population size. So, we have to establish a proper mechanism to facilitate the process of invention commercialisation. As the inventor's commission, we are doing our best to help innovators to commercialise their new ideas, but we would be able to do more if we have a much more powerful organisational mechanism for facilitating inventors to commercialise their ideas.[62]

Speaking on 'Innovation and the Importance of IP in Moving the Sri Lankan Economy Forward', an official at COSTI commented[63]:

Patents can serve as an important indicator on how much a nation engages in innovation. As an emerging economy if Sri Lanka can reach towards USD 7000 per capita income, there must be visible changes taking place in both the industry and the economy. This is not limited simply to strengthening Sri Lanka's current industries but requires a change in the economic landscape itself. Therefore, Sri Lanka should not be a hub for knowledge transfer but should instead aspire towards knowledge creation as well. Reaching USD 7000 per capita income will not be a difficult target for Sri Lanka to achieve, especially considering the fact that Sri Lanka already has a high literacy level on par with any developed nation. However, what is lacking is the utilisation of this knowledge towards achieving our economic goals.

---

[60] Interviewee # 14.

[61] Kumara (2020).

[62] Interviewee # 14.

[63] De Alwis (2015).

The official further stated:

> So, our mindset needs to be in a different alignment and bring out the creativity spark among all individuals and then looking at the creativity, the ideas should be realised in innovation and the inventions should follow-up, resulting in innovations. It is the innovation that matters to the economy at the end through IP. Having an idea is not sufficient. You need to translate the idea into action.

Therefore, establishing an environment for the acceptance of IP as a basis to innovation for start-ups or SMEs is very important to a developing country such as Sri Lanka. Although proper IP protection to an innovation can add value to a company globally, IP value is not regarded as a value addition to the company. This was stated by the scientist at NSF[64]:

> In 2017, NSF has facilitated 10 PhDs and 10 patents but in the standard accounting system, we don't have a method to calculate the patent value as a profit but only as an investment. It is there as something we have delivered. Hence, for decision-makers, a patent does not have a direct social community impact. But in applied research, one cannot directly convert into rupees and cents. These are intrinsic values.

The statement of the Principal Scientific Officer, NSF, that 'we don't have a method to calculate the patent value as a profit but only as an investment' was reiterated by the DG of WIPO. He stated the perception that a patent is not regarded as an asset is a global challenge that every country is facing, and it is important to find solutions where patents could be considered a collateral in monetary terms.'[65] This is a discourse yet to be recognised.

In contrast, recent government policies introduced from 2009 have emphasised aspirational biotechnology/nanotechnology push as key to the new approach to IP. Acknowledging that Sri Lanka should go forward in high-technology sectors initiatives have taken to develop biotechnology and nanotechnology industries in Sri Lanka. Biotechnology requires sophisticated knowledge and infrastructure, which Sri Lanka started building with investment in a biotechnology park and several scientific institutes such as SLINTEC.[66] The SLINTEC vision is to build a futuristic nanotechnology and science park that has advanced facilities to support all interested stakeholders in pursuing their R&D and to embark on new areas of research relevant to the development of the industrial base in Sri Lanka within an internationally competitive landscape.[67] The nanotechnology push will be discussed later in this chapter.

The documentation of the discourse from the interviews in this book supports that the ST discourse in Sri Lanka is a more of a local story than an international story even with the nanotechnology push. Most ST policies aim to influence local innovation rather than to promote international innovation, via IP and TT. Patents are an

---

[64] Interviewee # 6.

[65] Tang (2021).

[66] SLINTEC (2021).

[67] Ibid.

identifiable primary output of the R&D activity in the sense that more R&D investment will encourage more inventions and more innovations lead to more patents,[68] but as will be discussed later in the chapter, whether patents can be regarded as a driver for economic development in the context of Sri Lanka depends on many mitigating factors that indicate that the international high-technology approach is not sufficiently supported to enable it to be effective. These mitigating factors identify inconsistencies of approaches, a lack of clarity and issues relating to how IP is to be used locally.

5.2.5 Mitigating Factors for Declining Interest in IP in Sri Lanka

From the investigations and interviews conducted for this book, an interesting discourse on the declining interest in IP was raised by interviewees. These include university priorities, and issues about patent ownership, assignment, licensing and drafting and the commercialisation of inventions.

5.2.5.1 University Priorities

University academics had different views regarding the above observations. A senior academic of University of Colombo made it very clear that the priority should be undergraduate education and other activities that are conducted should not affect education. This leads to the second observation that research is secondary and can only be undertaken in an academic's spare time. This thinking differs from that of universities in developed countries where research and publications are identifiable as knowledge impact and this output has priority over teaching. In developed countries, the research output of a university influences its ranking. With regard to inadequate resources and funding, a senior academic at University of Colombo had a different view. She made the following point[69]:

> Not only lack of resources, because when we started, we did not have anything but managed to put something into the market, even though it is not high-tech, with limited funding. The awareness of scientific research has to be improved because some industries are very keen to have strong partnerships with universities. Developed countries find funding through industry collaborations.

This situation is mainly due to the Sri Lankan industry's perception that Sri Lanka lacks the research capability that it needs, which has thus sought to have its research needs met in countries such as India and Singapore.[70]

---

[68] Sener and Saridogan (2011).

[69] Interviewee # 13.

[70] Mendes, *Integrating Intellectual Property* (n 51) 28.

The discourse revealed that since all major universities that engage in research are funded by the government, additional issues, such as ownership of research produced and ways to commercialise it, are issues researchers have little or no knowledge about.

5.2.5.2 Ownership of Patents

Moreover, researchers stated there was little incentive to encourage them to apply for patents owing to the unclear nature of ownership under the provisions of the *Universities Act 1978*. Section 28(1) of this Act establishes each university as a separate legal entity, with broad powers to acquire and dispose of property and, therefore, to have power to enter into commercialisation contracts by which it may, for example, license IP. Section 29 of the Act suggests that each university's major focus is upon teaching and education and receiving fees for this, but the only mention that would relate to commercialisation is the incidental powers provision of s 29(1)(t), namely 'to do all such other acts and things, whether incidental to the powers aforesaid or not, as may be requisite in order to further the objects of the University'.

This incidental power for the university would cover research and commercialisation of research, but the discourse indicates there is confusion because of a lack of understanding of who owns the IP when commercialised. Fortunately, given that all universities are government funded, there is a perception that universities have no mandate to commercialise. In this regard, a senior academic of University of Colombo stated[71]:

> Although we are told to do research and have patents, the Act doesn't have anything on commercialisation. From the 2017 Budget, there is an expectation to change the *Universities Act* about who owns the IP in research. The Act is silent on this aspect.

Owing to this lacuna, there is confusion about the extent to which universities and individual academics are allowed to commercialise the fruits of their research.[72] The ownership and distribution of IPR in academia has been a controversial issue even in the US, the UK and Australia.[73] The lack of clarity regarding IP ownership operates as an obstacle to research collaborations between universities and industry. International best practice is that the ownership of IP arising from research undertaken from research funds granted by the government needs to rest with the grantees of those funds.[74] Ownership gives the power to license others; for example, the NSF presently adopts international best practice by having the ownership of IP arising

[71] Interviewee # 13.

[72] Mendes, *Integrating Intellectual Property* (n 70).

[73] Monotti and Ricketson (2003). See also Monotti (2018).

[74] Mendes, *Integrating Intellectual Property* (n 72).

from research it funds vest in the grant recipient,[75] but the *Universities Act 1978* has not been amended to support this best practice.

Moreover, universities and research institutes need to have an IP policy.[76] An IP policy usually clarifies and prescribes issues of IP ownership, commercialisation choices and options, the distribution of commercialisation revenue among IP inventors and creators, TT arrangements, the manner of disclosure of inventions, the assignment of IP and the criteria for applying for local and international patents.[77]

At present, the University of Colombo, the University of Moratuwa, the University of Peradeniya, the University of Ruhuna and ITI have IP policies. All these policies have clear sections on IP ownership, commercialisation and TT. Moreover, the University of Moratuwa became the first Sri Lankan university to formulate a product commercialisation policy with a view to encourage and incentivise the commercialisation of its IP assets that are being developed for the mutual benefit of this University and industry.[78]

5.3 Assignment, Licensing and Drafting of Patents

Another concern of the researchers was about assigning IP. Most researchers were of the view that when they assign the IP created by them to a foreign assignee, the benefits of the IP would be lost to Sri Lanka.[79] This is correct, but what they were unaware about is that IP assignment is the last commercialisation option and arises because of the lack of capacity to produce or stimulate the local uptake of patents or that unutilised IP represents the loss of potential economic benefits, such as employment opportunities, an increase in the tax base, growth of Sri Lanka's manufacturing sector, export opportunities and foreign revenue opportunities. Further, the researchers did not know that the preferred commercialisation pathway is to license in order to ensure ongoing economic benefits. In this regard, Mendes has argued that the preferred option for Sri Lanka would be a Sri Lankan company that has the

[75] However, it retains the right to require the grantee to grant patent rights to a third party or the NSF in circumstances in which, for instance, the invention was not brought to practical use within a reasonable time or two years, if health or safety issues arose, if public use of the invention was required or if other legal requirements were not satisfied.

[76] Mendes, *Integrating Intellectual Property* (n 74).

[77] Ibid 45–6. The importance of having an IP policy for universities was recognised, and in 2017, a university IP policy workshop was held in Colombo, which was attended by universities, research institutes and private companies. This workshop was sponsored by the US Commercial Law Development Program in coordination with the University Grants Commission of Sri Lanka, NIPO, USPTO, WIPO and the US Embassy Colombo, and was funded by the US State Department and USPTO. Faculty of Engineering, University of Jaffna (Website, 24 April 2017), Faculty staff participated to the Sri Lanka University Intellectual Property Policy Workshop - Faculty of Engineering, University of Jaffna (jfn.ac.lk) .

[78] The Economic Times (2021).

[79] Mendes, *Integrating Intellectual Property* (n 76).

capability to exploit, and desirably, the capability to do so in a way that accrues the greatest economic benefit to the country.[80]

Nevertheless, there will always be occasions when IP assignment will be necessary. For example, the IP may be such that there is no capability in Sri Lanka for its exploitation, nor likely to be. Likewise, in Australia, often local companies do not have the capital or the scale to commercialise, certainly not without government support. For example, to develop the mRNA vaccines, the Australian government has allocated AU$5 million from an AU$50 million mRNA fund to the Monash Institute of Pharmaceutical Sciences.[81] However, IP gives IP holders something to bargain with. If this is the situation, then, for practical reasons, IP assignment should be considered the only available strategy or even the preferred strategy.[82]

A senior academic from the University of Moratuwa confirmed the above statement[83]:

> Sadly, the policymaking people in universities, who are not inventors, do not know the difference between licensing and assigning. Many developed universities go for licensing owing to two reasons. One is they will give the technology but will hold the ownership. But in assigning, you give the whole technology to some institution and lose the opportunity to develop it. Therefore, universities always try to go for licensing since they want to keep a hold on the technology. But the industry knows the difference and is simply not providing the correct information.

The lack of patent drafting skills among researchers in Sri Lanka undermines innovation.[84] The drafting of patent claims is a highly skilled and specialised task. For effective patent claims to be drafted, ideally, the drafter should have scientific skills in the field of science, but researchers lack the technical skills required for drafting patents. Assistance is being developed at present through the establishment of TISC, which will provide free service on patent drafting in every university and research institute in Sri Lanka.

5.4 Commercialisation of Innovations

The local discourse also reveals that researchers did not understand how commercialisation of research could be achieved through the university, which raised discussions that university research was haphazard and universities themselves did not understand how to coordinate and manage research for commercialisation. The WIPO Report identified the lack of technology management offices ('TMOs') to assist in commercialisation.[85] TMOs play the critical role of bringing research outcomes from

---

[80] Ibid.

[81] Dunstan and Choahan (2021).

[82] Ibid.

[83] Interviewee # 14.

[84] Moir (2021).

[85] Mendes, *Integrating Intellectual Property* (n 79) 43–45.

the lab to the market and, as a result, benefitting the community and the economy.[86] TMOs are the interface between researchers and industry, which facilitate research collaborations, research alliances and commercialisation agreements.[87] Without a TMO to undertake these tasks, research remains research, without any benefit to the community and without any economic benefits being realised.[88] Hence, a TMO acts as a crucial node to communicate with other actors in the research community to facilitate R&D. TMOs are not yet established in Sri Lanka, which is a bottleneck for the commercialisation of innovations.

5.5 Commercialisation Readiness

In the Sri Lankan context, in determining the type of research to focus on, one criterion could be the time that it takes to reach commercialisation readiness. Information technology, for example, as a rule, has a very rapid time to commercialisation readiness and to the point of economic impact. Protection is often more through first-mover advantage than codified IP. Sri Lanka's information technology and business process outsourcing sectors are among the country's most dynamic sectors, which have tripled exports and doubled the workforce in a little more than five years, from 2015 to 2020.[89] Hence, to gain positive economic impact in this field, that is, from the time of conception, through to R&D, the entire process should be completed within a very short duration, that is, in one to two years. However, due to the bottlenecks in the Sri Lankan system, sometimes, the time frame to commercialisation readiness is difficult to achieve. For example, commercialisation readiness is delayed owing to the lack of access to equipment, delays in the NIPO process,[90] prolonged processes to approve funds and delays in obtaining special types of state-of-the-art chemicals.[91]

5.6 Examination of Mitigating Factors to the Effectiveness of Patents in Sri Lankan Discourse

The mitigating factors identified in the local discourses indicate a bifurcation of rhetoric between government policy that is focused on high-technology approaches for enabling development, and local discourses that identify Sri Lanka has not reached a stage for high-technology protection. This is further demonstrated by an examination of who has applied for patents and registered, since the end of the civil war in

[86] Ibid.

[87] Ibid.

[88] Ibid 43.

[89] International Trade Administration (2021).

[90] Interviewee # 5.

[91] Interviewee # 6.

2009. Patent applications data thus are a proxy of what investors and industry think or perceive that the patent system provides.[92] Chap. 3 outlined the difficulties experienced with the patent system, whereas in this chapter, the analysis focuses on the actors identified in the local application data as those who are utilising the system and the associated reasons. Are the applicants and registrations predominately international applicants seeking high-level rights for foreign industries or does the analysis tell a uniquely local story disjointed from the international and government policy rhetoric? For this analysis, statistical data for 2010–20 were used.[93]

5.6.1 Local Patent Applications and Registrations

Figure 5.1 provides an overview of the number of patent applications and patent registrations lodged in Sri Lanka. The number of filings has increased from 460 in 2010 to 600 in 2020, which, by the standards of the developed world, is not large, and supports interviewees' comments that the knowledge and use of patents for commercialisation by industry is not prominent. There is an upward trend, given that patent applications have increased over the period.[94] The anomaly here is a slight decline in 2011 to 429, which may be attributed to the economic slowdown that swept across every region in the world owing to the 2008 global financial crisis.[95] The discourses reveal that the annual fluctuations in patent application numbers can be attributed to the industry's underutilisation of the patent system.[96] In addition, the overall increase in the number of patent applications may be attributable to the knowledge diffusion by local actors, such as COSTI, TISC and SLIC, and collaborations arising from government policies and initiatives, which will be discussed later in this chapter.

Second, with regard to the patent registration trends, as can be observed from Fig. 5.1, in 2010, there were 504 grants, which is the highest number recorded during 2010–2020. However, the number of patent grants declined sharply in this period, which, according to the discourses, may be attributable to the difficulties revealed by interviewees in using the patent system and the NIPO.[97]

Although patent statistics are used as a proxy for knowledge creation, the discourse in Sri Lanka indicates that because most forms of innovations do not meet the international standards for patenting, domestic firms pursue other methods, such as 'imitative' or 'dependant technological strategies', rather than relying on patents.[98] Hewage's study conducted in 2011–2012 has confirmed that many industries in

[92] Falvey and Foster (2006).

[93] National Intellectual Property Office (2022); Also see, 2018 National Science Foundation (2018).

[94] See discussion of the problems in the patent office and registration system in Sect. 3.6 as possible explanations for the reduction in patent applications.

[95] Hewage (2015).

[96] Ibid.

[97] See Chap. 3 in this book.

[98] Hewage (2015).

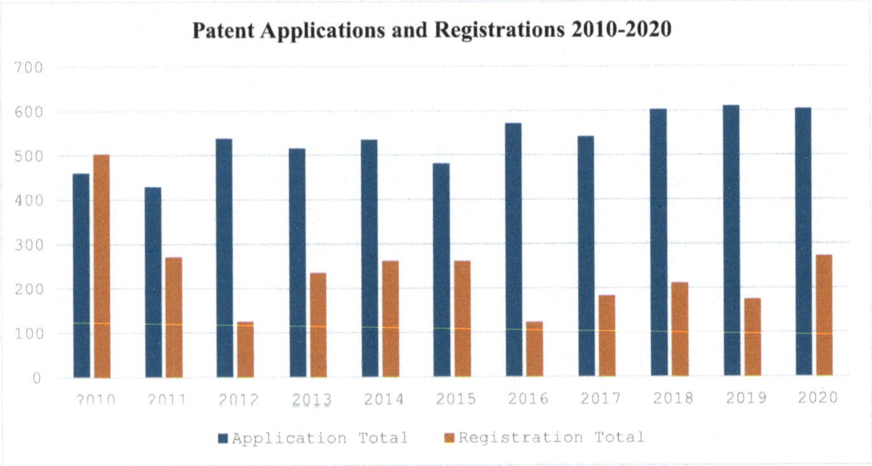

Fig. 5.1 Patent applications and registrations 2010–2020. *Source* Based on statistics from NIPO, Sri Lanka

Sri Lanka often use alternative mechanisms (non-IP strategies), such as lead-time advantage, secrecy and complementary sales, rather than patents.[99] The study further indicated that most small industries in Sri Lanka do not consider patent protection as something that is important or necessary for their business owing to the level of innovations they create,[100] and that most patents granted in Sri Lanka are for domestic products in low-technology areas, such as mechanical, electronics, agricultural tools and equipment, domestic appliances, and food and beverages.[101]

Further, this study revealed that in the SME sector, 59% were not aware of patents. Out of the remaining 41% who were aware of patents, 56% did not use patents and only 44% used patents in their business.[102] Thus, only 18.04% of the SME sector use patents in their business, and this includes not only the use of local patents but also the licensing of foreign patents. This study is of particular interest because the international discourse promoted by WIPO has targeted the adoption of IP (particularly patents) by SMEs, but this has not been adopted by the local SME industry. The low level of patent applications and patent registrations implies a lack of enthusiasm, confidence and awareness of the patent system. This further reiterates that the patent system has not contributed to Sri Lanka's development owing to a lack of discourse between the two sectors because the innovation system does not cater to the Sri Lankan industries. The reason for this lack of engagement between the two sectors was the absence of a prominent node to influence IP in the SME sector in Sri Lanka. This will be examined later in this chapter.

---

[99] Ibid 108.

[100] Ibid.

[101] Ibid 106.

[102] Ibid 108–9.

Interestingly, as in the Sri Lankan context, the Australian Patent Accessibility Review of 2021 also concluded that Australian SMEs do not make much use of the patent system, and it appears that they do not export much IP,[103] which may indicate this is not just a Sri Lankan issue but an SME-specific problem internationally. Moir revealed similar findings for developed countries,[104] and she concluded that a patent policy does not confer net economic benefits. She further stated that in the US, other than in the chemical and pharmaceutical industries, small firms have reported the patent system does not induce innovation.[105] These studies found that the most common reasons that firms in developed countries choose patents are to prevent copying, block rivals, prevent infringement suits, and in negotiating access to other firms' patented technologies.[106] As discussed in Chap. 3 and will be discussed in this chapter, IP lawmaking in Sri Lanka has not reached a stage to use these strategies as reasons for having a patent policy. Hence, as will be discussed in the following sections, it is not surprising that firms in Sri Lanka are reluctant to use patents and hence adopt a low-technology approach to IP.

5.6.2 Who is Applying for Patents in Sri Lanka?

A further discourse illuminates the patent discussion by examining who is applying for patents, namely, are the filings by local actors (resident applicants) located in Sri Lanka or international corporations, filing to protect their international (non-resident) patent interests.

Figure 5.2 illustrates the trends in resident[107] and non-resident[108] patent applications in Sri Lanka. Resident (domestic) and non-resident (foreign) are defined by the country of origin of the application. Phirouzabadi and Nikzad concluded that on the basis of the close relationship between resident and non-resident patents and GDP, countries could be categorised as developed, mid-developed and developing.[109] This implies that annual patent filings may be an indicator of optimism about the strength of a jurisdiction's patent system and its underlying economy.

How does this relate to Sri Lanka? According to Fig. 5.2, from 2010 to 2016, except in 2013, resident patent filings have declined compared with international filings. However, from 2017 to 2020, resident patent filings have increased from 282 to 351, but international filings have declined slightly from 260 to 253. The reason

[103] Mortley (2021).

[104] Moir (2013).

[105] Ibid.

[106] Ibid.

[107] A resident filing in the IP data refers to an application filed by applicants at their national IP office.

[108] Similarly, a non-resident filing refers to an application registered by an applicant at a foreign IP office.

[109] Phirouzabadi and Nikzad (2013).

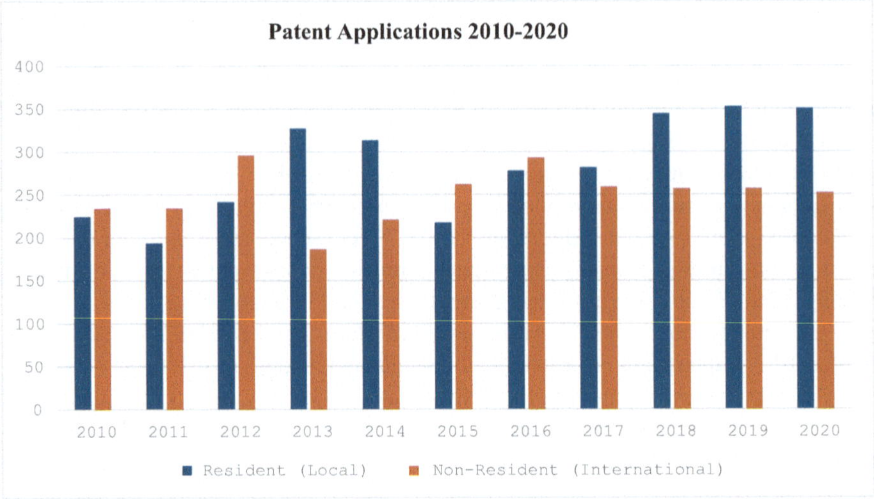

Fig. 5.2 Patent applications 2010–2020. *Source* Based on statistics from NIPO, Sri Lanka

for the increase in resident filings could be the initiatives introduced through TISCs that encouraged local innovators to draft patent claims free of charge rather than by hiring lawyers for large fees. However, the increase was not a real outcome that is expected from a knowledge society, for there were no data to evaluate the nature of patents granted in terms of whether or not they were scientific and whether or not they were commercial.[110]

However, the overall majority of patent applications in Sri Lanka are filled by foreign applicants. Does this mean that the majority of foreign entrepreneurs and inventors want to file patents in Sri Lanka because the Sri Lankan market has become attractive to foreign patent holders for commercialising their inventions or is it a defensive strategy to cement rights to prevent infringement? Hewage's study suggested that non-resident patent filing can be interpreted as defensive patenting to prevent possible infringement by local firms.[111]

5.6.2.1 Patent Registration

As evident from Fig. 5.3, foreign patent grants exceed domestic patent grants. For example, in 2020, the total number of foreign patents granted was 226, of which 204 patent registrations were by way of the *PCT* and only 22 by other countries, but these NIPO figures do not provide details of the number of foreign grants given to Sri Lankan overseas.[112]

---

[110] Hewage (2015).

[111] Ibid 101.

[112] NIPO Statistics (n 93).

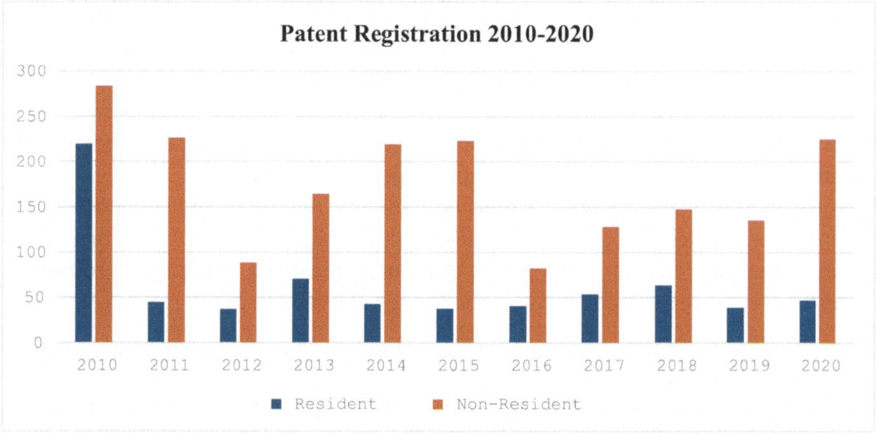

Fig. 5.3 Patent registration 2010–2020. *Source* Based on statistics from NIPO, Sri Lanka

Resident patent grants, in contrast, have not exceeded 100, except in 2010, which is very low by international standards. The reason for this low number, as discussed earlier, is the number of rejections of patent applications. For example, the rejection rate of patent applications in 2018–2020 was considerably high about which an official of NIPO, stated: 'The main reason for this is the inventions do not satisfy the patentable criteria under the IP Act.'[113]

However, the increase in foreign registrations do provide indicators about development in Sri Lanka. First, the increase implies that the Sri Lankan patent system is attractive for foreign patent holders. Second, foreign patent registrations may provide an instrument of TT to Sri Lanka.[114] TT is beneficial to the host country because, for example, if an inventor in a foreign country files a patent application in Sri Lanka it signals willingness to deploy that technology in the country.[115] That means a patent provides a direct (licensing) as well as an indirect (data in patent application) source of TT. Patents may be used exclusively on a standalone basis but often are a means to structure cross-licensing and collaborative ventures.[116] On occasions when it is defensive, the patent holder may need the impetus of financial incentives or performance requirements, for instance, to partner with local firms. This aspect will be discussed later in the chapter.

In contrast, the patent statistics have shown there is a significant percentage of independent inventions in the national patent system of Sri Lanka. Of the total resident patent applications, 77% were submitted by independent inventors. It indicates an increase of up to 80% and 85% in 2017 and 2018, respectively. Hewage concluded that the reason for this increase in the individual patent applications was the application

[113] Interviewee # 23.

[114] Hewage (2015).

[115] Ibid.

[116] Gilson (1999).

fee, which is double for patents filled by a company.[117] Individual inventors have been the driving force of the Sri Lankan innovation system.[118] Approximately 75% of the local independent inventors who were the award winners of SLIC[119] have been recognised to be among the best inventors in the world.[120] However, these award winners have not achieved commercial success because, as stated earlier, the business community in Sri Lanka has not supported local inventors.[121]

However, the data collection for this book revealed that some independent innovators are not interested in registering patents or pursuing marketing of their inventions because of several reasons. An official at Dilmah Tea Pvt Ltd made the following interesting revelation about the reluctance to register patents[122]:

> I have invented a Bio Cha machine because we have a problem with our tea waste. Bio Cha is a soil amendment. Our soil is not doing well at the moment because decades of unsustainable agricultural practices have deteriorated it. So, the plants that grow on those soils are not healthy and not doing well, and with tea waste, we designed an equipment to burn this continuously and we are trying to revive the soils using Bio Cha.

The official further stated[123]:

> Bio Cha was invented using thermodynamics, a subject in which I have a degree from Colombo University. Thermodynamics is about getting heat into that chamber, which is my area. Finally, we managed to succeed and registered the patent. If anyone is interested and wants to try, we are willing to give it free of charge. If somebody gets the same patent, then that person may prevent others—that is the only reason that we have patented it. There are a couple of other things we have done, but we are not applying for a patent. We have no interest in patents. If you want to protect something, not taking a patent is the best you can do. For me, it's a double-edged sword. Many people hide their components and lodge the patent, which doesn't make sense. Patents are picked up from the NIPO, and it goes out.

The above statements indicate the level of distrust in the innovation community. As an innovator, he does not trust NIPO or the disclosure criteria in the patent system owing to the fear of industrial espionage. This is a serious lacuna in the system that will demoralise innovators. He said that patent registration is not performed properly at NIPO and that some patented inventions have been manufactured many times worldwide.[124] This implies that NIPO does not check the international registries properly, and apparently, the registered patents can be considered technically invalid. As discussed in Chap. 3, this discussion reveals that NIPO has become the biggest bottleneck to foster IP and innovators in Sri Lanka, and until the system is streamlined, the patent system will not influence an innovation culture. This is not only because

---

[117] Hewage (2015).

[118] Wickramasinghe and Ahamed (2012).

[119] Sri Lanka Inventors Commission (2022).

[120] Ibid.

[121] Dasanayaka et al. (2020).

[122] Interviewee # 3.

[123] Ibid.

[124] Ibid.

local protection is absent, but also because the patents are not technically secure enough to assign/license to an industry partner.

The interviews have indicated a lack of discourse between innovators and industry, and of innovators with focal nodes, such as NIPO, which, significantly, does not seem to be connected with COSTI and the STP. It also illustrates that the discourse is not solely about knowledge creation but involves additional issues about the impact and diffusion of knowledge and not just that the patent system does not appeal to the local industries as an indicative tool for knowledge creation. Thus, discourse theory illuminated the wider debate occurring in the community about the relevance of patents and patent statistics as an indicator of innovation and that innovations do occur but are not always registered. This is because the policy has had an unrealistic focus on locals making 'breakthrough' inventions (e.g. the push for nanotechnology) when it would be more useful to strengthen the collaboration, transfer and spin-off aspects and considerations that low-technology approaches to IP can advance. To advance this discussion, a brief overview of the current Sri Lankan industrial sector is required.

5.7 Overview of Sri Lankan Industrial Sector

Sri Lanka's outward-oriented economy has historically been based on the export of agricultural products, including tea, rubber, coconut and spices. Currently, these still account for a large proportion of Sri Lanka's economic activity, with agricultural products contributing approximately 21% to GDP and providing employment to 38% of Sri Lanka's workforce.[125] The largest exports by value are of apparel (~18%), followed by tea (~13%). In addition, refined oil, gems and processed agricultural products are also exported.[126]

Over time, Sri Lanka's manufacturing and service sectors have grown. These include mining, energy, transportation and construction. Tea, rubber and coconut accounted for 90% of export earnings in the 1950s, but in 2021 accounted less than16%, and manufactured products accounted for 1% of export earnings in the 1950s but in 2021 accounted for more than 60%. The manufacturing sector contributes 19% to Sri Lanka's GDP and employs 17% of the workforce.[127] A large part of R&D activities in Sri Lanka relate to traditional industries and low-technology manufacturing, such as the apparel industry, and rubber-based products for export. Even the apparel sector is predominately focused on low value-added products that appeal to mass-market consumers rather than elite customers. Thus, Dasanayaka described this as technological development to a low equilibrium trap

---

[125] Central Bank Sri Lanka (2021).

[126] Ibid.

[127] Ibid.

position.[128] Hence, most technologies are limited to assisting the existing technologies in improving process productivity and diversification or improving the quality of existing products, and not for developing innovative value-added products.[129]

Further, most of these industries are labour intensive and use imported raw materials where little value addition is provided through technology. The Chief Executive Officer ('CEO') of Micro Ltd Mr Lawrence Perera stated that importing technology is cheaper in Sri Lanka because of the size of the market.[130] Although Sri Lanka has the capabilities to design new technology, investing in new technology is not viable in the Sri Lankan context, which means its technological output is low.[131]

However, the government policy statements focus on developing a fast-growing information technology export sector, including software development, knowledge process outsourcing and information-technology-enabled services. Dasanayaka has argued that even with this focus, the country still lags far behind its more dynamic South Asia counterparts, due to the lack of a proper technology policy framework integrated with an industrial development framework.[132]

Hence, if Sri Lanka wants to become progressively competitive in the innovation era, it will first have to focus on strengthening business innovation and commercialising R&D, including creating a customised platform to facilitate the integration of the capabilities of research institutions with companies and the private sector agencies to deliver innovative solutions to industry.[133] In this regard, an IP policy will help to create a framework that incentivises value creation, particularly through patents within a STP.

5.7.1 Does the SME Sector Promote IP in Sri Lanka?

The Government of Sri Lanka recognises SMEs as the backbone of the economy, for this sector accounts for more than 75% of the total number of enterprises as well as for 45% of the employment and 52% of the GDP. Within the Sri Lankan context, the SME sector is regarded as not merely a sector for 'protection and promotion' but, more importantly, a driving force for 'growth and development.'

The government started focusing on SMEs in 1952 following the World Bank's suggestion that it should develop SMEs rather than promote large industries[134] In the 1960s, the government focused on developing cottage industries and SMEs for the dual purposes of saving foreign exchange through import substitution and increasing local employment. It was not until 1977 with the post-liberalised economy that the

[128] Dasanayaka (2013).

[129] Perera and Dasanayaka (2004).

[130] Interviewee # 9.

[131] Ibid.

[132] Dasanayaka (2013).

[133] Poh (2016).

[134] Institute of Policy Studies (2002).

SME sector was developed to drive the export market and thus became the backbone of the economy.[135] Subsequent to this development, a multitude of government agencies and private sector banks were established to provide the necessary institutional support to the sector.

Nevertheless, the SME sector has lacked a regulatory framework. In 2017, the National Policy Framework for SME Development recognised the importance of R&D as a powerful process to develop modern technologies through increased partnership between industries, research institutes and universities for developing cost-effective technologies.[136] However, the document does not specify how this is to be implemented in the industry, unlike the South Korean policy that has developed IP through the SME sector.[137] Many interviewees[138] believed that because Sri Lanka's well-established SME sector could utilise innovation in a broader sense, the current lack of discourse on policy implementation mechanics between government and industry has resulted in yet another missed opportunity in the Sri Lankan system. This suggest that government as a governing node has failed to use the SME sector to develop IP in Sri Lanka.

5.7.2 Commercialisation of Innovations in Different Sectors

The discussion above does not mean that innovation does not occur in Sri Lankan industry. The NSF handbook on the National Research and Development Survey divides the sectors relevant to innovation as Government, R&D Institutes; Business Enterprises (combining all businesses including SMEs) and Higher Education. An examination of the most recent data available, that is, for 2018, indicate that more innovation has been occurring than suggested by the aforementioned number of patent applications and registrations.

The National Research and Development Survey has a broader interpretation of innovation, which includes the development of design prototypes, import substitutes and new products services and processes, and improvements to existing products and services. Table 5.1 presents the aggregate figures for each sector category in each relevant innovation type and the total identified for each innovation type. The data in Table 5.1 demonstrate that business enterprises may not be patenting their developments for various reasons, as discussed above, but are producing new products, services and processes, improving existing products and developing import substitutes, all of which indicate there is a grassroot ability to innovate, even if IP is not the primary method of implementation. However, the data in Table 5.1

---

[135] Ibid.

[136] Ministry of Industry and Commerce (Sri Lanka) (2017).

[137] OECD (2020). Korean delegations visited Sri Lanka a few times on the invitation of Sri Lanka's Ministry of Industry and Commerce to provide advice on methods to develop IP through SMEs.

[138] Interviewee # 1; Interviewee # 14.

Table 5.1 Sector-wise Innovation: 2018

Innovation type	Government R&D institutes (% of total)	Business enterprises (% of total)	Higher education sector (% of total)	Total (total %)
Development of new products/services/processes	97 (6)	1499 (91)	42 (3)	1638 (100)
Existing products/services significantly improved	86 (3)	2645 (96)	15 (1)	2746 (100)
New plant varieties/hybrids developed	24 (24)	75 (75)	1 (1)	100 (100)
Import substitutes developed	18 (9)	189 (90)	3 (1)	210 (100)
Design/prototypes developed	21 (7)	284 (89)	14 (4)	319 (100)

Source National Research and Development Survey of Sri Lanka, 2018

confirm the belief expressed by interviewees[139] that collaboration between sectors is vital because except in the areas of commercialisation for new plant varieties or hybrids, the government was not a dominant force in the utilisation or development of innovations.

Compared with the figures for developed and developing countries, these figures are not at all encouraging. For example, 6% of the development of new product and services was by the government and 3% by the higher education sector, which is very disappointing. The lack of innovation in the government sector is confirmed by most interviewees in this study, who stated the reason is the lack of funding and appropriate policy implementation. In contrast, in Singapore, public sector research institutes have grown significantly through increased government funding.[140]

In contrast, Table 5.2 sheds light on the commercialisation of innovations by sectors. Not all innovations have been commercialised. Business enterprises are the highest contributors and utilisers of innovations, and the government and the higher education sector are not fulfilling the perceived potential that their R&D should provide towards developing the economy.

Sri Lanka is categorised as a lower middle-level innovation system in the Global Innovation Index[141] because of its low-level ST activity, limited science–industry linkages, low absorptive capacity of firms and constrained entrepreneurship. The low level of ST activities has negative effects on localised R&D, TT through technological and commercial innovations, FDI and IP licensing. These aspects are important innovation indicators, which will be discussed in the following section.

---

139 Ibid.

140 Poh (2016).

141 WIPO (2021).

Table 5.2 Commercialisation of innovation by sectors: 2018

Innovation type	Government R&D institutes (% of total)	Business enterprises (% of total)	Higher Education sector (% of total)	Total (total %)
Commercialisation of new products/services/processes	32 (3)	1058 (96)	16 (1)	1106 (100)
Commercialisation of improved existing products/services/processes	26 (2)	1252 (97)	11 (1)	1289 (100)
Commercialisation of new plant varieties/Hybrids	42 (52)	39 (48)	0 (0)	81 (100)
Commercialisation of import substitutes	4 (6)	63 (88)	4 (6)	71 (100)
Commercialisation of design/prototypes	10 (10)	94 (89)	1 (1)	105 (100)

Source National Research and Development Survey of Sri Lanka, 2018

5.8 Bottlenecks to Local R&D

The high-end value-added industries that utilise and foster IP are underdeveloped in Sri Lanka. This is a factor that interviewees recognise as a prominent bottleneck to fostering innovation, but the discourse identifies that the elements of knowledge impact and diffusion are interconnected stories about how to encourage and connect industry with knowledge developers. Universities and higher education centres are regarded as the repositories for the development of knowledge, as well as industry itself. The difficulty in assessing the ability of a society to innovate lies in capturing the communication and knowledge diffusion between these repositories—the one of knowledge and solutions and the other of problems requiring resolution. This fact was reiterated by many stakeholders. A scientist at John Keels,[142] stated[143]:

> Innovators should have some kind of nexus between inventions and industry. How to bring this invention out? That is where we are not doing very well. As I said, there are many people who are coming here annually for inventors' commission exhibition, and we hear about many good inventions, but we never hear that these things come into the market. Why? May be a lack of knowledge, a lack of facilities, no person to support: no entrepreneur, no company or no industry to support to this inventor. The inventor sells this for $3–4,000, which they think is a lot of money, but [do not realise] they could earn royalties forever [by licensing].

[142] John Keels Holdings PLC, Sri Lanka, http://www.keels.com, John Keels Holdings PLC is Sri Lanka's premier diversified conglomerate company focused on seven industrial sectors, including logistics, tourism and transport, and investment with a portfolio of international clients, MNCs, SMEs, educational institutions, NGOs and governmental organisation.

[143] Interviewee # 5.

He further stated that the underlying reason is the lack of collaboration between inventors and industry[144]:

> There is a trust issue and a lost in translation issue. Scientists are not in a situation to explain an idea to a businessperson. There is a knowledge difference between the two, and their vantage points are different. They can't understand each other, so there is a lost in translation issue.

5.9 Interactions Between University and Industry: Problems and Successes

RN Weerasinghe and AK Jayawardane's study of university–industry partnerships conducted in 2018 found SMEs are reluctant to visit universities for knowledge exchange for they are unaware of the university capabilities and believe that universities are unable to solve industrial problems.[145] Moreover, V Wickramasinghe and K Malik's study claimed that universities and industries in Sri Lanka 'speak different languages' and are disconnected, not knowing what they can offer each other.[146]

A senior academic from the University of Moratuwa made a similar statement[147]:

> The first issue is the industry, not the education or the innovation system. We don't have a mature industry that needs innovation. In other developed countries, the industry brings the money, and we provide the intellectual knowledge; finally, the product is owned by both parties based on a certain percentage. But in Sri Lanka, the situation is sad because we don't have a developed industrial base in the country. And on the other side, we have an SME sector that is looking for options. They are looking for jobs and new ideas. We have about 2,000 patents and then we have an SME sector. But there is no link created for communications between the two. This is a big issue in the country.
>
> Second, most industries don't understand what an innovation is. We have a lot of companies, both local and international. International companies know about IP, but local companies are not aware of what IP is and how to deal with the professionals or the intellectuals in the country. This is a big issue. Also, we don't have a good R&D culture in industries. Even though most of the companies have an R&D section, those are not really performing.
>
> The third is the trust issue. The SMEs do not trust the inventor, and the inventor does not trust the real people who can pump in money. This must be broken up. If we can do this, in a few years we can reach the goals. Because there are many inventions being created.

The Chairman of NASTEC made a disturbing statement about the lack of support for local innovators[148]:

> After getting the innovation certificate, they don't get sufficient support from the industry, and after that, they don't know where to take it. Even though we have innovations done by local innovators, most of these innovations are not supported by the local industry, but foreign

---

[144] Ibid.

[145] Weerasinghe and Jayawardane (2018).

[146] Wickramasinghe and Malik (2018).

[147] Interviewee # 14.

[148] Interviewee # 7.

industries have approached some of these innovators. For example, Manju Gunawardena of SLINTEC who innovated a bulb. No local industries were interested, but an Indian industry has approached him.

The non-recognition of local innovation by local industry is a matter of concern and confirms a lack of engagement between creators and users. Even when an innovation is a success, it is produced or sold overseas, for local industry does not support the local product. The absence of a prominent local node to push local innovation suggest a failure in the IP eco-system.

Over the past 10 years, studies by Sridharan Govindaraj in 2010,[149] RN Weerasinghe, AKW Jayawardane and AL Deshani in 2016[150] and C Wijesinghe et al. in 2018[151] have examined the lack of university–industry partnerships and its implications for supporting or fostering advances in high-technology IP. These studies identified not only cultural issues, such as a lack of trust, a lack of communication channels, university management directives, academic or student culture, and a lack of personal relationships with industry, but also structural issues in industry and universities, such as a lack of funding and infrastructure for research and a lack of consistency in government policy. These studies identified the importance of university industry partnerships the support for high-technology IP, but the implementation of this required a discourse with each actor within the universities and the industry, which currently has not succeeded owing to the difficulties identified.

The methods identified in the international discourse to foster stronger university industry partnership relationships include the development of patent information centres. A former WIPO official stressed the importance of establishing patent information centres in universities to foster innovation[152]:

> We wanted a network of patent information centres to be established in Sri Lanka, but we failed in doing so because NIPOs didn't encourage WIPO to establish these centres in the universities, particularly in the University of Moratuwa where most of the inventions are created. I see the great potential in getting the university linking up with industry and entrepreneurs—those who are in a position to provide venture capital for these things. This is not happening in Sri Lanka.

The present research has identified a governing nodal failure by NIPO (discussed in Chap. 3) to be a primary linkage between universities and industry, but as will be discussed in this chapter, when a nodal blockage occurs, other local actors develop separate systems of communication and 'workaround solutions.' WIPO has been involved in establishing TISCs at universities, and universities as actors within the local discourse have also been active, as the following section identified grassroot developments and advances in communications have been fostered locally, through stakeholders such as the universities themselves, together with public–private partnerships, the government, industry organisations and private company initiatives.

---

149 Govindaraj (2010).

150 Weerasinghe et al. (2016).

151 Wijesinghe et al. (2020).

152 Interviewee # 21.

This book identifies that the local discourse is encouraging IP development. These stakeholders will be examined next.

5.10 Stakeholder Alliances in ST

The following section highlights the good practice examples from stakeholder alliances in Sri Lanka's ST ecosystem that push innovation and IP.[153]

5.10.1 Universities Initiatives

Universities have developed methods to commercialise and interact with industry, and the local discourse has highlighted the following examples.

5.10.1.1 The University of Moratuwa

The University of Moratuwa's successful engagement with industry has resulted in it registering many patents beneficial to Sri Lanka.[154] It has six research centres wholly funded by industry that undertake industrially relevant applied research.[155]

5.10.1.2 University of Colombo

The University of Colombo established the Colombo Science and Technology Cell in 2013, with funding that it received from the World Bank for an initial three-year period, but this Cell is currently self-funding through contract research with industry.[156] It is a joint venture company limited by guarantee established by seven science departments[157] in the university and is intended to act as the interface with industry. It focuses on creating opportunities for research collaborations between the university and industry. It hopes over time to extend its operations to include a TMO to undertake assessments of IP outcomes arising from the research undertaken at the

[153] Mendes, *Integrating Intellectual Property* (n 85) 43–5.

[154] University of Moratuwa, Intellectual Property Advisory Committee, *Patent Databases: Patents Granted,* Patent Granted | University of Moratuwa (uom.lk).

[155] Dialog-UoM Mobile Communication Research Laboratory, DSI-UoM Rubber Production and Process Development Incubator, High Performance Computing Laboratory, Premium International-UoM Research Laboratory for Biomedical Technologies, UoM-Cargills Food Process Development Incubator, Zone 24 × 7-UoM Electronic Systems Research Laboratory.

[156] Mendes, *Integrating Intellectual Property* (n 153).

[157] DepartmentS of Chemistry, Mathematics, Nuclear Sciences, Physics, Plant Science, Statistics and Zoology.

university and to seek out commercialisation partners.[158] A similar company was also formed to serve the similar needs and objectives of the School of Computing at the University of Colombo.[159]

The Colombo Science and Technology Cell, with the support of industry, was successful in launching Bioclean[160] (the first and only biodegradable toilet bowl cleaner in Sri Lanka) in 2016; Mosguard, a non-sticky and synthetic free insect repellent lotion in 2017[161]; the first ever 3D printer in Sri Lanka in 2018; and filter technology developed in Sri Lanka that uses aluminium waste to treat wastewater in the textile industry.[162]

However, a senior academic at University of Colombo stated that all these ventures are licence agreements but no-IP[163] is attached to these products and processes.[164] Thus, these successes are grassroot collaborations, which indicates that the local community discusses and develops solutions that do not mirror the requirements of the demanded high-technology IP in the government rhetoric or international discourse. The interaction and local discourse identify the discussions and solutions are low-technology ones.

5.10.1.3 University of Peradeniya

The University of Peradeniya has an Engineering Design Centre within its Faculty of Engineering. It was established in 1993 with funding from the Asian Development Bank and is now self-funding.[165] Its mission is to strengthen its R&D capabilities by forming partnerships with industry, focusing on the national interest. It aims to use the latest advanced technologies for engineering design, manufacturing, material and product testing and for conducting short courses and certificate courses, while serving as the commercial arm of the Faculty of Engineering and as the bridge between the Faculty and industries.[166] The commercialisation of products and processes will be the final project outcome.

---

158 Mendes, *Integrating Intellectual Property* (n 156).

159 Ibid.

160 *Daily FT* (2016). See also Science and Technology Cell (2016).

161 *Daily FT* (2007).

162 Al Circle (2019).

163 Interviewee # 13. The meaning of the the term no-IP is that the products and processors are not patentable. Hence, everyone can use the IP underlying the products free of charge.

164 Ibid.

165 Perdeniya (2021).

166 Ibid.

5.10.1.4 Industrial Technology Institute

Another example of close engagement between a research organisation and industry is the ITI, a wholly owned government research institute that functions under the MSTR. ITI has a broad mandate in its IP policy to encourage and sustain creativity and undertakes much of its work at the request of industrial partners, to assist them in finding technical solutions to problems.[167] ITI performs R&D in the areas of food and nutrition, environment, materials, natural products and traditional knowledge, which have societal value for the local industry and also explores the areas of biotechnology and nanotechnology.[168] Over the past five years, more than 20 technologies developed by ITI have been commercialised successfully in the food, herbal, material, environmental and biotechnology areas.[169] ITI's output has significantly improved during 2010–19 in terms of annual revenue, publications in refereed journals, research communications, major technologies transferred and awards received.[170]

This discussion indicates that universities are reaching out to industry and industry is connecting to universities, but these advances are still in their infancy and require nurturing to enable ST development. This discourse reinforces that, presently, the demands for industry and the interactions with universities confirm low-technology IP is being considered rather than high-technology IP.

Nevertheless, the local discourse is not solely about universities and the higher education sector's interaction with industry—the government has also been involved through policies and initiatives identified earlier in this chapter and has established public–private partnerships and partnerships with industry organisations. In addition, the local discourse identifies a private company initiative in the car industry as an example of the IP discourse occurring in the wider STI sector at a local level. These three will be examined next.

5.10.2 Public–Private Partnerships

As discussed earlier, discourse in the area of knowledge does not conveniently divide between those that produce and those that use; rather, it is a conversation between individuals, and between government, industry and higher education as stakeholders in economic development as a wider construct. Governments in Sri Lanka have been involved not only in their nodal capacity as policy creators but also as participants in the establishment of public–private bodies to foster both knowledge creation and diffusion and the discourses arising will now be examined.

---

[167] Industrial Technology Institute Sri Lanka (2014), and specifically Industrial Technology Institute, *Intellectual Property Policy* (2012), http://iti.lk/images/stories/pdf/ippolicy.pdf.

[168] Ibid.

[169] Industrial Technology Institute (2014).

[170] Interviewee # 4.

5.10.2.1 Sri Lanka Institute of Nanotechnology

SLINTEC is the first public–private partnership in Sri Lanka, in which the government has partnered with eight leading private sector companies.[171] This government ST initiative commenced in 2008 and specialises in nanotechnology R&D to make innovative products and add value to natural resources. The NSF oversees the Government's involvement in SLINTEC. SLINTEC research commenced in 2009 with a team of top-class scientists from Sri Lankan universities and with state-of-the-art labs in place. Research at SLINTEC is primarily in six areas, namely, sustainable agriculture, smart textiles, printable electronics and sensors, energy, minerals and composites, and medical diagnosis and preventive medicine, but it also attempts to identify new areas of research relevant to the development of the country's industrial base within an internationally competitive landscape.[172] During 2008–2021, a total of 13 technologies were developed and transferred to local and overseas firms,[173] and 15 patents were filed locally and internationally as identifiable outputs.[174] Of these, six patents are pending currently and seven have been obtained.[175] Further, 37 research papers have been published thus far in international scientific journals.[176] Within the Sri Lankan context, the use of nanotechnology in agriculture has the potential to reduce crop waste and to monitor crops more effectively by redesigning the DNA structure in plants.[177]

A senior official of SLINTEC made the following statement about the change in the country's R&D culture[178]:

> SLINTEC is about creating an R&D mentality in the country, and it has a far bigger emphasis on young people interested in science and engineering to give them an opportunity to conduct high-end research. Which means you need the facility, because today, those in the country are moving out and the reason is there are no opportunities in the country. Thus, creating such an infrastructure is critical in the science field because without relevant equipment and access to relevant chemicals, one can't embark on something like that. This was the real focus.

The official also emphasised the importance of the SLINTEC Endowment Trust Fund[179] in strengthening the innovation culture in Sri Lanka by encouraging qualified people in the age group of 40–50 years, who are willing to take a risk to return from overseas to add some value and contribute to Sri Lanka, by giving them incentives.[180]

---

[171] SLINTEC, 'Our Partners', https://www.slintec.lk/about-OurPartners,us/our-partners/<us/our-partners/>, Browns and Company, MAS Holdings, Brandix Lanka Ltd, Camso Loadstar (Pvt) Ltd, Hayleys Ltd, Dialog Axiata, Lankem Ceylon PLC, Lanka Orient Leasing Company.

[172] SLINTEC (2021).

[173] SLINTEC (2022a).

[174] SLINTEC (2022b).

[175] Ibid.

[176] SLINTEC (2022c).

[177] Dasanayaka (2013).

[178] Interviewee # 8.

[179] SLINTEC (2022d).

[180] Wijesinha (2011).

The Endowment Trust Fund is a classic example of how a governing node can influence individuals through communication and interaction to invest in ST. Hence, SLINTEC has shifted the discourse in innovation by focusing not only on leading-edge research, but also on endowment in order to add value and thus foster the country's economic development.

5.10.3 *Government–Industry Partnerships*

5.10.3.1 Sri Lanka Inventors Commission

As discussed earlier, the innovation culture in Sri Lanka is not mature. The main reason for this is the lack of knowledge about innovation even among innovators and of a platform to promote innovation in the country. SLIC was established to narrow this gap and provide prospective innovators a one-step forum for learning about the importance of innovations.[181] For example:

1. SLIC provides patent, financial, technical and commercialisation support for investors to promote their inventions.
2. It has introduced national events, such as the annual National Invention and Innovation competition, to encourage the creation of inventions by Sri Lankan citizens.[182] The competition involves activities that engage schools in an annual exhibition where students can showcase their innovations. This competition is open to international and local inventors as two separate events.
3. In 2019, SLIC won 108 awards in international competitions.[183]
4. SLIC also facilitates the Young Inventor Entrepreneur Lead Development Program, inventor clubs, exhibitions, ceremonies, international inventor competitions and incubator centres.

Moreover, the SLIC, under the State Ministry of Skills Development, Vocational Education, Research & Innovations, has introduced new initiatives to popularise innovations at the village level whereby the conversion of small-scale inventions to commercial-level products will be facilitated.[184] Hence, over the years, SLIC has become a governing node within the ecosystem, which influences inventors to invent by providing the necessary infrastructure. This organisation supports and promotes knowledge and interaction from grassroots level, which often is a low-IP level.

---

[181] Sri Lanka Inventors Commission (2022).

[182] Ibid.

[183] Sri Lanka Inventors Commission (2022).

[184] Interviewee # 14.

5.10.3.2 National Science Foundation

NSF is Sri Lanka's premier driving force in promoting STI for economic development. Accordingly, the NSF facilitates research, development, innovation and TT through funding, knowledge creation, capacity building, partnerships, information dissemination and popularising science in the community. In line with this vision, the NSF mandate is to initiate, facilitate and support basic and applied scientific research by universities, ST institutions and scientists to strengthen the scientific research potential.[185] NSF provides funds for conducting R&D, but only a very low percentage of research is commercialised via IP. According to a scientist at NSF[186]:

> If the research is completed, as per our policy, IP remains with the researcher. However, if the researcher doesn't act for economic benefits, the NSF has march-in rights, and so, we can acquire the patent and work on it. This has never happened for we always encourage to commercialise.

Hence, NSF is a governing node connecting the entire scientific community in Sri Lanka through discourse to push STI in Sri Lanka. However, a lack of resources, delays in transferring funds, cumbersome procedures and a lack of consistent vision in the government has become a major bottleneck to continuing the good practices of NSF.[187]

5.10.3.3 Coordinating Secretariat for Science, Technology and Innovation

COSTI was established on 1 February 2013 as mandated by the Cabinet Decision of September 2011 with the specific aim of coordinating and monitoring STI activities in Sri Lanka.[188]

The establishment of COSTI was timely, for up to 2012, STI was under 20-line ministries and no single institution or ministry had the mandate to coordinate STI, which was the greatest bottleneck to the development of STI. COSTI's main objectives include establishing an Inter-Ministerial Steering Committee for Science, Technology and Innovation to coordinate all STI-related activities, including funding with relevant ministries' institutional support and monitoring activities.[189]

An officer at COSTI explained the origins of this institution as follows[190]:

> COSTI was the brainchild of Prof Sirimali Fernando, the former chairperson of NSF. At that time, she was the advisor to the former Minister of ST &R Prof Tissa Vitharana.[191] Prof

---

[185] National Science Foundation (2022).

[186] Interviewee # 6.

[187] Ibid.

[188] COSTI (2021b).

[189] Mendes, *Integrating Intellectual Property* (n 158) 13.

[190] Interviewee # 2.

[191] Doctor of Medicine in Clinical Medicine from the University of Ceylon; Diploma in Bacteriology from the London School of Hygiene & Tropical Medicine; PhD in Virology from the University

Fernando explained to the Minister the need for a higher authority that would bring all those activities together. The ex-Minister, who has a scientific background, understood the need and helped her to implement the plan.

This relationship indicates how a governing node within a system can influence the government (a Minister) who possesses similar grammar to achieve a common goal (foster innovation) though communication and interaction.

The implementation of COSTI created a shift in Sri Lanka's ST ecosystem. The ST ecosystem, which was haphazard and fragmented with many actors owing to a lack of discourse, suddenly became decentralised and had the right people acting as governing nodes to streamline ST. The COSTI aim was coordinated research in focus areas directed to nationally viable sectors in Sri Lanka.[192] COSTI indicates how a governing node could influence the IP policy making within the nodal governance theory.

TISCs is another initiative launched as a WIPO-funded project to provide innovators in Sri Lanka with access to locally based, high-quality technology information and related services. The centres will help the innovators to exploit their innovative potential and to create, protect and manage their IPR. The TISC@COSTI was launched on 18 December 2014 and its target is to facilitate the IP ecosystem of the country.[193] Detailed information on the TISCs has been provided in Chap. 3.

Another innovative outcome of COSTI was the introduction of the National Innovation Dashboard in 2015. This is an opportunity for Sri Lanka to develop and maintain a national database on research and scientists, with a complete list of those engaged in research and innovation activities and their outputs. This database was urgently needed because of the absence of a one-stop location for obtaining information on national ST. A COSTI official stated[194]:

> Sri Lanka's achievements have never been reflected fully at the international level, although our innovators, scientists and researchers have made some significant contributions towards the development of science, technology and innovation in the country. Unfortunately, these contributions are not captured in our data. The global indices do not highlight all our achievements because of the unavailability of proper data.[195]

Hence, the Dashboard will become one of its own kind, the first national-scale portal for recording of all R&D and STI activities in Sri Lanka. Moreover, the Dashboard will connect and network all those involved in R&D and the commercialisation of innovations within the innovation ecosystem to find solutions for local issues.[196]

---

of London; head of Virology in the Medical Research Institute from 1972 to 1994; Director of the Medical Research Institute from 1983 to 1994; consultant virologist at the Edinburgh City Hospital's Regional Virus Laboratory in the 1980s; deputy director of the Victoria Infectious Diseases Reference Laboratory in Melbourne from 1991 to 1993; professor of microbiology at the University of Sri Jayewardenepura from 1995 to 2000; advisor to the World Health Organization on virology for years.

[192] Interviewee # 13.

[193] COSTI (2021a).

[194] Interviewee # 2.

[195] Ibid.

[196] COSTI (2021a).

5.11 Private Company Initiative: Micro Car Company

Within the government/industry/higher education discourse about the development of businesses that utilise IP is the automobile industry. It has been used by Japan and China as a basis for developing and launching an innovative society. The automobile industry utilises high-technology protection and innovative technologies that attract consumers. Sri Lanka was not known for automobile manufacture and assembling because the market is very small compared with that of other countries, but in the 1960s, the late Mr Upali Wijewardaena, a well-known businessman, assembled cars for local sale under licence from foreign manufacturers, Mazda and Fiat. Mazda and Fiat both recognised his achievements, but the government did not support the industry and the investment became unproductive.

In 1995—35 years later—an automobile engineer, Dr. Lawrence Perera established the Micro Cars Limited (Micro) with 20 employees and one factory. The objective was to engineer and design Sri Lanka's first truly homegrown low-cost automobile utilising local resources and labour. Hence, in the discourse on science and development, Micro is a completely local discourse. Micro is the first national automobile in Sri Lanka to win an international patent and an industrial design for its unique design. Dr. Perera's first vehicle launched in 2001 was manufactured for 10 to 12 years and led to the belief that Sri Lanka can manufacture high-quality vehicles. From 2004 onwards, Micro has received many local and international awards for industrial excellence and innovation.

The interesting factor in this discourse is that the creation of the initial vehicle led to Micro manufacturing SsangYong SUVs in 2008 under licence as a value add for sale locally. Further, in 2011, Micro obtained the rights to export locally made SsangYong vehicles to Pakistan, Bangladesh and Nepal.[197] Hence, following this international recognition, the discourse changed from a local to an international one, that is, from a local creation of a vehicle to licenced manufacturing for export, and this change shows that local innovation can lead to the development of an export industry. Moreover, exporting to foreign markets is very important to Sri Lanka since it is a mechanism to increase FDI to Sri Lanka. This aspect will be discussed later in the chapter.

The CEO made the following comment regarding the change of discourse[198]:

> I was recognised by some giants in the car industry who are capable of car assembly. So, we created that recognition because Sri Lanka is only known to produce primary products. I showed to the international market our capability in a different sector.

Manufacturing under license involves dual branding,[199] that is, the new brand is Micro-SsangYong, whereas the original Micro was the outcome of exclusive patent rights held by Dr. Perera. Interestingly, the SsangYong brand is itself the outcome

---

[197] Micro Car Pvt Ltd, *Company* (Web Page), https://www.microcars.lk/company.html.

[198] Interviewee # 9.

[199] Ibid. Also see, Nguyen et al. (2018).

of a mix of IP from different countries, given that it uses technology licensed from Mercedes-Benz AG along with homegrown technology.

This transition demonstrates that development and IP are both a local and an international discourse because the vehicles created are partly Sri Lankan and Korean and partly European. Moreover, under the dual branding requirement, local government regulation requires a minimum of 30% local value addition, and thus implements a local performance requirement.[200] Dr. Perera explained this further[201]:

> It's our labour and our time, and the components that go into the car that should be equal to the 30% minimum requirement. When we achieve that, we are given certain concessions. That's how the concessions work. With that recognition we have created as a national car manufacturer. But if we are to export Micro-SsangYong from Sri Lanka, then we need to come to an understanding under which name we are exporting. We haven't come to that stage.

The story behind Micro is an interesting discourse, considering that it originated as a local developer with a specific goal of creating a local brand, which involves high-technology transfer through licensing from SsangYong, and Mercedes. Nevertheless, car assembly remains a low-technology activity, which was usually the case for most innovations in Sri Lanka. However, the following statement by the CEO indicates how the governing nodes, such as the government, ministries and banks did not support the car industry because the government did not understand the needs of the car industry, was afraid to take risks in unknown areas and underestimated the potential of Sri Lanka:

> The car was presented in 2002. The right framework was not there for the legislation required for a local car manufacturer. The Ministry of Industries didn't know about the automobile industry because they were used to spices and garments. That's the industry they were looking after at that time. I met the National Development Bank, but the banks were not ready to lend money for a car industry. When I started, there was no support from the then government.

Dr. Perera also identified problems with the training of staff to manufacture the Micro-SsangYong car. They had problems retaining staff once they were trained for about 50% of the trained staff emigrated for better paying jobs once they developed the required skills. As discussed earlier, emigration is a reason for the declining interest in ST. Emigration is a very common occurrence in many developing countries. For example, in India, talented people have gone overseas for post-graduate studies and then work for foreign companies in Silicon Valley, but the country has benefited eventually from their return to work in local industries and start-up businesses once the country's economic condition improved. Unfortunately, the situation is not similar in Sri Lanka. Most people who migrate from Sri Lanka rarely return, except after retirement, which significantly reduces their contribution to their country's development.[202]

---

200 Although the Sri Lanka *IP Act* is silent with regard to the local working of patents, the Micro example suggests that there is a government regulation that requires a minimum local value addition in local manufacturing sectors. See Marsoof (2021).

201 Ibid.

202 See additional comments made by CEO SLINTEC that confirm this point at Sect. 5.10.2.1 on endowment program of SLINTEC.

Moreover, even with the success of Micro in creating an industry, Sri Lanka is a small market, where 97% of the cars are imported and only 3% are locally made, and it was difficult to develop a long-range strategy for the government continually changed its policies with respect to the industry. Dr. Perera made the following statement[203]:

> Every year in the budget, we are affected by policies. Most developed countries set up their policies for 10 to 15 years. In Sri Lanka, policies last only for a year. Policies change. Policies change from government to government and Minister to Minister. This is the reason that Sri Lanka is still a third-world country. Things have changed, but not in the right way. For example, if the tax on imported cars goes up, the tax on local industry goes up as well. This happened in the 2017 Budget. Technically, tax on local industries should go down to support the local industry. The politicians need to be educated.

The above examples demonstrate that the discourse for ST in Sri Lanka has shifted from low-technology protection to high-technology protection, especially in the nanotechnology and biotechnology sectors because, as discussed earlier, the discourses of the government, universities and industry are focusing on the development of higher technology leading-edge research. The above interview data confirm the establishment of new networks, such as the inter-university collaboration, public–private partnerships, collaborations between government institutions and the private sector, has resulted in the emergence of a new discourse, and these networks together function as a node to develop a network of influence because of NIPO's failure to do so. Systems theory thus has given the structure to respond to these new discourses on which the interviewees have elaborated.

However, these examples are pockets of excellence, within a wider discourse on development that Sri Lanka is still in the early stages of innovation, and this has implications for Sri Lanka's ability to attract FDI and TT in order to make the leap to the high-technology protection desired by the government and international discourse. These aspects will be discussed next.

5.12 Role of FDI in Stimulating IP and Innovation

FDI refers to an international investment made by a resident entity in one country (direct investor) for establishing a lasting interest in an enterprise (the direct investment enterprise) located in another country. 'Lasting interest' implies the existence of a long-term relationship and a significant degree of influence by the direct investor on the management of the direct investment enterprise.[204] It can also support local industry upgradation in host economies and facilitate their participation in the global value chain.[205] FDI contributes to sustainable development, directly by increasing capital investment, exports, employment and tax revenue and indirectly through its

---

[203] Interviewee # 9.

[204] Samapappuli and Tharanga (2009).

[205] Adikari et al. (2021).

impact on local suppliers, TT, productivity, innovation and good governance.[206] Most importantly, FDI inflows include knowledge about new technologies and materials, production methods and organisational management skills.[207]

FDI decisions are not homogeneous in nature; rather, they depend on the individual country's broader objectives regarding trade and economic growth, such as market openness and deregulation, competition regimes, development policies and IPR. Further, it is dependent upon investors aiming to exploit proprietary advantages and the relevant industrial base within a country to satisfy these objectives. Thus, the aim of FDI discourse is to achieve technological advantages and protection of their investments via IP, which focusses on high-level protection. In other words, FDI will not be feasible without the development of patented technologies and strong IPR protection, which are considered a necessity, a precondition for FDI to materialise.

For Sri Lanka, although it is critical to increase FDI inflows, it is more important to focus on the types of FDI it attracts and the conditions attached to such investments, rather than on the quantum of FDI. Adikari's study in 2021 demonstrated that Sri Lanka has a weak tendency to accelerate its innovation capabilities by utilising foreign sources because of the lack of R&D capabilities in local firms, whereby even though the monetary value of FDI increased from US$47 million in 1979 to $758 million in 2019, the investment was in lower-technology goods and services, such as textiles and apparel, electronic assembly, distribution and hospitality.[208] Little FDI occurs in high-technology industries, such as aircraft and spacecraft, pharmaceuticals, computers, semiconductors and communication equipment owing to a lack of investment in these industries locally.[209] Thus, although FDI appears to be a mechanism for obtaining advanced technology from developed countries,[210] currently, there is little incentive because investors do not see existing industries that can support the investment. In this argument about FDI, a familiar question arises: Which comes first, the 'chicken or the egg'? What the discourse does disclose though is Sri Lanka's lack of commitment to fostering FDI.

5.12.1 Current Backwardness on FDI in Sri Lanka

Against this background, the following narrative will examine the impact on FDI of Sri Lanka's economic development. Sri Lanka has missed many opportunities to attract foreign investment in industry owing to the ethnic conflict. The late Dr. Saman Kelagama, an economist, stated[211]:

---

[206] Ibid.

[207] Ibid.

[208] Ibid.

[209] Sanderatne (2011).

[210] Adikari et al. (n 943).

[211] Kelegama (2000).

> 1983 was a turning point regarding missing big international investors, and all hopes of becoming the new investment centre of Asia faded away. In the mid-1980s, Sri Lanka missed the chance of attracting some portion of the Japanese surplus due to the war-related uncertain political climate. The Southeast Asian economies really made a kickstart from this recycling surplus during the mid-1980s.

Kelagama very specifically identified the impact of the civil war on foreign investment. During the civil war period, two major electronic MNCs—Motorola and Harris Corporation—withdrew from Sri Lanka after the 1983 ethnic riots.[212] This discourse shows how superstructural nodes, such as MNCs, can influence the investment climate in Sri Lanka.

Even after the end of the civil war, FDI in high-technology industries has not commenced. What are the explanations for the current backwardness on FDI in Sri Lanka? First, by 2022, as a percentage of GDP, FDI stands at a mere 0.6% and lags behind Malaysia, where it is 3–4% and Vietnam, where it is 5–6%. The main reason for Sri Lanka's low FDI percentage is that FDI has skewed away from high value-added global production networks to investment in tourism and low value-added markets of apparel, surgical gloves, tyres and low-value software,[213] resulting in an increasing trade deficit.[214] The investment in tourism infrastructure, for example, may boost jobs and growth temporarily during the construction period, but these investments have little long-term impact on FDI.[215]

Higher levels of FDI would also strengthen exports, foster growth and assist the country to put its debt on a more sustainable footing. Faris Hadad-Zervos, World Bank Country Director for Sri Lanka, Nepal and Maldives stated[216]:

> We believe this is entirely doable given the country's rich natural resources, strategic location, highly literate workforce, and opportunities for investment. We have identified that in some sectors such as high value-added textile and clothing, IT and manufacturing Sri Lankan firms have been expanding their footprint and have been able to become very competitive globally and move up the value chain to more sophisticated products and markets. Here you are showing your potential, so I think the discussion we need to have is clear.

However, Mr Hadad-Zervos stated that for Sri Lanka to leverage these competitive advantages, it needs to focus on comprehensive reforms to increase productivity and competitiveness through value addition.[217]

Second, the current government policies imposed on importers to Sri Lanka result in high barriers. According to a World Bank study, Sri Lanka's import regime is one of the most complex and protectionist in the world.[218] US stakeholders have raised concerns that the government does not adequately consult with the private sector prior to implementing new taxes or regulations—citing the severe import

[212] Ibid.

[213] Nenova (2018).

[214] *Daily FT* (2018).

[215] Nenova (n 213).

[216] Ibid.

[217] US Department of State (2020).

[218] Ibid.

restrictions imposed as a reaction to the COVID-19 pandemic. Sri Lanka ranks poorly in World Bank's Doing Business Indicators 2020 in a several areas, including contract enforcement (164 out of 190); paying taxes (142/190); registering property (138/190) and obtaining credit (132/190). Sri Lanka ranks well in protecting minority investors, coming in at 28/190.[219]

Faris Hadad-Zervos, World Bank Country Director for Sri Lanka, Nepal and Maldives, in June 2021, made the following statement regarding the regulatory barriers[220]:

> The Government needs to set in place a collective set of policies and practices that make up an investment ecosystem, ranging from improvements of the investment climate, elimination of unnecessary regulatory burdens to enhancing predictability of laws and responsiveness of bureaucracy to deliver effective FDI services, Mr Faris Hadad-Zervos told the online gathering. What we have seen in other countries is that investment promotion is the beginning of the game and not the end. The name of the game is attracting and retaining efficiency seeking FDI.[221]

Third, the World Bank study further emphasised that Sri Lanka is a challenging place to do business, with high transaction costs aggravated by an unpredictable economic policy environment, inefficient delivery of government services and opaque government procurement practices. However, the study did not mention IP. US stakeholders and potential investors have expressed particular concern about corruption in large infrastructure projects, and in government procurement, which is a constraint on foreign investment. While the country generally has adequate laws and regulations to combat corruption, enforcement is weak, inconsistent and selective. Historically, the main political parties do not pursue corruption cases against each other after gaining or losing political positions.[222]

The fourth relates to the Board of Investment ('BOI').[223] BOI is a regulatory body for potential foreign investors, which informs them about laws and regulations that affect business operations in Sri Lanka, including new regulations and policies that are frequently developed to protect specific sectors or stakeholders. However, effective enforcement mechanisms are lacking, and investors cite coordination problems between BOI and relevant line agencies. The lack of sufficient technical capacity within the government to review financial proposals for private infrastructure projects also creates problems during the tendering process.[224] However, BOI does not deal with IP-related issues.

---

[219] Ibid.

[220] World Bank (2021).

[221] Ibid.

[222] Ibid.

[223] BOI (2022). BOI can grant project incentives such as tax holidays or preferential tax rates, exemption from customs duty, and foreign exchange controls; arrange utility services; assist in obtaining resident visas for expatriate personnel; and facilitate import and export clearances. The share of industrial exports by enterprises with foreign equity participation that number approximately 600 is 54%

[224] US Department of State (n 217).

Last, in addition to the enforcement concerns, other important factors in the country have deterred substantial FDI. For example, tax concessions, financial incentives and assurances hardly offset this drawback of insecurity. The fact that Japan, the highest aid provider to Sri Lanka and an important trading partner, is not a large FDI investor in Sri Lanka is a telling example, since it is counter to the usual practice of aid, trade and investment moving in tandem. This lost opportunity has been very costly because it is more difficult to attract FDI currently when many countries are offering attractive incentives.[225] This means that the concessions offered by BOI are not an effective mechanism to attract foreign investors.

This discussion suggests that although Sri Lanka has the necessary regulation framework to foster investment, there has been lack of discourse among the relevant sub-actors to coordinate activities to promote investment. In other words, no central authority, such as COSTI, has the mandate to coordinate the investment procedure. BOI is the central body, dependent on ministerial line management that is outdated, administratively rigid and unpredictable because of bureaucratic discretion, since even after the investment procedures have been streamlined through BOI, Sri Lanka is not an attractive investment destination to many foreign and domestic investors, according to the US Department of State.[226] This indicates according to nodal governance, the BOI does not have necessary mentalities, resources and technologies to influence policy making. The current economic crisis in Sri Lanka in 2022 has meant that plans and debates about reform of the investment regulatory environment are in a complete state of flux. In this context, after the economic crisis is resolved, Sri Lanka can perhaps change the discourse on investment by being more assertive and placing performance requirements on public funding and foreign investment, such as IP licensing, TT requirements, local sourcing or export platforms.

Within the above context, as FDI is regarded as one of the effective channels of TT across borders, the next section will examine the role of TT in attracting FDI, as a mechanism to stimulate ST and high-technology IP in Sri Lanka.

5.12.2 Role of TT in Attracting FDI in Sri Lanka

The *TRIPS Agreement* emphasises the importance of TT as follows:

> protection and enforcement of intellectual property rights should contribute to the promotion of technological innovation and to the transfer and dissemination of technology, to the mutual advantage of producers and users of technological knowledge and in a manner conducive to social and economic welfare, and to a balance of rights and obligations.[227]

---

[225] Kelegama (2000).

[226] US Department of State (n 224).

[227] *TRIPS Agreement* art 7. The obligation for developed countries to provide incentives for TT is in art 66.2.

Twenty-eight years later, it is still a subject of vigorous debate whether standalone IP standards facilitate or impede TT,[228] and whether increasing IPR from low technology to high technology in Sri Lanka would foster further TT. The answer might be a mix of rights and obligations for the primary objective of TT is to enhance productivity at project, firm and industry level and to promote long-run economic growth in the host country.

5.12.3 Status of TT in Sri Lanka

The first experience of TT in Sri Lanka was in 1960–1977, through donations from the Soviet bloc in the form of investment in mega factories that focused on local assembly and import substitution. Later, politicisation almost wiped out the competitiveness of these low-technology industries and they became a burden to the public for they were inefficient.[229]

However, with limitations, external technological knowledge acquisition has been taking place in Sri Lanka via international TT.[230] The literature has indicated that at present, mechanisms such as international joint ventures and subcontracting arrangements are widely used in the building materials and construction industry in Sri Lanka.[231] In whatever form, TT is a mechanism to establish or develop missing technological and managerial competence within firms in developing countries and to reduce their dependence on foreign capital, skill and technology in the long run,[232] since often, international TT relates to high technologies whereas local TT involves low technologies. Domestically, TT facilitates the growth of domestic industrial capacity, to bridge the gap in advanced technologies experienced in emerging economies, enhance productivity and industrial capacity for new construction and maintenance, and potentially contributes to infrastructure development, industrialisation and development in developing countries.[233] However, the government policies aim to develop Sri Lanka through an innovation economy, which will require access to high technology, but such TT currently faces[234] bottlenecks and will be examined next.

Devapriya and Ganesan examined the problems and prospects of domestic TT within the local construction sector as a mechanism to boost the indigenous construction capacity in Sri Lanka.[235] They found TT through single projects cannot be a major vehicle to effectively diffuse knowledge within the domestic industry unless

[228] Gentile (2013).

[229] Dasanayaka (2013). See also Perera and Dasanayaka (2004).

[230] Malik (2013).

[231] Ganesan and Kelsey (2006).

[232] Devapriya and Ganesan (2002).

[233] Ibid.

[234] Schaaper (2019).

[235] Ganesan and Kelsey (2006).

advanced knowledge is gained through such projects. In other words, TT that targets domestic industries through low TT are not economically viable since such mechanisms do not attract FDI to boost the economy.

In contrast, Ganesan and Kelsey's study in 2002 examined the TT in international collaborations in Sri Lanka.[236] They revealed that despite the presence of favourable conditions in the projects examined, there was negligible real productivity changes in construction in Sri Lanka owing to stagnation in the growth of local absorptive capacity. One reason for this stagnation could be the absence of a 'local working' requirement for foreign registered owners to maintain their IPR as a condition in the *IP Act* 2003.[237] While not explicit, art 31 of *TRIPS* may allow members to require that international registrations be worked locally and that, otherwise, the rights would be subject to a compulsory licence. The threat of a compulsory licence if the owner does not use the patent locally is thought to encourage or induce voluntary licensing by the foreign owner. Non-recognition of a 'local working requirement' has significant disadvantages to Sri Lanka, for it impedes the TT being established in local industrial factories. In contrast, the Ganesan and Kelsey pointed out that China has placed a balanced emphasis on upgrading building materials and equipment, design and construction and on building up an impressive local absorptive capacity, by modernising entire industries.[238] They suggested performing advance planning for TT in foreign-funded projects to ensure the greater participation of local firms (via the local working condition) together with a balanced focus on efficient and timely execution of projects, the profitability of participants and the realisation of TT goals.[239]

5.12.3.1 Difficulties in Promoting TT Via IP

IP can be a vehicle for TT in many ways. First, a stronger IPR regime can have a significant impact in open economies, thus relying more on foreign patents and reducing domestic patenting, and international trade can transmit knowledge across borders. A reason for providing stronger IP protection for developing countries is the belief that it is safe for foreign corporations to invest in a developing country and provide high-technology transfer because stronger IPR increases the difficulty for competitors to imitate or infringe.[240] This implies that weak IP protection deters foreign investors from investing in technology-intensive sectors because they rely heavily on IPR.[241] Hence, IPR and FDI go hand in hand and the importance of attracting FDI in high-technology sectors is part of the Sri Lankan discourse.[242]

---

[236] Ibid 276.

[237] Marsoof (2018).

[238] Ganesan and Kelsey (2006).

[239] Ibid.

[240] Glas and Saggi (2002).

[241] Javorcik (2004).

[242] 'Prof Ananda Jayawardena', 'Industry University Collaboration' (n 969).

Moreover, IPR leads to increased trade flows and acts as a substitute for the products domestically available, thus leading to less domestic patent filing and increased foreign patent filing.[243] According to Keith Maskus, countries tend to acquire international technology more readily if domestic firms have R&D programs, domestic research laboratories and universities, and a sound basis of technical skills and human capital, while the host countries offer security, grants and tax incentives.[244]

That expectation encourages the host country to make conditions attractive enough to induce FDI. Some countries will go further, however, to apply some conditions for FDI, such as using local R&D, local licensing and local working of patents, when acquiring international technology.[245] These factors reduce the cost of imitation, adaptation and follow-on innovation. A country such as Sri Lanka with low IPR protection does not offer a conducive environment since the STI ecosystem lacks the abovementioned performance requirements identified by Maskus.[246] It is true that international treaties tend to proscribe these performance requirements, but the WTO *TRIMS* only applies to trade in goods, not FDI, and Sri Lanka has not agreed to the kind of FTAs that do contain such investment chapters.

Second, case studies suggest that substantial technology diffusion occurs because of FDI.[247] Therefore, most MNCs evaluate the strength of IPR before making investments, including the adequacy of the legal infrastructure, the laws pertaining to the particular technology and the government agencies' treatment of foreign entities. When transferring technologies, MNCs generally differentiate between countries on the basis of their level of IPR; MNCs are more likely to transfer newer technologies to host countries with stronger IPR protection, while they use older technologies in subsidiaries located in economies with weak IPR regimes.[248] Khaleel Malik's study of Sri Lanka confirmed this practice and also found that the technology provider would retain higher margins on critical spare parts even though it was older technology.[249]

Moreover, as discussed earlier, the level of IPR protection and patent registration activity is often perceived as a measure of FDI received by the host country in the high-technology sectors.[250] Thus, there is a positive relationship between FDI and IP enforcement. In developing countries, FDI is focused on distribution activities owing to weak IP laws. In addition, most MNCs conduct their R&D in weak IP enforcement countries because these countries have low-cost researchers, but the innovation is integrated with the company's knowledge and resources abroad to realise the return on investment in high-protection countries. Therefore, the low-cost advantage and the country's risk are also important factors to be considered in making

243 Bhutani (2016).

244 Maskus (2016).

245 Marsoof (n 237).

246 Maskus (n 244).

247 Ibid.

248 Glas and Saggi (2002).

249 Malik (2013).

250 Ibid.

FDI. Further, firms should make informed decisions while making investments by considering factors such as market size, existing resources and production costs.

Third, technology licensing is considered the most important factor for TT. Most developed countries have adequate resources to spur innovation and growth through technology diffusion, unlike developing countries. A stronger patent regime not only encourages licensing opportunities to firms in developing countries but also leads to technology spillovers to local technology companies.[251] Positive spillovers may arise because of labour turnover and vertical linkages. Negative horizontal spillovers may occur if MNCs siphon off domestic demand or bid away high-quality labour.[252]

The risk is higher when developing countries have the requisite innovative capacity to develop imitative products and tailor the technology to suit local requirements and standards. Thus, most technology firms embrace imports instead of establishing a local presence. Hoekman et al. argued that foreign firms may prefer direct turnkey FDI to external licensing owing to its in-house confidentiality mechanism, and this results in foreign firms' decisions not to license to local firms at all or perhaps transfer lagging technologies.[253] Hence, successful TT normally requires the capacity to learn and the investment to apply technologies into local production processes. For these reasons, countries with substantial engineering skills and R&D programs for adaptation and learning are greater recipients of licensing flows than other countries that lack these factors.[254] For example, countries such as Sri Lanka face many barriers, such as those of language, human resources and training, in the international TT process.[255]

The local TT process in Sri Lanka is different. For example, the ITI in Sri Lanka uses a non-exclusive contractual know-how agreement, and it retains the right to transfer technology to more than one industrial enterprise or it partners with an SME by securing minority holdings, which is in the interest of both the ITI and the firm.[256]

Fourth, labour turnover, the movement of people and imitation are informal channels for technology diffusion. Little attention is given to their impact on TT, given that there is more labour exchange in countries where local firms are close to MNCs. Thus, the ability of local firms to absorb new technologies is a determinant of whether labour turnover is a means of diffusion.[257] Hence, international TT continues to be a key catalyst to economic growth in a developing country such as Sri Lanka, but within the Sri Lankan context, international TT is non-existent, locals are not hired, and hence, policies that stimulate intra-firm TT to affiliates of foreign corporations may have no effect on local SMEs.[258] Some TT occurs when locals study and work abroad and then return home.

---

[251] Hoekman et al. (2005).

[252] Ibid.

[253] Ibid.

[254] Ibid.

[255] Malik (2013).

[256] Liyanage (2008).

[257] Ibid.

[258] Gentile (2013).

In Sri Lanka, mechanisms such as the purchase of patents, the careful study of scientific papers, the importation of new technology-embedded capital goods, and the process of reverse engineering, which involves the dismantling and reproduction of a technology, are used.[259] All these mechanisms come under innovation outputs within a NIS, but they are low-technology approaches to industry in a country that is interested in high-technology solutions. In the Sri Lankan context, it is very important to facilitate TT for the management of IP assets through TMOs. In developed countries, TT is managed by TMOs that have the experience and expertise for processing TT agreements, determining patentability, evaluating the commercial potential of the invention, obtaining patent protection, searching for commercial partners and negotiating and managing licences.[260] As discussed earlier, none of the universities and research institutes has employed a TMO to facilitate TT and most of the procedures relevant to TT are performed by research staff.[261]

Regarding this lack of expertise in TT, a senior official of SLINTEC stated[262]:

> TT is an area in which we are looking for expertise. One of the weaknesses is that there are no TT experts available in Sri Lanka. The volume of activities that require TT is also limited because of the limited number of transactions taking place on a regular basis. As a result, we do not have a full-fledged TT team, but we are trying to build one over the next 18 months. Now, we are beginning to see a larger volume of research and it is also becoming commercially relevant. Now, we need to move to the next level, which is the technology readiness level, and we are looking for someone to guide us.

This discussion reveals that TT is an area in which Sri Lanka has limited potential owing to its lack of infrastructure, resources and expertise. Currently, 90% of the technologies are imported into Sri Lanka.[263] Only 1% of these are developed in the country, and as a result, the developed technologies are based on low-technology innovations that do not facilitate economic development or satisfy the demands and desires to develop the country into a high-technology innovator. Sri Lanka is dependent on the adaptation of foreign technology to drive local innovation, rather than on the acquisition of high-technology innovations; thus, a more nuanced approach to IP is needed to address the technological lag in the country.

Two major reasons that Sri Lanka is left behind in TT are its inability to face the fierce global competition and to adopt technology at the right time. However, the lack of technology adoption is not the only reason for this underperformance. In Sri Lanka, technology adoption mainly occurs in agricultural practices and through ICT adoption in SMEs, to boost business.[264] These technological adoptions are not supplanted by ramping up the domestic innovation capacity. Consequently, Sri Lanka does not attract foreign knowledge and technology, maximise spill overs, attract or

[259] Dasanayaka (2013).

[260] Liyanage (2008).

[261] Ibid.

[262] Interviewee # 8.

[263] National Science Foundation (2018).

[264] Athapaththu and Nishantha (2018). See also Madushanka et al. (2016).

retain mobile talent and design smart and strategic innovation and IP policies.[265] These negative aspects affect the innovation input in Sri Lanka.

5.13 Conclusion

To sum up, as discussed in this chapter, the STI ecosystem has undergone a series of shifts over the past few decades—many STI government policies have been introduced in Sri Lanka, and these policies have aimed to promote and foster low-technology innovations, from local or foreign firms, rather than to encourage high-technology innovations that would compete in the global economy. This implies the STI discourse is local and conservative, and although it has been subject to some global discourse (WIPO, for instance), the international discourse has been rhetorical rather than substantive. The question that arises is whether policymakers have been successful in constructing a local innovation policy in Sri Lanka through IP by linking the country's research capabilities and industry structure to foster an innovation ecosystem.

As discussed, on the basis of the data collected and statistics, amid the numerous policies, the IP discourse in Sri Lanka has not moved forward, compared with the discourses in other developing countries in the region. The main reason behind the backwardness of the STI discourse is that policies are statements of intent without practical implementation strategies; they are not demand-side innovation policies that make a difference at the national and the international level.[266] None of the policies emphasised mechanisms to drive economic development via high-technology solutions to boost national and local needs and tackle the major global challenges.[267] In other words, policymakers did not shift the focus towards promoting a culture of innovation as a matter of policy and the policies that were introduced did not reflect Sri Lanka's socio-economic and cultural context.[268] Accordingly, the STI discourse in Sri Lanka has not gained the strength to develop high-technology IP clusters and activities, resulting in the development of industries that have low-technology IP requirements, such as manufacturing and service industries. Low technology places less emphasis on business innovation and R&D commercialisation and lacks openness to foreign investment, which results in low inflows of FDI and TT; limited access to international production networks, export markets and international aid; and the import of useful products.[269]

In other words, ST did not align with the industrial policy goals in Sri Lanka to boost the innovation economy. As discussed in this chapter, there has been a lack of discourse convergence between policymakers, innovators and industry, especially

[265] Ibid.

[266] Elder (2016).

[267] Ibid.

[268] Marsoof et al. (2022).

[269] Poh (2016).

the SME sector that the Sri Lankan economy is highly reliant upon because there was no governing node to align all these sectors. Moreover, most of the IP-related technologies that are created are for the local market and are not attractive to the international market. As a result, Sri Lankan firms rely on technology adoption and imitation rather than pursuing international TT. This is because the R&D base in Sri Lanka is the lowest in the region in terms of expenditure and outputs.[270] Crucially, as shown in this book, IP has rarely featured in the local ST policy discourse, despite the place it has in the global development discourse, which largely favours its protection, albeit with conditions sometimes, to ensure its benefits are spread.

To sum up the chapter, ST discourse consist of two levels: national and global. The national level is more prominent within ST mainly because (unlike in the other two case studies), ST discourse is predominantly a local story since all policies and lawmaking are designed locally with local actors in the ST field to drive innovation through IP. The global discourse mattered to some extent, that is, in terms of WIPO's technical assistance, but WIPO's assistance is demand driven and not mandatory and there was no evidence of coercion.

As discussed in this chapter, due to the lack of awareness and expertise on IP, STI remains low-technology protection but new local discourses emerged through university collaborations, public–private partnerships, government institutions and the private sector. These new networks like the SLINTEC have shifted the discourse from low- to high-technology innovation by emphasising leading-edge research and creation of infrastructure to facilitate scientific research.

Systems theory, nodal governance and discourses were the appropriate mode of study in this chapter, because the theories identified illuminated that ST discourse is constituted by nodes like the Ministry of Science, Technology, and Research (MSTR), COSTI and SLINTEC have power dynamics within the networks to exert influence in Sri Lanka to foster innovation. Although local lawmaking and processes assisted the discourse on STI, dialogue and communication between the influential actors were more powerful tools to examine the involvement in science, innovation and IP than documentary research.

This is highlighted through the interviews conducted for this book, revealing good practice examples of communications between actors pushing the STI ecosystem to a better position in Sri Lanka. The discourse though identifies STI ecosystem is lagging and can be developed only though progressive, achievable reforms that emphasise high-end research in the STI field. Notably, the theoretical analysis from the interviews identify that NIPO stands outside this conversation, which is a crucial challenge for Sri Lankan policymakers, as NIPO should be a governing node for providing support for implementation of patent related issues in STI policies.

Competing Interests The author has no conflicts of interest to declare that are relevant to the content of this chapter.

[270] 'Prof Ananda Jayawardena' 'University Industry Collaboration' (n 214).

References

Abeyratne S (2010) Road to realise "Mahinda Chinthana vision. Sunday Leader (Sri Lanka)

Adikari AMH, Liu H, Marasinghe MMSA (2021) Inward foreign direct investment: induced technological innovation in Sri Lanka: empirical evidence using RADL approach. Sustainability 13

Al Circle (2019) New technology to developed to use aluminium waste to waste water management. New technology developed to use aluminium waste for treating waste water in textile industry; Aluminium Extrusion, Profiles, Price, Scrap, Recycling, Section (alcircle.com)

Athapaththu JC, Nishantha B (2018) Information and communication technology adoption in SMEs in Sri Lanka: current level of ICT usage and perceived barriers. Int J E-Entrepreneursh Innov 8:1

Bhutani K (2016) Role of intellectual property in transfer of technology. Linkedin. https://www.linkedin.com/pulse/role-intellectual-property-technology-transfer-karan-bhutani

BOI (2022) Invest Sri Lanka. http://www.investsrilanka.com

Central Bank Sri Lanka (2021) Economic and social infrastructure. Annual Report 2020 | Central Bank of Sri Lanka (cbsl.gov.lk)

Chandrasekera (2017) Sri Lanka wants rs 10 million bio technology park in Homagama. Lanka Business Online. https://www.lankabusinessonline.com/sri-lanka-wants-rs100mn-biotechnology-park-in-homagama/

COSTI (2021a) Innovation dashboard. https://costi.gov.lk/index.php/en/32-uncategorised/86-innovation-dashboard

COSTI (2021b) COSTI home. https://www.costi.gov.lk/index.php/en/

Daily FT (2007) Hemas manufacturing launches safe and natural Mosguard lotion to provide protection against mosquito. Daily FT. https://www.ft.lk/Healthcare/Hemas-Manufacturing-unches-safe-and-natural-Mosguard-lotion-to-provide-protection-against-mosquito/45-641369

Daily FT (2016) Bioclean blazes pathway for corporate-university research collaboration. Daily FT. https://www.ft.lk/Business/bioclean-blazes-pathway-for-corporate-university-research-collaboration/34-557277

Daily FT (2018) Prof Ananda Jayawardena calls for university-industry collaboration. Daily FT. https://www.ft.lk/Opinion-and-Issues/Prof-Ananda-Jayawardena-calls-for-university-industry-collaboration/14-662913

Dasanayaka S (2003) Technology, poverty, and the role of new technologies in eradication of poverty: a case study of Sri Lanka. In: South Asian conference on technologies for poverty reduction

Dasanayaka S (2013) Poverty eradication through technology integration approach: a case study of Sri Lanka. J pro Poor Growth 1:1

Dasanayaka WSB et al (2020) Identification of factors for the success of the Sri Lankan independent investors. Int J Bus Glob 25:2

De Alwis A (2015) International association for the protection of intellectual property. COSTI Sri Lanka

Devapriya KAK, Ganesan S (2002) Technology transfer through subcontracting in developing countries. Build Res Inf 30:2

Drahos P (2010) The global governance of knowledge: patent offices and their clients. Cambridge University Press

Dructer P (1992) The age of discontinuity. Taylor and Francis

Dunstan J, Choahan N (2021) Australia's first locally made COVID-19 mRNA vaccine candidate is set for clinical trials. ABC News. https://www.abc.net.au/news/2021-06-20/mrna-covid-19-vaccine-trials-in-australia-variant-booster/100229294

EDC Perdeniya (2021) Engineering Design Centre, Faculty of Engineering, University of Peradeniya. http://eng.pdn.ac.lk/pages/Centers/edc/?page_id=62

Elder J (2016) Local needs, global challenges: the meaning of demand-side policies for innovation and development. The Global Innovation Index. https://www.wipo.int/edocs/pubdocs/en/wipo_pub_gii_2016.pdf
Falvey R, Foster (2006) The role of intellectual property rights in technology transfer and economic growth: theory and evidence. United Nations Industrial Development Organization
Ganesan S, Kelsey J (2006) Technology transfer: international collaboration in Sri Lanka. Constr Manage Econ 24
Gentile E (2013) Intellectual property rights and foreign technology adoption in developing countries: an empirical investigation. National University of Singapore. https://doi.org/10.2139/ssrn.2290507
Gibbons LJ (2011) Do as I say (not as i did): putative intellectual property lessons from emerging economies from the not so long past of the developed nations. SMU Law Rev 64
Gilson RJ (1999) The legal infrastructure of high technology industrial districts: silicon valley, route 128, and covenants not to compete. New York Univ Law Rev 74
Glas AJ, Saggi K (2002) Intellectual property rights and foreign direct investment. J Int Econ 56
Govindaraj S (2010) A study of the national innovation system in Sri Lanka. Master's Dissertation, University of Moratuwa
Hewage NS (2015) Promoting a Second-tier protection regime for innovation of small and medium-sized enterprises in South Asia: a case of Sri Lanka. Nomas
Hoekman BM, Maskus KE, Saggi K (2005) Transfer of technology to developing countries: unilateral and multilateral policy options.World Dev 33:10
Indraratna ADV de S (2012) Export growth and sustained development. Colombo Telegraph. www.colombotelegraph.com/index.php/export-growth-and-sustained-development/5/
Industrial Technology Institute Sri Lanka (2014) Our capabilities. Ministry of Technology and Investment Promotion. http://iti.lk/images/iti/home/Our_capabilities_for_web.pdf
Institute of Policy Studies (2002) White paper on national strategy for small and medium enterprise sector development in Sri Lanka. IPS. https://www.ips.lk/national-strategy-for-small-and-medium-enterprise-sector-development-in-sri-lanka-white-paper/
International Trade Administration (2021) Sri Lanka—country commercial guide: telecommunications and information technology. https://www.trade.gov/country-commercial-guides/sri-lanka-telecommunications-and-information-technology
Javorcik BS (2004) The composition of foreign direct investment and protection of intellectual property rights: evidence from transition economies. Eur Econ Rev 48
Jaysuriya GCN, De Silva M (1972) The national science council of Sri Lanka. J Natl Sci Council Sri Lanka 1
Kelegama S (2000) Development in independent Sri Lanka: what went wrong? Econ Pol Wkly 35:17
Kumara S (2020) 101: Sri Lanka's rank in the global innovation index 2020. The Sri Lankan Scientist. https://scientist.lk/2020/09/07/101-sri-lankas-rank-in-the-global-innovation-index-2020/. Accessed
Liyanage C (2008) Technology Transfer in Government Research Institutes: A Case of Industrial Technology Institute. Master's Dissertation University of Moratuwa
Madushanka LS, Weerasinghe KS, Weerakkody WJSK (2016) Adoption of information communication technology in cashew sector: a case in Puttalam District of Sri Lanka. In: International conference on advances in ICT for emerging regions
Malik K (2013) International technology transfer and its impact on innovation enhancement for firms based in Sri Lanka. Int J Technol Transf Commercialization 12(1–3)
Marsoof A (2018) Local working of patents: the perspective of developing countries. In: Bharadwaj A, Gupta VI (eds) Multi-dimensional approaches towards new technology. Springer. https://doi.org/10.1007/978-981-13-1232-8_15
Marsoof A (2021) Exclusive patent rights and local working requirements: a developing country's perspective. Working Paper

Marsoof A, Kariyawasam K, Thalagala C (2022) Reframing intellectual property in Sri Lanka: lessons from the developing world and beyond. Springer

Maskus KE (2016) Patents and technology transfer through trade and the role of regional trade agreements. In: East-West center working papers: innovation and economic growth series

Mendes P (2015) Integrating intellectual property into innovation policy formulation in Sri Lanka. WIPO. https://www.wipo.int/edocs/pubdocs/en/wipo_report_inn_lk.pdf

Micro Car Pvt Ltd. https://www.microcars.lk/company.html

Ministry of Education Sri Lanka (2022) National science and technology commission. http://www.nastec.gov.lk/reports/nrdf

Ministry of Finance and Planning (2010) Mahinda Chintana: vision for the future. Law and Environment Assistance Platform. https://www.preventionweb.net/files/mahinda_chintana_vision_for_the_future_eng%5B1%5D.pdf

Ministry of Finance and Planning (2020) Unstoppable Sri Lanka

Ministry of Industry and Commerce Sri Lanka (2017) National Policy Framework for Small and Medium Enterprise (SME) Development. http://www.industry.gov.lk/web/images/pdf/framew_eng.pdf

Ministry of Science and Technology of Sri Lanka. *National Biotechnology Policy* http://www.nsf.ac.lk/images/stories/STPRD/biotechnology_policy.pdf

Ministry of Technology and Research, Sri Lanka (2022) Science, technology and innovation strategy (2011–2015). Yumpu. https://www.yumpu.com/en/document/view/49242730/science-technology-innovation-strategy-for-sri-lanka-ministry-of-

Moir HVJ (2013) Patent policy and innovation: do legal rules deliver effective economic outcomes? Edward Elgar

Moir HVJ (2021) Empirical evidence on patents and data protection: response to the productivity commission's issues paper on intellectual property arrangements. Issue Paper

Monotti AL (2018) Employment law and intellectual property law: attempts to resolve issues at the points of convergence. In: Monotti (ed) Employment law and intellectual property law. Edward Elgar Publishing. https://ssrn.com/abstract=3430158

Monotti AL, Ricketson S (2003) Universities and intellectual property: ownership and exploitation. Oxford University Press

Mortley R (2021) Patent Accessibility Review. Final Report of Australia, Department of Industry, Science, Energy and Resources Australia

Mudalige D (2019) The government to set-up national innovation agency. Daily News. Govt. to set-up National Innovation Agency | Daily News

National Intellectual Property Office (2022) Statistics. https://www.nipo.gov.lk/web/index.php?option=com_content&view=article&id=8&Itemid=130&lang=en

National Science Foundation (2018) Statistical handbook on research and development of Sri Lanka technology and innovation. National Science Foundation

National Science Foundation (2022) National science foundation. http://Home(nsf.ac.lk)

Nenova T (2018) Six ways Sri Lanka can attract more foreign investment. World Bank Blogs. https://blogs.worldbank.org/endpovertyinsouthasia/six-ways-sri-lanka-can-attract-more-foreign-investments

News First (2019) Sri Lanka's ancient "Wewa" water system recognised as global heritage system. https://www.newsfirst.lk/2018/04/19/sri-lankas-ancientwewa-water-system-recognised-as-global-heritage-system-by-un/

Nguyen C, Romaniuk J, Faulkner M et al (2018) Are two brands better than one? Investigating the effects of co-branding in advertising on audience memory. Mark Lett 29. https://doi.org/10.1007/s11002-017-9444-3

OECD (2020) Economic surveys: Korea. OECD. https://www.oecd.org/economy/surveys/korea-2020-OECD-economic-survey-overview.pdf

OECD/Eurostat (2018) Oslo manual 2018: guidelines for collecting, reporting and using data on innovation. OECD. https://doi.org/10.1787/9789264304604-en

Parliament of Sri Lanka (2016) Parliamentary debates

Perera C, Dasanayaka S (2004) Technology development: key issues in productivity. In: Kelegama S (ed) Economic policy in Sri Lanka: issues and debates. Sage Publications
Phirouzabadi, Nikzad N (2013) An analysis of relation between resident and non-resident patents and gross domestic product: studying 20 countries. Int J Conceptions Manage Soc Sci 1:2
Poh LC (2016) From research to innovation enterprise: the case of Singapore. The Global Innovation Index
Samapappuli N, Tharanga GCR (2009) Compilation of foreign direct investments in Sri Lanka. Central Bank of Sri Lanka 66
Sanderatne N (2011) New law add to the gloom over FDI. Sunday Times (Sri Lanka)
Schaaper M (2019) The human factor in innovation. The global innovation index
Science and Technology Cell (2016) Bio clean, product with Darley Butler. Bio Clean – Science and Technology Cell (cmb.ac.lk)
Sener S, Saridogan E (2011) The effects of science-technology-innovation on competitiveness and economic growth. Procedia Soc Behav Sci 24
De Silva MAT, Amaradasa RAW (2001) Science and technology in industry proceedings. In: First Biennial conference on science and technology in national development. National Science and Technology Commission Sri Lanka
SLINTEC (2021) Sri Lankan institute of nanotechnology. http://slintec.lk/
SLINTEC (2022a) Technologies developed-transferred-commercialized details from 2008–2021. http://www.slintec.lk/commercialized-technologies/
SLINTEC (2022b) Patents. https://www.slintec.lk/our-innovations/patents/
SLINTEC (2022c) Research papers. https://www.slintec.lk/our-innovations/research-papers/
SLINTEC (2022d) Endowment. https://www.slintec.lk/slintec-endowment/
Sri Lanka Inventors Commission (2022) Statistics. http://slic.gov.lk/statistics/
Sri Lanka Investors Commission. https://slic.gov.lk/
Tang D (2021) The future of intellectual property and WIPO in a time of crisis and opportunity. Francis Gurry Lecture on Intellectual Property
The Economic Times LK (2021) Moratuwa university become first university in Sri Lanka to formulate a product commercialization policy. The Economic Times LK. https://economictimes.lk/index.php/2021/06/01/moratuwa-university-become-first-university-in-sri-lanka-to-formulate-a-product-commercialization-policy/
University of Moratuwa Intellectual Property Advisory Committee. Patent databases: patents granted. Patent Granted | University of Moratuwa (uom.lk)
US Department of State (2020) 2020 Investment climate statement: Sri Lanka. https://www.state.gov/reports/2020-investment-climate-statements/sri-lanka/
Weerasinghe RN, Jayawardane AKW and Deshani AL (2016) Systematic View of Innovation: Role of Universities in National Innovation System of Sri Lanka. Conference Paper
Weerasinghe RN, Jayawardane AK (2018) University-industry partnerships for innovation: Sri Lankan experience. Ann Spiru Haret Univ Econ Ser 8:1
Wickramasinghe CN, Ahamed N (2012) Influence of demographic and technical profile on success of independent investors in Sri Lanka. J World Intellect Prop 15
Wickramasinghe V, Malik K (2018) University-industry collaboration in Sri Lanka: a developing country perspective. Int J Innov Technol Manag 15:4
Wickremesinghe R (2018) Sri Lanka PM: this is how i will make my country rich by 2025. World Economic Forum. https://www.weforum.org/agenda/2018/08/this-is-how-we-will-make-sri-lanka-rich-by-2025/
Wijesinghe C et al (2020) Influential factors for ICT innovations in Sri Lanka university-industry collaboration: a systematic literature review. J Res Innov Impl Educ 4:4
Wijesinha A (2011) Dynamic growth in Sri Lanka: the innovation imperative. Talking Economics. http://www.ips.lk/talkingeconomics/2011/10/13/dynamic-growth-in-sri-lanka-the-innovation-imperative/
WIPO (2017) Using IP for development: success stories from around the world. https://www.wipo.int/edocs/pubdocs/en/wipo_pub_using_ip_dev.pdf

WIPO (2021) Global innovation index 2021: Sri Lanka. WIPO, SRI LANKA (wipo.int)
World Bank (2017) Vision 2025: Sri Lanka's path to prosperity. https://www.worldbank.org/n/news/feature/2017/10/17/vision-2025-sri-lankas-path-to-prosperity
World Bank (2021) Foreign investment can help Sri Lanka build better. World Bank. https://www.worldbank.org/en/news/feature/2021/06/10/foreign-investment-can-help-sri-lanka-build-back-better.

Chapter 6
Conclusion

Abstract This concluding chapter discusses how the lawmaking discourses have contributed to the IP ecosystem to foster innovation in Sri Lanka based on the theoretical framework of this book. First, it reviews the main findings from the case studies, consider the answers to the inquiries and examines the strengths of the conclusions, and then, it concludes by presenting the overall implications of those findings.

6.1 Introduction

This book explored IP lawmaking discourses and processes in Sri Lanka and attempted to identify the IP setting they regard as necessary to foster an innovation economy in the country. In this book, theories such as nodal governance, systems theory and discourses have been employed to identify actors, processes and crucially competing discourses. To pursue this inquiry three case studies were conducted, namely, the patent administration, PVR and STI discourses, to identify how different actors within the IP ecosystem communicate with each other and the discourses that have influenced the lawmaking.

Findings from the competing discourses identified in this book show that, thus far, the patent administration, PVR and STI discourses align with low-technology IP protection in contrast to the high-technology IP protection that most developed and developing countries have perceived as crucial for an innovation economy. Reasons for low-technology IP protections are employed in the thee case studies will be explained later in Sects. 6.2 and 6.3 based on of this book. Then, to explain this state of play, the book has argued that the key actors' perceptions worked to approve or disapprove the competing discourses on IP and innovation. For example, why do we find that IP is not considered important to innovation or is it too early to predict this? If IP is considered important for innovation, what are the areas that Sri Lanka should emphasise and are there any bottlenecks within the system that hinder progression and are to be reformed?

Having described the law, this book turns to the findings in order to characterise and explain the IP lawmaking process. Both available documentary sources and

A. Perera, *Dilemmas of Intellectual Property Discourse in Sri Lanka*,
https://doi.org/10.1007/978-981-97-6117-3_6

interviews were obtained in the field, in Sri Lanka and abroad, with policymakers, scientists, industrialists, research institutes, government functionaries, ministry officials and WIPO and UN officials. It should be understood, at times, that the findings are presented on the basis of the evidence on the absence and silence of IP lawmaking.

When mapping the findings, the book has illuminated who are the actors, what they have been communicating, which actors are more influential than the others, their position and power dynamics, education, and status in the society, and how they communicate with each other to exert influence over the choice between high- and low-technology protection. Drawing on the findings of this study, the discussion will then predict how the lawmaking discourses can be strengthened to introduce reforms to the IP ecosystem in Sri Lanka.

The following section will explain the policy implications of the analysis undertaken to answer the two research inquiries.

6.2 Has IP Law Discourse in Sri Lanka Favoured Low-Technology Rather Than High- Technology IP Protection?

To characterise the legal state of play in Sri Lanka, this book identified that the actors had the power dynamics to influence the discourses surrounding IP promotion and implementation. Several actors locally and globally have been governing nodes who influenced the lawmaking over time through communicating and interacting with each other within the PGA and PVR lawmaking ecosystems. However, this study found that some local actors were more influential in exercising considerable power dynamics over official discourses on patent administration PVR and STI and consequently their low-technology views often prevailed because according to these nodes, based on the infrastructure, expertise and skills, financial resources in these sectors discourages introducing high-technology IP protection.

As discussed in Chap. 3, patent law discourse in Sri Lanka emerged with the implementation of the 1979 *IP Code* in Sri Lanka, which was the first IP legislation enacted after Sri Lanka gained independence. As discussed in Chap. 2, Mr. Lakshman Kadirgamar, the first WAPBD, was a pioneer in instigating the 1979 Code, which was based on the WIPO *Mode! Law*, and the late Minister of Trade and Shipping Mr Lalith Athulathmudali was influenced by Mr Kadirgamar, thus becoming at the time a governing node for the enactment of the *IP Code* to promote commercial activities in the county.

This discourse was influential in shaping and commencing the local IP law in Sri Lanka. This indicates that even in 1979, patents were regarded as an instrument of commercial policy, while the enactment of the *IP Code* was implemented to preserve and enhance the competitiveness of local low-technology innovations.[1] In other words the policy makers in Sri Lanka like the late Ministers, believed that

---

[1] Sri Lanka Parliament (2003).

patents drove economic development, but strongly believed that innovation in Sri Lanka is based on low-technology due to the status of STI in Sri Lanka. However, he acknowledged that by promoting and implementing IP in that era, in the long run will be beneficial to Sri Lanka. Thus, both Ministers became prominent local nodes by exerting their power dynamics to introduce a novel piece of legislation to Sri Lanka.

How did the various groups of actors form shared interpretations about the policies and laws regarding the patent administration, PVR and STI ecosystems in Sri Lanka.? As discussed in Chap. 2, in the absence of coercion, discourses are the foundation for lawmaking. In Chap. 2, identified that there are individual actors and groups of local actors within the IP ecosystem, such as the UN representative, Ministers, the NIPO officials, COSTI officials, academics, scientists and CEOs, who appear to share a similar interpretation about how IP fits in to foster innovation in the light of systems theory. They belong to an interpretive community because they share similar epistemological assumptions, beliefs and preferences and interpret and respond in similar ways to IP development in Sri Lanka. For example, the UN representative and COSTI officials communicate with each other on IP-related matters and possible solutions mainly because they have a similar educational qualification, have known each other for a long time, were both beneficiaries of free education in Sri Lanka and believe that IP could foster innovation in Sri Lanka. Hence, to achieve this target, they interpret and respond to legal processes on the basis of their epistemological framework, thus becoming nodes of influence in the IP who exert power-dynamics in Sri Lankan IP policy development Yet, as discussed in Chap. 3 there were others such as the NIPO senior officials and most past and present Ministers, who were important nodes, but did not regard the law as an important discourse for influencing IP to foster innovation because of their lack of discourse with each other thus creating a significant bottleneck in the patent administration. Furthermore, this research found that if Sri Lanka desires to be a part of the global patent network, by activating the *PCT* and links with other patent offices for instance, it should contemplate reforms to the existing *IP Act* to remedy the weaknesses in the current system with assistance from local and global actors.

What were the discourses between the local policy makers with society in general regarding IP policy making? The discourses between these actors give impetus to lawmaking. As discussed in Chap. 3, the establishment of COSTI as a mechanism to mandate STI in the country was the brainchild of the former chairperson of NSF. As a scientist, the former chair identified that the lack of a central authority to coordinate STI was a bottleneck in the system and the former chair, as the Secretary to the Minister, communicated with the former Minister and emphasised the need for such an authority. The discourse was positive because both were scientists, who were important local nodes in the IP ecosystem and recognised the importance of having such a body. Both were policymakers; thus, COSTI was implemented. Similarly, SLINTEC, which is a successful public–private partnership, was established with the involvement of the NSF. NSF, having realised the potential of nanotechnology, interacted with the private sector to secure funds for the project.[2] NSF convinced the

---

[2] Govindaraj (2010), p. 163.

private sector of the immense opportunities offered by nanotechnology, and therefore, this sector decided to contribute to the project.[3] Both NSF and the private sector are subsystems under systems theory, operating on social discourses according to their own codes and programs to perceive a common goal, namely, to foster innovation in nanotechnology, which is strongly connected to IP.

Moreover, the implementation of the 10 PAP is another example of nodal influence and discourse between interpretive society and the government. When the WIPO DG visited Sri Lanka in 2013 to deliver the Kadirgamar memorial address, the UN representative in consultation with the Sri Lankan Government, converted the visit to an official visit for creating a platform to discuss IP-related issues. The 10 PAP, which WIPO quickly designed for the visit, later became a model for developing countries. These social discourses and dialogues and learning among actors have contributed to the implementation of the 10 PAP.[4] A WIPO study conducted on 2015 on *Integrating Intellectual Property into Innovation Policy Formulation in Sri Lanka*[5] is another example of how communication coexisting with other subsystems, such as NIPO, COSTI and government, could influence the policymaking discourse in Sri Lanka to strengthen its innovation ecosystem.

In addition to local nodes, global nodes too influenced IP policy making in Sri Lanka. WIPO is a global actor, but unlike the WTO, is based on the demand-driven concept, meaning that it recommended the WIPO *Model Law*, with certain changes to suit Sri Lanka because the country was keen to have an *IP Code* in late 1970s. Hence, WIPO did not coerce Sri Lanka to transplant the *Model Law* in 1979, or to modify the *Model Law* to respond to the local industry or its specific needs. However, it later continued to offer Sri Lanka considerable technical assistance with its patent system.[6]

In contrast, as discussed earlier, the main reason for introducing the *IP Act* in 2003 was to comply with the WTO *TRIPS Agreement* high-technology obligations and an expressly stated objective linked IP with the promotion of national creativity and protection of consumer interests.[7] Yet, again, as discussed previously local low-technology protection prevailed due to the STI status in Sri Lanka. The *IP Act* did not drastically reform the IP law as per TRIPS Agreement, because the local innovators at this time was making innovations for the local market, based on low-technology protection. Therefore, the policy makers had to balance the changing the IP Act in compliance with the TRIPS requirements taking into consideration the active promotion of individual innovators' or creators' rights and to adhere formally to the requirements of the global node, the WTO, who has power dynamics to coerce any developing country into changing IP laws. The interview data reveal Sri Lanka was compliant in providing the laws 'on the books' rather than 'rocking the boat' to promote local interests.

---

[3] Ibid.

[4] Gillespie (2006), p. 24.

[5] Mendes (2015).

[6] Refer to Chap. 3 in this book.

[7] Parliamentary Debates (n 1).

This compliance means that the WTO has not exerted power dynamics over Sri Lanka relating to IP, unlike in the case of some developing countries, such as India, mainly because Sri Lanka by providing compliant legislation and by not breaking any rules 'appears to be flying under the radar' on issues of how complete the implementation of *TRIPS* is in a local environment. Further, the WTO is ultimately an international node of government-to-government member actions rather than a hands-on developer of local rights and interests, such as WIPO.

Furthermore, while IP and STI is not considered strong in Sri Lanka, the country is less attractive economically for other reasons to MNCs, than are other developed or developing countries, and is certainly less attractive to high-technology industries. Thus, during this period, the local high-technology IP discourse is present, but it is not prominent and so did not undergo substantial shifts to promote development and awareness. Sri Lanka was not the target of bilateral pressures, such as from the US Government. Hence, due to the above reasons, within the context of nodal governance, the WTO nor the US Government has not exerted power-dynamic with the aim to change the existing IP legislation.

However, from 2010, as discussed in Chap. 3, a shift in the IP discourse was very visible owing to a prominent set of local actors who pioneered changes in the IP ecosystem in Sri Lanka with WIPO's technical assistance. For example, MSTR's establishing of COSTI to mandate, promoting the WIPO 10 PAP to streamline IP, sending the right people for overseas IP training and interacting, and following up on the relevant IP matters with stakeholders, were the changes introduced and implemented positively. However, this change did not affect the low-technology IP protection due to the weak IP settings discussed in Chap. 3.

Thus, local actors with the modalities and knowledge sought to link the local discourse through the influence of assistance, such as that of WIPO, to develop the structure for providing the appropriate local administration for IP. However, the data in Chap. 3 revealed that the main obstacle to ensuring an effective patent regime is the archaic nature of the patent grant administration system. Unlike the systems in other countries in the region, the Sri Lankan system lacks features to attract local or foreign high-technology innovators.[8] For example, patent grant examination is based on low-technology criteria known as the formality of examination, which is a very outdated system. This suggest, even though the influence of the WTO TRIPS on IP, which is based on high-technology IP protection, Sri Lankan IP system did not change, nor were reforms introduced to shift from low-technology to high technology IP protection, because the TRIPS did not change the policy makers perception on IP in Sri Lanka due to the under develop status of NIPO. This issue is discussed in Chap. 3.

Moreover, interviewees identified that the present patent examination system does not motivate local investors either because the level of innovation required is low with the current system, as discussed in Chap. 5 shows, there is a reluctance among local innovators and SMEs to register their patents. A utility model system has been recommended but unfortunately, as discussed in Chap. 3, this has not been

[8] Perera (2014), p. 344.

implemented yet. Neither has the IP system modified the examination process to offer rigorous and defensible high-technology patent grants to foreigners, despite the assistance available to it from WIPO and patent offices in other countries, such as Japan and India. Hence, policies and discourses in Sri Lanka are rather neglected, unlike in certain other countries, and have allowed space for imitation until locals create their own inventions.

This finding indicates that without the continuous influence of governing nodes and their interaction within the IP sub system, the desired outcomes will not materialise in Sri Lanka. In this regard, not only the present but also the previous NIPO senior officials have been unable to influence the government to promulgate suitable patent reforms as a governing node. Hence, for promoting IP, NIPO remains a major bottleneck in the patent system in Sri Lanka, and without any development, it is difficult to predict whether IP could boost high-technology economic development in Sri Lanka in the near future.

Turning to the findings from Chap. 4 on the PVR discourse, PVR is the topic of an unresolved debate for the past 21 years in Sri Lanka. NIPO and DoA have been prominent local nodes to promote the PVR Bill, but, as discussed in Chap. 4, there has been a huge grassroot power-dynamics, through alliances between stakeholders such as farmers, environmentalists and NGOs, against the implementation of the PVR Bill because it does not favour Sri Lankan farming communities.

As discussed in Chap. 2, legal transfers should be socially constructed.[9] In other words, once a global script is transferred, recipient states construct and reinterpret the meaning of the global script to suit their local conditions.[10] With regard to PVR, *TRIPS* mandated PVR in every member state, either patents or sui generis, and then, the *UPOV Act* (mainly the 1978 version) has been a global script and a governing node that has influenced most developed and developing countries as a sui generis law on PVR under nodal governance. As a result, UPOV has been a key actor in the PVR discourse globally.

However, as regards Sri Lankan legislation of the PVR law, the UPOV model was not reinterpreted to suit local conditions. For example, the first Draft in 2001 on PVR in Sri Lanka was a verbatim transcription of the *UPOV 1991* version that favours high-technology PBR for breeders of new varieties and disregarded the rights of farmers. This element is still visible in all the subsequent PVR Bills. Either there is no mechanism to recognise FR or the majority of the farmers are not happy with the mechanism adopted by the policymakers. Hence, there was a lack of discourse by either party.

Unless these two groups reach a consensus, the PVR will not be implemented. However, the data reveal that neither the WTO nor MNCs have exerted power dynamics on Sri Lanka to implement it, unlike in the case of countries such as India. Meanwhile, laws have been introduced to recognise and reward farmers (imperfectly) for their stewardship of plant resources such as seeds, which is not the emphasis of TRIPS nor UPOV This aspect has been discussed in Chap. 4.

---

[9] Lessing (1995), p. 992.

[10] Ibid.

As discussed in Chap. 5, amid the conscious effort by some of the governing nodes to push STI in Sri Lanka, the data reveal that the STI lawmaking discourse has not achieved its objective. The vast volume of policies relating to STI, IP, R&D, FDI and TT do not align with the economic and industrial strategies of Sri Lanka nor provide mechanisms for the implementation of change. In this sense, the STI lawmaking discourse has been limited again to the law on the books, and evidence is lacking about significant application to the task of crafting the law to assist the economic development of the country either through local innovation or FDI. In other words, the STI national lawmaking policies and discourses, attempted to achieve high-technology protection, has failed to achieve its objectives due to the weak STI infrastructure system in Sri Lanka.

Owing to these bottlenecks in the system, the country has not progressed in the field of STI. This decline has affected the development of the patent system significantly, although the lack of development also relates to other factors needed to establish conditions conducive to innovation, such as TT and local upskilling. This suggests, Sri Lanka IP still remains low-technology protection.

6.3 What Are the Reasons that Sri Lanka Favours Low-Technology Protection for IP Law?

Section 6.2 identified that while there may have been genuine effort by some local nodes to introduce high-technology patent protection in some sectors like Nanotechnology that would benefit the country, the implementation of law, a lack of concerted and coordinated discourse, as revealed in all case studies conducted in this book, have discovered that IP regulatory framework in Sri Lanka remain low-technology protection due to other extraneous factors, such as a lack of political will, bureaucratic interference, changes of government, interdepartmental rivalries, haphazard decision-making, civil war and economic crises. These factors have delayed, or led to the neglect of, IP lawmaking in Sri Lanka. In Chaps. 3, 4 and 5, it was explained which factors have influenced the IP implementation process and which of these factors differ and diverge according to the pluralism of different actors.

As discussed in Chap. 3, the patent administration of Sri Lanka has been the major bottleneck for the underdevelopment of IP in Sri Lanka. The patent examination system, which is based on formality of examination is an outdated system which is based on low-technology protection. No attempt has been taken to change this system because to introduce a standard patent examination requires reforms to the entire IP system. This was not feasible due to lack of expertise, skills and financial restrictions.[11] This implies that there is no power dynamics within the patent administration system to push for change and also the actors in the IP sub system are not

[11] Refer to Chap. 3 in this book.

willing to listen to the nodes who recommends reforms. For example, the recommendations to introduce the utility model system has been not taken seriously by any actor in the IP subsystem, even though this reform will benefit the local innovators in Sri Lanka.[12]

As discussed in Chap. 4, the PVR Bill has not been implemented because of an impasse between the pro-IP regime, such as the agents of the biotechnology industry in Sri Lanka who support IP for PVR, and the anti-IP regime, which does not favour high-technology IP on plant varieties, namely, farmers, NGOs, environmentalist and academics. Therefore, for example, even after 20 years of debate Sri Lanka is yet to implement PVR since it is yet to achieve an appropriate balance between the interests of commercial breeders and traditional farmers due to the power dynamics of both sectors. Unless, these competing interests are balanced, PVR will never be implemented in Sri Lanka, regardless of the international obligations stated in the discourse. As discussed in Chap. 4, when implementing the PVR law, legitimate concerns of farmers like the farmers' rights that are deeply rooted in cultural settings cannot be overlooked by the government who is a governing node. Simultaneously, policymakers need to consider the advantages Sri Lanka would gain from implementing the PVR, considering that the country's major agricultural exports are limited to tea, rubber, coconut and spices and it still has a large community of subsistence farmers.[13]

Further, the STI sectors in any country are directly linked with its IP ecosystem, because the objective of an STI policy is to enhance an innovation economy through IP. Sri Lanka is considered a middle-income country and the discourse of policymakers was that IP could boost innovation in the long run only by developing high-technology innovations, and not through low-technology innovations. This was identified under the first inquiry. All policymakers were of the view that a patent can be an economic policy instrument via commercialisation of inventions. Hence, as discussed in Chap. 5, a sound STI ecosystem is a contributory factor to fostering innovation in Sri Lanka.

However, as discussed in Chap. 5, the ST discourse in Sri Lanka has not yet reached the maturity or innovation level of the discourses in developed countries. The data reveal that a strong R&D based on STI is lacking in Sri Lanka.[14] Within the Sri Lankan context, the IP system, in general, and patent law, in particular, were developed on the basis of the above objective, and practically all interviewees in different sectors shared this view. However, as discussed in Chap. 5, although the majority of the government's STI policy discourses were aimed at fostering high-technology research, in practice, this was not achievable because the policies were over-ambitious and did not align with the available resources, expertise and the weak R&D base in Sri Lanka. For example, as discussed in Chap. 5, the National Science, Technology, and Innovation Strategy 2011-2015 was the most comprehensive and futuristic framework implemented in Sri Lanka to address the promotion of science-industry linkages and

[12] Ibid.

[13] Refer to Chap. 4 in this book.

[14] Perera and Dasanayake (2004), pp. 244–245.

university-industry collaborations, which is crucial for fostering innovation and IP promotion.[15] However, this strategy was not embraced within a broader framework of the NIS, including not only the ST sector but connecting with other government and private sector organisations, such as SLINTEC who could disseminate and implement this agenda.

This implies that economic policymaking plays a critical role in facilitating innovation or hindering it and within the Sri Lankan context, but due to the non-alignment of policies and lack of nodal affect STI sector remains low- technology because implementation has been hampered by a lack of discourse between relevant groups about what the effects of these policies would be and how the industrialisation strategies would enable users to be involved in having a greater impact on the economy of Sri Lanka.[16]

As this book has demonstrated, in Sri Lanka, there is lawmaking discourse for IPR protection locally, but it has not achieved a consensus and hence a trajectory, even though on the surface the legislation itself appears to have been proposed to comply with the international discourse on IP. These discourses, both local and global, have been examined through three case studies: patent administration, PVR and the STI sectors. These case studies revealed competing discourses between low-technology protection and high-technology protection. These competing discourses indicate different outcomes for the IP lawmaking in Sri Lanka. The strong IPR high-technology protection argument would conclude that IP lawmaking has not contributed to innovation in Sri Lanka because the country adopts a low-technology criterion for patents and PVR and its R&D capabilities are insufficient to foster its STI sectors. However, the alternative argument is that the low-technology protection method is appropriate for the local farming and SME sectors because these sectors have still not embraced high-technology production, unlike their counterparts in developed countries.

These findings reveal that the IP lawmaking discourse in Sri Lanka is a complex interrelated problem, and not solely an argument based on the implementation of strong IP laws and STI policies. This book has demonstrated that legal discourses and processes are greatly affected by nodal failures within the IP system. Power dynamics affects the wider Sri Lanka legal and business community as users, which prevents the development of IP. According to the researcher's view, this is a sad situation because Sri Lanka gained independence in 1948, but after 75 years, it is still a developing country with poor economic statistics, no way near becoming an upper-middle income country and the local discourse demonstrates there is IP, but it is in its infancy in developmental terms.

Competing Interest The author has no conflicts of interest to declare that are relevant to the content of this chapter.

---

[15] Wijesinha (2011).

[16] Athukorala (2021).

References

Athukorala PC (2021) Rethinking Sri Lanka's industrialisation strategy: achievements, lost opportunities and prospects. School of Public Policy ANU College of Asia and the Pacific. https://crawford.anu.edu.au/sites/default/files/publication/acde_crawford_anu_edu_au/2021-06/acde_td_athukorala_2021_14.pdf>

Gillespie J (2006) Transplanting commercial law reform: developing a 'rule of law 'in Vietnam. Ashgate

Govindaraj S (2010) A study of the National Innovation System in Sri Lanka. Master of Business Management Thesis. University of Moratuwa Sri Lanka

Lessing L (1995) The regulation of social meaning. Univ Chicago Law Rev 62:3

Mendes P (2015) Integrating intellectual property into innovation policy formulation in Sri Lanka. WIPO

Perera A (2014) The administration of patent system in Sri Lanka: a critical appraisal. Common Law World Rev 43

Perera C, Dasanayake S (2004) Technology development: key issues in productivity. In Kelegama S(ed) Economic policy in Sri Lanka: issues and debates. Sage Publications

Sri Lanka Parliament (2003) Parliamentary debates

Wijesinha A (2011) Dynamic growth in Sri Lanka: the innovation imperative. https://www.ips.lk/talkingeconomics/2011/10/13/dynamic-growth-in-sri-lanka-the-innovation-imperative/

SPRINGER NATURE

GPSR Compliance

The European Union's (EU) General Product Safety Regulation (GPSR) is a set of rules that requires consumer products to be safe and our obligations to ensure this.

If you have any concerns about our products, you can contact us on ProductSafety@springernature.com

In case Publisher is established outside the EU, the EU authorized representative is:

Springer Nature Customer Service Center GmbH
Europaplatz 3
69115 Heidelberg, Germany

The manufacturer's authorised representative in the EU is Springer
Nature Customer Service Centre GmbH, Europaplatz 3, 69115 Heidelberg,
Germany. If you have any concerns regarding our products, please
contact ProductSafety@springernature.com

Printed and bound by CPI Group (UK) Ltd, Croydon, CR0 4YY
01/10/2026
02225859-0003